Protein Structure

Protein Structure

Determination, Analysis, and Applications for Drug Discovery

edited by

Daniel I. Chasman

Variagenics, Inc.
Cambridge, Massachusetts, U.S.A.

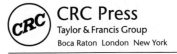

CRC Press
Taylor & Francis Group
Boca Raton London New York

CRC Press is an imprint of the
Taylor & Francis Group, an **informa** business

CRC Press
Taylor & Francis Group
6000 Broken Sound Parkway NW, Suite 300
Boca Raton, FL 33487-2742

First issued in paperback 2019

© 2003 by Taylor & Francis Group, LLC
CRC Press is an imprint of Taylor & Francis Group, an Informa business

No claim to original U.S. Government works

ISBN-13: 978-0-8247-4032-0 (hbk)
ISBN-13: 978-0-367-39534-6 (pbk)

Library of Congress Cataloging-in-Publication Data
A catalog record for this book is available from the Library of Congress.

To my father
and the
memory of my mother

Preface

It has been about 80 years since James B. Sumner first crystallized urease to suggest the discrete structure of proteins and J. D. Bernal and Dorothy M. Crawfoot (later Hodgkin) demonstrated that protein crystals of pepsin were sufficiently ordered to diffract X-rays. In this time, protein structure has been transformed from a topic of speculation and monumental experimental challenge to a field with the aspirations and the technological capacity for enumerating the full diversity of protein folds in the biosphere. Throughout its development, the field has been guided by a single enduring principle—that to understand a protein's structure is to begin to understand its function in molecular detail.

Structural studies have indeed discovered much about proteins and their functions. They have revealed the secondary structural elements and a shared hierarchy of structural elements common to all proteins as well as the physicochemical basis of their thermodynamic stability. The framework for describing the catalytic mechanisms of enzymes derives from structural studies as do insights linking structural mutability to biological function. Structure has been used to show how the interactions of proteins with DNA and other macromolecules can regulate processes in biological development and differentiation. Large assemblies of proteins performing a broad spectrum of biological roles outside the cell, within the membrane, and inside the cell can only be understood adequately in the context of the descriptions provided by structural analysis.

This volume is intended as a reference for the researcher with a basic knowledge of protein structure who would like to understand more about determining, analyzing, and using structural information, especially in conjunction with a genomics perspective. In the selection of topics, the main goal was to be comprehensive so that this single reference could organize and help initiate in-depth study. Each group of authors surveys a field and supplies an extensive reference list for pursuing aspects of the topics that are not covered explicitly. The theme of structural genomics throughout the volume emphasizes high-throughput methods, automation, and computation. Many of these technological advances are relatively new to the protein structure field and had only been explored superficially as recently as one or two decades ago. One of their crucial ramifications is the freedom to imagine insights derived from a greatly expanded knowledge of protein structural diversity.

This book is divided into four parts, with Part I providing an introductory chapter on structural genomics. Part II describes methods for producing proteins in structural studies, experimental approaches for solving structures by crystallography and NMR, and computational strategies for determining structural information. The unique challenge of crystallizing membrane proteins is addressed in this part (in Chapter 3). Part III describes analysis—mostly computational in nature—for gaining a deeper understanding of proteins from their structures. This part includes procedures for detecting errors in protein structures, finding functionally important links between protein sequence and structure, and identifying biological properties from structure. It also contains descriptions of the database repositories of protein structures and the standards used to curate them. Part IV illustrates some potential uses of protein structure in the drug discovery process. This part of the book also includes discussions of structure-based drug design, refining protein pharmaceuticals using structure, and the impact of genetic variation on protein function and pharmacology.

I would like to express my gratitude to my colleagues at Variagenics, in particular Vince Stanton and Mark Adams, for providing the opportunity to complete this volume in a commercial environment. Anita Lekhwani at Marcel Dekker, Inc., first suggested the project to me and provided unfailing encouragement throughout its development. Of course, the authors of the chapters were essential to the realization of the original concept and I gratefully acknowledge their efforts.

The current genomic sequencing initiatives are generating a complete catalog of proteins in a wide variety of well-studied organisms. All of the resources are in place for a companion effort in protein structure. I hope this volume can help sustain and intensify interest in the renewed effort to learn about protein structure and its role in biology.

Daniel Chasman

Contents

Part III   Analysis

Part IV Applications for Drug Discovery

Contributors

Ruben A. Abagyan, Ph.D. Department of Molecular Biology, The Scripps Research Institute, La Jolla, California, U.S.A.

Pedro M. Alzari, Ph.D. Département de Biologie Structurale et Chimie, Institut Pasteur, Paris, France

Cheryl H. Arrowsmith, Ph.D. Affinium Pharmaceuticals and Ontario Center for Structural Proteomics, Toronto, Ontario, Canada

Susan M. Baxter, Ph.D. Research and Genome Analysis, GeneFormatics, Inc., San Diego, California, U.S.A.

Helen M. Berman, Ph.D. Department of Chemistry and Chemical Biology, Rutgers, The State University of New Jersey, Piscataway, New Jersey, U.S.A.

Philip E. Bourne, Ph.D. Department of Pharmacology and San Diego Supercomputer Center, University of California, San Diego, La Jolla, California, U.S.A.

Marvin Cassman, Ph.D. Institute for Quantitative Biomedical Research, University of California, San Francisco, San Francisco, California, U.S.A.

Daniel I. Chasman, Ph.D. Variagenics, Inc., Cambridge, Massachusetts, U.S.A.

Omoshile Clement, Ph.D. Catalyst Department, Accelrys, San Diego, California, U.S.A.

Dimitris Dimitropoulos Macromolecular Structural Database Group, EMBL–European Bioinformatics Institute, Hinxton, Cambridgeshire, United Kingdom

Aled M. Edwards, Ph.D. Affinium Pharmaceuticals and Banting and Best Department of Medical Research, University of Toronto, Toronto, Ontario, Canada

Ann E. Ferentz, Ph.D.[*] Department of Biological Chemistry and Molecular Pharmacology, Harvard Medical School, Boston, Massachusetts, U.S.A.

Jacquelyn S. Fetrow, Ph.D. GeneFormatics, Inc., San Diego, California, U.S.A.

András Fiser, Ph.D. Laboratory of Molecular Biophysics, The Rockefeller University, New York, New York, U.S.A.

R. Michael Garavito, Ph.D. Department of Biochemistry and Molecular Biology, Michigan State University, East Lansing, Michigan, U.S.A.

Kim Henrick, Ph.D. Macromolecular Structural Database Group, EMBL–European Bioinformatics Institute, Hinxton, Cambridgeshire, United Kingdom

Trevor W. Heritage, Ph.D. Discovery Informatics, Tripos Inc., St. Louis, Missouri, U.S.A.

Liisa Holm, Ph.D. Department of Biosciences, University of Helsinki, Helsinki, Finland

Raymond Hui, Ph.D. Affinium Pharmaceuticals, Toronto, Ontario, Canada

John Ionides, Ph.D. Macromolecular Structural Database Group, EMBL–European Bioinformatics Institute, Hinxton, Cambridgeshire, United Kingdom

---

[*] *Current affiliation*: Variagenics, Inc., Cambridge, Massachusetts, U.S.A.

Charles D. Kang, MBA Licensing Department, Invitrogen Corporation, Carlsbad, California, U.S.A.

Michael Karpusas, Ph.D. Department of Basic Sciences, University of Crete Medical School, Heraklion, Crete, Greece

Peter A. Keller, B.Sc., M.Sc. Macromolecular Structural Database Group, EMBL–European Bioinformatics Institute, Hinxton, Cambridgeshire, United Kingdom

S. Roy Kimura, Ph.D. Variagenics, Inc., Cambridge, Massachusetts, U.S.A.

Stacy Knutson Research and Genome Analysis, GeneFormatics, Inc., San Diego, California, U.S.A.

Eugene Krissinel, M.Sc., Ph.D. Macromolecular Structural Database Group, EMBL–European Bioinformatics Institute, Hinxton, Cambridgeshire, United Kingdom

Fabien Marino Affinium Pharmaceuticals, Toronto, Ontario, Canada

Brian D. Marsden, M.A., D.Phil. Department of Molecular Biology, The Scripps Research Institute, La Jolla, California, U.S.A.

Philip McNeil, B.Sc., M.Sc., Ph.D. Macromolecular Structural Database Group, EMBL–European Bioinformatics Institute, Hinxton, Cambridgeshire, United Kingdom

Duncan E. McRee, Ph.D. Crystallography, Syrrx, Inc., San Diego, California, U.S.A.

Adrea T. Mehl, Ph.D. Scientific Services, Accelrys, San Diego, California, U.S.A.

Jorge Navaza, Ph.D. Laboratoire de Génétique des Virus, Centre National de la Recherche Scientifique, Gif-sur-Yvette, France

John C. Norvell, Ph.D. Protein Structure Initiative, National Institute of General Medical Sciences, National Institutes of Health, Bethesda, Maryland, U.S.A.

David J. Osguthorpe, Ph.D. Centre for Protein Analysis and Design, University of Bath in Swindon, Swindon, United Kingdom

Christos A. Ouzounis, Ph.D. Computational Genomics Group, EMBL–European Bioinformatics Institute, Hinxton, Cambridgeshire, United Kingdom

Burkhard Rost, Dr. rer. Nat. Department of Biochemistry and Molecular Biophysics, Columbia University, New York, New York, U.S.A.

Andrej Sali, Ph.D. Laboratory of Molecular Biophysics, The Rockefeller University, New York, New York, U.S.A.

Alexei Savchenko, Ph.D. Ontario Center for Structural Proteomics, Toronto, Ontario, Canada

Sophia Tsoka, Ph.D. Research Programme, EMBL–European Bioinformatics Institute, Hinxton, Cambridgeshire, United Kingdom

Sameer S. Velankar, Ph.D. Macromolecular Structural Database Group, EMBL–European Bioinformatics Institute, Hinxton, Cambridgeshire, United Kingdom

Frank von Delft, Ph.D. Crystallography, Syrrx, Inc., San Diego, California, U.S.A.

John Westbrook, Ph.D. Department of Chemistry and Chemical Biology, Rutgers, The State University of New Jersey, Piscataway, New Jersey, U.S.A.

Adrian Whitty, Ph.D. Department of Quantitative Biochemistry, Biogen, Inc., Cambridge, Massachusetts, U.S.A.

Ken Yamazaki Affinium Pharmaceuticals, Toronto, Ontario, Canada

Adelinda Yee, Ph.D. Ontario Cancer Institute and Department of Medical Biophysics, University of Toronto, Toronto, Ontario, Canada

Christine Zardecki, Ph.D. Department of Chemistry and Chemical Biology, Rutgers, The State University of New Jersey, Piscataway, New Jersey, U.S.A.

Protein Structure

1

Structural Biology and Structural Genomics: A Federal Agency Perspective

John C. Norvell
National Institutes of Health, Bethesda, Maryland, U.S.A.

Marvin Cassman
University of California, San Francisco, San Francisco, California, U.S.A.

The first protein structure took about three decades to complete, and all protein structures solved in the early years required Herculean efforts. Most aspects of the process were difficult, time consuming, expensive, labor intensive, and problematic. But during the past decade, technological breakthroughs in protein production, crystallization (still the most trying step), data collection, structure solution, and refinement have dramatically altered this picture. Although it is difficult to pick the most significant advance, development of user-friendly synchrotron beamlines for protein crystallography is high on the list. Of course, many classes of proteins—notably, large protein complexes and membrane proteins—often still require years of intense effort and imagination to solve. On the other hand, many soluble globular proteins can now be solved almost routinely. The power of structural studies to advance biological understanding was obvious from the start. Three-dimensional structures have already provided unique insight into macromolecular function and mechanism. Structure has also become an important aid for targeted drug design. Additionally, a "complete" set of structures can provide insights into the architecture of proteins and its relationship to function, as well as protein folding and evolution.

An inspection of National Institute of General Medical Sciences (NIGMS) research grant programs reveals the growth of structural biology. The NIGMS and all the other institutes of the National Institutes of Health (NIH) provide research support through several mechanisms, especially investigator-initiated, hypothesis-driven individual research grants (the R01s). The success and maturation of structural biology over the past decade has resulted in major changes in the focus of these crystallographic grants. Initially, almost all of the crystallographic awards were made to "card-carrying" crystallographers, i.e., the experts in the field. Now the awards focus more on biological significance and less on crystallographic technique. The number of crystallographic-related grants (i.e., those that contain at least one major structure project) awarded to principal investigators that are not experienced crystallographers is now twice the number awarded to the expert crystallographers.

Sources of funding in structural biology have also changed over the years. In the early 1980s, NIGMS provided most of the research support for structural biology in the United States and about two-thirds of the total NIH support. Today, NIGMS contributes only about half of the NIH support for structural biology. As protein structure studies became more integral to the research mission of other institutes, the relative percentage of NIGMS funding decreased. Even so, about 15% of the institute's current research budget is awarded to projects that involve high-resolution protein structure determination by crystallography or nuclear magnetic resonance (NMR) spectroscopy. Funding for protein crystallography by the Department of Energy (DOE), National Science Foundation (NSF), and other agencies and foundations has also grown significantly. The NSF and DOE support of user-based synchrotrons and numerous protein crystallographic beamlines has been essential to the growth of the field. In addition, the Howard Hughes Medical Institute has provided substantial support for many investigators in structural biology.

In about 1998, motivated by the successes and recent technical advances of structural biology and the results and demonstrated value of genome-sequencing projects, scientists began to consider national and international effort in structural genomics. The field of "structural genomics" can be defined many ways, and all of them are justified. In the broadest sense, it can be defined as high-throughput structure determination guided by genomic information to identify targets. Currently, there are federally funded structural genomics efforts under way in a number of countries, including the United States, Japan, Germany, Canada, France, the United Kingdom, and Italy. The U.S. effort, called the Protein Structure Initiative (PSI), is spearheaded by the NIGMS. In addition, numerous industrial efforts focus on high-throughput structure determination for targeted drug design.

The goals and approach of the Protein Structure Initiative vary significantly from many of the other structural genomics programs. The main goal of the PSI is to arrive at a complete description of protein structures. In contrast, the goal of many of the international programs and most of the private efforts is to obtain structures of select proteins based on medical interest or other biologically important issues. These programs do not have any explicit interest in completeness, nor do they address this goal in their target selection strategies, although both approaches rely on genomic data. This chapter will focus on the basic research goals and approaches of the NIGMS program. The PSI is a large-scale, high-throughput effort to increase the number of structures of unique, nonredundant proteins, permitting the study of a broad range of protein structures. The PSI is expected to provide a minimum of 10,000 selected structures in 10 years.

Many scientists had initially agreed on the value of a complete set of all protein structures found in nature, but such an undertaking seemed impossible. Since the numbers of proteins are (as we now know) much larger than the number of genes in an organism (perhaps by an order of magnitude), it is neither feasible nor affordable to consider one-by-one structure determination of the universe of protein structures. However, as many experts in the field have discussed, computational analyses of sequence data permit the classification of proteins into structural families and thus provide a "shortcut" method to reach for this completeness: experimentally determining the structure of a representative of each family, followed by modeling of the homologous proteins in the family. This approach should make the problem more manageable.

Although the production of protein structures is increasing at a dizzying rate (with over 15,000 structures now deposited in the Protein Data Bank), most of these structures are not unique—instead, they are many variants of the same structures and sequences. Such variants, while they are important for studying the details of biological mechanisms at the atomic level, do not significantly expand our knowledge of protein structure space. The goal and major rationale for an organized structural genomics project, specifically the NIGMS Protein Structure Initiative, is to focus on structures chosen as family representatives and on methodology development, leading to a comprehensive and efficient coverage of protein structure space. In other words, this effort would form an inventory of all the protein structures in nature. This inventory would be a public resource freely available to the scientific community.

However, unlike the Human Genome Project, defining *completeness* in a structural genomics project is not at all obvious. *Completeness* might be defined in terms of the number of structures that could be both experimentally determined and modeled by homology. This still leaves plenty of room for interpretation. A recent paper concludes that the goal is "obtaining a set (of protein structures) such that accurate atomic models can be built for almost all functional domains" (1). Other goals are possible, and *completeness* is likely to be understood as the project advances and our understanding increases of what the global array of structures looks like.

Experimental details and strategies of structural genomics have been discussed in numerous meetings and scientific articles over the past few years. An excellent collection of summary articles can be found in a recent review (2). The first major meeting to discuss large-scale structure determination was held at the Argonne National Laboratories in January 1998. organized by the DOE. This meeting was initiated because of a general feeling among a number of investigators and federal science administrators that the time was ripe to consider developing the same global understanding of protein structure that was being accomplished for gene sequence. Some small pilot programs had already been established at the DOE and the NIGMS. Although the discussants by no means uniformly approved of an organized national program, enough enthusiasm was generated to prompt further consideration. The enthusiasm arose from the importance of protein structures and the perceived benefits of a program of global structure discovery to biologists of all kinds.

Following the Argonne meeting, the NIGMS spent over a year examining the need for a national program in structural genomics. Three workshops and several advisory meetings were held that included many experts in the various fields involved, with representation from a wide range of backgrounds and opinions. These were designed to assess whether a large-scale effort of the kind proposed was timely and appropriate. The three workshops were held between April 1998 and February 1999. Participants concluded that the technology was available, the goals were feasible, and the benefits justified the effort. Attendance at these workshops included representatives not only from the U.S. research community but also from Europe, Israel, and Japan. It became clear that interest extended beyond the United States, and that the scale of the program required an international effort.

Several international meetings have addressed scientific and policy issues for this field. The First International Structural Genomics Meeting was held in the United Kingdom in April 2000, followed by a number of workshops and meetings, including an Organization for Economic and Cooperative Development conference in Florence, Italy, in June 2000; the International Conference on Structural Genomics in Yokohama, Japan, in November 2000; and the Second International Structural

Genomics Meeting at the Airlie Center, Virginia, in April 2001. This last meeting focused on international cooperation and policies such as data release, publication, coordinate deposition, and intellectual property. Information on this and other meetings can be found at the NIGMS PSI website (3).

The first stage of the NIGMS PSI is the creation of several research centers that serve as pilots for a future production stage. Each research center must include all components of structural genomics so that it can test strategies for large-scale high-throughput structure determination by X-ray crystallography and/or NMR as well as new computational, experimental, and management approaches. Target selection is left to the individual groups, but it must be genome driven. The strategies must focus on obtaining the maximum number of novel structures as protein family representatives, but can also include other selection criteria: known function, unknown function, eukaryotic proteins, pathogenicity, phylogenetic relationships, minimal genomes, etc. Some classes of proteins, such as membrane proteins, are not suitable for high throughput at this time and are thus seldom considered for targets. This could change in the future, with technical improvements under way, including special projects in several PSI research centers.

Since these PSI grants are intended to prepare the way for a public resource, grant-related requirements are more stringent than with individual research grants. Data release and coordinate deposition cannot be delayed until publication but instead must be completed within four to six weeks of structure completion. In addition, the identity and status of target proteins must be made available on each center's publicly available webpage. Employment of graduate students and postdoctorals must be justified. The centers do retain intellectual property rights, but only those consistent with the data release policy.

Seven PSI research center awards were announced in September 2000. These centers spent the first year organizing themselves into cohesive units and hired staff and acquired robotic equipment for protein production and sample preparation. Two additional research center awards were made in September 2001, bringing the institute's support of these centers to $40 million annually. The NIGMS is planning further efforts in support of the PSI, including workshops on technical bottlenecks, a centralized target registration Website at the Protein Data Bank, electronic publication of structures, a facility for storage of resulting physical materials, and an experimental results database.

The NIGMS expects these research centers to provide guidance for the future of the project. The structures produced should provide a more realistic idea of what will be required to achieve complete coverage of protein structures in nature. One outcome is already apparent and should benefit all structural biologists—the development of new high throughput methods and automated equipment for protein production and crystallization. The institute hopes that this inventory of structures of protein family representatives will serve as a public resource for research scientists from both the public and private sectors and will be a crucial body of knowledge for studies of protein structure, folding, and evolution. The modeled structures should also serve for subsequent studies of the relationship of structure to function and as the starting place for studies of targeted drug design.

Because of its emphasis on large data sets and completeness, the PSI can be considered a branch of *proteomics*, which has been defined as "the analysis of complete complements of proteins" (4). For example, the incentive is not simply to increase the number of enzymes known, but rather to achieve in an organized manner a complete assessment of some biological systems, usually by itemizing their molecular components and defining their interactions. Why this interest in large-scale data collection, which had previously been denigrated as "fishing expeditions" or "stamp collecting"? The Human Genome Project clearly demonstrates the value of completeness in the understanding of biological systems. It is not merely the identification of new genes but the ability to view the architecture of the genome that has provided a novel understanding of the organization and evolutionary history of biological systems. Increasingly, it is the ability to contrast and compare entire genomes from different organisms, rather than just to examine the differences between a few individual genes, that underlies the project's great new insights.

It is incumbent on us, however, to view the new enthusiasms for large-scale data collection with a grain of skepticism. From antipathy to such data-collection efforts in the early 1990s, we have now swung over to the view that any global data collection is worth doing. Although it is hard to argue that data are not, or may not be, useful, these undertakings are expensive in manpower and dollars, and need to submit to cost–benefit analyses. The primary issue that should govern any such effort is simple— who benefits? Large-scale programs should have large-scale benefits, both in the breadth of the scientific community that is affected and in the potential applicability to many biological questions of interest. The structural genomics programs are no exception. It is our belief that the compendium of complete protein structures that is planned by the NIGMS Protein Structure Initiative will be of value not only to structural biologists, but also to the increasing number of scientists in all branches of biology who find structural information essential in the course of their research.

REFERENCES

1. D Vitkup, E Melamud, J Moult, C Sander. Completeness in structural genomics. Nat Str Biol 8:559–566, 2001.
2. Nature Structural Biology, Supplement 7S, November 2001.
3. http://www.nigms.nih.gov/funding/psi.html.
4. S Fields. Proteomics in genomeland. Science 291:1221–1223, 2001.

2

Producing Proteins

Aled M. Edwards
Affinium Pharmaceuticals and University of Toronto, Toronto, Ontario, Canada

Cheryl H. Arrowsmith
Affinium Pharmaceuticals and Ontario Center for Structural
Proteomics, Toronto, Ontario, Canada

Raymond Hui, Fabien Marino, and Ken Yamazaki
Affinium Pharmaceuticals, Toronto, Ontario, Canada

Alexei Savchenko
Ontario Center for Structural Proteomics, Toronto, Ontario, Canada

Adelinda Yee
Ontario Cancer Institute and Department of Medical Biophysics,
University of Toronto, Toronto, Ontario, Canada

1 BACKGROUND

Genomics has both captivated and disenchanted the pharmaceutical industry: captivated in that the sequence information will doubtless provide molecular explanations and therapeutic targets for all human diseases, yet
disenchanted in that it has proven to be difficult to translate the sequence
information into drug discovery. The difficulty arises largely from two factors. First, the pharmaceutical infrastructure has not been developed to
process the hundreds of new targets in an efficient and cost-effective manner.
The many targets revealed by the genomic technologies must still be pared
down to a handful that can be processed using traditional strategies. Second,
genomic information is useful for drug discovery only if expressed in structural and functional terms, and it is still impossible to predict protein structure, function, and disease relevance from sequence information.

9

In this chapter, we will address the current and future approaches to translate sequence into structural information. We will briefly review the procedures to generate purified proteins for structural studies and focus the chapter on the application of these standard protein purification methods in high-throughput biology.

2 STRUCTURAL BIOLOGY AND DRUG DISCOVERY

Structural biology has historically been used to expedite the drug discovery process by facilitating lead optimization. Over the past few years, with the increased availability of structural information for therapeutic targets, the pharmaceutical researcher has been able to use the improving methods of virtual screening to reduce the cost of high-throughput screening. Now, with the completion of the human genome–sequencing effort, it will be possible to generate structural information for all therapeutic targets, and this is expected to improve target validation/invalidation, screening and lead optimization.

Structural proteomics, which is the field focusing on high-throughput structure determination, aims to determine the three-dimensional (3D) structures of all proteins using either experimental or computational approaches (1–3). Most of the international effort in this area is taking place in the public sector, with major efforts under way in Canada, Germany, Japan, and the United States (4–6). Private sector efforts are focused primarily on the fraction of proteins that are current targets for therapeutic intervention.

The information from the combined public and private efforts is expected to generate valuable clues to the rules for predicting protein folding, to the understanding of biochemical function, and for facilitating structure-based drug discovery. The development of better and faster methods to clone, express, and purify proteins, which is essential for structural proteomics, is also expected to generate new methods and reagents (clones, proteins, and purification procedures) that will benefit the general biological community as well as structural proteomics researchers.

3 CHALLENGES FOR STRUCTURAL PROTEOMICS

Rapid progress of the structural proteomics efforts will require major advances in several areas, including protein expression, protein purification, protein crystallization, and NMR sample preparation. Most progress is required in the steps prior to generating an excellent sample for structural biology, because with current structural methodologies, given an excellent structural sample, it is virtually guaranteed that a 3D structure will be rapidly achieved. Accordingly, improvements in the throughput of NMR data collection, in NMR data processing, and in X-ray diffraction methods will be helpful to the effort, but these are unlikely to be the rate-determining steps for the foreseeable future.

Generating large numbers of excellent structural samples will require increased throughput in the methods for cloning, expression, purification, and screening for crystallization or NMR conditions. In most of these areas, the technologies that are being applied to structural proteomics are not novel. Rather, the novelty in the areas of high-throughput cloning, expression, and purification is the engineering component that converts what are standard methods into parallel processes. Structural proteomics must therefore be considered an engineering problem as much as a scientific one. One aspect of this review will describe the approaches that are being used to convert these routine molecular biological processes into high-throughput platforms.

This review will also outline the equally important challenge of integrating individual experimental technologies into an efficient process. The process optimization discussion will describe the software and hardware needs as well as the requirement for excellent information management.

4 CLONING, EXPRESSION, AND PURIFICATION: THE OBLIGATE STEPS

Since the inception of structural proteomics research, a number of academic research groups and biotechnology companies have developed high-throughput protein preparation systems (2,7,8). Although each group has had different objectives and methodology, the key steps involved are common, and typically include

Making expression constructs from genomic DNA or cDNA

Testing and optimizing the level of expression of soluble proteins

Scale-up of cell growth

Protein purification, commonly by affinity chromatography

We will describe the state of the art in each of these areas along with the strategies that are employed at Affinium Pharmaceuticals (Toronto) to accomplish the rapid purification of protein targets.

4.1 Cloning

Producing an expression construct for those genes without introns is a matter of conventional recombinant DNA technology. For intron-containing genes, the rate at which expression constructs are created will be dictated only by the availability of full-length cDNA clones. This should not be a significant issue for structural proteomics because libraries of full-length cDNA clones are easily created and because several are commercially available. There are also many kits available to facilitate the construction of full-length clones. One can also be confident in assuming that full-length cDNAs for at least one splice variant of every gene will be commercially available in the coming years. With full-length clones in hand, the generation of expression constructs will be a matter of implementing conventional cloning methods.

With the imminent commercial availability of full-length cDNA clones, there will be a need for high-throughput sub-cloning cloning in structural proteomics research. Over the past decade, structural biologists have gained an appreciation that rarely does the first expression construct for any given protein generate a protein preparation that will crystallize or behave well in NMR experiments. The basis for this observation is that the probability of generating a suitable structural sample is thought to increase if the unstructured parts of the protein are eliminated and, without modification, the first protein expressed usually contains peptide segments that lack discrete structure. As a result, it is common to have to screen dozens of variants of a given protein to identify one suitable for structural determination. These include sequence variants or variants with different N- and C-termini. As one example, several fragments of the DNA-binding domain from the EBNA1 protein from Epstein–Barr virus form crystals, but only the fragment lacking the unstructured, acidic C-terminal domain formed well-ordered crystals suitable for structure determination (8). Thus, the focus of cloning efforts in structural proteomics will not be to generate cDNA clones but will be to develop cloning systems that can rapidly generate multiple constructs for a variety of forms of any given protein.

There are currently two cloning strategies to create expression constructs; both are in common practice. The first involves the cloning of PCR products into expression vectors that supply either an N- or a C-terminal fusion protein. The PCR primers are appended with restriction sites in order to facilitate directional cloning. The restricted PCR product can be cloned into a series of different expression vectors that supply different fusion proteins. One of the most popular vector series suitable for this strategy is the pET vector family commercially available from Novagen (Madison, WI), which uses the power of bacteriophage T7 transcription machinery (9). Alternatively, the PCR fragments are cloned into the vectors that take advantage of the ability of Taq polymerase to modify the $3'$ end of a PCR fragment with an additional adenosine (10). These vectors [commercially available from Invitrogen (Carlsbad, CA), Novagen, Promega (Madison, WI), etc.] provide thymidine residues linked into the $3'$-ends of linearized plasmid DNA, which will allow some annealing to occur between the vector and the A-tailed PCR product to be ligated (11). These vectors are generally referred to as *T-vectors*, and the process is called *TA cloning*. Commonly, the vectors also supply the sequence for a selective protease, which allows for the removal of the tag protein from the purified fusion protein. The advantages of this method are:

Simplicity and speed: The PCR-cloning method has been used for a decade or more, and each step has been optimized. After optimizing the process, it is relatively straightforward to create hundreds of expression vectors per person per week.

Availability of vectors: There are dozens of commercially available expression constructs that have been designed to accommodate PCR products with a variety of restriction sites.

Proven success: This strategy has been tried and tested; hundreds of protein structures have been determined from clones generated using this approach.

Fidelity of protein sequence: The strategy allows for the expression of near-native protein; after protease treatment, the final product has only a few non-native amino acids at the N- or C-termini.

Cost: Using this strategy, the cost per expression clone is usually lower than $US50, including labor.

Versatility: The restricted PCR product can be cloned into expression vectors designed for bacterial, yeast, insect, or human cells.

The second strategy for subcloning genes into expression vectors makes use of the recombination machinery from prokaryotic phage (12). In these systems, the cDNA is amplified into a PCR product or cloned into a plasmid in which the gene of interest is flanked by recombination sequences. In the presence of the appropriate, commercially available enzymes, the gene can be shuttled from one PCR product or plasmid into another vector that has the appropriate recombination sites by recombination in vitro. This extraordinarily facile set of reactions allows for the shuttling of a gene into an assortment of different plasmids without having to transform bacterial cells. The advantages of this method are:

Simplicity and speed: The recombination machinery is highly specific and very robust. The reactions can be carried out quickly and with a high degrees of success.

Fidelity: Once the initial construct is created and sequenced, the subsequent constructs can be generated without the need to resequence.

Accepted practice: There is an increasingly large panel of expression constructs that are being created to accept input clones from recombination cloning strategies.

For the near future, these cloning approaches will be the most commonly used in the structural proteomics area. Since most of the manipulations involve liquid handling, they are attractive targets for automation; many of the structural proteomics efforts are directed to this end.

4.1.1   The Use of Affinity Tags

Automated protein purification, probably an essential aim of structural proteomics, almost certainly requires that the recombinant proteins be fused to a protein or peptide tag that can be used for affinity purification (*affinity tag*). It is commonly believed that the expression and solubility of a given protein can be affected quite significantly by the choice of the fusion protein. Studies that systematically compare the efficacy of the commonly used affinity tags, in terms of expression and solubility, are now being reported (13). In a set of small human proteins, fusions to maltose-binding protein were more highly expressed and more soluble than other tags, including the polyhistidine tags (14). The propensity to form well-ordered crystals can also be affected dramatically by the choice of the fusion protein. Large fusion proteins, such as maltose-binding protein, are likely to inhibit the formation of well-ordered crystals. Smaller fusion proteins, such as hexahistidine tags, are less likely to adversely affect crystallization. There has not yet been a systematic study to identify the optimal fusion protein for protein structure determination.

One commonly used strategy is to select a single type of affinity tag and quickly identify the proteins that are amenable to structural biology. In this strategy, the recalcitrant proteins could then be fused with an alternative affinity tag(s) for subsequent analysis. It appears that the polyhistidine fusions are the most popular for the initial construct.

Most fusion proteins are linked to the recombinant protein via a sequence of amino acids that are recognized and cleaved by a specific protease. The removal of the fusion protein adds significant complexity to the protein purification process, and thus there is a tendency to attempt crystallization or NMR studies with the fusion protein intact. However, it is commonly believed that unstructured portions of proteins, such as a polyhistidine tag, interfere with protein crystallization. A large-scale, well-controlled study will be required to determine if it is advisable to leave or remove the fusion protein prior to crystallization or NMR studies. At the present state of knowledge, it is probably advisable to try both forms of the protein.

4.2 Protein Expression

Our analysis of over 1000 proteins, derived from all three biological Kingdoms, has revealed that approximately 20% of small (< 50 kDa) non-membrane proteins will be able to be purified and concentrated for structural studies (2). These proteins can be studied with current technologies, and they represent the first phase of the structural proteomics projects. Many groups are studying these more tractable proteins, not only because they provide the opportunity to determine new structures but also because they provide a large sample of proteins for scientists seeking to increase the throughput of downstream technologies, such as data collection, data processing, and structure determination and analysis.

In the first phase of the structural proteomics projects, *E. coli* is being used almost exclusively as an expression system because of its ease of use and low cost, the ready availability of suitable expression vectors, and the ease with which proteins can be labeled metabolically with selenomethionine for crystallography or with ^{15}N and ^{13}C for NMR studies. As such, it is most desirable for the structural biologist to modify the protein so expression in *E. coli* is possible.

There are certain proteins that will be more difficult to express in soluble form in *E. coli*. For the most part, these fall into five classes:

Those proteins that are not expressed because they are encoded by a set of codons not commonly used in *E. coli*

Those proteins that are not good substrates for the bacterial-folding machinery, in which case there is an aggregation of folding intermediates

Those proteins that are insoluble because of an intrinsic property of a protein, for example, those that aggregate due to a very hydrophobic patch on the surface

Those proteins that require an obligate cofactor or additional protein for proper folding

Those proteins that require post-translational modifications that do not occur in *E. coli*

There are some relatively simple solutions to each of these problems. For proteins whose codon composition varies from that used in *E. coli*, the cells can be supplemented with genes encoding tRNAs that recognize the low-abundance codons (15). There are now engineered bacterial strains, such as the Codon Plus system from Stratagene, that are augmented with genes for rare tRNAs (16). The strategy has proven remarkably effective in many instances. For proteins that do not fold well in *E. coli* and that are produced in an insoluble form, one strategy is to induce them to fold properly by the coexpression of chaperones in the bacterial cell (18,19). More often than not though, this process has not proven effective, and the proteins ultimately must be expressed in a different system. The same is true for those proteins that require post-translational modification that does not occur in *E. coli*. Finally, a protein that requires another protein for expression and folding can be coexpressed in the same bacterial cell from the same plasmid (19). The proteins are encoded either in a single RNA or by a set of tandem genes. The coexpression strategy is highly effective, but it requires considerable knowledge of the protein target's biochemical properties.

4.2.1   Emerging Approaches to Generate Structural Samples From More Challenging Targets

Screening for the Most Soluble Orthologue.   Many recombinant proteins are insoluble when expressed in *E. coli* or other heterologous systems. It is currently impossible to predict the degree of solubility of the encoded protein from its gene sequence. It is known, however, that even subtle changes in amino acid sequence can dramatically affect protein solubility (20,21). Thus, for proteins that have many orthologues, a common strategy is to clone and express many and select the orthologue with the best solubility properties. This approach is proving to be quite productive. We initially studied 68 pairs of orthologous proteins from *Thermatoga maritima* and *E. coli*, hyperthermophilic and mesophilic bacterias, respectively. Proteins of thermophilic origin are usually more stable than their mesophilic orthologues. There is also a prevailing belief that orthologous proteins from thermophilic organisms are more amenable to structural biology methods, presumably because they are predicted to have fewer disordered regions and a higher proportion of salt bridges on the surface (22). We decided to test this hypothesis by comparative analysis of the recombinant expression, the solubility, and the suitability for structural analysis by NMR and/or X-ray crystallography of thermophilic and mesophilic orthologue proteins (23).

A sample suitable for structural studies was obtained for 62 of the 68 pairs of orthologues under standardized growth and purification procedures. Fourteen (eight *E. coli* and six *T. maritima* proteins) samples generated NMR spectra of a quality suitable for structure determination and 30 (14 *E. coli* and 16 *T. maritima* proteins) samples formed crystals. Only three (one *E. coli* and two *T. maritima* proteins) samples both crystallized and had excellent NMR properties. We concluded that the inclusion of even a single orthologue of a protein will increase the number of structural samples dramatically. We also discovered that there was no clear advantage to the use of thermophilic proteins to generate structural samples. We have yet to determine what, if any, additional benefits will be accrued by the addition of more orthologues.

Protein Domains. Proteins that comprise multiple domains are difficult targets for structural proteomics efforts, for three reasons. First, multidomain proteins are difficult to express in *E. coli*. Second, these proteins exhibit conformational heterogeneity, which decreases the probability of crystallization. Third, multidomain proteins are relatively large, which increases the difficulty of using NMR to determine their structure.

A general and powerful strategy that simplifies the analysis of complex proteins is to produce and study them as individual domains. Experience has shown that a single domain of a protein can often be expressed in bacteria, whereas the intact, multidomain protein cannot. Over the past decade, this approach has yielded structural information for dozens of eukaryotic proteins, and we expect that a similar strategy on a proteome-wide scale will be necessary in order to complete the project.

Experimental analysis by limited proteolysis coupled with mass spectrometry (24) is an excellent indicator of domain boundaries. This method is successful because protein domains are relatively more stable to proteolysis than are unstructured portions of proteins. As a result, protein domains can be identified because they are stable intermediates during the proteolysis of a protein. To identify the borders of the stable intermediates, protease-resistant protein fragments can be isolated for mass spectrometry and their masses determined. Once the masses have been determined, the corresponding portion of the protein can be identified using computational methods and an open reading frame encoding the stable fragment subcloned for recombinant expression.

Sequence-based approaches to predict protein domains can also be used, particularly with the advent of genomic information for sometimes dozens of homologues. In this method, a multiple sequence alignment is used to identify highly conserved portions of proteins. The boundaries of the areas of sequence conservation are thought to indicate the boundaries of the functional domains, which can also correspond to structural domains. Secondary structure predictions are also used to guide the selection of the exact N- and C-termini of the conserved protein fragment. The exceptions to the correspondence of functional and structural domains are when functionally conserved regions of proteins do not adopt a stable tertiary structure (such as a protein-interaction motif that folds only when bound to its partner).

In our experience, the experimental approach more often identifies the structural domains than does the sequence-based methods. Accordingly, at Affinium Pharmaceuticals, the process of domain mapping using limited proteolysis and mass spectrometry was automated. Using Affinium's DomainHunter platform, the domain structure of dozens of proteins can be determined automatically in a few days. The use of the DomainHunter™ platform has enabled Affinium scientists to generate new constructs and 3D structures for proteins that had proven intractable by conventional technologies.

Genetic Selection.   The use of orthologues increases the number of samples suitable for structural biology, because they differ from one another predominantly in surface properties, which can dramatically affect the propensity to crystallize. Many crystallographers have now used directed mutagenesis of surface residues to induce crystallization of a given protein.

One emerging strategy to increase the solubility and propensity of a protein to crystallize is to set up genetic screens to select for proteins that both express well and are soluble when produced in *E. coli.* In one example of this strategy, Waldo and colleagues (25) fused a variety of coding sequences N-terminal to the coding region of the green fluorescent protein (GFP), which is known to fold poorly in *E. coli.* Insoluble proteins were found to inhibit the folding of GFP; proteins that were soluble did not affect the folding of GFP. The solubility of the fusion protein could therefore be monitored by measuring the fluorescence of the bacterial colonies after transformation. A similar strategy used chlorampheticol acetyl transferase as the fusion protein and antibiotic resistance as the readout (26). Although elegant in design, it is unclear how successful these methods will be in practice. These methods have now been in practice for several years, yet they have been applied in relatively few reported structure determinations. It is not clear whether this is because there are unexpected difficulties in the methods or whether they have not yet been put into widespread use.

Cell-Free Expression.   Bacterial cell-free expression was developed as an alternative to bacterial expression decades ago, but cell-free methods were unable to accomplish the production of sufficient amounts of recombinant protein to rival intracellular expression. There is now a resurgence of interest in its use because the problem with inefficient expression has been overcome by incorporating continuous-flow methods (27). This is a significant advance because cell-free expression may allow for the soluble expression of those proteins that are unable to fold properly in bacteria. However, before the cell-free protein expression method is adopted for widespread use as a primary protein production method, it will need to be compared directly with bacterial expression for a large number of proteins.

4.3 Protein Purification and Generation of Structural Samples

Structural proteomics projects require the purification of thousands, if not tens of thousands, of proteins and/or protein fragments. This goal cannot be met with current technology because protein purification currently demands considerable user intervention and expert decision-making abilities. Thus, the success of structural proteomics depends on the development of automated or semiautomated, robust, and inexpensive methods for protein purification.

4.3.1 Different Requirements for NMR and Crystallization

Purification strategies are routine for proteins that are highly expressed for use in NMR or X-ray crystallography, and they usually involve an affinity chromatography step using a removable tag, such as hexahistadine. For NMR studies, one or two simple chromatographic steps yield protein samples that are sufficiently pure for acquisition of an initial HSQC NMR spectrum. The small hexahistidine tag is advantageous in samples destined for NMR samples, because its presence greatly simplifies purification but does not usually interfere with the spectrum. For crystallization, removal of the tag and an additional purification step may be required. Greater purity increases the probability that crystals will grow and enhances the reproducibility among crystallization trials. The main concern for both crystallization and NMR is usually the elimination of contaminating proteases from protein samples.

4.3.2 High Throughput Protein Expression and Purification

Cloning and Test Expression. The success of structural proteomics may require the automation of subcloning, test expression, and protein purification. The automation of subcloning and small-scale expression, which are mainly liquid-handling operations, can be achieved in 96-well format by customizing any of a number of existing automation platforms (such as Beckman–Coulter and Qiagen). Commercially available systems are also available for the ancillary cloning operations, such as vacuum filtration, spreading the bacteria on plates, and picking the bacterial colonies. The amount of soluble protein expression is most often monitored using denaturing gel electrophoresis, although capillary methods are now also becoming available (28–30).

Most of the processes of cloning through test expression have been automated. Both Structural Genomix (SGX) and Affinium Pharmaceuticals have adopted remarkably similar strategies. At SGX, 96-well-format liquid-handling systems are used for all steps of the cloning system. Automated colony picking for each expression construct candidate enables rapid 96-well-format screening of individual clones for soluble expression. At Affinium, the cloning and expression system combines an extensively modified, off-the-shelf liquid-handling robot with customized robots for colony picking and for spreading bacterial cells on plates. At SGX, plate cell lysis permits rapid small-scale Ni-ion affinity purification. Production of the desired protein is confirmed via mass spectrometry. At Affinium, the use of a mass spectrometer also allows a quantitative output of the level of protein expression. In addition, the use of mass spectrometry rather than gel electrophoresis allows results from the cloning to be incorporated directly into the laboratory information database. The Affinium platform can generate about 500 new clones per week while at the same time providing quantitative information about the amount of soluble protein that is produced from each expression clone.

Protein Purification. There are two main strategies for automated protein purification: to completely automate the process and to automate selectively. Perhaps the champions of the first approach are the Genomics Institute at the Novartis Research Foundation, the Scripps Institute, and Syrrx Genomix (San Diego), who collaborated to develop an impressive high-throughput protein expression and purification pipeline. This system accomplishes the fermentative growth of 96 cultures in parallel, in 65–70-mL volumes. The integrated system then harvests and lyses the bacteria, clarifies the lysate, and performs the column chromatography. Ninety-six to 192 proteins can be partially purified in a single day. These proteins, which have been purified over a single affinity column, are then ready for further purification steps.

At Affinium Pharmaceuticals, the "flexible automation" approach has been adopted. The ProteoMax^{TM} system is highly modular and was developed to process bacterial extracts to purified, concentrated protein suitable for protein crystallization. ProteoMax^{TM}, which fits on a benchtop, clarifies the bacterial lysate, performs the column chromatography steps, and concentrates the protein for structural studies.

Table 1 Strategies for Optimizing Sample Production for Structural Biology

Production problem	Strategy to resolve problem
Poor expression[a]	• Compensate for codon usage in host strain • Alternative host organism (baculovirus) or strains (*E. coli*) • Alternative expression conditions (temperature/medium) • Alternative fusion tag • Coexpress with required partner protein, if known • Alternative expression construct (small deletion mutants or subdomain of protein) • Select homologous protein as target
Poor solubility[a]	• Purify with GdCl and refold (for small His-tagged proteins) • Alternative host organism (baculovirus) or strains (*E. coli*) • Alternative expression conditions (lower temperature) • Alternative fusion tag • Coexpress with required partner protein, if known • Alternative expression construct (small deletion) mutants or domain of protein) • Select homologous protein as target • Genetic selection of soluble mutants
Failure to crystallize and/or diffract X-rays	• Remove fusion tag • Optimize buffer conditions for stable, nonaggregated protein • Include known ligand(s) or cofactors in sample mutants or subdomain of protein) • Select homologous protein as target • Coexpress with required partner protein, if known
Poor-quality NMR spectrum	• Remove fusion tag • Optimize buffer conditions for stable, nonaggregated protein • Coexpress with required partner protein, if known • Include known ligand(s) in sample • Alternative expression construct (small deletion mutants or domain of protein) • Select homologous protein as target

[a] Associated strategies are best explored in parallel, on a small scale preferably with automation.

Structural Genomix (SGX, San Diego) has developed a modular automated platform that produces large quantities of purified soluble proteins for crystallization. Wherever possible, commercially available robotic systems were incorporated into the technology platform. Highly parallel large-scale purification is carried out using automated serial column chromatography (Ni-ion affinity, ion exchange, and gel filtration). Current production capacity at all three companies supports large-scale purification of thousands of proteins per year.

5 SUMMARY

In the naissance of structural proteomics, it was impressive to clone, express, and produce hundreds of proteins per year. There are now established methods to clone and purify thousands of proteins per year. However, the reality is that from these thousands of purified proteins, there will be only dozens of structures. The historical success rate for determining structures from high-throughput protein purification studies has been 1–5%. It is therefore apparent that the challenge facing protein purification specialists is not simply to produce purified proteins, but to develop rapid methods to engineer and produce proteins that crystallize or that are good NMR samples. Table 1 summarizes many of the strategies that are useful for optimizing protein samples for structural biology. To date, the most productive approach has been to develop methods to identify protein domains, protein–ligand complexes, and protein assemblies, all of which offer advantages in forming excellent structural samples. Some of these methods have already been adapted for high throughput, such as Affinium's DomainHunter™ robot for automated domain mapping. Other approaches will doubtless appear in the near future. With increased technological capabilities in NMR and X-ray crystallography, though, it will be a long time before the production of crystals or NMR samples ceases to be the rate-determining step in the structural proteomics pipeline.

REFERENCES

1. Yee, A., Chang, X., Pineda-Lucena, A., Wu, B., Semesi, A., Le, B., Rameelot, T., Lee, G.M., Bhatacharyya, S., Gutierrez, P., Denisov, A., Lee, C.H., Cort, J., Kozlov, G., Liao, J., Finak, G., Chen, L., Wishart, D., Lee, W., McIntosh, L.P., Gehring, K., Kennedy, M., Edwards, A., Arrowsmith, C.H. An NMR approach to structural proteomics. Proc. Natl. Acad. Sci. USA 99:1825–1830, 2002.

2. Christendat, D., Yee, A., Dharamsi, A., Kluger, Y., Savchenko, A., Cort, J., Booth, V., Mackereth, C., Saridakis, V., Ekiel, I., Kozlov, G., Maxwell, K., Wu, N., McIntosh, L.P., Gehring, K., Kennedy, M., Davidson, A., Pai, E.F., Gerstein, M., Edwards, A., Arrowsmith, C.H. Structural proteomics of an archeon. Nat. Struct. Biol. 7:903–909, 2000.
3. Chance, M.R., Bresnick, A.R., Burley, S.K., Jiang, J., Lima, C., Sali, A., Almo, S., Bonanno, J.B., Buglino, J., Boulton, S., Chen, H., Eswar, N., He, G., Huang, R., Ilyin, V., McMahan, L., Peiper, U., Ray, S., Vidal, M., Wang, L. Structural genomics: a pipeline for providing structures for the biologist. Prot. Sci. 11:723–738, 2002.
4. Terwilliger, T.C. Structural genomics in North America. Nat. Struct. Biol. 7 Suppl:940–942, 2000.
5. Yokoyama, S., Matsuo, Y., Hirota, H., Kigawa, T., Shirouzu, M., Kuroda, Y., Kurumizaka, H., Kawaguchi, S., Ito, Y., Shibata, T., Kainosho, M., Nishimura, Y., Inoue, Y., Kuramitsu, S. Structural genomics projects in Japan. Prog. Biophys. Mol. Biol. 73:363–376, 2000.
6. Heinemann, U. Structural genomics in North America. Nat. Struct. Biol. 7 Suppl.:940–942, 2000.
7. Heinemann, U., Frevert, J., Hofmann, K.P., Illing, G., Maurer, C., Oschkinat, H., Saenger, W. An Integrated approach to structural genomics. Prog. Biophys. Mol. Biol. 73:347–362, 2000.
8. Bochkarev, A., Bochkarev, E., Frappier, L., Edwards, A. The 2.2-Å structure of a permanganate-sensitive DNA site bound by the Epstein–Barr virus origin binding protein, EBNA1. J. Mol. Biol. 284:1273–1278, 1998.
9. Studier, F.W., Rosenberg, A.H., Dunn, J.J., Dubendorff, J.W. Use of T7 RNA polymerase to direct expression of cloned genes. Meth. Enzymol. 185:60–89, 1990
10. Clark, J.M. Novel non-templated nucleotide addition reactions catalyzed by procaryotic and eucaryotic DNA polymerases. Nucleic Acid Res. 16:9677–9686, 1988
11. Kovalic, D., Kwak, J.H., Weisblum, B. General method for direct cloning of DNA fragments generated by the polymerase chain reaction. Nucleic Acids Res. 16:4560, 1991.
12. Palazzolo, M.J., Hamilton, B.A., Ding, D.L., Martin, C.H., Mead, D.A., Mierendorf, R.C., Raghavan, K.V., Meyerowitz, E.M., Lipshitz, H.D. Phage, lambda cDNA cloning vectors for subtractive hybridization, fusion-protein synthesis and Cre-loxP automatic plasmid subcloning. Gene 88:25–36, 1990.
13. Kapust, R.B., Waugh, D.S. *Escherichia coli* maltose-binding protein is uncommonly effective at promoting the solubility of polypeptides to which it is fused. Protein Sci. 8:1668–1674, 1999.
14. Hammarstrom, M., Hellgren, N., Van den Berg, S., Berglund, H., Hard, T. Rapid screening for improved solubility of small human proteins produced as fusion proteins in *Escherichia coli*. Protein Sci. 11:313–321, 2002.

15. Kane, J.F. Effects of rare codon clusters on high-level expression of heterologous proteins in *Escherichia coli*. Curr. Opin. Biotechnol. 6:494–500, 1993.

16. Carstens, C.P., Waesche, A. Codon bias-adjusted BL21 derivatives for protein expression. Strategies 12:49–51, 1999.

17. Luo, Z.H. & Hua, Z.C. Increased solubility of glutathione S-transferase-P16 (GST-p16) fusion protein by co-expression of chaperones GroES and GroEL in *Escherichia coli*. Biochem. Mol. Biol. Int. 46:471–477, 1998.

18. Hayhurst, A., & Harris, W.J. *Escherichia coli* skp chaperone coexpression improves solubility and phage display of single-chain antibody fragments. Protein Expression Purification 15:336–343, 1999.

19. Bochkarev, A., Bochkareva, E., Frappier, L., Edwards, A.M. The crystal structure of the complex of replication protein A subunits RPA32. and RPA14 reveals a mechanism for single-stranded DNA binding. EMBO J. 18:4498–504, 1999.

20. Dale, G.E., Langen, H., D'Arcy, A., Stuber, D., Improving protein solubility through rationally designed amino acid replacements: solubilization of the trimethoprim-resistant type S1 dihydrofolate reductase. Protein Eng. 7:933–939, 1994.

21. Nieba, L., Honegger, A., Krebber, C., Pluckthun, A. Disrupting the hydrophobic patches at the antibody variable/constant domain interface: improved in vivo folding and physical characterization of an engineered scFv fragment. Protein Eng. 10:435–444, 1997.

22. Wesson, L, Eisenberg, D. Atomic solvation parameters applied to molecular dynamics of proteins in solution. Protein Sci. 1:227–235, 1992.

23. Savchenko, A., Yee, A., Khachatryan, A., Skarina, T., Evdokimova E., Pavlova, M., Semesi, A., Northey, J., Beasley, S., Lan, N., Das, R., Gerstein, M., Arrowmith, C.H., Edwards, A.M. Strategies for structural proteomics of prokaryotes: quantifying the advantages of studying orthologous proteins and of using both NMR and X-ray crystallography approaches. Proteins, accepted, 2002

24. Koth, C., Botuyan, M., Moreland, R., Jansma, R., Conaway, J., Conaway, R., Chazin, W., Friesen, J., Arrowsmith, C., Edwards, A. Elongin from *Saccharomyces cerevisiae*. J. Biol. Chem. 275:11174–11180, 2000.

25. Waldo, G.S., Standish, B.M., Berendzen, J., Terwilliger, T. Rapid protein-folding assay using green fluorescent protein. Nature Biotech. 17:691–695, 1999.

26. Maxwell, K.L., Mittermaier, A.K., Forman-Kay, J.D., Davidson, A.R. A simple in vivo assay for increased protein solubility. Protein Sci. 8:1908–1911, 1999.

27. Spirin, A.S., Baranov, V.I., Ryabova, L.A., Ovodov, S.Y., Alakhov, Y.B. A continous cell-free production translation system capable of producing polypeptides in high yield. Science 242:1162–1164, 1988.

28. Landers, J.P., ed. CRC Handbook of Capillary electrophoresis: Principles, Methods, and Applications, CRC Press: Boca Raton, FL, 1993.

29. Braddock, R.J., Bryan, C.R., Burns, J. Capillary electrophoresis analysis of orange juice pectinesterases. J. Agric. Food Chem. 49:846–850, 2001.
30. Grady, J.K., Zang, J., Laue, T.M., Arosio, P., Chasteen, D. Characterization of the H- and L-subunit ratios of ferritins by sodium dodecyl sulfate-capillary gel electrophoresis. Anal. Biochem. 302:263–268, 2002.

3

Crystallization of Membrane Proteins

R. Michael Garavito
Michigan State University, East Lansing, Michigan, U.S.A.

1 INTRODUCTION

Since the early 1990s, an increasing number of crystal structures of integral membrane proteins have appeared in the literature, many of which have been hailed as stunning breakthroughs (1,2). Nonetheless, the crystallographic analysis of membrane proteins still remains difficult, for one simple reason: Straightforward and routine methodologies for obtaining X-ray-quality crystals are still rudimentary. This sobering statement contrasts markedly with the current state of structural analysis for soluble proteins, where "high-throughput" crystallography is in vogue in this postgenomic era. Nonetheless, integral membrane proteins represent at least 25% of the proteins encoded in the genomes of most organisms (3), and they include many potential sites for drug development. This has spurred new efforts to crystallize integral membrane proteins.

This chapter attempts to highlight the maturing methods and strategies for obtaining crystalline preparations of integral membrane proteins for single crystal X-ray diffraction analysis. Several general reviews (4–10) have covered the field of membrane protein crystallization, more or less extensively. As with any difficult methodology, many rules, dogmas, and bits of lore have arisen. However, recent crystal structures and crystallization stu-

dies have shed new light on the problem and have altered the way researchers approach membrane protein crystallization.

2 BACKGROUND TO THE PROBLEM: CRYSTALLIZING A GREASED BALL

The successful crystallization of soluble proteins and nucleic acids essentially depends on preparing samples of the desired macromolecules that are
pure as well as structurally and chemically homogeneous (11,12). With an
isotropic, nonaggregated sample, standard screening methods for potential
crystallization conditions will yield suitable crystals without substantial
effort in most cases. The primary obstacle in dealing with membrane proteins is that they exist in the quite anisotropic, amphipathic environment of
biological membranes. To remain stably integrated within a lipid bilayer, a
significant portion of their surface has a hydrophobic character. Once
removed from the bilayer, membrane proteins are not readily soluble in
simple aqueous or apolar environments.

Techniques for handling membrane proteins in a manner suitable for
crystallization experiments place the target protein in a nonbiological detergent environment during isolation from the membrane. These detergents
first disrupt the bilayer and allow the extraction of the protein as a protein–detergent complex (PDC). Generally, nonionic detergents have provided a general and efficacious means to solubilize and manipulate
membrane proteins. However, a poor choice of a solubilization detergent
can often lead to metastable solubilization and subsequent, nonspecific
aggregation. Moreover, the activity and/or physical stability of a membrane
protein may be compromised by its removal from the lipid bilayer (13,14).
Hence, finding solubilization conditions for integral membrane proteins,
which are also compatible with most crystallization protocols, remains a
major and primary obstacle. Understanding how detergents and PDCs actually behave has helped push forward the critical developments in the field of
membrane protein crystallization. Many new detergents for membrane biochemistry have been synthesized over the last decade, and the characterization of their solution and phase behavior has given us a better idea of their
usefulness in crystallization experiments.

In this chapter, I will briefly discuss the basic aspects of detergent
chemistry and PDC structure that are relevant to protein crystallization.
For more detailed information on detergent chemistry, the reader is directed
to several earlier sources. Comprehensive reviews by Helenius and Simons
(15), Tanford and Reynolds (16), Helenius et al. (17), Kühlbrandt (7), and
Zulauf (18) cover the action and behavior of detergents from a biochemical
viewpoint. Two excellent monographs by Tanford (19) and Rosen (20), as

well as a review by Wennerström and Lindman (21), describe the physical chemistry of detergents and surfactants in detail.

2.1 Surfactant Properties of Detergents and Lipids

Detergents are surface-active molecules that can self-associate and bind to hydrophobic surfaces in a concentration-dependent manner (18,20,21). The amphipathic character of detergents is evident in their structures (Fig. 1), which consist of a polar (or charged) head group and a hydrophobic tail. Most detergents fall into three categories, depending on the type of head group: ionic (cationic or anionic), nonionic, and zwitterionic (both anionic and cationic). The behavior of a specific detergent is dependent on the character and stereochemistry of the head group and tail.

In the broader sense, lipids are the same as detergents: They are both surfactants. What distinguishes one from the other are the concentration regimes for self-association and the kinds of multimolecular structures each can make. The problem of isolating native membrane proteins from lipid bilayers and then subsequently manipulating them is, in essence, a problem of dealing with mixed surfactant systems. In membrane protein crystallization, the most common question is whether a "magic bullet" detergent

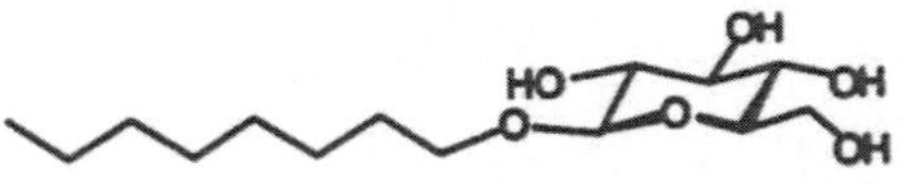

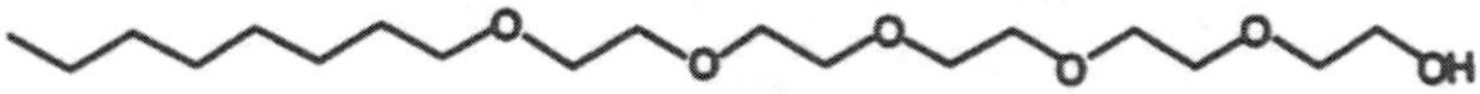

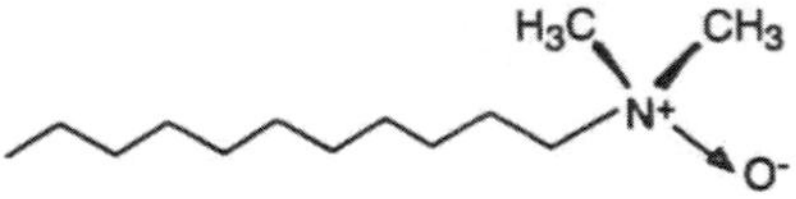

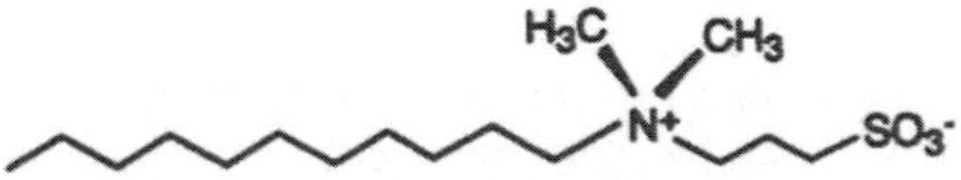

Figure 1 Structure of some typical detergents. Detergent monomers of β-D-octyl glucoside (β-OG), octyl-pentaoxyethylene (C_8E_5), lauryl-dimethylamine-oxide (LDAO), and zwittergent 3-12 (Z3-12) are shown; each consists of a polar head group and N-alkyl tail.

exists. The simple answer is no, but successful strategies for detergent use can be developed if one understands how detergents and lipids impact the physical nature of a PDC and its behavior.

2.2   The Nature of Detergent Micelles

Detergent monomers in aqueous solutions are involved in two kinds of basic phase transitions. First, monomers can crystallize in aqueous solution (20), although the majority (*but not all*) of detergents used in membrane biochemistry do not (7,15–17). Second, detergent monomers self-associate to form structures called *micelles* (18,20,21). At the broad threshold of monomer concentration called the *critical micelle concentration*, or CMC (Fig. 2), self-association occurs and micelles form. Ideally, the concentration of detergent monomers stays constant above the CMC as more detergent is added to the solution; only the concentration of micelles increases (22).

When the detergent concentration exceeds the CMC, hydrophobic and amphipathic solutes, such as lipids, can be solubilized into mixed micelles and micellar aggregates (18,21). The complete and stable solubilization of many integral membrane proteins also occurs above the CMC. In a manner similar to their self-association into micelles, detergent monomers associate

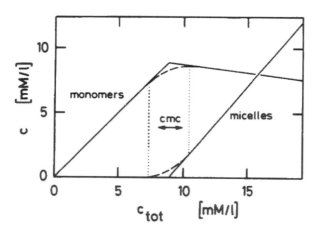

Figure 2   Change in concentration of monomer and micellar fractions with the total detergent concentration. As the total detergent concentration increases, the monomer concentration increases until micelles begin to form (the critical micelle concentration, or CMC). After the CMC is passed, the ambient concentration of detergent monomers does not generally increase. The CMC is not really a sharp boundary, but a broad transition. Thus, the CMC is often taken as the midpoint of the concentration range for the transition. (Adapted from Ref. 22.)

with the hydrophobic surfaces of membrane proteins to create water-soluble PDCs (23–25).

Micellarization is a common phenomenon with many surfactants. The average size and shape of micelles depend on the type, size, and stereochemistry of the surfactant monomer (20,21,26) as well as the solvent environment. The size of a micelle can be described by its average molecular weight, hydrodynamic radius, or aggregation number (the average number of monomers per micelle). The majority of nonionic detergents used to crystallize membrane proteins (4,6,7) form relatively small spherical or oblate ellipsoidal micelles (18,27,28). The physical and chemical characteristics of a detergent determine micelle size and shape as well as the size and shape of the detergent layer in a PDC.

Contrary to the simplistic cartoon of spherical micelles we see in the literature (Fig. 3a), the detergent monomers do not assume ordered conformations in micelles and in PDCs. The more realistic picture of a detergent micelle (Figs. 3b and 3c) has the hydrophobic tails packing in a very compact but disorganized fashion. This packing arrangement results in micelle radii that are about 10–30% smaller than the fully extended length of the detergent monomer (18). Three important conclusions arise from molecular dynamic studies on short-chain detergents (i.e., a tail length of 8–12 carbons) (29–31). First, the micelle surface is quite rough and inhomogeneous in character, and not all of the hydrophobic tails are buried. This allows the detergent tails to have considerable contact with water and solutes. Second, micelle shape is very dependent on aggregation number (Fig. 3), which in turn depends on the solvent environment. Finally, the concept of a "spherical" micelle really denotes only a small, *average* shape that may occur under only a very limited set of environmental conditions.

The concept of a compact, disordered micelle (Fig. 3) also suggests that packing defects could radically affect the size, shape, and behavior of micelles. Furthermore, the formation of mixed micelles with lipids, another detergent, or an amphipathic solute could introduce *or* eliminate packing defects in micelles. By extrapolation, the bound detergents in a PDC are unlikely to be well ordered and efficiently packed. Perhaps, the inability of a specific detergent to solubilize or stabilize some membrane proteins may arise from the unstable, defect-ridden packing of detergent monomers on the protein's surface.

Micelles are also not static and uniform structures. The term *monodisperse* is often applied to colloidal systems to signify a uniform size and shape of a population of particles. For detergents, monodispersity is better perceived to be a *lack of detectable* heterogeneity in the *average* micelle size and shape (32). The experimental evidence suggests that micelles are quite fluid and rapidly exchange micellar components with the solvent

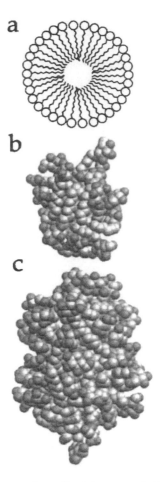

Figure 3 A classical representation of a detergent micelle compared (a) to space-filling models of β-D-octyl glucoside micelles in a 20-monomer micelle in (b) and 50-monomer micelle (c). The 20-monomer and 50-monomer micelles shown in (b) and (c), respectively, were derived from 40-ns molecular dynamics simulation data (29); note the nonspherical and nonuniform shapes. The polar portions of the detergents (oxygen, lighter gray; carbon atoms, dark gray) do not cover completely the micelle surface. Hence, substantial portions of the core are exposed to bulk solvent, including alkyl chains lying along the micelle surface.

(20,21,33,34). Micelles will deform, split, and fuse over time to form some complex detergent structures (20,21,29–31,35). Molecular dynamic studies on small detergent micelles (29–31) show clear and dramatic fluctuations in micellar shape.

Appreciable changes in micelle aggregation number, size, and shape may also occur as the total detergent concentration rises (36–38). This can be an important aspect of micelle behavior because the micelle must alter its shape (Fig. 3) as new monomers are incorporated into the aggregate (29–31). Thus, the shape can change from spherical to ellipsoidal or even to rodlike, depending on temperature, the presence of solutes, and detergent concentration. This phenomenon may be rather pronounced when a detergent is mixed with another detergent, lipid, or protein (39).

In a PDC, how a membrane protein behaves will be influenced by detergent–protein and detergent–detergent interactions as well as by interactions with any remaining lipid. The fluidity and packing efficiency of the detergent monomers bound to the protein will affect the deformability and stability of the detergent layer. Thus, detergent behavior will impact how a membrane protein will behave during isolation (23,24,40), characterization (23,25,41), and crystallization (6,7,10).

2.3 Detergent-Phase Behavior

Self-association and crystallization are only two of many possible phase transitions that surfactant solutions may exhibit (18,20). Phase diagrams of detergent behavior in aqueous solutions are generally simple for the nonionic detergents used in membrane biochemistry. However, some phase changes involve micellar growth and/or fusion to form mesophases with distinct structural properties (18,20,26). One common detergent phenomenon is called the *cloud point* (18,26), where a clear, homogeneous detergent solution turns turbid upon heating. The formerly single liquid phase (L_1) eventually separates into two immiscible solutions ($L_1' + L_1''$), one detergent-rich and the other detergent-poor. The boundary between the isotropic detergent phase and the coexistence of the two liquid phases (Fig. 4) is called a *consolute boundary* (18,26). Bordier (42) recognized that this phase phenomenon could be exploited for membrane protein purification.

Nonionic and zwitterionic detergents with N-alkyl tails of 12 carbons or longer tend to exhibit much more complex phase behaviors (Fig. 4, middle panel). These phase phenomena clearly show the structural and physical relationships between detergents and biological lipids. The phase transitions exhibited by a particular surfactant are determined by its structure (shape) as well as its chemistry (18,26), e.g., its ionization state or capacity for hydration. Changes in the hydration of a surfactant can also alter the nature of surfactant aggregation (18,43). In Figure 4, the detergent $C_{12}E_8$ exhibits the hexagonal H_1 phase (hexagonal packing of rodlike micelles) at 50% (w/w) mixture with water at 30°C. When the detergent

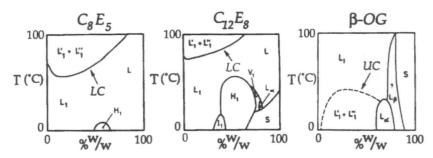

Figure 4 Detergent-phase diagrams for octyl-pentaoxyethylene (C_8E_5), dodecyl-octaoxyethylene ($C_{12}E_8$), β-D-octyl glucoside (β-OG). While the phase diagram for C_8E_5 is quite simple, the equivalent diagram for $C_{12}E_8$ shows several additional phases (see Refs. 18 and 26 for details). For C_8E_5 and $C_{12}E_8$, detergent-phase separation is often seen in membrane biochemistry, for salts and polymers can depress the lower consolute (LC) boundary to below room temperature. For β-OG in water, only the lamellar L_α and gel L_β phases are observed, aside from solid detergent (S). However, the addition of PEG causes the appearance of an upper consolute (UC) boundary, which rises with increasing polymer or salt concentration (Refs. 4 and 18).

concentration increases to above 70% (w/w), bicontinuous cubic (V_2) and lamellar (L_α) phases are seen (18,26).

Although many of the detergent-phase transitions occur at relatively high detergent concentrations (18,26), the addition of salts or polar solutes to a detergent solution can radically alter the phase boundaries. In mixed solute systems, phase phenomena can appear at much lower temperatures and at the lower detergent concentrations typically used for membrane proteins. The detergent-dependent phase separation is a frequent problem during membrane protein crystallization (4,6,7). For example, the octyl-oligo-oxyethylene (C_8E_m) detergents display a *lower* consolute boundary (*LC*, Fig. 4, left-hand panel), which is depressed to *lower* temperatures in the presence of high salt and other crystallization agents (18,43). As the temperature rises, micelles become increasingly dehydrated and begin to aggregate into clusters (18,38). When the lower consolute boundary is crossed, the micelle clusters phase out and form a new aqueous, detergent-rich phase (L_1''). Some polymer crystallization agents, like polyethylene glycol (PEG), also radically alter the phase behavior of nonionic detergents (4,18), particularly the alkyl glycosides detergents, such as β-D-octyl glucoside and β-D-decyl maltoside (β-OG and $C_{10}M$, respectively). Addition of PEG to a β-OG solution causes an *upper* consolute boundary to appear (*UC*, Fig. 4, right-hand panel). The take-home lesson is that solution and environmental parameters do not affect only the basic detergent phenomenon; they in turn can significantly impact membrane protein crystallization.

2.4 Mixed Micelles, Protein–Detergent Complexes, and Crystallization

What makes understanding surfactant-phase phenomena so important is that the mere use of detergents with membrane proteins forces us to confront them, from protein isolation to crystallization. Considering only detergents and lipids, mixed systems *will not behave* like solutions of the pure components (20,21). Changes in micelle shape and size, CMC, and phase behavior all occur, and they are not easily predicted. For simple solutions containing two detergents, nonideal mixing of components and perturbed CMCs can complicate something as simple as detergent exchange. How detergent behavior impacts the solubility, stability, and structure of protein–detergent complexes (PDCs) is then important to know.

For membrane protein crystallization, a major emphasis was initially placed on creating simple, lipid-free PDCs (6,7). In these "simple" systems, the shape, size, and behavior of the PDC were controlled by using nonionic detergents that produced small, almost spherical micelles (4,7,44). It was recognized quite early that detergent-dependent phase transitions had an enormous impact on crystallization. Unwanted phase behavior could prevent crystal growth (45) and even denature the protein (46). However, exploitation of detergent-dependent phase transitions soon began after it was discovered that crystal growth often occurred as conditions approached an upper or lower consolute phase boundary (6). Several studies have focused on how the detergent-dependent phase behavior of the PDC affects crystal growth (25,41,47) and how different detergents (28,45,48,49) can tailor the PDC for successful crystallization.

Information about the shape and structure of the detergent layer in a PDC has also been derived from the characterization of membrane protein crystals by single-crystal neutron diffraction and D_2O/H_2O density matching (50–54). The detergent complexes of OmpF porin from *E. coli* revealed some interesting aspects of detergent behavior. Pebay-Peyroula et al. (50) studied the tetragonal crystal form of OmpF porin containing decyl-dimethylamine-oxide (DDAO) or β-OG. With DDAO, the porin–detergent complex behaved as a "hard-sphere" complex (Fig. 5A). While there were substantial interactions between detergent surfaces in the crystal, the detergent layer appeared as a discrete and continuous torus about the protein. In contrast, the porin/β-OG complex revealed that a partial fusion of the detergent torus with its neighbor (Fig. 5B) seemed to occur. Penel et al. (51) looked at the trigonal crystal form of OmpF porin containing octyl-

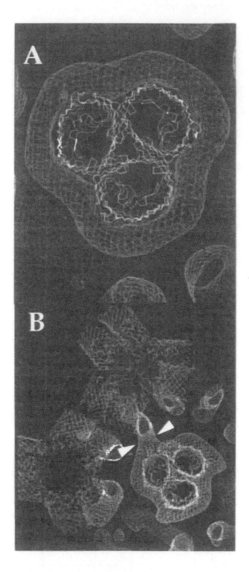

Figure 5 Views of the detergent layer about a membrane protein. The single-crystal neutron diffraction structure of OmpF porin is seen at 100% D_2O in (A) decyldimethylamine oxide (DDAO) or (B) β-OG (Ref. 50); the scattering-length map was contoured to reveal the bound detergent layer (dark gray). When overlaid on the C-alpha wire model (light gray in panels A and B) of OmpF porin in the crystal, the relationship between the protein and a torus of detergent is evident. For DDAO, the detergent layer does not merge with neighboring layers. In contrast, the β-OG layer about one porin trimer apparently fuses (arrows) with a detergent layer around another porin trimer.

hydroxyethyl-sulfoxide (OHES; Table 1). Here, the detergent torus about each porin molecule had completely fused with its nearest neighbors to create continuous detergent phase within the crystal. Clearly, detergents, which should normally produce just small spherical or ellipsoidal micelles, can be induced to form more complex structures at concentrations below 50% (w/w). Moreover, detergent–detergent interactions were *an integral part* of the long-range structure in these membrane protein crystals.

2.5 Lipid Interactions as Observed in Membrane Protein Crystals

The crystal structures of bacteriorhodopsin (55,56) and bovine cytochrome *C* oxidase (57) showed a remarkable feature: A layer of lipid molecules was resolved on the protein surface. The nature of the lipids, originating from their native membranes, and their positioning in the proteins' grooves and crevices suggests a structural role. The functional significance of this "annular layer" of lipid has been much debated, but the bilayer was generally considered as a hydrophobic solvent, albeit complex in its properties (58). With the advent of high-resolution crystal structures of membrane proteins, the observation of protein-bound lipid molecules now appears to be becoming a rule rather than an exception. Moreover, these crystalline complexes of membrane proteins and lipid do not contain just unusual lipids, such as cardiolipin (59) and diether lipids (56), but also more common phospholipids. The structure of bovine cytochrome *C* oxidase at 2.8-Å resolution revealed five phosphatidylethanolamine and three phosphatidylglycerol molecules per 200-kD monomer (57). These recent crystallographic results imply that lipid may stabilize membrane proteins in a more homogeneous conformation at the molecular level.

In some cases, the maintenance of some lipid–protein interactions may be critical for procedures like crystallization. Nussberger et al. (60) document the requirement for four molecules of digalactosyl diacyl glycerol per molecule of plant light-harvesting complex to allow two-dimensional crystallization. The crystal structures of rhodopsin [61] and the sarcoplasmic Ca^{++} pump (62) also emphasize this point. In the case of rhodopsin, minimal purification was used, including a single detergent extraction step (63), while the crystallization of the Ca^{++} pump involved readdition of lipid (62).

The significance of these findings could be profound in terms of how we approach the use of detergents in purification. For membrane protein crystallization, the complete removal of lipid to obtain monodisperse, homogeneous PDCs was an early goal. The reason for doing so was that the retention of significant amounts of phospholipid generally promotes self-association into insoluble, polydisperse aggregates (40). However, com-

Table 1 Common Detergents Used in Membrane Protein Crystallization[a]

Detergent name	Common name	Source	Formula	Formula weight	CMC (mM)
n-Octyl-β-D-glucoside	Octyl Glucoside	Anatrace[b]	$C_{14}H_{28}O_6$	292.4	20
n-Decyl-β-D-maltoside	Decyl Maltoside	Anatrace	$C_{22}H_{42}O_{11}$	482.6	1.8
n-Dodecyl-β-D-maltoside	Dodecyl Maltoside	Anatrace	$C_{24}H_{46}O_{11}$	510.6	0.17
Cyclohexyl-pentyl-β-D-glucoside	CYMAL-5	Anatrace	$C_{23}H_{42}O_{11}$	494.5	2
Tetraethylene glycol monooctyl ether	C_8E_4	Fluka[c]	$CH_3(CH_2)_{17}(OCH_2CH_2)_4OH$	306.2	7
Heptaethylene glycol monodecyl ether	$C_{10}E_7$	Fluka	$C_3(CH_2)_9(OCH_2CH_2)_7OH$	466.7	1
n-Decyl-N,N-dimethylamine-N-oxide	DDAO	Fluka	$C_{12}H_{27}NO$	201.4	10
n-Dodecyl-N,N-dimethylamine-N-oxide	LDAO	Anatrace	$C_{14}H_{31}NO$	229.41	1.5
2-Hydroxyethyloctylsulfoxide	OHES	Bachem[d]	$C_{10}H_{22}O_2S$	206.3	20
Decanoyl-N-hydroxyethylglucamide	HEGA-10	Anatrace	$C_{18}H_{32}NO_7$	379.5	7
N-Decylphosphocholine	Fos-Choline-10	Anatrace	$C_{15}H_{34}NO_4P$	323.4	11

[a] These are the author's preferences only. Bachem and Anatrace also provide custom synthesis for new detergents.
[b] Anatrace, Maumee, Ohio; www.anatrace.com; 1-800-252-1280.
[c] Fluka (a Sigma-Aldrich company); www.sigma-aldrich.com; 1-800-325-3010.
[d] Bachem AG, Bubendorf, Switzerland; www.bachem.com; +41/61/935 23 33.

plete removal of bound lipid from many membrane proteins is not only difficult and often detrimental to structure and function (23,64,65), but it is also rarely achieved. The trend now is to isolate partially delipidated PDCs that are monodisperse and homogeneous but that still contain a full complement of critical lipids. Hence, understanding the specificity of detergents for solubilizing protein *and* lipid is an important consideration in designing purification procedures with the aim of structure determination (40).

3 CRYSTALLIZATION STRATEGIES FOR PROTEIN–DETERGENT COMPLEXES

The information and concepts presented in the previous sections are merely the groundwork for approaching the crystallization of membrane proteins from detergent-solubilized protein preparations. To date, there are two successful methods for crystallizing membrane proteins. The first method applies conventional crystallization techniques for proteins (6,7,10) directly to a preparation of detergent-solubilized membrane protein. In most cases, crystals are obtained by the addition of standard precipitation agents such as ammonium sulfate (AS) and PEG. This method has been quite successful for growing large, X-ray-quality crystals of integral membrane proteins. The second method utilizes unique bicontinuous cubic phases of surfactant that can absorb membrane proteins in PDCs into a bilayer-like environment (66,67). In this method, the mechanism by which crystallization occurs and crystals grow is not yet understood, although crystals of microbial 7-helical membrane proteins are easily obtained (68–71). The essential aspects of each method are discussed in this section.

3.1 The Choice of Protein Target for Crystallization

While choosing a membrane protein target for study seems to be a trivial endeavor, it is a surprisingly critical step from the practical and technical viewpoints. For example, channel or receptor "X" may be the desired target, but it may not be readily crystallizable. For several recent structure determinations, success was achieved only after considerable effort was placed on surveying target homologs from various species. Suitable crystals of the mechanosensory channel MscL (72) were found after screening nine prokaryotic homologs. Chang and Roth (73) recently determined the structure of MsbA, an *E. coli* homolog of eukaryotic multidrug-resistance (MDR) transporters. However, this successful structure determination arose from extensive crystallization screens of 20 MDR transporters from 12 different bacterial species.

To determine the structures of some membrane proteins, e.g., OmpA (74) and the bacterial potassium channel KcsA (75), the expression of appropriately truncated versions of the target protein was necessary. Privès and colleagues (76,77) have proposed engineering in genetically large polar loops to increase the extramembranous surface of a membrane protein to enhance the possibility of crystallization. While this has not yet proven routinely feasible, Michel and coworkers (78,79) have used F_v fragments from monoclonal antibodies to create F_v–protein complexes that are crystallizable. The rationale here is that any increase in the extramembranous surface of a membrane protein could enhance the possibility of crystallization. The monoclonal antibody technique has produced successful structure determinations in many (80–82), though not all, cases.

3.2 The Choice of Detergent

To reiterate a major point from Section 2, the choice of which detergent(s) to use has a critical impact in the crystallization process. This effect can start at the moment of protein solubilization (6,83). However, choosing a suitable detergent remains a trail-and-error process and is complicated by the fact that not all membrane proteins are stable in the best detergents for crystallization. What complicates the situation further is that a "two-detergent" isolation procedure may be needed to obtain crystallizable protein (83): a detergent for protein isolation and initial purification steps, followed by exchange into a second detergent before crystallization. Hence, careful studies on the effect of detergent type and detergent-to-protein ratio on the extraction of specific lipids and protein and the resultant protein activity (see Ref. 13) are advised. Crystallization trials with protein isolated using different detergents may also result in markedly different levels of crystal appearance and space groups (6,83). Table 1 lists several of the pure, well-characterized detergents suitable for the purification and crystallization of membrane proteins. Several less pure detergents (e.g., octyl-POE, Tween-20, and Triton X-100) can also be used for protein purification *if* they can be quantitatively exchanged for a "crystallization" detergent at the final stage of sample preparation.

3.3 Crystallization of Protein–Detergent Complexes from Isotropic, Detergent-Containing Solutions

Once a protein has been prepared in a suitable detergent system, the "classical" methods for protein crystallization can be used (12,84) to induce the protein–protein interactions needed for crystallization. These methods require the addition of a precipitant to the detergent-solubilized protein solution to initiate crystal growth. The most common precipitants, such as AS and PEG are effective crystallization agents in the presence of low concentrations (0.1–1.0% by volume or weight) of detergent. However, the presence of precipitants will modify the physical properties of the detergent in the crystallization system, as mentioned in Section 2, and unwanted precipitant-induced protein–detergent and detergent–detergent interactions must be watched for.

3.3.1 Precipitant System

Large X-ray-quality crystals have grown in the presence of salts (e.g., AS, sodium citrate, and sodium formate) or polymers (e.g., PEG, PEG monomethylether, and polyvinylpyrrolidone), although crystals have occurred more often with PEG as the precipitant. An important criterion for choosing one precipitant system over another is whether the detergent/salt/buffer system allows one to reach high enough precipitant concentrations to induce crystal growth in the absence of detergent-phase separation. I recommend that one first determine at which precipitant concentrations phase transitions occur with the detergent system being used (47,85). This is important because some zwitterionic detergents not only will phase-separate at high precipitant concentrations, but also can form birefringent liquid crystal phases (J. A. Jenkins and R. M. Garavito, unpublished observations). Because of this phenomenon, one must view the appearance of "protein" microcrystals with a certain amount of skepticism until they are analyzed.

3.3.2 Additives or Small Amphiphiles

The behavior of the detergent is significantly affected by the addition of amphiphilic compounds. These cosolutes or cosurfactants interact directly with micelles and protein–detergent aggregates by partitioning into the detergent layers (25,27,86) and creating mixed micelles. These compounds can also alter the apparent CMC, micelle size, and phase transitions of a detergent solution. While contamination by amphiphilic compounds (e.g., detergent impurities) is undesirable, judicious use of an additive can suppress detergent-phase separation or select a particular crystal form. In the simplest system, a second well-defined detergent component is added to the crystallization experiments at a low molar or weight ratio with respect to the primary detergent (45,48,87).

Amphiphilic compounds other than a detergent (i.e., no observable CMC below 0.1 M) can also act as cosolutes and have allowed the growth of large X-ray-quality crystals of certain membrane proteins (88,89). Examples of such compounds are alcohols (45), alkyl-diols, alkyl-hydroxyethanol (48), and the "small amphiphiles," such as heptane-1,2,3-triol (44,88). These amphiphilic compounds must be added at relatively high concentrations (1–5% w/v) to have an influence on the crystallization process and the detergent-phase transitions. Recent studies have confirmed that heptane-1,2,3-triol addition can alter the apparent micelle size and behavior (25,27,44,86). The crystallization experiments on protein complexes from photosynthetic bacteria still provide the best examples for the use (and drawbacks) of additives in crystallization protocols (88–91). The drawbacks of small-amphiphile use (protein denaturation, irreproducible nucleation, and crystal metastability) are a result of the high concentrations needed to induce crystallization. Often, supersaturating concentrations of the small amphiphiles are reached, which results in amphiphile crystallization; if protein crystals have already grown, they sometimes degrade when the amphiphile crystallizes. Because crystals are often obtained without resorting to adding such compounds, additives may best be used as a means to fine-tune existing crystallization conditions.

3.3.3   Crystallization System

Virtually all crystallization systems work on membrane proteins. Large X-ray-quality crystals of membrane proteins have been grown using bulk methods, vapor diffusion (hanging and sitting drop), microdialysis, and free-interface diffusion. The microscale method of hanging-drop vapor diffusion affords a quick and economical way to test different crystallization conditions. The free-interface diffusion method (12,84) has also been quite successful for screening crystallization conditions for membrane protein on a microscale (92). However, some physical modifications to a crystallization system might be necessary to accommodate detergent-induced physical changes in the protein solution behavior. With the hanging-drop method, it should be noted that the reduction in surface tension of the protein solution, due to the presence of detergent, limits the drop size to much less than 10 μL.

3.3.4   Temperature

The phase transitions of detergents are very temperature sensitive (18,21) and membrane protein crystallization often displays similar temperature sensitivity (6,45). We have often needed to control the temperature of the crystallization environment to within ±1°C to ensure good crystal growth and stability (D. Picot and R. M. Garavito, unpublished observations). It is wise to maintain adequate temperature control throughout the crystallization experiment for reproducible results. However, because temperature is a critical variable in detergent-phase behavior, the use of temperature as a crystallization variable is also possible (Q. Ling and R. M. Garavito, unpublished observations).

3.3.5 Purity and Homogeneity of the Protein Preparation

Successful crystallization often depends on the preparation of pure, homogeneous protein (11,12,93), and thus all factors that create chemical heterogeneity must be minimized or eliminated. The improvement in protein purity for OmpF porin (45), bacterial RC (90, 94), prostaglandin H synthase (83,95), and bacterial LH2 complexes (96) was a critical factor in the growth of large X-ray-quality crystals. Posttranslational modifications (e.g., glycosylation and phosphorylation) that create a heterogeneous population of protein must also be dealt with. While the chemical modifications themselves do not necessarily affect crystallization, the heterogeneity they introduce will. Thus, a wise choice of expression systems and expression conditions will dramatically improve the chances of successful crystallization.

3.3.6 Lipid Content

A question arises about the effect of lipids on crystallization, as the discussion in Section 2 addresses. While heterogeneous native lipids can have adverse effects on crystallization (45), one might ask if crystallization could occur with a homogeneous complex of protein and native lipids or in the presence of pure lipids. Because most aqueous systems of phospholipids exist not as monodisperse micellar solutions but as bilayer structures, crystal formation probably would not occur unless detergents are added to create a micellar solution. However, Eisele and Rosenbusch (92) have examined this hypothesis, using *E. coli* OmpF porin and short-chain lipids as a model system, and observed good crystal growth. This was extended further in the crystallization and structure determination of sarcoplasmic Ca^{++}-dependent ATPase (62), where crystals were obtained after the readdition of lipid (62). Thus, the ability of pure surfactants, whether a detergent or a lipid, to form an appropriate PDC may be an important physical criterion for crystallization. Heterogeneity due to lipid content and detergent exchange can be conveniently monitored by a number of techniques (97), such as thin-layer chromatography and gas chromatography.

3.4 In Cubo Crystallization of Protein–Dependent Complexes

If detergent interactions and structure play a role in membrane protein crystal growth and integrity, could a more lipid-like surfactant environment induce membrane protein crystallization? Landau and Rosenbusch posed this question and came up with a novel way of crystallizing membrane proteins using monoacyl glycerols (66,67). In essence, a preformed surfactant phase with a more bilayer-like structure is used to partition membrane proteins into an environment that could favor close interactions suitable for nucleating and sustaining crystal growth. The bicontinuous cubic surfactant phases (26,98) seem ideal for this purpose because continuous regions of solvent and surfactant extend throughout the phase and can coexist with a bulk solvent phase. Hence, detergent-solubilized membrane protein, added externally, can easily partition into the bicontinuous cubic phase, and the solvent channels allowed the manipulation of the aqueous environment to initiate crystallization. While many of the assumptions made by Landau and Rosenbusch are not confirmed, their technique allowed the high-resolution structure determination of bacteriorhodopsin (55,56), halorhodopsin (68), and sensory rhodopsin (70). Because of its initial success, a great deal of effort is being made to understand the process of in cubo crystallization (67,99,100) and to study the effects of crystallization variables on bicontinuous cubic phases (101).

4 SEARCHING FOR CRYSTALLIZATION CONDITIONS

The search for successful crystallization conditions is the most intimidating and exhausting part of the research for determining a membrane protein crystal structure. A careful look at the conditions under which X-ray-quality crystals of membrane proteins grow demonstrates that while crystallization conditions for similar proteins are similar, they are also uniquely different. A systematic search of conditions will always be necessary, and the number of variables in the system is large. The crystallization experiments on bacteriorhodopsin (91), Rdb. spheroides (90,102,103), and prostaglandin synthase-1 (83) show how subtle changes in conditions can cause dramatic changes in crystal quality. The porins from *E. coli* and photosynthetic bacteria also show how similar proteins crystallize under roughly similar conditions of salt and PEG (5). Nonetheless, the precise conditions for the growth of X-ray-quality crystals differ distinctly from protein to protein.

The dilemma one faces in setting up crystallization trials is how to search all the possible combinations of variable. Once a set of initial conditions has been defined, searching this potential "crystallization" space is the next obstacle. A number of options are available as far as search strategies are concerned (104–107). The most intriguing method is the "sparse matrix" method (108) which has been modified by a number of groups (109,110). The basis of the sparse-matrix strategy is that only a limited set of (50–100) extreme crystallization conditions are searched for crystallization "potential" (e.g., microcrystal formation or formation of globular, birefringent material). It is common that the first screen with a combination of a sparse matrix and hanging-drop vapor diffusion will yield small, well-formed crystals from soluble proteins (108–110).

Unfortunately, the use of commercially available sparse-matrix screens with detergent-containing samples often yields numerous occurrences of detergent-phase separation. This phenomenon is not important for crystallization, as discussed in Section 2. However, the micellar interactions underlying this detergent-phase separation seemingly play a role in crystal nucleation and growth (5); this is being verified experimentally (47). In most cases, the phase region open to crystallization experiments is dependent on *where* the phase separation boundary is and *how* the phase separation boundary and the crystallization boundary change as the crystallization conditions vary. Hence, before crystallization experiments are set up, it is highly recommended to prescreen all possible buffer–detergent–precipitant conditions for undesirable phase behavior and to define the region open to crystallization experiments. This labor-intensive step need be done only once and henceforth used as a laboratory database. Such a strategy has recently yielded crystals of the plasma membrane H^+-ATPase from Neurospora crassa (85).

Gouaux and coworkers have used this approach to adapt the sparse-matrix method for use with membrane proteins (111). They prescreened the buffer–detergent–precipitant combinations in a "standard" sparse-matrix array of Jancarik and Kim (108) to weed out undesirable phase behavior. They then altered some of the conditions to make them compatible with a chosen detergent (in this case, C_8E_4). Loll and colleagues (47) have taken this approach further and have begun to optimize sparse-matrix screens for use with several detergents (P. J. Loll, personal communication). The sparse-matrix strategy can provide a powerful and rapid means to screen potential crystallization conditions for membrane proteins, as well as being adaptable to high-throughput robotic technologies (112).

For those researchers interested in using in cubo crystallization methods (67,100), the current methodology is not applicable to rapid screening. For most experiments, setup of the bicontinuous lipidic phase is time consuming, and the amounts of sample needed per experiment is still enormous. Recognizing these deficits in the method, Peter Nollert (University of California, San Francisco) and Emerald Biostructures (Bainbridge Island, Washington) have begun adapting the in cubo crystallization method for microscale screening that would be suitable for high-throughput robotic technologies. The initial results are encouraging (P. Nollert, personal communication), and we may see an advance in this methodology in the near future.

5   HANDLING MEMBRANE PROTEIN CRYSTALS

The crystallization conditions for prostaglandin synthase-1 (6,83) are highly reproducible from preparation to preparation, but the yield of good crystals is never outstanding: Most of the crystals are either too small or not single. Moreover, several physical and environmental factors resulted in a low success rate in mounting crystals for data collection, particularly in the early phase of the project. First, because the crystallization occurs near a detergent-phase boundary, phase separation often occurs either during or after crystallization. Because the small drops contain precipitate and (owing to the detergent-phase separation) two liquid phases, the drops contain little homogeneous mother liquor for crystal manipulation. Second, the crystals are quite fragile and often adhere strongly to the precipitate and/or the cover slip. These are not uncommon problems encountered when working with membrane protein crystals (7,46,49).

Far more difficult to control are the environmental factors that can lead to disorder or nonisomorphism. Significant nonisomorphism between crystals, arising from slight changes in the salt and precipitant concentrations, can noticeably alter the quality of the diffraction data (D. Picot and R. M. Garavito, unpublished observations). Compounding this problem, subtle changes in the detergent environment can influence the stability of the crystal, and the uncontrolled variation of the detergent concentration of the mother liquor can easily destroy membrane protein crystals. For example, soaking solutions with β-OG concentrations just above the CMC will slowly dissolve prostaglandin synthase-1 crystals; the rate of crystal dissolution increases substantially as the β-OG concentrations exceed the CMC. Increasing the PEG concentration retards but does not stop this process.

Two factors are at work here: the detergent is an integral part of the protein crystal (Fig. 5), and a substantial amount of protein-bound detergent is brought into the crystals during crystal growth. In a hanging-drop vapor diffusion experiment, the protein–detergent ratio remains constant, even though the detergent concentration increases as crystallization proceeds. Hence, the *free* detergent concentration in the mother liquor may not increase as significantly. Adding artificial mother liquor with a detergent concentration equal to the total detergent concentration in the drop can markedly disturb the detergent monomer–aggregate equilibrium and change the amount of detergent within the crystal. The packing arrangement in OmpF crystals (Fig. 5) clearly shows how a change in the structure of the detergent interface could easily disrupt crystals contacts.

Similar observations have been made with other membrane proteins (5,7,46,49,88), consistent with the hypothesis of an active role for detergent interactions in the crystallization process. In the case of *E. coli* OmpF porin, an extreme sensitivity to changing detergent concentration, particularly during crystal mounting, made data collection on vapor diffusion–grown crystals (49) nearly impossible. Upon shifting to microdialysis methods (45), where the ambient detergent concentration could be better controlled, these crystals could be easily handled. Hence, an investigator must be ready to alter crystallization conditions and method not only to grow better crystals, but also to handle them successfully for X-ray diffraction experiments.

6 FINAL COMMENTS

If a membrane protein can be obtained as a pure, stable preparation of PDCs, there are no *a priori* reasons that preclude its eventual crystallization. However, a substantial effort must be put into obtaining an appropriate protein preparation. For the crystallization of many membrane proteins, much of the effort was focused on dealing with the biochemical parameters related to crystallization: protein stability, homogeneity and monodispersity. Often, this means conceptually combining the purification optimization and initial crystallization screening as one surveys different detergents. Hence, setting up 10,000–40,000 crystallization experiments is not unexpected in an effort to crystallize a membrane protein. This not only underscores the often hidden, seemingly heroic effort needed to bring such a project to fruition, but also stresses the need for improved high-throughput methodologies for membrane protein expression, purification, and crystallization.

ACKNOWLEDGEMENTS

Some of the work discussed in this chapter was supported in part by P01 GM57323 and R01 HL56773. The author would like to thank Drs. S. Bogusz, R. M. Venable, and R. W. Pastor for allowing access to their molecular simulation data on the β-D-octyl glucoside micelles. The author would like to thank those collaborators who have provided unpublished observations.

REFERENCES

1. W Kühlbrandt, E Gouaux. Membrane proteins. Curr Opin Struct Biol 9:445–447, 1999.
2. M Saraste, JE Walker. Membrane proteins. Channels, pumps and charge separators. Curr Opin Struct Biol 8:477–479, 1998.

3. E Wallin, G von Heijne. Genomic-wide analysis of integral membrane proteins from eubacterial, archean, and eukaryotic orgainisms. Protein Sci 7:1029–1038, 1998.

4. RM Garavito, Z Markovic-Housley, JA Jenkins. The growth and characterization of membrane protein crystals. J Crystal Growth 76:701–709, 1986.

5. RM Garavito, D Picot. The art of crystallizing membrane proteins. Methods: A Companion to Methods in Enzymology 1:57–69, 1990.

6. RM Garavito, D Picot, PJ Loll. Strategies for crystallizing membrane proteins. J Bioenerg Biomem 28:13–27, 1995.

7. W Kühlbrandt. Three-dimensional crystallization of membrane proteins. Quart Rev Biophys 21:429–477, 1988.

8. H Michel. General and practical aspects of membrane protein crystallization. In: H Michel, ed. Crystallization of Membrane Proteins. Boca Raton, FL: CRC Press, 1991, pp 73–88.

9. C Ostermeier, H Michel. Crystallization of membrane proteins. Curr Opin Struct Biol 7:697–701, 1997.

10. F Reiss-Husson. Crystallization of membrane proteins. In: A Ducruix, R Giege, eds. Crystallization of Nucleic Acids and Proteins: A Practical Approach. New York: IRL Press, 1992, pp 175–193.

11. B Lorber, R Giege. Preparation and handling of biological macromolecules for crystallization. In: A Ducruix, R Giege, eds. Crystallization of Nucleic Acids and Proteins: A Practical Approach. New York: IRL Press, 1992, pp 19–45.

12. A McPherson. Preparation and Analysis of Protein Crystals. New York: Wiley, 1982.

13. P Banerjee, JB Joo, JT Buse, G Dawson. Differential solubilization of lipids along with membrane proteins by different classes of detergents. Chem Phys Lipids 77:65–78, 1995.

14. WJ De Grip. Purification of bovine rhodopsin over concanavalin A—sepharose. Methods Enzymol 81:256–265, 1982.

15. A Helenius, K Simons. Solubilization of membranes by detergents. Biochim Biophys Acta 415:69–79, 1975.

16. C Tanford, JA Reynolds. Characterization of membrane proteins in detergent solutions. Biochim Biophys Acta 457:133–170, 1976.

17. A Helenius, DR McCaslin, E Fries, C Tanford. Properties of detergents. Methods Enzymol 56:734–749, 1979.

18. M Zulauf. Detergent phenomena in membrane protein crystallization. In: H Michel, ed. Crystallization of Membrane Proteins. Boca Raton, FL: CRC Press, 1991, pp 54–71.

19. C Tanford. The Hydrophobic Effect. New York: Wiley, 1980.

20. MJ Rosen. Surfactants and Interfacial Phenomena. New York: Wiley, 1978.

21. H Wennerström, B Lindman. Micelles. Physical chemistry of surfactant association. Phys Reports 52:1–86, 1979.

22. G Gunnarsson, B Jönsson, H Wennerström. Surfactant association into micelles. An electrostatic approach. J Phys Chem 84:3114–3121, 1980.

23. L Haneskog, L Andersson, E Brekkan, AK Englund, K Kameyama, L Liljas, E Greijer, J Fischbarg, P Lundahl. Monomeric human red cell glucose transporter (Glut1) in nonionic detergent solution and a semielliptical torus model for detergent binding to membrane proteins. Biochim Biophys Acta 1282:39–47, 1996.

24. M le Maire, S Kwee, J Andersen, J Møller. Mode of interaction of polyoxyethyleneglycol detergents with membrane proteins. Eur J Biochem. 129:525–532, 1983.

25. PA Marone, P Thiyagarajan, AM Wagner, DM Tiede. Effect of detergent alkyl chain length on crystallization of a detergent-solubilized membrane protein: correlation of protein–detergent particle size and particle–particle interaction with crystallization of the photosynthetic reaction center from *Rhodobacter sphaeroides*. J Crystal Growth 207:214–225, 1999.

26. DJ Mitchell, GJT Tiddy, L Waring, BT, MP McDonald. Phase behaviour of polyoxyethylene surfactants in water. J Chem Soc Faraday Trans 79:975–1000, 1983.

27. PA Timmins, J Hauk, T Wacker, W Welte. The influence of heptane-1,2,3-triol on the size and shape of LDAO micelles. Implications for the crystallisation of membrane proteins. FEBS Lett. 280:115–120, 1991.

28. PA Timmins, M Leonhard, HU Weltzien, T Wacker, W Welte. A physical characterization of some detergents of potential use for membrane protein crystallization. FEBS Lett 238:361–368, 1988.

29. S Bogusz, RM Venable, RW Pastor. Molecular dynamics simulations of octyl glucoside micelles: structural properties. J Phys Chem B 104:5462–5470, 2000.

30. J-P Maillet, V Lachet, PV Coveney. Large-scale molecular dynamics simulation of self-assembly processes in short- and long-chain cationic surfactants. Phys Chem Chem Phys 1:5227–5290, 1999.

31. DP Tieleman, D van der Spoel, HJC Berendsen. Molecular dynamics simulation of dodecylphosphocholine micelles at three different aggregate sizes: micellar structure and chain relaxation. J Phys Chem B 104:6380–6388, 2000.

32. FM Menger. On the structure of micelles. Accounts Chem Res 12:111–117, 1979.

33. MJ Thomas, K Pang, Q Chen, D Lyles, R Hantgan, M Waite. Lipid exchange between mixed micelles of phospholipid and Triton X-100. Biochim Biophys Acta 1417:144–156, 1999.

34. C Zhou, MF Roberts. Diacylglycerol partitioning and mixing in detergent micelles: relevance to enzyme kinetics. Biochim Biophys Acta 1348:273–286, 1997.

35. Y Rharbi, MA Winnik. Solute exchange between surfactant micelles by micelle fragmentation and fusion. Adv Colloid Interface Sci 89-90:25–46, 2001.

36. M Corti, C Minero, V Degiorgio. Cloud point transition in nonionic micellar solutions. J Phys Chem 88:309–317, 1984.

37. P-G Nilsson, H Wennerström, B Lindman. Structure of micellar solutions of nonionic surfactants. Nuclear magnetic resonance self-diffusion and proton

relaxation studies of poly(ethylene oxide) alkyl ethers. J Phys Chem 87:1377–1385, 1983.

38. M Zulauf, JP Rosenbusch. Micelle clusters of octylhydroxyoligo(oxyethylenes). J Phys Chem 87:856–862, 1983.

39. O Lambert, D Levy, JL Ranck, G Leblanc, JL Rigaud. A new "gel-like" phase in dodecyl maltoside–lipid mixtures: implications in solubilization and reconstitution studies. Biophys J 74:918–930, 1998.

40. U Kragh-Hansen, M le Maire, JV Moller. The mechanism of detergent solubilization of liposomes and protein-containing membranes. Biophys J 75:2932–2946, 1998.

41. C Hitscherich, J Kaplan, M Allaman, J Wiencek, PJ Loll. Static light-scattering studies of OmpF porin: implications for intrgral membrane protein crystallization. Protein Sci 9:1559–1566, 2000.

42. C Bordier. Phase separation of integral membrane proteins in Triton X-114 solution. J Biol Chem 256:1604–1609, 1981.

43. K Weckstrom, M Zulauf. Lower consolute boundaries of a poly(oxyethylene) surfactant in aqueous solutions of monovalent salts. J Chem Soc Faraday Trans 81:2947–2958, 1985.

44. H Michel. Crystallization of membrane proteins. Trends Biochem Sci 8:56–59, 1983.

45. RM Garavito, JP Rosenbusch. Isolation and crystallization of matrix porin (OmpF) from *E. coli*. Methods in Enzymol. 125:309–328, 1986.

46. H Michel. Characterization and crystal packing of 3-dimensional bacteriorhodopsin crystals. EMBO J 1:1267–1271, 1982.

47. PJ Loll, M Allaman, J Wiencek. Assessing the role of detergent–detergent interactions in membrane protein crystallization. J Crystal Growth 232:432–438, 2001.

48. RM Garavito, U Hinz, J-M Neuhaus. The crystallization of outer membrane proteins from *E. coli*: studies on lamB and OmpA gene products. J Biol Chem 259:4254–4257, 1984.

49. RM Garavito, JA Jenkins, JN Jansonius, R Karlsson, JP Rosenbusch. X-ray diffraction analysis of matrix porin, an integral membrane protein from *E. coli* outer membrane. J Molec Biol 164:313–327, 1983.

50. E Pebay-Peyroula, RM Garavito, JP Rosenbusch, M Zulauf, PA Timmins. Detergent structure in tetragonal crystals of OmpF porin. Structure 3:1051–1059, 1995.

51. S Penel, E Pebay Peyroula, J Rosenbusch, G Rummel, T Schirmer, PA Timmins. Detergent binding in trigonal crystals of OmpF porin from *Escherichia coli*. Biochimie 80:543–551, 1998.

52. M Roth, B Arnoux, A Ducruix, F Reiss-Husson. Structure of the detergent phase and protein–detergent interactions in crystals of the wild-type (strain Y) *Rhodobacter sphaeroides* photochemical reaction center. Biochemistry 30:9403–9413, 1991.

53. M Roth, A Lewitt-Bentley, H Michel, J Deisenhofer, R Huber, D Oesterhelt. Detergent structure in crystals of a bacterial photosynthetic reaction centre. Nature (London) 340:659–662, 1989.

54. PA Timmins, E Pebay Peyroula. Protein–detergent interactions in single crystals of membrane proteins studied by neutron crystallography. Basic Life Sci 64:267–272, 1996.

55. H Belrhali, P Nollert, A Royant, C Menzel, JP Rosenbusch, EM Landau, E Pebay Peyroula. Protein, lipid and water organization in bacteriorhodopsin crystals: a molecular view of the purple membrane at 1.9 Å resolution. Structure Fold Des 7:909–917, 1999.

56. H Luecke, B Schobert, HT Richter, JP Cartailler, JK Lanyi. Structure of bacteriorhodopsin at 1.55 Å resolution. J Mol Biol 291:899–911, 1999.

57. T Tsukihara, H Aoyama, E Yamashita, T Tomizaki, H Yamaguchi, K Shinzawa-Itoh, R Nakashima, R Yaono, S Yoshikawa. The whole structure of the 13-subunit oxidized cytochrome C oxidase at 2.8 Å. Science 272:1136–1144, 1996.

58. SH White, WC Wimley. Membrane protein folding and stability: physical principles. Annu Rev Biophys Biomol Struct 28:319–365, 1999.

59. KE McAuley, PK Fyfe, JP Ridge, NW Isaacs, RJ Cogdell, MR Jones. Structural details of an interaction between cardiolipin and an integral membrane protein. Proc Natl Acad Sci U S A 96:14706–14711, 1999.

60. S Nussberger, K Dorr, DN Wang, W Kuhlbrandt. Lipid–protein interactions in crystals of plant light-harvesting complex. J Mol Biol 234:347–356, 1993.

61. K Palczewski, T Kumasaka, T Hori, CA Behnke, H Motoshima, BA Fox, I Le Trong, DC Teller, T Okada, RE Stenkamp, M Yamamoto, M Miyano. Crystal structure of rhodopsin: a G protein-coupled receptor. Science 289:739–745, 2000.

62. C Toyoshima, M Nakasako, H Nomura, H Ogawa. Crystal structure of the calcium pump of sarcoplasmic reticulum at 2.6 Å resolution. Nature 405:647–655, 2000.

63. T Okada, I Le Trong, BA Fox, CA Behnke, RE Stenkamp, K Palczewski. X-Ray diffraction analysis of three-dimensional crystals of bovine rhodopsin obtained from mixed micelles. J Struct Biol 130:73–80, 2000.

64. B De Foresta, F Henao, P Champeil. Cancellation of the cooperativity of Ca^{2+} binding to sarcoplasmic reticulum $Ca^{(2+)}$-ATPase by the nonionic detergent dodecylmaltoside. Eur J Biochem 223:359–369, 1994.

65. S Lund, S Orlowski, B de Foresta, P Champeil, M le Maire, JV Moller. Detergent structure and associated lipid as determinants in the stabilization of solubilized Ca^{2+}-ATPase from sarcoplasmic reticulum. J Biol Chem 264:4907–4915, 1989.

66. EM Landau, JP Rosenbusch. Lipidic cubic phases: a novel concept for the crystallization of membrane proteins. Proc Natl Acad Sci USA 93:14532–14535, 1996.

67. P Nollert, A Royant, E Pebay Peyroula, EM Landau. Detergent-free membrane protein crystallization. FEBS Lett 457:205–208, 1999.

68. M Kolbe, H Besir, LO Essen, D Oesterhelt. Structure of the light-driven chloride pump halorhodopsin at 1.8 Å resolution. Science 288:1390–1396, 2000.

69. H Luecke, HT Richter, JK Lanyi. Proton transfer pathways in bacteriorho-dopsin at 2.3-angstrom resolution. Science 280:1934–1937, 1998.

70. H Luecke, B Schobert, JK Lanyi, EN Spudich, JL Spudich. Crystal structure of sensory rhodopsin II at 2.4 angstroms: insights into color tuning and transducer interaction. Science 293:1499–1503, 2001.

71. E Pebay-Peyroula, G Rummel, JP Rosenbusch, EM Landau. X-ray structure of bacteriorhodopsin at 2.5 angstroms from microcrystals grown in lipidic cubic phases [see comments]. Science 277:1676–1681, 1997.

72. G Chang, RH Spencer, AT Lee, MT Barclay, DC Rees. Structure of the MscL homolog from *Mycobacterium tuberculosis*: a gated mechanosensitive ion channel. Science 282:2220–2226, 1998.

73. G Chang, CB Roth. Structure of MsbA from *E. coli*: A homolog of the multidrug-resistance ATP binding cassette (ABC) transporters. Science 293:1793–1800, 2001.

74. A Pautsch, GE Schulz. High-resolution structure of the OmpA membrane domain. J Mol Biol 298:273–282, 2000.

75. DA Doyle, J Morais Cabral, RA Pfuetzner, A Kuo, JM Gulbis, SL Cohen, BT Chait, R MacKinnon. The structure of the potassium channel: molecular basis of K^+ conduction and selectivity. Science 280:69–77, 1998.

76. G Privès, HR Kaback. Engineering the lac permease for purification and crystallization. J Bioenerg Biomembr 28:29–34, 1996.

77. G Privès, GE Verner, C Weitzman, KH Zen, D Eisenberg, HR Kaback. Fusion proteins as tools for crystallization: the lactose permease from *Escherichia coli*. Acta Cryst D50:375–379, 1994.

78. G Kleymann, C Ostermeier, B Ludwig, A Skerra, H Michel. Engineered F_v fragments as a tool for the one-step purification of integral multisubunit membrane proteins. Biotechnology 13:155–160, 1995.

79. C Ostermeier, S Iwata, B Ludwig, H Michel. F_v fragment–mediated crystal-lization of the membrane protein bacterial cytochrome *C* oxidase. Nat Struct Biol 2:842–846, 1995.

80. C Hunte, J Koepke, C Lange, T Rossmanith, H Michel. Structure at 2.3 Å resolution of the cytochrome bc(1) complex from the yeast *Saccharomyces cerevisiae* co-crystallized with an antibody F_v fragment. Structure Fold Des 8:669–684, 2000.

81. S Iwata, C Ostermeier, B Ludwig, H Michel. Structure at 2.8 Å resolution of cytochrome *C* oxidase from *Paracoccus denitrificans*. Nature 376:660–669, 1995.

82. C Ostermeier, A Harrenga, U Ermler, H Michel. Structure at 2.7 Å resolution of the *Paracoccus denitrificans* two-subunit cytochrome *C* oxidase complexed with an antibody F_v fragment. Proc Natl Acad Sci USA 94:10547–10553, 1997.

83. M Malkowski, S Ginell, W Smith, R Garavito. The productive conformation of arachidonic acid bound to prostaglandin synthase. Science 289:1933–1937, 2000.

84. A Ducruix, R Giege. Methods of Crystallization. In: A Ducruix, R Giege, eds. Crystallization of Nucleic Acids and Proteins: A Practical Approach. New York: IRL Press, 1992, pp 73–98.

85. GA Scarborough. Large single crystals of the *Neurospora crassa*plasma membrane H$^+$-ATPase: an approach to the crystallization of integral membrane proteins. Acta Cryst D50:643–649, 1994.

86. P Thiyagarajan, DM Tiede. Detergent micelle structure and micelle–micelle interactions determined by small-angle neutron scattering under solution conditions for membrane-bound protein crystallization. J Phys Chem 98:10343–10351, 1994.

87. KA Stauffer, MGP Page, A Hardmeyer, TA Keller, R Pauptit. Crystallization and preliminary X-ray characterization of maltoporin from *Escherichia coli*. J Mol Biol 211:297–299, 1990.

88. H Michel. Three-dimensional crystals of a membrane protein complex. The photosynthetic reaction centre from *Rhodopseudomonas viridis*. J Molec Biol 158:567–572, 1982.

89. MZ Papiz, AM Hawthornwaite, RJ Cogdell, KJ Woolley, PA Wightman, LA Ferguson, JG Lindsay. Crystallization and characterization of two crystal forms of the B800-850 light-harvesting complex from *Rhodopseudomonas acidophila* strain 10050. J Molec Biol 209:833–835, 1989.

90. SK Buchanan, G Fritzsch, U Ermler, H Michel. New crystal form of the photosynthetic reaction centre from *Rhodobacter sphaeroides* of improved diffraction quality. J Molec Biol 230:1311–1314, 1993.

91. GFX Schertler, HD Bartunik, H Michel, D Oesterhelt. Orthorhombic crystal form of bacteriorhodopsin nucleated on benzamidine diffracting to 3.6 Å resolution. J Molec Biol 234:156–164, 1993.

92. J-L Eisele, JP Rosenbusch. Crystallization of porin using short-chain phospholipids. J Molec Biol 206:209–212, 1989.

93. MC Robert, B Capelle, B Lorber, R Giege. Influence of impurities on protein crystal perfection. J Crystal Growth 232:489–497, 2001.

94. J Deisenhofer, Epp, K Miki, R Huber, H Michel. Structure of the protein subunits in the photosynthetic reaction center of *Rhodopseudomonas viridis* at 3-ångstrøm resolution. Nature (London) 318:618–624, 1985.

95. D Picot, PJ Loll, RM Garavito. The X-ray crystal structure of the membrane protein prostaglandin H2 synthase-1. Nature (London) 367:243–249, 1994.

96. G McDermott, SM Prince, AA Freer, Hawthornthwaite-Lawless, MZ Papiz, RJ Cogdell, NW Isaacs. Crystal structure of an integral membrane light-harvesting complex from photosynthetic bacteria. Nature (London) 374:517–521, 1995.

97. M Kates. Techniques in Lipidology. New York: Elsevier, 1986.

98. J Briggs, H Chung, M Caffrey. The temperature–composition phase diagram and mesophase structure characterization of the monoolein/water system. J Phys II France 6:723–751, 1996.

99. M Caffrey. A lipid's eye view of membrane protein crystallization in mesophases. Curr Opin Struct Biol 10:486–497, 2000.

100. ML Chiu, P Nollert, MC Loewen, H Belrhali, E Pebay Peyroula, JP Rosenbusch, EM Landau. Crystallization in cubo: general applicability to membrane proteins. Acta Crystallogr D Biol Crystallogr 56:781–784, 2000.

101. X Ai, M Caffrey. Membrane protein crystallization in lipidic mesophases: detergent effects. Biophys J 79:394–405, 2000.

102. JP Allen, G Feher, TO Yeates, K Komiya, DC Rees. Structure of the reaction center from *Rhodobacter sphaeroides* R-26: the protein subunits. Proc Nat Acad Sci USA 84:5730–5734, 1987.

103. C-H Chang, M Schiffer, D Tiede, U Smith, JR Norris. Characterization of bacterial photosynthetic reaction center crystals from *Rhodopseudomonas sphaeroides* R-26 by X-ray diffraction. J Molec Biol 186:201–203, 1985.

104. CW Carter Jr. Efficient factorial designs and the analysis of macromolecular crystal growth conditions. Methods: A Companion to Methods in Enzymology 1:12–24, 1990.

105. RL Kingston, HM Baker, EN Baker. Search designs for protein crystallization based on orthogonal arrays. Acta Cryst D50:429–440, 1994.

106. EA Stura, AC Satterthwait, JC Calvo, DC Kaslow, IA Wilson. Reverse screening. Acta Cryst D50:448–455, 1994.

107. PC Weber. A protein crystallization strategy using automated grid searches on successively finer grids. Methods: A Companion to Methods in Enzymology 1:31–37, 1990.

108. J Jancarik, S-H Kim. Sparse matrix sampling: a screening method for crystallization of proteins. J Appl Cryst 24:409–411, 1991.

109. R Cudney, S Patel, K Weisgraber, Y Newhouse, A McPherson. Screening and optimization strategies for macromolecular crystal growth. Acta Cryst D50:414–423, 1994.

110. A D'Arcy. Crystallizing proteins—a rational approach? Acta Cryst D50:469–471, 1994.

111. L Song, JE Gouaux. Membrane protein crystallization: application of sparse matrix to alpha-hemolysin heptamer. Methods in Enzymol. 2761995.

112. RC Stevens. High-throughput protein crystallization. Curr Opin Struct Biol 10:558–563, 2000.

4

Prospects for High-Throughput Structure Determination by X-Ray Crystallography

Frank von Delft and Duncan E. McRee
Syrrx, Inc., San Diego, California, U.S.A

Charles D. Kang
Invitrogen Corporation, Carlsbad, California, U.S.A.

1 GENERAL

1.1 The Need for High Throughput

Visualization has always been central to advancing knowledge, because it supplies the most explicit kind of model: the light microscope revealed the cell, the electron microscope exposed the organelle, and with X-ray crystallography we have penetrated the realm of molecules, which has opened up to direct view the mechanisms of proteins and nucleic acids in all living processes, from metabolism to signaling and to transcription, expression, and heredity.

Structural genomics, the systematic structural analysis of the protein universe, is the attempt to apply the power of structural insights to answering the questions that have arisen from the vastly successful genome sequencing projects: assigning functions to the many gene products that have now been identified. Generating structures for large numbers of novel genes should not only help understand individual functions, but shed light on entire metabolic and signaling pathways in different organisms.

Such insights have direct applicability, for rational drug design in particular: if the three-dimensional structure of a defective or infecting protein is available, compounds can be designed to bind specifically to the active site and modulate or interfere with its undesired action (1). This approach holds the promise of new, more effective, and cheaper drugs, due to potentially fewer side effects and shorter development times; it has already had notable successes, e.g., in the treatment of HIV (2), and is now being applied in almost all therapeutic areas.

Despite its power, traditional crystallography remains laborious, costly, and inefficient; however, it has also become evident that this need not be the case. With the demands of the public structural genomics efforts, the desire in the private sector to repeat the early successes of structure-based drug design, and driven by recent advances in technology, both public and private efforts have been initiated to develop high-throughput (HT) structure determination platforms, in order to streamline and automate the process and speed it up by orders of magnitude.

1.2 Requisites

The traditional crystallographic process includes cloning, expression, protein purification, crystallization, X-ray diffraction, data collection, and, finally, structure determination (3). Each of these operations alone is complex, with a limited success rate; it is their combination that makes crystallography a difficult endeavor. Current methods usually take months or even years to solve a single structure, and the costs have been estimated at $300,000 per structure; one of the primary goals of the various structural genomics efforts is to develop high-throughput technologies that make the structure determination process more effort and cost efficient (4).

Developing a high-throughput X-ray crystallography system requires expertise across many diverse areas of science and technology, including molecular biology, protein chemistry, crystallography, physics, engineering, robotics, and information technology, to name a few. This multidisciplinary system must work seamlessly in order for the entire system to work. Anecdotes of protein structures determined in a matter of hours are limited to favorable cases and reflect only the time after data collection; the preceding steps—cloning, expression, purification, crystallization—require far more effort than data collection and analysis. If macromolecular crystallography is to reach a timeline and scale that can be truly termed "high throughput," new techniques must be developed and, more importantly, new ways of problem solving must be implemented.

1.3 High-Throughput Philosophy

High-throughput (HT) does not merely constitute speed; it requires success as well. "Success" includes scientific quality, which must be emphasized, since it implies that it is more than a matter of automation using expensive machines. Automation helps, of course, but can in theory be replaced by hosts of technicians. Instead, HT makes use of tried-and-tested experimental techniques, but with a fundamental shift in strategy towards two basic and complementary principles: parallelization and orthogonality.

1.3.1 Parallelization

Although parallelization can be applied in any context and is not particularly novel, it is central to achieving the sort of efficiencies needed in the HT context. Instead of samples being treated separately at each step they traverse in the process, all samples passing through the same step are bunched together and treated as a single batch, of whatever size is convenient. Thus, a step needs to be set up and managed only once, not 10, 20, or 96 times, with a corresponding increase in speed and simplification of management. Of course, handling 20 samples in one step takes somewhat longer than doing just one sample, but not longer than doing one step 20 times sequentially.

1.3.2 Orthogonality

Orthogonality is the "whatever works" component. Since it is clear that one generic approach will not work for all targets, many alternative avenues are pursued simultaneously for a given project or target, rather than exhausting one approach before turning to another. Which particular approach is successful for a particular target does not matter; what is important is ultimate success. Thus, rather than maximizing the probability of success for each procedure, the number of alternative procedures is maximized.

This influences both logistics and experimental design, because migration between or adaptation to various approaches to the same step must be relatively painless for a given target; for instance, the use of vectors compatible with different expression systems. It also implies a low tolerance for failure: For a given target, as soon as a given approach proves problematic, it is abandoned in favor of its alternatives. Of course, for targets of special importance, if all approaches prove to be problematic, nonstandard approaches can always be followed on a case-by-case basis.

Orthogonality applies at different levels. For instance, at the level of target selection, it is a luxury afforded by the overall goal to solve representative (of a fold, ortholog, etc.), rather than all, structures, which loosens the success criteria.

1.3.3 Tools

Naturally, automation is a major factor in HT crystallography. The realization that the tedium of the traditional crystallographic process is unnecessary has recently been increasingly converted into real technical solutions (e.g., Ref. 5), resulting in vastly accelerated process times, e.g., for culture growth, crystallization, and crystal screening. Less obvious, but just as important for the HT operation, are the concomitant elimination of human experimental variability (i.e., repeatability), gain of data integrity, and the ability to carry out systematic quality control.

It is information technology, however, that forms the backbone of the HT process. One of traditionalists' often-stated (or -implied) objections to HT crystallography, that it does not allow one to "get intimate" with the target, is indeed valid, unless robust process- and data-management tools are in place. There is a huge number of targets and samples to track and assess in various contexts, and only if all available information about each is instantly accessible where needed, and viewable in the appropriate form, can a target or sample be given the same human, scientific evaluation that is afforded to projects in conventional laboratories and that will always remain essential to sustain success rates.

Beyond that, the whole process must be continuously monitored for bottlenecks and the many different procedures assessed for relative usefulness, in order to identify trends and allow continuous refinement and optimization of the process. Such learning requires not only managed data, but also data integrity, which is a problem for nonautomated procedures, because of human involvement. While integrity can be enforced by data entry interfaces, it is vital that they do not encumber the experimenter. On the other hand, careful design will not only ensure data integrity, but also present the interfaces as tools that allow even greater efficiency.

1.3.4 Technological Advances

Apart from the shift in experimental design, specific, recent technological advances have set the stage for HT. Examples include powerful synchrotron radiation that reduces the requirements on crystal size. Smaller crystals require less protein and therefore reduce the demands on protein expression. Synchrotrons allow multiwavelength anomalous dispersion (MAD) phasing of seleno-methionine protein by virtue of their tunability (6), and this has made solving new structures fast and easy. Computer applications for crystallography are more sophisticated and robust than in past decades, allowing faster structure solution and refinement (7).

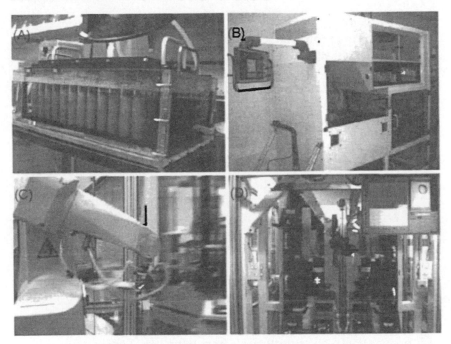

Figure 1 A selection of robotic solutions in use at Syrrx: (A) 96-well fermenter. (B) Combined sonicator and centrifuge: a multihead sonicator inserts into tubes that are still in the centrifuge bucket. (C) The crystallization robot in action: a robotic arm transfers plates between stations responsible for various steps, such as preparing well solutions, dispensing protein, and sealing drops. (D) The plate storage and imaging system. Plates are stored in shelves, and a robotic arm retrieves them for imaging, management, etc. The imager (inset: screenshot) can image a plate in less than a minute.

1.4 Target Selection

Considering the sheer number of known or putative proteins, even highly efficient HT crystallography is not up to the task of pursuing every protein from even just one complete genome; some form of target selection is needed, even if it is random. There are various goals that can be considered: complete coverage of fold space; elucidation of specific pathways, such as glycolysis, in several organisms; a focus on a protein family, such as kinases, phosphatases; or exploration of a broader class of proteins, e.g., those involved in cell signaling. The selection may also be guided by practical considerations, such as the exclusion of membrane proteins based on hydro-phobicity analysis, and targeting genomes of thermophilic organisms because of the ease of purification of their proteins once expressed in *E. coli*.

For bacterial genomes, where a large number of related genomes are available for comparison, target criteria can be extended to include homologs and orthologs; and since bacterial genomes contain homologs of human genes, this has applicability to the human genome as well. In general, bacterial proteins are more soluble, stable, and easier to express in *E. coli*, and thus have higher success rates for crystallization, than the corresponding human constructs. Such approaches have been used often in the past, for instance, in the case of bacterial P450s (8) that were crystallized as examples of the human microsomal enzymes, which have important roles in drug toxicity.

As one of its goals (4), the NIH Protein Structure Initiative aims to establish the number of unique folds that form protein space. For this aim, targets are selected by considering protein sequence families and pursuing representative members only of new sequence families, which maximizes the probability that each structure will represent a new structure.

Target selection is complicated by the need to pursue a number of putative members of a fold to guarantee success for at least one member, since the downstream success rate cannot be known at the outset. Intuition and literature still guide the selections, but as projects advance, better criteria should emerge based on real success rates. Indeed, on their own such observations will constitute an important contribution of structural genomics projects to HT crystallography. On the other hand, considerable attrition rates are likely to remain a reality, so comprehensive coverage of fold-space coverage will require considerable front-end loading of the process.

Apart from the bioinformatic approaches already outlined, more direct means can be used, such as employing gene chips to find genes regulated by certain stimuli or expressed differentially in various cell lines or tissue types. Homologs from various species of target genes thus identified can then be included in the pipeline.

1.5   Diversity

In the context of HT crystallography, diversity is used to increase the success rate by increasing the number of targets; it is orthogonality applied to the sample. Diversity may be natural or induced: The former was exploited by protein crystallographers from the very first, when Kendrew et al. selected sperm whale myoglobin (9) simply because it crystallized easily and was abundantly available, not because sperm whales had been identified as a target of the national health plan. The modern equivalent would be to clone simultaneously a number of myoglobin genes from a number of mammalian species, working on all of them in parallel.

Diversity may, however, also be induced, specifically by random or specific mutagenesis of a target, to yield a family of slightly different proteins. The very concept of *homolog* implies that protein structure is highly tolerant to most small changes in sequence, particularly to surface residues; whereas proteins frequently have loose ends and loops that complicate crystallization by introducing microheterogeneity and can be removed without altering the fold or activity. Selected (but usually unpredictable) point mutations on the surface can also dramatically impact the protein's solubility and ability to crystallize.

1.6 The Evolutionary Approach

An operating HT pipeline opens up the unprecedented possibility of applying an evolutionary approach to improve the success rate of crystallography. Evolutionary algorithms are an established optimizing approach in computer programs, deriving from the principles of evolution: Random variation in the "genetic material" of a population makes some members of the population more fit to succeed—as measured by some calculated score— which are selected for the next generation, after the "genetic material" is randomly shuffled and mutated a bit. The process is repeated for as many generations as necessary or desired, depending on which—the desired optimization or excessive boredom—is first achieved.

The "genetic material" can in general be completely abstract, as long as it directly influences "fitness." Of course, crystals consist of protein, so it is rather straightforward: The genetic material is simply the sequence of the target; and the fitness is the protein's solubility, stability, ability to crystallize, diffraction quality, or whatever else is relevant.

What the HT pipeline now provides is the ability to continue the evolution for several generations, because time and effort have been reduced to realistic levels. At each generation, the most soluble (or best diffracting, etc.) samples are selected, shuffled and randomly mutated, and retransformed; this is repeated, until, say, the integral membrane protein dissolves in 2M NaCl solution or the proteosome diffracts to a resolution of 1.3 Å.

While many targets may not justify the expense and effort involved, some important systems may prove unsolvable by any other approach.

1.7 Challenges

The biological challenges in HT crystallography are not much different from those in conventional crystallography: membrane proteins, solubility, expression, and stability. This is largely *because* there is no satisfactory, general solution to any of these problems. Only a few membrane proteins have been crystallized (e.g., Refs. 10 and 11), usually by using a number of specific detergents, additives, or other tricks that were chanced upon. Solubility, expression, and stability are addressed with a plethora of approaches, which often depend significantly on the experimenter's skill and experience.

On the other hand, the HT pipeline provides opportunities that were difficult to exploit before: diversity and orthogonality. Many expression systems can be tried simultaneously; a large number of mutants and variants can be tested for solubility and stability, especially in the case of membrane proteins; the evolutionary approach adds breadth to the search. How successful this is remains to be seen, but, on the other hand, there will always be cases solvable only by individual attention and conventional treatment; crystallographers are not about to become obsolete.

Scale (of expression and purification) initially appears to be a potential pitfall: High yields are frequently difficult to achieve, even in conventional experiments, quite apart from the material costs involved. However, the problem is not only circumvented by exploiting miniaturization; the use of smaller experimental volumes solves other problems along the whole pipeline, as discussed later.

2 MOLECULAR BIOLOGY

2.1 Cloning

Critical to HT X-ray crystallography is the efficient production of highly purified recombinant proteins. Protein expression and purification techniques have typically been optimized for individual proteins on a case-by-case basis, but the comprehensive and HT nature of structural genomics requires a more robust process for producing crystallographic-quality protein, beginning with DNA cloning.

The ideal cloning vector for high-throughput crystallography would be easily moved between expression systems, allow for multiple tags to be constructed simply, and allow tight regulation over induction and produce similar amounts of protein for any gene that is inserted. The TOPO® vector system (11a) with an arabinose promoter system has produced good results.

Once the gene of interest and its DNA sequence are identified, full-length cDNAs are amplified via (PCR), amplified cDNAs are cloned into the appropriate expression vector. However, because protein expression and solubility are highly dependent on the specific protein sequence as well as on the vector, host cell, and culture conditions, adequate expression can be difficult, especially when working with novel or poorly characterized proteins. It may therefore be necessary to try many different expression vectors in *E. coli*, yeast, and/or baculovirus expression systems. Recloning cDNAs into each specific vector is extremely labor intensive, but the use of recombinatorial cloning can greatly simplify this process. In recombinatorial cloning, the gene of interest is cloned only once into a donor vector and from there can be moved into any number of recipient plasmids for expression in different hosts, significantly reducing time and effort (12–14).

More specific to crystallography, cloning and molecular biology are especially important since the native protein will often have certain regions, such as loops or specific sequence patterns, that are not conducive to crystal lattice packing. Trying to determine whether a particular region is responsible for poor lattice packing would be extremely difficult and could take years to perform. The high-throughput approach assumes that some level of mutagenesis will be required, typically including amino- or carboxy-terminal truncations, point mutations, and orthologs of the protein from different species (15).

Another important consideration is the use of fusion tags to facilitate more efficient and selective downstream purification as well as protein detection. A fusion tag such as the commonly used His-tag (15a, 15b) enables a single-step protein purification using standard immobilized metal affinity chromatography (15c) and eliminates the need for developing and optimizing unique purification conditions. As part of the integration strategy, the use of fusion tags that facilitate downstream purification and even protein detection should be considered and must be incorporated into the cloning step (16).

2.2 Constructs

Several tag constructs can be done in parallel, to increase the likelihood of successfully expressing and purifying a given protein. Poly-His tags can be added to both the N- and C-termini of the protein, and fusions with maltose-binding protein (16a) or Glutathione-S-transferase (16b) are commonly used. The poly-His tags are especially attractive because they simplify protein purification with the use of a nickel-affinity resin. There is a possibility that any given tag will interfere with crystallization. If crystals cannot be obtained with tag-purified protein, a tagless construct can be tried. This should be done last because the effort for purification will generally be greater for tagless protein.

2.3 Mutations

In order to increase solubility, a number of options are available. One approach would be to use random mutagenesis and to express proteins in 96-well plate format to look for soluble protein. The success rate for this could be quite low, and in many cases a bioinformatics analysis of the protein could point to a knowledge-directed approach, such as removing a putative membrane-spanning region. Particularly challenging to identify are membrane-associated proteins that bind to one side of the membrane and have loops or amphipathic helices attaching them to the membrane; only a few structures exist for such proteins. It could be argued that these proteins are rare, but a more likely explanation is that they present difficulties in expression and have been historically intractable. An example of such a protein class are microsomal cytochrome p450 enzymes, of which it is estimated that there are over 50 such genes in humans, and over 3000 genes have been identified in all species. However, only one crystal structure has been done of the membrane-bound form (17), and that was done by removing a putative N-terminal membrane-spanning helix and performing mutagenesis on a loop that in hindsight formed part of a monofacial membrane anchor.

A similar challenge exists for proteins that are normally part of a complex in the cell. Without its partner, such a protein may expose a large hydrophobic face that makes it insoluble. One strategy for this is coexpression of the protein with its partner, if known. Often the partner will not be known, in which case, if a pathway for the protein is known, it may be possible to use a combinatorial expression approach. Again, this could be done in small-scale expression trials.

2.4 Truncation and Fragmentation

A number of proteins can be naturally divided into separable domains that can be crystallized individually. This has been a common approach for a number of membrane proteins that have a soluble cytoplasmic domain attached to a membrane-spanning domain. A challenge for bioinformatics is to find algorithms that can reliably predict the extent of such domains and provide information on where to divide the sequence. It may still be necessary to try a number of constructs, moving the ends of the domain plus and minus a few residues to yield good expression and solubility. Another approach would be to systematically cut the protein into pieces every 10 or 15 residues. For a good-size protein this will yield hundreds of constructs that can be tested for solubility on a microscale.

2.5 Random Mutagenesis

In order to yield crystals it has been proposed to change surface residues to provide new crystal contacts and remove others. Lysine residues are particularly attractive candidates in this regard (18). They are very likely to be on the surface and rarely appear in protein–protein contacts, leading Bell et al. (19) to suggest that one role of lysines is to keep proteins apart. In order for a crystal to grow, it is necessary to bring proteins together at a few specific points.

3 PROTEIN PRODUCTION

3.1 Scale Issues

Building a scalable and reproducible protein purification scheme presents a difficult technological challenge. Like children, every protein is unique and presents its own problems, whereas finding conditions that will work with a large variety of proteins is a prerequisite to a successful high-throughput crystallography experiment. However, in keeping with the high-throughput philosophy, the goal is not to get every protein attempted expressed and purified, but to find systems that maximize the success rate of a large group of proteins or constructs.

3.2 Expression Systems

The best choice of expression system depends on the protein target being solved. *E. coli* expression systems, which are comparatively cheap, work well for most prokaryotic as well as some eukaryotic genes. However, mammalian genes often express poorly or are insoluble in such systems, and it will be necessary to turn to more expensive alternatives, such as the baculovirus/insect cells system or yeast cells. A plethora of systems are commercially available, and cost issues become truly significant.

The selection of expression system can be approached through a hierarchy of approaches: *E. coli* is tried first, being both the cheapest and simplest, both at 30° and 15°C; if unsuccessful, it can be attempted in some type of eukaryotic expression system, *etc. E. coli* expression screening is a good idea even when success seems unlikely: Even a small percentage of successes will be a substantial boost to the overall program, at little cost.

3.3 Microexpression and Prescreening

Microexpression, coupled with prescreening, provides a powerful logistical tool that enables the planning of subsequent macroexpression. Clones are initially grown and protein expressed in milliliter cultures, which allows expression and solubility, among other properties, to be assessed. This allows the clones to be broadly classified—for refolding, for size-exclusion, for charge-based chromatography—and dealt with in parallel during scale-up of expression and purification.

3.4 Purification Systems

In order to make it practical to do a large number of protein purifications, the volume of starting material must be minimized, since the cost and time of a purification scales with the volume of liquid being handled. If the volumes can be kept small enough to use analytical columns, then the final purity that can be achieved will be higher, due to the superior separation characteristics of these columns relative to the larger preparative columns. Careful estimates need to be made of the volume that will yield sufficient material for crystallization trials.

3.5 Parallel Purification

Purification should be done in parallel, for maximum efficiency and throughput. It may be possible to bin proteins to be purified on a given day by first doing a small-scale characterization to determine if the protein sticks to positively charged or negatively charged resin. Proteins with similar purification profiles can be then done without changing columns between runs. At Syrrx, up to 96 proteins can be expressed at once is a 96-tube fermentor (Fig. 1A). At the end of the fermentation, all 96 tubes are transferred to a 96-tube automated centrifuge (Fig. 1B). The centrifuge can spin down the cells, resuspend in lysis buffer, and then sonicate four samples simultaneously. The cell debris is spun down and the supernatants aspirated and run over a nickel column (for poly-His–tagged proteins). The eluate of the nickel column is then either directly crystallized or further purified as needed. If desired, the pellet with inclusion bodies can be solubilized in a detergent buffer and saved for refolding experiments.

3.6 Protein Concentration

Surprisingly, concentration is one of the trickier bottlenecks. In order to crystallize a protein, it usually must be brought up to a concentration of 10 mg/mL or greater. A number of proteins will fail to concentrate to this point without precipitating from solution. Also, the rate at which a protein concentrates depends on a number of factors, and it can be difficult to accurately control the endpoint of a concentration run. For a single protein, careful monitoring of the concentration apparatus works well, but this can become a logistical problem if 96 samples are being concentrated at the same time.

3.7 Protein Characterization

It is desirable to do a microcharacterization of the purified samples. Such characterization will be an aid in reconciling differences with future batches. A particularly useful method is mass spectrometric characterization of the protein, to identify the molecular weight of the protein that has been purified. This will help diagnose cases where ends were proteolyzed and, in extreme cases, that the wrong protein entirely was purified. It has happened that a minor protein native to *E. coli* that sticks to Ni^{++} columns has been purified and crystallized instead of the intended protein.

3.8 Incorporation of Selenomethionine

One of the best methods for solving protein structures in high-throughput mode is MAD phasing with selenomethionine (Se-Met) (see Sec. 5.1.1); first, however, selenomethionine must replace the methionines in the native protein. The reason the technique is so powerful is that most expression systems can be tricked into using Se-Met in the place of methionine, either by reverting to a system deficient in methionine synthesis (20) or by inhibiting methionine synthesis with metabolic feedback inhibition by additionally added amino acids (21). The latter method has been made to work in *E. coli*, in yeast (22), and even in insect cells (23).

Although most selenomethionine proteins can be purified like their wild-type counterparts, the protocol often needs adjusting, because selenomethionine protein expression yields are as a rule lower than for the wild type (e.g., Ref. 24). Selenomethionine proteins are more susceptible to oxidation, which can destroy the crystal in unfavorable cases, and occasionally the selenomethionine version will aggregate and precipitate upon concentration.

4 CRYSTALLIZATION

Proteins are crystallized by bringing the protein solution to a state of supersaturation, usually by adding a precipitant. If the conditions are right, a protein may crystallize; at other times it will form an amorphous precipitate. There is no way to know the conditions that will cause a crystal to grow *a priori*. However, over the years the cumulative experience of protein crystallography has come up with a number of criteria and methods that will increase the odds of growing a protein crystal (24a).

The protein needs to be concentrated—generally 10 mg/mL or greater.

The protein should be 90% pure or better.

The protein must be stable for a period of days in the crystallization conditions.

Many, if not most, of the known precipitants should be tried.

pH, salts, cofactors, and temperature are all factors that must be controlled.

The drops should be small, to allow as many trials as possible with a given sample.

In general, a precipitating agent, such as polyethylene glycol, is added to the protein solution until the protein precipitates or crystallizes while the other factors, such as temperature, are held constant.

4.1 Methods

4.1.1 Vapor Diffusion

Vapor diffusion is the most widely used method for bringing proteins to supersaturation. A large volume of precipitating solution (0.5 mL) at the final concentration is placed in one well of an apparatus and a small drop of protein (typically 2–4 microliters) is mixed with an equal volume of the well solution in a second chamber connected to the first such that water vapor can equilibrate between the two. The apparatus is sealed (with a clear glass cover so that it can be observed through a microscope) and the system allowed to equilibrate. The protein solution, being a small fraction of the other well, will dry until it reaches the concentration of the well. This results in a 2× concentration of the protein and the precipitant. If the experiment is arranged correctly, the protein solution will start out below saturation and will slowly concentrate until it is supersaturated, at which point it crystallizes (or forms a precipitate).

Two types of apparatus are used for vapor diffusion, hanging drop and sitting drop. In hanging drop, the protein drop is placed on a cover slip that is then inverted. This method is popular because the cover slip then forms an optically clear window in which the drop can be observed, much as diver's mask works. The variant to this is the sitting drop, in which the drop sits on a small shelf or depression. Proponents of this method cite the superior insulation to small temperature variations by having the drop isolated in the center of the apparatus. In practice, both methods work well, the differences are a matter of preference.

At Syrrx, we use a patented sitting-nano-drop method: The drops are simpler to set up robotically because they don't need inverting of the cover slips; the drops can be sealed with a clear tape instead of using the more difficult glass and silicone grease seal; and the crystals are easy to harvest by cutting the tape and fishing with a small nylon loop. The crystal sits off to one side on a small polished shelf that makes optical imaging easy. The plates are standard 96-well footprint, half-height plates with a well that holds about 0.1 mL. The robot sets up a drop of 50 nanoliters protein and then adds another 50 nanoliters of well solution. In using such a small drop size it is important that the drops be sealed quickly to avoid excessive drying. The Syrrx robot takes about 30 seconds from the time the first protein drop is laid down until the plate is sealed with tape.

4.1.2 Microbatch

Another technique that is amenable to small drop sizes is the microbatch method, where a small drop of protein solution is set up under a layer of silicone oil. The protein dries very slowly under the layer of oil. The method has a very small footprint. A plate used by DeTitta and coworkers has 1536 individual experiments per plate (25). The drawbacks are that the crystals are hard to observe and difficult to harvest, so the technique is mainly a screening method.

4.2 Screens

A number of approaches exist for discovering and optimizing the chemical conditions that drive crystal growth.

In a *grid screen*, an array of drops that differ only slightly in concentration or pH are set up to search for the best crystallization conditions. The technique is the best for finding the ideal conditions for crystal growth, but it can be wasteful of protein because a large number of drops are needed. Practically speaking, there is never enough protein to set up a grid screen for every precipitant that needs to be explored. The method is therefore used to zero in on conditions once a hit has been found or to set up on the most successful precipitant, such as PEG 6K or ammonium sulfate.

In order to explore a large number of conditions when it is not possible to sample all conditions, *an incomplete factorial* of the conditions, instead of a complete grid, is used, randomly picking a number of conditions. These screens are often called *coarse* screens. The method takes advantage of the fact that small crystals often grow under conditions a fair distance away from the ideal conditions. Once the small crystals are found, a finer screen around any coarse-screen hits are set up to grow crystals large enough for X-ray characterization.

4.3 Storage and Imaging

In a small lab, storage of the crystal trays is a large problem. In a high-throughput setting where thousands of proteins are being crystallized, storage is a tremendous issue. In fact, it can be quickly shown that unless a project is willing to invest huge resources in the rental of space, a time limit on storage of plates must be decided upon. At Syrrx, we use an automated storage "fort" to store and image crystal experiments (Fig. 1C). The fort has a central gantry with an arm that moves plates to any number of storage racks. Each plate has a barcode, and the fort schedules each plate to be imaged periodically. The crystallographer can ask for a plate to be harvested, and the fort will remove that plate from its storage location to an output station. After 28 days, the plates are disposed of into a dustbin (the plates must be treated as hazardous waste, as with any other laboratory solution).

4.4 Crystal Harvesting

4.4.1 Importance of the Mount

The most crucial step in the crystallographic analysis, given that a crystal is available, is the quality of the crystal mount. The equation is simple, and it is not particular to crystallography: The better mounted the sample, the better the data and the quicker, more straightforward, and less ambiguous the analysis—and thus the more automatable.

On the one hand, because of its vital role in the success of the experiment, this is probably the step one can least afford to automate. On the other hand, repetition is the name of the game: It is not uncommon that tens (even hundreds) of mounted crystals must be screened before commencing data collection (Sec. 5.4), and without automation the need to mount so many crystals has the potential to become a major bottleneck.

4.4.2 Automation

The standard mounting procedure currently relies on the dexterity of the experimenter, who manually fishes the crystal from the drop with a small rayon loop (26). Such a procedure is clearly not directly automatable: wielding a mounting loop with a robot arm would involve a vast artificial intelligence (AI) effort, since it is difficult to predict the crystal's behavior during mounting. In addition, because of mechanical stresses applied during transfers, it is unlikely to be the best way to treat the fragile crystals.

Automation is more likely to employ a nonlooping approach. NASA is developing a system for the International Space Station that relies on pipetting the solution together with the crystal onto a loop (27); this has the added advantage of reduced stress, because it does not involve breaking a meniscus. Another approach is to grow the crystals in the mounting loop.

4.4.3 Mounting Nanocrystals

The routine use of nanocrystals has been shown to provide an unexpected benefit: their apparent resilience to abuse during mounting. The majority of nanocrystals can be flash-soaked in cryoprotectant, and they are generally less sensitive to the cryoprotectant than are large crystals; a low surface-to-volume ratio means that nanocrystals experience changes in osmotic pressure more uniformly throughout the crystal, as pointed out by Garman and Schneider (28). In addition, the mechanical stresses acting on the crystal are lower, since the crystals are of similar or smaller size than the natural radius of curvature of a water droplet, particularly on a loop.

4.5 Sample Handling

4.5.1 The Role of Cryogenics

Cryogenic crystal mounting has greatly facilitated high-throughput crystallography (HTC) (29). With room-temperature crystallography, whenever a crystal in the X-ray beam looked promising, a full data set would be collected, without knowing whether a better crystal was available in the same batch. This is unfeasible for the large numbers of crystals produced by high-throughput operations, simply due to time constraints. However, when crystals are cryomounted (28), they can be exposed, retrieved, stored, and accessed again at a later time, which makes it possible to screen every mounted crystal and then to select only the very best for time-expensive data collection.

Cryogenic crystal mounting resolves not only this methodological problem of HTC, but also the logistical ones of crystal management, by transforming the crystal from a fragile, microscopic, transient entity into a robust, manageable, virtually immortal one. Crystals can be prepared long before they are exposed, decoupling crystal growth from the availability of synchrotron beam time, both of which are often sporadic. Expensive synchrotron beam time can be reserved for actual data collection, since crystals can be screened in advance for quality at the home source. Labor can be divided, because the team responsible for crystal mounting does not need to be involved in data collection as well. Inconvenient synchrotron data-collection trips may be minimized, since crystals can be shipped around the globe by courier and data collection remotely controlled (provided the infrastructure is in place).

4.5.2 Storage and Transport

A difficulty with cryogenically mounted crystals is that they must be stored and handled exclusively at liquid nitrogen (lN_2) temperatures. The traditional solution of storing crystals in individual labeled vials is wholly inadequate for hundreds of crystals. Instead, a storage cassette that would hold multiple crystals and be identifiable by bar-coding is required.

At Syrrx, we have adopted the "puck" as our unit of handling. Developed at the Advanced Light Source (ALS) under commission from Syrrx, it is an aluminum disk that resembles and ice hockey puck, with 16 wells that hold the mount pins and a magnetic lid that locks over the top; seven such pucks fit into the standard dry shipping dewar. The simplification to crystal handling has been sensational. Unlike vials, its size allows it to be clearly labeled and easily manipulated, but it is not so large that it is unwieldy. It can be immersed in lN_2 in a shallow dewar, without other special devices needed for adding and retrieving crystals, and heat exchange with air is slow enough that it can be exposed to room temperature for minutes without affecting the samples inside. Individual crystals are tracked by their position in the puck

Storage at liquid nitrogen temperatures does not guarantee crystal survival. Residual water in the liquid nitrogen appears to migrate to samples in long-term storage, leading to icing.

4.5.3 Robohutch

In the HT context, where tens to hundreds of crystals must be screened prior to data collection, the need for an automated way to load and retrieve samples into and from the X-ray beam is self-evident: The manual procedure has a heavy time penalty, especially at synchrotron sources, where entering and exiting the experimental hutch is tedious. An automated system can be operated remotely and potentially run unsupervised continuously, particularly when immediate judgment calls are not vital (i.e., when screening for diffraction); equally importantly, it allows the tracking of samples to be automated.

The first automated system was described by the crystallography group at Abott Laboratories (30) and is now being manufactured by Rigaku-MSC. Other system are being built by SSRL (31) and ALS at their beamlines. All the systems make use of a robotic arm that retrieves the crystal from storage and places it on the goniometer while keeping it immersed in lN_2; both storage and goniometer positions are flexible. In the Abott and ALS systems, sample pins point upward from a magnetic base under lN_2, and a gripper closes down from above, rotates to the horizontal position, and mounts the crystal on the horizontal goniostat. The use of a mounting robot in the hutch has had a huge impact on the screening process at Syrrx; 50–100 crystals can now be assessed in a single morning at the Syrrx beamline at ALS.

In order to allow completely automated screening, the mounted crystal must be automatically centered in the beam. Centering the loop itself is doable, and this has been implemented; however, the center of the loop is not the center of the crystal, and identifying the crystal in the frozen solvent is decidedly nontrivial, sometimes even for experienced crystallographers, and edge-detection algorithms are only partly successful. Other proposals have included scanning the sample with a small, low-intensity beam and testing natural fluorescence; but currently, beamlines have addressed the issue by providing clickable user interfaces (31a), which does speed up the operation tremendously.

5 X-RAY ANALYSIS

5.1 De novo Phasing

5.1.1 Anomalous Dispersion: Multiwavelength Anomalous Dispersion (MAD) and Single-Wavelength Anomalous Dispersion (SAD)

High-throughput crystallography might never have been considered feasible without anomalous dispersion (AD)-based phasing, pioneered by Karle (32) and Hendrickson (33), which has in recent years clearly established its experimental superiority over other phasing techniques, by routinely producing electron density maps of exceptional quality, even for low-resolution structures. This naturally vastly simplifies map interpretation, increases the reliability of automated map interpretation (34), and greatly reduces the data-to-structure time. Equally significant, the experimental phases can be included in structure refinement, leading to more accurate final structures (as evidenced by smaller discrepancies between R and R_{free}), speeding up convergence of refinement, and increasing the convergence radius.

The pioneering MAD experiments were based on the premise that both anomalous and dispersive differences are necessary to generate unambiguous phase distributions (35). Since crystals were at room temperature and prone to radiation decay, it was vital to record all measurements of the same reflection close in time, which was achieved by orienting the crystal so that anomalous pairs were collected on the same image and by collecting the same small wedge of data at all three different wavelengths before proceeding to the next wedge.

It is now clear that, provided they are accurately measured, only one set of differences is usually sufficient to obtain unambiguous phases (36): Even though a single set of differences necessarily leads to perfectly ambiguous phases, there is inherent orthogonal phase information in the known heavy-atom substructure, so phase ambiguities can be partially resolved, allowing a solvent envelope to be defined and thence phase resolution to be completed by solvent flattening and other density modification techniques (37).

Of the two sets of differences, anomalous differences are the easiest to measure accurately, by measuring a data set at a single wavelength (hence "SAD") with high observational redundancy (allowing accurate estimation of experimental uncertainties), and treating anomalous reflection pairs independently. Rice et al. (36) have shown this approach to be very general; at Syrrx, this is our primary approach to de novo phasing.

Of course, measurements at additional wavelengths will always improve phase estimates, but in HT operations, efficiency is important and short-cuts welcome.

Such SAD phasing does not work very well when the ratio of anomalous to total scattering is very small so that both the anomalous signal is weak and the heavy-atom substructure too small to resolve phase ambiguities convincingly. In such cases, it is vital to measure dispersive differences as well, i.e., to collect data at different wavelengths.

5.1.2 Anomalous Dispersion vs. Isomorphous Replacement

The success of MAD has not made more traditional isomorphous replacement approaches (multiwavelength isomorphous replacement–MIR; single-wavelength isomorphous replacement—SIR) superfluous. Anomalous dispersion and isomorphous replacement are merely variants of the same principle: Perturbation of diffraction intensities leads to measurable intensity differences that are used to calculate phases once the atomic structure of the perturbation (heavy-atom model) is known (38). This has been most rigorously implemented in the SHARP program (39), in which the heavy-atom models of all derivates are refined simultaneously, using all measured data, resulting in a single "best" phase.

On the other hand, finding isomorphous derivatives has always been the Achilles heel of isomorphous replacement, even if parallelization and automation should permit more effective screening of heavy-atom soaking conditions. Thus, a more promising use of heavy-atom derivatives is to treat promising soaks—those with evidence of derivatization—as SAD experiments and to include any other data sets in phasing if they happen to be isomorphous.

5.1.3 Substructure Solution

Soaked heavy atoms typically bind to the crystal in fewer than 10 positions, which can often be located, with relative ease, by manual Patterson interpretation or else by various Patterson-based or direct methods programs.

However, in selenomethionine-labeled protein, substructures of 20–40 selenium atoms or larger are common, and solving them becomes nontrivial. While the various Patterson-based search algorithms in CNS (40), Solve (41) or Xhercules (42) have successfully solved such large substructures (43), they suffer the serious drawback of being computationally extremely expensive, in practice placing an upper limit to the size of problems solvable. Moreover, these algorithms rely on multiple-wavelength data for cross-comparison of Patterson maps. These algorithms are therefore nonideal for HT operations, not least because the success of an experiment can only be assessed once data collection has been completed (as discussed later).

Shake-and-Bake direct methods, pioneered in SnB (44) and subsequently also implemented in ShelxD (45), have completely transformed the situation: With sufficiently accurate data from a single wavelength, substructures are solved within seconds to minutes—at worst hours for obscenely large ones. (Sufficient accuracy is best achieved through high observational redundancy, reducing exposure times to offset crystal decay.) Moreover, it is not clear that substructure size is limiting: The current largest successful substructure, 160 selenium atoms (46), did not in retrospect pose any fundamental problems and was solved simply by very high redundancy and a long computation.

We have found that, in many cases, once the substructure has been solved, the structure as a whole can be considered phased: If anomalous differences are accurate enough for substructure solution, they're accurate enough for SAD phasing too, so the success of an experiment can be gauged even before the first wavelength has been collected to completion! (The exception occurs when the substructure is small—and solvable even with noisy data—but the anomalous signal is weak: Additional wavelengths are then required. Pseudocentric, heavy-atom substructures are also problematic.)

5.1.4 Anomalous Scatterers

In the past, due to limited experimental sensitivity, derivatives and anomalous scatterers had to have very strong signals to be useful, and the very heavy 5th and 6th period atoms were used as a rule. These were usually introduced to the crystal by soaking, but there was always uncertainty as to whether atoms have been bound. More recently, more sensitive detectors have made possible the detection of very small signals from different scatterers that have other conveniences that make them much better suited to HT operations.

Selenomethionine. Selenium is now the most popular scatterer used for de novo phasing (47), and it is excellently suited for HT operations, because protein labeling is highly automatable. It is incorporated into proteins with relative ease in the form of selenomethionine, and most proteins have sufficient methionines to ensure a favorable anomalous signal, while even large substructures are solvable using modern direct methods (Sec. 5.1.3). Crucially, the presence of selenomethionine can be confirmed by mass spectrometry *before* committing the protein to waste time and resources in crystallization or at the synchrotron. Moreover, its absorption peak lies at an energy accessible to hard X-ray synchrotrons.

Two significant drawbacks are cost, which can become considerable for large-scale production, and that its incorporation in nonbacterial expression systems is tricky, though possible.

Halide Soaks. The halide ions bromide and iodide have recently come to prominence as cheap and universally applicable anomalous scatterers for SAD (48). When crystals are briefly soaked in submolar halide solutions, ions bind noncovalently but specifically and extensively to protein surfaces. While the fluorescence edge of bromide is close to that of selenium, iodide introduces a significant anomalous signal (six electrons) for CuK_α radiation. Although the halide substructure is typically large (> 20), it is solvable by direct methods, just as are large selenium substructures, with good, redundant data.

In cases for which this works with iodide in particular, the economy is astounding: At the cost of (at most) a few days' exposure on a home source, a completely unknown structure may be phased de novo; the technique is the most likely solution to the problem of limited synchrotron beam time.

Native Sulfur. It has been shown possible to solve *de novo* lysozyme from a single SAD data set using the (weak: 0.5 electrons) anomalous signal of sulfur using synchrotron at the CuK_α radiation wavelength (49) as well as on an in-house source (49a). It remains to be seen whether this procedure is general enough to be useful for HT operations; the question mark lies over the ability to solve typically large sulfur substructures with a weak anomalous signal.

This sulfur signal has been demonstrated to be useful for resolving SIR phase ambiguities: The sulfur positions in the native crystal are bootstrapped using the derivative phases for cross-phasing anomalous Fourier maps (49b).

5.2 Molecular Replacement

5.2.1 Suitability for High Throughput

Purely experimentally, molecular replacement (MR) (50) is by far the most efficient and cheapest technique: If a crystal diffracts satisfactorily, even only to low resolution, a single data set is sufficient—even an incomplete one may work—and the X-ray analysis can proceed. There is no need for expensive reagents or complicated or time-consuming labeling procedures. New methods, such as the MOLREP program (51), are making the procedure more automated.

The trade-off in efficiency, however, comes from the downstream analysis, and the problems are well known: Identifying an MR "hit" is often difficult, and phase bias gives rise to artifacts (52)—especially when starting from more distant homologs—that require some experience to identify and remove. This leads to expensive, time-intensive cycles of manual rebuilding and refinement, a problem especially at low resolutions. Because of this cost, at Syrrx we attempt MR as soon as particular native data are available, but if it proves problematic, it is shelved and the problem approached by de novo phasing, in particular, selenomethionine MAD.

On the other hand, for high-resolution data and a good hit, the ARP/wARP procedure (34) using maximum-likelihood refinement (53) has transformed MR: Even hits with relatively low homology are used to yield information-rich, easily interpretable maps, which can often be built automatically as well, with a cost of only a few hours' or days' automatic computations.

5.2.2 Finding the Molecular Replacement Hit

As more homolog structures become available for a given target—as will occur increasingly with structural genomics efforts—the probability of finding an MR "hit" is greatly increased. Other problems are unrelated to the search model and may continue to make the MR search more effort than alternative, de novo phasing: Multiple copies or domains in the asymmetric unit; unpredictable conformational changes; high-symmetry space groups; small or nonglobular search models. It is important to identify these problems early so that little time is spent on them except as a last resort.

5.2.3 Molecular Replacement vs. Anomalous Dispersion Single-Wavelength

One of the implied benefits of structural genomics is that, once representatives of all folds are available, crystallography will be reduced to simple MR. Whether that is likely (or indeed desirable) is still an open question. But until such time, de novo phasing, in particular SAD/MAD, will remain a mainstay of any HT operation. This will be true even for many structures that appear on paper to be facile MR problems: While the effort for foolproof MR algorithms is ongoing, unforeseeable problems will always arise and require a de novo approach.

On the other hand, even for structures that appear solvable by MR, the efficiency of the analysis can be greatly improved if phase information is available: Using even weak phases makes a large difference both to the sensitivity of the MR search and to subsequent structure refinement. The SAD phases, especially weak ones that may be insufficient to solve the structure on their own, are not necessarily hard to come by, e.g., from the anomalous signal from halide soaks or native sulfur, as discussed earlier; alternatively, a monochromatic beamline fixed near the selenium edge is often adequate to obtain SAD SeMet phases. Such design decisions can allow experimental phasing to be attempted as a matter of course, with little additional experimental overhead, thereby improving the overall through-put for novel structures.

5.3 Automated Phasing

Several software systems are available that will attempt to generate phases automatically, given only the raw or integrated data. The most widely used is *SOLVE*, a self-contained, script-driven software system that accepts inte-grated data and will automatically attempt to solve the heavy-atom/anom-alous substructure, generate phases, and assess their quality.

ELVES (54) is a suite of scripts written in minimal C-shell, for max-imum portability in UNIX. It contains considerable intelligence to make installation and operation of third-party software transparent and will accept simple natural-language commands to execute the steps from proces-sing to phasing. Its appeal lies in its simplicity of interaction and installa-tion, but it is not yet as widespread as it probably should be.

The Buster Development Group has recently released *AUTOSHARP* (55), which aims to produce a largely refined model given integrated reflec-tions; it is based on *SHARP* and *BUSTER* for phasing and refinement.

Such methods can be great time savers; however, the single biggest drawback of all these methods is that, at the time of writing, none imple-mented any Shake-and-Bake direct methods for substructure solution. While this is planned for at least *ELVES* and *AUTOSHARP*, until such time the substructure will remain the weak link in these procedures, which will therefore continue to produce a significant proportion of garbage results and thus fail to allay completely crystallographers' (somewhat harsh) suspi-cions.

5.4 Data Collection

5.4.1 Optimizing Data Collection

The most important factor in X-ray structure analysis is the data, since that is what distinguishes protein crystallography from protein modeling. In the HT context, collecting diffraction data is a trade-off between data quality and time constraints: The improved counting statistics that result from longer exposures *vs.* the finite lifetime of the crystal in the X-ray beam; or the improved signal that is obtained from high observational redundancy vs. the need to collect as many data sets as possible, something particularly important in an HT operation.

In monochromatic data collection—e.g., on a series of ligand soaks—it is sufficient that data are complete. In contrast, for SAD phasing it is important that the crystal survive long enough to yield redundant data, whereas measurement of the weak reflections at the resolution limit is merely a luxury, provided the strong, lower-resolution data have been observed; the exposure time may be therefore be drastically reduced.

Deciding on a collection strategy at the start of the experiment has in the past been largely left to the crystallographer's experience; whether this leads to a successful experiment could be confirmed only by a complete analysis of the data, i.e., sometime after data collection is over. Fast computers and algorithms, however, mean that the experimenter can now, in the course of data collection, repeatedly complete the data analysis to a stage where the experiment's success can be judged and then modify the strategy as necessary. This is crucial in HT operations, which require optimization of scarce resources, *viz.* synchrotron time.

Thus, for most SeMet AD experiments—certainly when there are no complications—thanks to the power of direct methods programs ShelxD or SnB, it is possible to solve the selenium substructure, and often have good phases calculated, even before the peak wavelength is completely collected. Collecting data at more wavelengths is then pointless and another crystal may be mounted. On the other hand, in radiation-sensitive crystals, premature radiation damage can be detected as soon as it occurs, so, if necessary, a new crystal can be turned to immediately, using shorter exposures.

Assessing crystal decay is especially important in AD cases that are expected to be problematic: large substructures, weak anomalous signal, merohedral twinning. These cases require very accurate diffraction amplitude estimates with small uncertainties, which is achieved by extremely high observational redundancy (at one or more wavelengths). Thus, crystal decay should be deferred as long as possible, since data are collected until the crystal decays, even though the substructure is unlikely to be solved before that happens.

In the case of ligand-soaked crystals, success is usually easier to judge: the presence or not of the bound ligand. The phases from a quick rigid-body refinement of the known structure can reveal this even when data are still significantly incomplete.

5.4.2 Automating Data Collection

While the real-time analysis discussed in the previous section has become a part of modern data collection, it remains work-intensive and in particular requires the attention of an experienced crystallographer, day and night. Automating the intimate feedback it allows requires not only remotely controllable (i.e., robotic) sample-mounting and data-collection hardware, but also software that allows direct coordination of the beamline hardware and the downstream analysis. Hardware issues have been discussed (Sec. 4.5.2); a nascent software system, designed with the generality that can embrace such heterogeneous components, is discussed in Section 6.2.2.

Such a system also streamlines the initial screening of crystals: Each crystal is placed in the beam in turn, and a few exposures are recorded (preferably 90° apart), which are analyzed and scored automatically for resolution limits, mosaicity, background, icing, diffuse scatter, anisotropy, etc. Thus, large numbers of crystals can be rapidly prioritized before data collection, and the use of beam time is optimized. Features such as the presence of anomalous scatterers or ligand and the absence of merohedral twinning can, however, be established only from significantly complete data sets.

5.4.3 Synchrotrons

While access to synchrotron radiation remains limiting for independent laboratories, many HT initiatives have addressed this problem by obtaining a dedicated beamline. Tunable beamlines offer the flexibility for MAD phasing, although they are significantly more expensive to build than monochromatic beamlines. Moreover, the potential of SAD phasing means that many existing monochromatic beamlines are suitable for *de novo* phasing, provided the wavelength is fixed sensibly, e.g., just shorter than the selenium peak. (This has the social side benefit of lowering the demand for tunable beamlines so that they become more accessible for non-SeMet MAD experiments).

The Syrrx-owned beamline, BL5.0.3 at the ALS, is a good example. It is monochromatic, thus reducing costs; the adjacent beamline, BL5.0.2, is tunable and for MAD cases may be accessed through the Syrrx agreement with the ALS. In any case the combination of a MAD-capable line with a monochromatic side station is a powerful combination for HTC: The monochromatic line can be used to screen rapidly for the best-diffracting crystals, and these can then be transferred to the MAD station for structure solution. Crystals that can be solved by MR (i.e., those for which a homolog exists with ~40% or greater sequence identity) can be collected on the monochromatic line.

5.4.4 In-House Source vs. Synchrotron

At first glance, it appears that the in-house source has no place in a high-throughput crystallography setup: Many orders of magnitude weaker than third-generation synchrotron undulator beamlines, with a comparatively poorly focused beam, and fixed wavelength, it does not appear to fit into the more–faster–better scheme. Nevertheless, it does retain a vital role, not merely for economic, but also for scientific reasons.

Crystal Screening. The sample—the crystal mount—remains the most crucial aspect of the entire crystallographic experiment, and screening conditions of crystal mounting for good diffraction are vital. However, using synchrotron radiation for this purpose is not only inconvenient but wasteful, since it remains expensive, sporadic, and off-site. The same is true for heavy-atom soaks: They must be screened not only for diffraction, but for successful derivatization as well.

Routine Data Collection. Modern in-house sources, such as the FRD produced by MSC, produce brilliance comparable to first-generation synchrotron sources; for well-diffracting crystals, exposures may be as short as one minute, and therefore not more than an order of magnitude slower than a beamline such as 5.0.3 at the ALS, Berkeley. On the other hand, even top-end in-house machines cost a fraction of a beamline, also in maintenance, are available 24/7, and are accessible without the inconveniences of travel and night shifts. If equipped with suitable robotics (e.g., the Abbott/MSC system), its throughput can approach or exceed that achievable even by regular visits to a synchrotron beamline.

In-house radiation applies especially to well-diffracting crystals and to ligand-soaks in particular, since these are usually attempted with optimized crystals.

5.5 Model Building

5.5.1 Current Reality

Model building, which includes both map interpretation and refinement, remains a hands-on procedure. All graphical modeling programs provide semiautomatic tools to speed up model building to various extents; some provide direct interfaces to refinement programs, significantly simplifying the rebuilding–refining cycle. Nevertheless, the process requires the dedicated attention of an experienced crystallographer.

A number of programs do offer truly independent, automated model building: ARP/wARP (34) is the oldest, while RESOLVE (55a) and MAID (55b) were released more recently; TEXTAL (55c) is only available through web submission. Given good starting maps, these programs can automatically build more than 90% of the protein backbone; however, success is highly dependent on data resolution and map quality. Realistically, data should extend to 2.3–2.5 Å; success has been reported for as low as 2.8 Å, but typically a much lower fraction is automatically completed. Even the most completely traced structures, however, invariably require confirmation and additional work by a crystallographer.

Because it is more time intensive to interpret poorly phased electron density than to improve experimental phases, especially in an HTC context where new derivatives, mutants, or orthologs are relatively easy to produce, the map interpretation stage need generally be entered only when good phases are available. Therefore, building the structure per se does not present the major bottleneck, even if it is not necessarily trivial, and will continue to require experts for the foreseeable future, especially for low-resolution structures.

What *is* the bottleneck, however, are the structural ambiguities that are found in most structures, frequently in biologically relevant regions, and that require often-painstaking work to resolve. It is doubtful that this will ever be fully automated: Structure interpretation is essentially the formulation of a scientific hypothesis and thus requires, almost by definition, human intellect.

5.5.2 A High-Throughput Approach to Structural Ambiguities

The HT context provides a promising approach to resolving structural ambiguities. Traditionally, electron density is generally calculated using data from the single "best" crystal. (The exception are crystals that can neither be cryomounted nor survive radiation, thus requiring several crystals for a data set.) However, the signal obtainable from one crystal is bound to be weaker than that from multiple ones. (This principle is used to great effect in multicrystal averaging.)

Simply merging data from different crystals can be problematic, however, since crystals are not perfectly isomorphous, especially when cryomounted; the nonisomorphism is implicit in the diffraction data and leads mainly to increased scatter in the merged data. On the other hand, nonisomorphism is explicit in real space, where the merging of information is much simpler and differences between crystals lead to an improved signal.

The problem of collecting and solving independently 10 (identical) crystal structures, usually daunting, becomes realistic in an HT context, where the process is streamlined so that it can be repeated at the figurative click of a button, with little intervention required. Thus, one is in a much better position to establish whether ambiguities are true disorder or merely variable from crystal to crystal.

5.6 Validation and Reporting

The question of what constitutes a competed structure depends on the goals of the HT operation. Structural genomics initiatives will tend to aim for fully refined structures; when considering ligand soaks, a simple qualitative assessment based on initial difference density may be sufficient. In either event, since several crystallographers are likely to be involved, criteria should be laid down at the outset; fortunately, there is broad consensus in the crystallographic community.

The type of validation needed for final structures is no different from that in conventional crystallography, and the standard tools should be used: cross-validation (56), Ramachandran angles (57), probe contact surfaces (58), residual difference density (59), and various knowledge-based tests (e.g., Ref. 60), etc.

Beyond that, the need for stringency does become more acute, because of the numbers of structures any individual crystallographer deals with and the time constraints under which she often operates. During conventional structure deposition at the PDB, the natural procedure includes validation by an independent party; this is a very wise model to emulate, even within a closed organization.

The HT context does make another type of independent validation possible: The same structure may be independently solved multiple times and the models compared directly. This is related to the principle outlined in Section 5.5.2 and would be extremely powerful for the same reasons. Whether it can be done on a routine basis will depend on time constraints in the pipeline, although it is likely that the benefits eventually outweigh the associated time penalty.

The deposition procedure in common use, as enforced by the PDB (61), is a tried-and-tested model, and indeed the public structural genomics initiatives are obligated to follow it.

More critically, there currently is no accepted system for annotating localized structural features and potential errors or ambiguities; HT operations are inherently collaborative, so such a system becomes vital. At Syrrx, we have developed an XML-based annotation scheme, with standard, machine-parsable annotations, that can be generated as sticky notes within Xfit and becomes an essential component of the model, as much a part of it as the atoms or temperature factors.

6 INFORMATION MANAGEMENT

6.1 Experiment Management

The single most important precondition to scalable high throughput is information management (IM). By definition, HT involves a large number of targets, which all must traverse the numerous steps from gene to structure, not necessarily linearly, and all with potential problems that require individual, nonstandard treatment. Not only must each step be directed and scheduled, but the observations and results must be stored in a standardized way so that they are easily accessible downstream wherever relevant and also to enable data mining and learning in order to improve efficiency and success rates. Moreover, the parallelization and diversification of targets made possible by an HT infrastructure only adds to the Babylonian confusion that ensues when the laboratory notebook—or any digital but decentralized record keeping—is used to manage tens to hundreds of targets passing through a dozen different hands.

In order to manage such vast amounts of data, data entry takes on a vital role: Interfaces must exist for every step in the HT operation so that data integrity can be enforced and maintained—this is particularly necessary for nonautomated steps, where human error can be introduced. More than that, well-designed user interfaces drastically increase the efficiency of such manual steps by facilitating experiment planning, speeding up data recording, and providing access to data relevant to the particular experiment, such as sample history.

6.2 X-Ray Analysis

6.2.1 The Problems for High-Throughput Analysis

Whereas all steps in the gene-to-structure pipeline upstream of the mounted crystal are experimental in nature, once data have been collected, the pipeline becomes mainly computational. These computations take the form of a series of steps in a loosely defined sequence, with several, separately developed programs available for each of the various steps. The programs are executed individually ("jobs") and judged for success, and the results are manually prepared for the following step.

This approach provides great flexibility to the analysis, but it is also the main reason why the analysis is still often slow: It carries a large management overhead, which has little to do with the analysis as such. Many programs are text-based, so scripts must be written or configured once the documentation has been deciphered; data must often be converted between formats; resources such as CPU time and disk space must be secured; program execution must be monitored, usually on several machines; and job sequence history must be explicitly recorded separately. Program suites [Shelx (62), XtalView (42), CCP4 (63), CNS (64)] have done much to alleviate the problem of incompatible formats; graphical user interfaces [XtalView, Sharp (39), CNS, CCP4] have, to varying extents, dealt with problems of program configuration, often with loss of flexibility; automated procedures [Solve (41), arpWarp (34), ELVES (54), AutoSHARP (55)] have tried to deal with many problems at once. Nevertheless, no such solution on its own encompasses all necessary steps, and all leave resource management to the user.

Most important, no currently available solution provides tools for HT operations, i.e., for managing large numbers of projects and facilitating collaboration on each. When analysis does proceed rapidly, it tends to be due to experience and various complicated scripts, either self-written or inherited. However, it leads invariably to long lists of files, named by the crystallographer's own unique logic, making the job sequence traceable by someone else only with considerable effort, and precluding any form of data mining and learning.

6.2.2 Automated Structure Analysis of Proteins (ASAP) Architecture

At Syrrx, a software system, CrystalNet, has been developed that specifically addresses the existing computational shortcomings just discussed, by exposing high-level work-flow management while hiding low-level job control. Based on the ASAP (automated structure analysis of proteins) concept, the software system envisioned by the JCSG, it streamlines and standardizes the X-ray analysis, allowing learning and thus leading eventually to a largely automated system.

The work-flow management allows the crystallographer high-level planning of sequences of crystallographic computations. In a graphical interface, icons, representing jobs or procedures, are arranged in a structured data flowchart that allows the sequence of calculations to be visually recognized by both the crystallographer and collaborators. At the same time, the interface allows the same flexibility available in the traditional scripting approach, since analyses often require nonstandard treatment. The progress of the computations is monitored on the same flowchart, which can be modified in real time, as necessary. All details of the calculations—location of input and output data, parameters, log output, context—are stored in a database, as is the flowchart, its ownership, and its execution status.

The job control aspect of CrystalNet handles the execution, scheduling, and data management of computations and is hidden from the user. It manages heterogeneous resources (i.e., CPU, data storage) through daemon processes, allocates computations, and monitors their execution, storing everything in the database. Crystallographic output data from each computation remains on the computer where it was generated, in order to optimize network traffic; the system schedules computations accordingly, to allow near-real-time computations, and moves data around as required; this is especially important for large data files on geographically remote resources (images at synchrotrons). For performance, communication is CORBA-based.

The system allows complete crystallographic flexibility because any crystallographic program—including interactive programs—can be made available to the system, provided it interacts with the system in a simple and well-defined way, usually best achieved by wrapping it in a script. Communication of meta-information between CrystalNet and a given (wrapped) program occurs in XML format, and expert user interfaces can be defined as XSL stylesheets. Naturally, the degree of functional granularity from a program depends on the wrapper, which may contain considerable intelligence, but the more atomic a wrapper, the more versatile it will be in general. Indeed, the programs do not have to be limited to computations but can include the likes of beamline operations, provided these have been sufficiently computerized.

The work-flow paradigm is very powerful: Many variations on the same protocol may be set-up easily in order to explore parameter space. Useful, general, or repeatable protocols may be stored and labeled for reuse by simply selecting the relevant items of the flowchart; tedious repeat-calculations, such as for ligand soaks, are then quick to set up by simply reassigning the input data. However, more than that, this opens up the path to extensive automation: Certain protocols will, in time, establish themselves as good choices in given situations, and these rules, if established, form the basis of automation.

7   STRUCTURAL GENOMICS INITIATIVES

7.1   Public Initiatives

The widespread success of the Human Genome Project has laid the groundwork for a very similar movement in structural genomics. In June 1999, the NIH announced $90 million in federal funding for the Protein Structure Initiative: These funds would be available to researchers focused on structural genomics and high-throughput structure determination. Currently there are seven public HT structure determination efforts, summarized next (4).

7.1.1   NIH-Funded Initiatives

The New York Structural Genomics Research Consortium is aiming to solve several hundred protein structures from a variety of model organisms, from bacteria to humans.

The Midwest Center for Structural Genomics is a consortium of seven institutions and will use targets from all three kingdoms, in particular unknown folds from pathogens; the aim is to reduce the cost of a structure to $20,000.

The Berkeley Structural Genomics Center is focusing on bacteria with very small genomes (*M. genitalium* and *M. pneumoniae*) and those proteins vital for independent life.

The Northeast Structural Genomics Consortium, consisting of groups from five states and Ontario, Canada, is targeting proteins from the model organisms *D. melanogaster*, *S. cereviciae*, and *C. elegans* and any human homologs; both NMR and X-ray crystallography are being used.

The TB Structural Genomics Consortium, a collaboration between scientists from six countries, is focusing exclusively on *Mycobacterium tuberculosis*. This consortium is cofunded by the National Institute of Allergy and Infectious Diseases, which hopes that it will lead to drugs and vaccines against tuberculosis.

The Southeast Collaboratory for Structural Genomics, based in Georgia and Alabama, is combining NMR and crystallography to target the genomes of *Caenorhabditis elegans* and *Pyrococcus furiousus* as well as the human genome.

The Joint Center for Structural Genomics is emphasizing high-throughput methods for all stages of the process and will focus on novel structures from the thermophile *Thermotoga maritima* as well as signaling proteins from *C. elegans*.

The Center for Eukaryotic Structural Genomics is based at the University of Wisconsin-Madison, but includes partners in Washington State, Tokyo and Israel; its initial focus is the genome of the eukaryotic *Arabidopsis* plant.

The Structural Genomics of Pathogenic Protozoa Consortium is based at the University of Washington, with other members at the HW MRI in Buffalo and the University of Rochester in New York; the focus is on a number of major global pathogenic protozoa.

7.1.2 European Union

The Protein Structure Factory in Berlin is a collaboration between structural biologists in the area and the German Human Genome Project; it aims to take human targets to structure, but automating the steps from sequence to structure.

The European Union funding "Framework 6" has made provision for structural genomics programs, enabling larger collaborations so that "critical mass" may be achieved. The outcome of such projects must contribute to common knowledge.

Yeast Structural Genomics is a collaboration between a number of French laboratories, with focus on yeast as a useful model organism.

7.1.3 Japan

The Institute of Physical and Chemical Research (RIKEN) is targeting a range of organisms, including *T. thermophilus*, *Mus musculus*, and *A. thaliana*, but only a subset of the latter two; emphasis will be placed on novel folds. Both crystallography and NMR are to be employed.

7.1.4 Others in North America

The Clinical Genomics Centre: Proteomics is based in Toronto, and uses X-ray crystallography along with NMR and other forms of protein characterization as part of a proteomics initiative.

The Montreal-Kingston Bacterial Structural Genomics Initiative uses both X-ray crystallography and NMR to study small and uncharacterized proteins from *E. coli*.

The Structure 2 Function Project is based at NIST in Maryland, making use of the IMCA beamline at the APS; targets are selected from the genome of *Haemophilus influenzae*.

7.2 High-Throughput Structure Determination in the Private Sector

Just as the Human Genome Project laid the foundation for an entirely new industry, the NIH Protein Structure Initiative has been accompanied by the creation of a number of private companies that pursue high-throughput structure determination with the aim of discovering lead compounds for drug development. As in the public initiatives, both X-ray crystallography and NMR are being used. TRIAD Therapeutics (San Diego, California) is using NMR exclusively, and Affinium Pharmaceuticals (Toronto, Canada) combines NMR and crystallography, but the majority are focusing on crystallography only:

Astex Technologies (Cambridge, UK)

Plexxicon, Inc. (San Fransisco, California)

Proteros Biostructures, GmbH (Martinsried, Germany)

Structural GenomiX, Inc. (San Diego, California)

Syrrx Inc. (San Diego, California)

8 CONCLUSIONS

High-throughput crystallography is no longer a pipe dream; it is already a reality. In particular, the kind of technology that had remained the wishful thinking of crystallographers for many years now either exists or is being developed—and, rather unsurprisingly, it works. Even so, it is still a new approach, and the vast possibilities, in particular as a tool for scientific enquiry, still lie open to exploration. The technology itself will also continue to evolve; the bar has been reset, however, and its usefulness will now be judged on a different scale.

The most publicized application of high-throughput crystallography is structural genomics and, in particular, the NIH goals of covering protein fold space (Sec. 7.1.1). Whether such results in themselves will be directly useful, as is frequently suggested, remains to be seen; skeptics argue persuasively that structural genomics alone will produce little of direct interest unless complemented by equivalent investments in functional studies.

The indirect impact of structural genomics on research, on the other hand, is easier to predict, and the frequent comparison with the Human Genome Project, its predecessor, certainly seems apt. The latter has provided molecular biologists with a powerful tool rather than necessarily with concrete answers; likewise, structural genomics will lead to a expansion of the knowledge pool that will greatly speed up more directed structural and functional investigations. Such applications range from obvious crystallographic uses in molecular replacement to permitting more sophisticated models of biological systems such as macroassemblies, thus enabling more informed experimental probing. The reliability of computational biology and bioinformatics—in particular structural and functional predictions—also can be expected to improve as the experimental data underlying these techniques become more extensive. Just as the Human Genome Project created an explosion of research and opportunity, we can expect that the structural genomics effort will also change the knowledge base and competitive landscape of life science research and business.

The technology developments that have been accompanying high-throughput efforts have broader applicability, and it is clear that this will impact crystallography as a whole. The biological systems being investigated are not getting simpler: Macroassemblies, membrane-spanning signaling systems, transcription machinery, and the like are already within reach of conventional approaches, but they remain nontrivial to solve. Human scientific input is hardly about to become redundant, and high-throughput technology and approaches will not change that; but they may make things just that little bit easier.

Of course, it is in drug discovery that HT crystallography has most direct applicability (65). The potential of structure-based drug discovery has long been recognized and has had a few notable successes (2). However, its broader use has been limited by the cost and low turnover rate of ligand complex structures, so other high-throughput screening techniques were preferred for lead compound discovery. This is now changing, and the structure-based approach is the focus of the private sector initiatives in particular: The attraction is not only the very direct access to the various cellular targets that underlie many First World ailments, but the approach may offer one of the few ways that will allow us to stay ahead of the spreading antibiotics resistance amongst pathogens.

REFERENCES

1. TL Blundell. Structure-based drug design. Nature 384:23–26, 1996.
2. J Greer, JW Erickson, JJ Baldwin, MD Varney. Application of the three-dimensional structures of protein target molecules in structure-based drug design. J Med Chem 37:1035–1054, 1994.
3. DE McRee, PR David. Practical Protein Crystallography, Academic Press, San Diego, CA, 1999.
4. NIH Structural Genomics Initiatives. http://www.nigms.nih.gov/funding/psi.html.
5. RC Stevens. High-throughput protein crystallization. Curr Op Str Biol 10:558–563, 2000.
6. WA Hendrickson. Determination of macromolecular structures from anomalous diffraction of synchrotron radiation. Science 254:51–58, 1991.
7. DE McRee. A brief history of crystallographic computing. Rigaku J 15:1–5, 1998.
8. JA Peterson, SE Graham. A close family resemblance: the importance of structure in understanding cytochromes P450. Structure 6:1079–1085, 1998.
9. JC Kendrew. Myoglobin and the Structure of Proteins (Nobel Lecture). 1962.
10. V Koronakis, A Sharff, E Koronakis, B Luisi, C Hughes. Crystal structure of the bacterial membrane protein TolC central to multidrug efflux and protein export. Nature 405:914–919, 2000.
11. K Palczewski, T Kumasaka, T Hori, CA Behnke, H Motoshima, BA Fox, I Le Trong, DC Teller, T Okada, RE Stenkamp, M Yamamoto, M Miyano. Crystal structure of rhodopsin: a G protein-coupled receptor. Science 289:739–745, 2000.
11a. S Shuman. Novel approach to molecular cloning and polynucleotide synthesis using vaccinia DNA topoisomerase. J Biol Chem 269(51): 32678–84, 1994.
12. SA Lesley. High-throughput proteomics: protein expression and purification in the postgenomic world. Prot Expr Pur 22:159–164, 2001.
13. Q Liu, MZ Li, D Leibham, D Cortez, SJ Elledge. The univector plasmid-fusion system, a method for rapid construction of recombinant DNA without restriction enzymes. Curr Biol 8:1300–1309, 1998.

14. JL Hartley, GF Temple, MA Brasch. DNA cloning using in vitro site-specific recombination. Genome Res 10:1788–1795, 2000.

15. KE Goodwill, MG Tennant, RC Stevens. High-throughput X-ray crystallography for structure-based drug design. Drug Disc Tech 6:S113–S117, 2001.

15a. R Janknecht, G De Martynhoff, J Lou, RA Hipskind, A Nordheim, and HG Stunnenberg. Rapid and efficient purification of native histidine-tagged protein expressed by recombinant vaccinia virus. Proc. Natl. Acad. Sci. USA 88, 8972, 1991.

15b. J Schmitt, H Hess, and HG Stunnenberg. Affinity purification of histidine-tagged proteins. Mol. Biol. Rep. 18, 223, 1993.

15c. E Hochuli, H Döbeli, and A Schacher. New metal chelate adsorbent selective for proteins and peptides containing neighbouring histidine residues. J. Chromatogr. 411, 177, 1987.

16. RC Stevens. Design of high-throughput methods of protein production for structural biology. Structure 8:R177–185, 2000.

16a. CV Maina, PD Riggs, AG Grandea 3rd, BE Slatko, LS Moran, JA Tagliamonte, LA McReynolds, CD Guan. An Escherichia coli vector to express and purify foreign proteins by fusion to and separation from maltose-binding protein. Gene 74(2): 365–73, 1988.

16b. DB Smith and KS Johnson. Single-step purification of polypeptides expressed in Escherichia coli as fusions with glutathione S-transferase. Gene 67(1): 31–40, 1988.

17. PA Williams, J Cosme, V Sridhar, EF Johnson, DE McRee. Mammalian microsomal cytochrome P450 monooxygenase: structural adaptations for membrane binding and functional diversity. Mol Cell 5:121–131, 2000.

18. KL Longenecker, SM Garrard, PJ Sheffield, ZS Derewenda. Protein crystallization by rational mutagenesis of surface residues: Lys to Ala mutations promote crystallization of RhoGDI. Acta Cryst D57:679–688, 2001.

19. S Dasgupta, GH Iyer, SH Bryant, CE Lawrence, JA Bell. Extent and nature of contacts between protein molecules in crystal lattices and between subunits of protein oligomers. Proteins 28:494–514, 1997.

20. WA Hendrickson, JR Horton, DM LeMaster. Selenomethionyl proteins produced for analysis by multiwavelength anomalous diffraction (MAD): a vehicle for direct determination of three-dimensional structure. EMBO J 9:1665–1672, 1990.

21. GD van Duyne, RF Standaert, PA Karplus, SL Schreiber, Y Clardy. Atomic structures of the human immunophilin FKBP-12 complexes with FK506 and rapamycin. J Molec Biol 229:105–124, 1993.

22. DA Bushnell, P Cramer, RD Kornberg. Selenomethionine incorporation in Saccharomyces cerevisiae RNA polymerase II. Structure 9:R11–14, 2001.

23. JJ Bellizzi, J Widom, CW Kemp, J Clardy. Producing selenomethionine-labeled proteins with a baculovirus expression vector system. Structure 7:R263–R267, 1999.

24. S Doublie. Preparation of selenomethyionyl proteins for phase determination. Meth Enzym 276:523–530, 1997.

24a. A McPherson. Crystallization of Macromolecules. Cold Spring Harbor Laboratory, 1999.

25. JR Luft, J Wolfley, I Jurisica, J Glasgow, S Fortier, GT DeTitta. Macromolecular crystallization in a high-throughput laboratory—the search phase. 2001. J Cryst Growth 232:591–595, 2000.

26. TY Teng. Mounting of crystals for macromolecular crystallography in a free-standing thin film. J Appl Cryst 23:387–391, 1990.

27. Oceaneering International Inc. Crystal Preparation Prime Item (CCPI). http:// www.oceaneering.com/adtech/space/adtech_space_crystalprep.htm.

28. EF Garman, TR Schneider. Macromolecular cryocrystallography. J Appl Cryst 30:211–237, 1997.

29. H Hope. Cryocrystallography of biological macromolecules: a generally applicable method. Acta Cryst B44:22–26, 1988.

30. SW Muchmore, J Olson, R Jones, J Pan, M Blum, J Greer, SM Merrick, P Magdalinos, VL Nienaber. Automated crystal mounting and data collection for protein crystallography. Structure 8:R243–246, 2000.

31. E Abola, P Kuhn, T Earnest, RC Stevens. Automation of X-ray crystallography. Nat Struc Biol 7 Suppl:973–977, 2000.

31a. G Snell, G Meigs, C Cork, T Earnest, R Nordmeyer, E Cornell, J Jaklevic, D Yegian, J Jin, RC Stevens. Automatic Sample Mounting and Alignment System for Macromolecular Crystallography at the ALS. Annual Meeting of the ACA, San Antonio, TX, 2002.

32. J Karle. Some developments in anomalous dispersion for the structural investigation of macromolecular systems in biology. In: International Journal of Quantum Chemistry: Quantum Biology Symposium. Vol. 7, pp. 357–367, 1980.

33. WA Hendrickson. Analysis of protein structure from diffraction measurement at multiple wavelengths. Trans Am Cryst Ass 21, pp. 11–21, 1985.

34. A Perrakis, R Morris, VS Lamzin. Automated protein model building combined with iterative structure refinement. Nat Struc Biol 6:458–463, 1999.

35. A Pahler, JL Smith, WA Hendrickson. A probability representation for phase information from multiwavelength anomalous dispersion. Acta Cryst A46:537–540, 1990.

36. LM Rice, TN Earnest, AT Brunger. Single-wavelength anomalous diffraction phasing revisited. Acta Cryst D56:1413–1420, 2000.

37. BC Wang. Resolution of phase ambiguity in macromolecular crystallography. Meth Enzym 115:90–112, 1985.

38. TC Terwilliger. MAD phasing: treatment of dispersive differences as isomorphous replacement information. Acta Cryst D50:17–23, 1994.

39. Ed La Fortelle, G Bricogne. Maximum-likelihood heavy-atom parameter refinement for multiple isomorphous replacement and multiwavelength anomalous diffraction methods. Meth Enzym 276:472–494, 1997.

40. RW Grosse-Kunstleve, AT Brunger. A highly automated heavy-atom search procedure for macromolecular structures. Acta Cryst D55:1568–1577, 1999.

41. TC Terwilliger, J Berendzen. Automated MAD and MIR structure solution. Acta Cryst D55:849–861, 1999.

42. DE McRee. XtalView/Xfit—A versatile program for manipulating atomic coordinates and electron density. J Struc Biol 125:156–165, 1999.

43. AM Deacon, SE Ealick. Selenium-based MAD phasing: setting the sites on larger structures. Structure 7:R161–R166, 1999.

44. CM Weeks, R Miller. The design and implementation of SnB version 2.0. J Appl Cryst 32:120–124, 1999.

45. GM Sheldrick, TR Schneider. Direct Methods for Macromolecules. In: D Turk, L Johnson, eds. Methods in Macromolecular Crystallography. IOS Press, 2001, pp. 72–81.

46. F von Delft, TL Blundell. The 160 Selenium Atom Substructure of KPHMT. Acta Cryst A58 (Supplement), C239.

47. CM Ogata. MAD phasing grows up. Nat Struct Biol 5 Suppl:638–640, 1998.

48. Z Dauter, M Dauter. Anomalous signal of solvent bromides used for phasing of lysozyme. J Mol Biol 289:93–101, 1999.

49. Z Dauter, M Dauter, E de La Fortelle, G Bricogne, GM Sheldrick. Can anomalous signal of sulfur become a tool for solving protein crystal structures? J Mol Biol 289:83–92, 1999.

49a. JE Debreczeni, G Bunkóczi, Q Ma and GM Sheldrick. In-house measurement of the anomalous signal of sulfur and its use for phasing. Acta Cryst A58 (Supplement), C83, 2002.

49b. C Yang, and JW Pflugrath. Applications of anomalous scattering from S atoms for improved phasing of protein diffraction data collected at Cu Kalpha wavelength. Acta Cryst D57(10):1480–90, 2001.

51. A Vagin, A Teplyakov. MOLREP: an automated program for molecular replacement. J Appl Cryst 30:1022–1025, 1997.

52. G Bricogne. A Bayesian statistical theory of the phase problem. I. A multi-channel maximum-entropy formalism for constructing generalized joint probability distrubutions of structure factors. Acta Cryst A44:517–545, 1988.

53. GN Murshudov, AA Vagin, A Lebedev, KS Wilson, EJ Dodson. Efficient anisotropic refinement of macromolecular structures using FFT. Acta Cryst D55:247–255, 1999.

54. J Holton. Elves. http://ucxray.berkeley.edu/~jamesh/elves/release.html.

55. GlobalPhasing. AutoSHARP. http://www.globalphasing.com.

55a. TC Terwilliger. Maximum-likelihood density modification using pattern recognition of structural motifs. Acta Cryst D57(12):1755–1762, 2001.

55b. DG Levitt. A new software routine that automates the fitting of protein X-ray crystallographic electron-density maps. Acta Cryst D57(7):1013–1019, 2001.

55c. T Holton, TR Ioerger, et al. Determining protein structure from electron-density maps using pattern matching. Acta Cryst D56 (6):722–734, 2000.

56. AT Brunger. Free R value—a novel statistical quantity for assessing the accuracy of crystal structures. Nature 355:472–475, 1992.

57. GN Ramachandran, V Sasisekharan. Conformations of polypetides and proteins. Adv Prot Chem 28:283–437, 1968.

58. JM Word, SC Lovell, JS Richardson, DC Richardson. Asparagine and glutamine: using hydrogen atom contacts in the choice of side-chain amide orientation. J Mol Biol 285:1735–1747, 1999.

59. F van den Akker, WG Hol. Difference density quality (DDQ): a method to assess the global and local correctness of macromolecular crystal structures. Acta Cryst D55:206–218, 1999.

60. RWW Hooft, G Vriend, C Sander, EE Abola. Errors in protein structures. Nature 381:272, 1996.

61. EE Abola, JL Sussman, J Prilusky, NO Manning. Protein Data Bank archives of three-dimensional macromolecular structures. Meth Enzym 277:556–571, 1997.

62. GM Sheldrick, TR Schneider. SHELXL: High-resolution refinement. In: RM Sweet, CWJ Carter, eds. Meth Enzym. Vol. 277. Orlando, FL, Academic Press, 1997, pp. 401–411.

63. Collaborative Computational Project, Number 4. The CCP4 Suite: programs for protein crystallography. Acta Cryst D50:760–763, 1994.

64. AT Brunger, PD Adams, GM Clore, WL DeLano, P Gros, RW Grosse-Kunstleve, JS Jiang, J Kuszewski, M Nilges, NS Pannu, RJ Read, LM Rice, T Simonson, GL Warren. Crystallography and NMR system: a new software suite for macromolecular structure determination. Acta Cryst D54:905–921, 1998.

65. TL Blundell, H Jhoti, C Abell. High-throughput crystallography for lead discovery in drug design. Nat Rev Drug Discov 1:45–54, 2002.

5

Prospects for High-Throughput Structure Determination of Proteins by NMR Spectroscopy

Ann E. Ferentz*
Harvard Medical School, Boston, Massachusetts, U.S.A.

I INTRODUCTION

Since the early 1990s, nuclear magnetic resonance (NMR) spectroscopy has developed into an extremely powerful tool for solving macromolecular structures. The combination of innovations in magnet and probe design, pulse programming, isotopic labeling, data analysis, and computational methods means that larger protein structures can now be solved more easily than ever before. Historically, NMR has been limited to very small proteins (initially those under ~ 10 kDa), but current methods allow for determination of structures as large as 30–40 kDa. This size limit is being pushed as new techniques challenge the fundamental resolution limit of NMR spectroscopy, enabling the acquisition of high-field spectra with better resolution than was previously possible (1). Solution structures of proteins in the 60-kDa range are now within reach (2), and systems larger than 100 kDa have been studied (3), although a complete structure of this size has not yet been reported. Since fewer than 6% of crystal structures in the Protein Data Bank (PDB) (4) are larger than 60 kDa, NMR and X-ray crystallography are both viable techniques for most protein structure determinations.

With the increased ease of solution structure determination, NMR structures currently constitute 15–20% of newly solved protein structures

Current affiliation: Variagenics, Inc., Cambridge, Massachusetts, U.S.A.

and 16% of all the depositions in the PDB (> 2100 structures). They still account for a disproportionate number of the small structures in the PDB, making up 37% of the structures under 10 kDa. This reflects both the limitations of early studies to these low-molecular-weight systems and relative rapidity of solving small structures by NMR today. The vast majority (~ 75%) of the NMR structures of proteins in the PDB do not have corresponding crystal structures, in large part because the proteins could not be crystallized (5). This exemplifies the complementarity of NMR spectroscopy and X-ray crystallography as approaches for solving protein structures. The future will likely include the two techniques working side by side, exploiting the unique strengths of each.

As structural biology enters the postgenomic era, high-throughput structure initiatives are gearing up. Several pilot projects in structural genomics have been initiated in which NMR spectroscopy plays a key role (5–7). One of the unique features of NMR that makes it particularly suitable for such endeavors is its ability to assess rapidly the folding state of a protein in solution. This could be extremely advantageous for screening samples prior to crystallization attempts or in delineating fragments of large, multidomain proteins that might be suitable for structural studies. Nuclear magnetic resonance is also uniquely capable of determining the structures of proteins that are partially unfolded, e.g., due to the absence of their binding partners. In addition, it can define weak interactions within complexes at atomic resolution, an ability that has provided a powerful approach to drug discovery and may play a critical role as the analysis of complexes comes to the forefront. The primary challenges for high-throughput applications of NMR spectroscopy are to reduce the amount of time required for data acquisition and to automate the now labor-intensive process of data analysis. State-of-the-art instrumentation and methodology, combined with automated or semiautomated data analysis and structure calculations, are having a major impact in this area and are dramatically reducing the amount of time required to solve a structure. This chapter will discuss current methods for solving protein structures by NMR spectroscopy and the prospects of the technique for high-throughput structure initiatives.

2   STATE-OF-THE-ART STRUCTURE DETERMINATION BY NMR

When the first protein structure was solved in 1985 (8), NMR instrumentation had already matured greatly from its infancy. By that time, superconducting magnets had been developed with field strengths high enough to provide the resolution and sensitivity needed to assign the spectra of a protein. Fourier transform spectroscopy, two-dimensional spectroscopy, and new computational methods allowed for acquisition and processing of data in a reasonable amount of time. Finally, the key insight that the nuclear Overhauser effect (NOE) at short mixing times could be used to obtain interproton distances within a protein brought the determination of a complete solution structure of a protein by NMR into the realm of possibility (9). However, the NOE could not be fully exploited until distance geometry methods were developed capable of deriving the fold of a protein from the distance data (10). With the capacity to solve macromolecular structures, NMR spectroscopy began to make major contributions to biology, taking its place beside X-ray crystallography as one of the two primary methods used by structural biologists.

Since then, developments in hardware, pulse programming, and computational methods have continued to leap forward. While the general approach for solving a protein structure by NMR has changed little since the early 1990s (Scheme 1), technological advances have affected the implementation of every step of the process. Today's state-of-the-art NMR spectrometer is equipped with four channels to allow detection of ^{1}H, ^{15}N, and ^{13}C nuclei with deuterium decoupling and a cryogenic probe that provides extremely high sensitivity. After preparation of a suitable isotopically labeled sample, multidimensional NMR data sets are acquired and processed to yield a set of NMR spectra for the protein being studied.

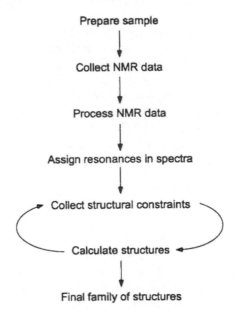

Scheme 1 General strategy for solving a protein structure by NMR spectroscopy.

Assignment of the resonances in the spectra to particular nuclei in the protein is accomplished in a semiautomated manner using interactive software packages. With the assignments in hand, additional NMR spectra are analyzed to derive experimental constraints (distances, dihedral angles, etc.) for structure calculations. Finally, structures are calculated that are consistent with the existing experimental constraints. These preliminary structures facilitate further data analysis to derive more experimental constraints that are used to recalculate the solution structure. This iterative process continues until the vast majority of experimental constraints are consistent with the structures calculated. The resulting bundle of structures represents the solution structure of the protein, with variations among the individual structures indicating the precision of the structure. The overall process is summarized in Scheme 1 and will be detailed in the following sections.

2.1 Sample Preparation

2.1.1 General Considerations

One distinct advantage of solving protein structures by NMR instead of X-ray crystallography is that NMR is carried out in aqueous solution and therefore does not require that protein crystals be grown. Moreover, NMR is an inherently insensitive technique, so NMR samples need not be as stringently pure as samples for crystallography, although they must be absolutely free from proteases to be stable. Another potential advantage of NMR is that small affinity tags (e.g., His_6) used during protein purification need not be removed prior to NMR studies. Thus, in many cases a simple one- or two-column purification procedure is quite adequate, and samples can often be prepared in a single day. Once milligram quantities of protein are in hand, final sample preparation for NMR is rapid and straightforward. The protein is exchanged into a suitable sample buffer (see later) and is concentrated as much as possible. This may be done in a stirred ultrafiltration device or by using a spun concentrator equipped with an appropriate molecular weight cutoff filter. The most efficient sample preparation is often a two-step procedure in which a stirred cell is first used to reduce larger volumes and exchange the buffer and a spun concentrator is used to bring the sample to its final volume.

The precise amount of protein needed for an NMR structure determination varies from protein to protein. In an ideal NMR sample, the concentration of protein is 1 mM or more, with higher concentrations being advantageous for some experiments. In general the concentration used is the highest that can be acheived without aggregating the sample. Approximately 500 μL of solution is sufficient for most experiments, although the exact sample volume required depends upon the probe and the sample tube being using. The minimum amount of material required has now been reduced to 300 μL of 0.1 mM protein, thanks to new types of NMR sample tubes (Shigemi tubes) and the increased sensitivity of cryogenic probes. This capacity to work at lower concentrations is invaluable for larger proteins and complexes that cannot be concentrated to the extent previously required. Smaller sample sizes will also make it possible to screen proteins in high-throughput applications while keeping growth culture volumes to a minimum. For structure determination, though, it is still preferable to work at higher concentration if possible, since this reduces the amount of experimental time, which in turn helps maintain the integrity of the sample.

2.1.2 Selection of Sample Buffer

The composition of the buffer can make a real difference in the solubility of a sample, its propensity to aggregate, its stability, and the overall quality of NMR data obtained. Sample conditions are typically derived in an iterative process, adjusting the pH, ionic strength, buffer type, concentration, and temperature of the sample until spectra with the best resolution and intensity are obtained. The most convenient buffers contain no exchangeable protons, avoiding complications of buffer resonances in the ^{1}H NMR spectrum. These may be inorganic buffers like phosphate, bicarbonate, or borate, or buffers available in fully deuterated form, such as Tris or acetate. A frequent starting point is a buffer containing phosphate ($\sim$ 50 mM) at neutral pH and a low concentration of sodium chloride (e.g., 20 mM) in H_2O/D_2O (19:1) along with a reducing agent (1 mM DTT) or metal chelating agent (0.1 mM EDTA), if needed. From this point, the pH may be lowered gradually or the salt concentration increased while the 1D ^{1}H NMR spectrum and the ^{1}H,^{15}N-HSQC are monitored for changes. Similarly, temperature can be stepped up to as high as $\sim$ 310 K and the effect on the spectra monitored. A new sample can then be made up at high concentration in the best buffer identified. The final sample may also contain protease inhibitors and sodium azide to inhibit microbial growth. The best conditions for the ^{1}H,^{15}N-HSQC generally yield the best three-dimensional spectra for structure determination.

2.1.3 Methods for Isotopic Labeling

Contemporary methods for structure determination of proteins by NMR spectroscopy rely heavily on the use of isotopically labeled samples. During the course of a typical structure determination four to five variously labeled samples may be prepared. ^{15}N and ^{13}C enrichment allows efficient detection of nitrogen and carbon nuclei within a protein and provides coherence pathways for the heteronuclear, multidimensional experiments that form the basis of today's assignment strategies (see Sec. 2.2). ^{2}H labeling sharpens the lines in heteronuclear spectra, which provides a vital improvement in the spectra of larger proteins (11). For proteins that are expressed at high levels in *Escherichia coli*, the preparation of uniformly labeled samples has become routine. Simply growing the bacteria on minimal medium made with ^{15}NH$_4$Cl and ^{13}C-glucose (or ^{2}H,^{13}C-glucose) will provide labeled protein, although adaptation of the cells to grow on D$_2$O may be required for production of a fully deuterated sample. If the protein fails to express well on minimal medium, labeled rich media are now available commercially. Similarly, feeding a single labeled amino acid to the *E. coli* (an auxotrophic strain may be required) will result in a sample enriched in that amino acid.

Newly emerging methods for isotope labeling are geared toward facilitating structural studies of larger proteins and streamlining the process of structure determination. While acquiring spectra on fully or partially deuterated samples has been essential for assigning proteins larger than ~ 20 kDa, the effect of deuteration is to remove the very same side-chain protons that provide NOEs to define the tertiary structure of the protein. To circumvent this problem, strategies are being developed for specific labeling of hydrophobic side chains, which comprise the core of a folded protein. The ability to examine only methyl and aromatic groups would mean that the most important NOEs, those within the core of the protein, could be identified at an early stage in structure determination, leading to rapid determination of the global fold of the protein without complete assignment of the side chains. Protonated methyl groups can be incorporated into the valine, leucine, and the δ1 methyl of isoleucine within a perdeuterated, ^{15}N,^{13}C-labeled protein by adding [3,3-^{2}H],^{13}C α-ketobutyrate and [3-^{2}H],^{13}C α-ketoisovalerate to the growth medium (12,13). *E. coli* are able to metabolize these precursors into isoleucine and valine/leucine, respectively, which are then incorporated into the overexpressed protein (Table 1). A more cost-effective strategy for labeling methyl groups is to use protonated α-ketobutyrate and α-ketoisovalerate in which only the methyls are ^{13}C-labeled (14) (Table 1). These precursors are synthesized by single or double alkylation of the *N,N*-dimethylhydrozone of pyruvate *t*-butyl ester with ^{13}C-methyl iodide, followed by hydrolysis to the α-ketoester and removal of the *t*-butyl group (14). The low cost of ^{13}C-methyl iodide means that this labeling method is comparable in cost to ^{15}N-labeling ($\sim$ \$30 per liter of growth medium).

Aromatic residues also tend to be located in the hydrophobic cores of proteins, and the identification of long-range NOEs involving aromatic residues can be key in defining the fold of a protein (15). To examine aromatic residues specifically, labeling schemes and new experiments have been developed side by side. The most popular method is reverse isotope labeling,

Table 1 Metabolites for Selective Isotope Labeling

Precursor	Incorporated as	Source	Refs.
[3, 3′-²H], ¹³C-α-ketobutyrate	(¹H-δ1 methyl)-Ile	Commercially available	13
[3-²H], ¹³C-α-ketoisovalerate	(¹H-δ methyl)-Leu (¹H-γ methyl)-Val	Solvent exchange of commercially available ¹³C α-ketovalerate in D₂O	12
[3-¹³C]-α-ketobutyrate	(¹³C-δ1 methyl)-Ile	Synthesize using ¹³C methyl iodide	14

Table 1 *Continued*

Precursor	Incorporated as	Source	Refs.
[3,3'-^{13}C]-α-ketoisovalerate	(^{13}C-δ methyl)-Leu (^{13}C-γ methyl)-Val	Synthesize using ^{13}C-methyl iodide	14
[ε-^{13}C]-L-phenylalanine	[ε-^{13}C]-Phe	Synthesize from commercially available ε-^{13}C-tyrosine	19

in which unlabeled (^{1}H,^{12}C,^{14}N) phenylalanine and tyrosine are added to labeled growth medium (16). When incorporated into an otherwise ^{13}C-labeled sample, NOEs to the ^{12}C-containing aromatic side chains can be assigned using ^{13}C-double-filtered or ^{13}C-filtered/edited experiments that detect NOEs between the unlabeled side chains and NOEs from the unlabeled side chains to other nearby protons, respectively (17). Incorporation of unlabeled aromatic residues into otherwise deuterated, ^{15}N-labeled proteins along with unlabeled threonine, isoleucine, and valine (FYTIV reverse labeling) provides a way to identify NOEs to FYTIV residues (18). ^{15}N filtering and editing can distinguish NOEs from carbon-bound protons in the FYTIV residues (all others residues are deuterated) to the amide protons of FYTIV residues from NOEs to non-FYVIT residues. This strategy has proved useful in assigning NOEs in a 47-kDa homodimer (18).

By combining the ^{13}C labeling of methyl groups with the incorporation of ^{15}N-labeled protonated phenylalanine and tyrosine in an otherwise ^{2}H,^{15}N-labeled protein, the Fesik laboratory has been able to simplify assignment of the NOEs involving valine, leucine, isoleucine, phenylalanine, and tyrosine (15). A ^{13}C-NOESY-HSQC is used to identify NOEs from methyl groups to other protons, while ^{15}N-filtered or edited NOESY spectra reveal NOEs from the amides to the protonated side chains. Looking at only the methyl and aromatic protons greatly simplifies the assignment process and focuses on the most important NOEs for structure determination.

One drawback to using aromatic resonances is the difficulty of assigning their side chains. Phenylalanine is particularly problematic because the aromatic ^{1}H and ^{13}C resonances are poorly dispersed, the proton linewidths tend to be large in ^{13}C samples, and the ^{13}C–^{13}C couplings are complex. These problems can largely be overcome by synthesizing phenylalanine with a ^{13}C label at only the epsilon position (19). This eliminates strong ^{13}C–^{13}C couplings, reduces linewidths of the δ and ζ protons, and allows one to resolve the aromatic protons using filtering and editing techniques. In the case of the 21-kDa DH domain, this labeling scheme allowed facile assignment of the protein's seven phenylalanines, which could not be assigned using a uniformly ^{13}C-labeled sample (19).

2.1.4 Alternate Expression Systems

All of the foregoing methods for producing labeled protein samples for NMR rely upon expression of the target protein in *E. coli*. Although this is by far the most economical system currently available, there is a wide range of interesting proteins that cannot be expressed in this host. Some genes may use codons that are rare in *E. coli*, other proteins may not fold correctly or may be toxic to the bacterium, still others might require post-translational modifications that do not take place in bacteria. Alternative systems for expressing proteins are being explored to overcome these limitations in NMR sample preparation. The most exciting prospects for expressing labeled proteins in systems other than *E. coli* include use of the yeast *Pichia pastoris* and the development of cell-free translation systems.

Proteins that require post-translational glycosylation or addition of lipids are good candidates for expression in the methylotrophic yeast *P. pastoris* (20). By using a signal sequence that targets the protein for secretion into the growth medium, protein purification is greatly simplified and the need to lyse the yeast cells, which are much more resilient than bacterial cells, is eliminated (21,22). Since yeast requires much more oxygen than *E. coli*, yields of protein are highest from cultures grown in a fermentor. Hundreds of milligrams of protein per liter of culture can be obtained under optimal conditions, and use of labeled glucose and/or ammonium chloride allows for production of glycosylated labeled proteins (23). Until the development of more economical small-scale fermentation instruments, growth in shaker flasks may be more economical, despite the lower yields. Indeed, a number of labeled samples, including a highly deuterated one (24), have been prepared from *P. pastoris* grown in shaker flasks, raising the possibility that deuterated, ^{15}N-,^{13}C-labeled samples can be produced in yeast systems. This will open up a range of larger, post-translationally modified systems to study by NMR.

Cell-free expression is particularly advantageous for proteins that tend to be insoluble, are particularly susceptible to proteolysis, to form inclusion bodies, or are toxic. Extract derived from wheat germ or bacterial cells provides most of the components required for expression (25). By using *E. coli* extract supplemented with ^{15}N,^{13}C-labeled amino acids ^{15}N,^{13}C-labeled proteins as large as 30 kDa have been prepared in yields up to 6 mg per mL of extract (26). Still larger proteins can be produced using wheat germ extract, which provides a particularly robust, high-yield system (27). The lower cost of wheat germ extract relative to previous cell-free systems (e.g., rabbit reticulocyte lysate) makes large-scale in vitro expression an economical and viable alternative to traditional in vivo systems. Additional factors can be introduced into the reaction mixture to facilitate folding, disulfide formation, or other post-translational processing that cannot be accomplished in bacterial systems and may proceed differently in humans and insect cells. T-cell receptor subunits have been correctly glycosylated in vitro (28), and a functional single-chain antibody can be produced in vitro without refolding when glutathione, chaperones, and protein disulfide isomerase are added to the reaction mixture (29). Complexes can even be formed in vitro: Six polypeptides have been coexpressed to generate a T-cell receptor–CD3 complex that could not be reconstituted by mixing components expressed separately (28). Because of the versatility of cell-free systems and the ease with which in vitro translation can be automated, cell-free expression will be the primary method for protein expression in the Japanese RIKEN Structural Genomics Initiative (6).

2.2 Data Acquisition and Analysis

Once a suitable NMR sample is in hand, the data-acquisition phase of structure determination can begin. This is a time-consuming step that generally requires weeks of instrument time. Structures of proteins up to ~ 25 kDa can be determined based on less than six weeks of data collection with standard technologies, although the use of cryogenic probes promises to reduce this time to under two weeks. Efficient streamlining of the structure determination process may shorten the data-acquisition time still further (Sec. 3.3). The experiments recorded fall into two categories: those required for assignment of the resonances of the protein and those that provide interproton distances for structure calculations. The former experiments are based on through-bond correlations of ^1H, ^{15}N, and ^{13}C spins in the protein, while the latter detect through-space interactions between protons. This section will outline a widely used scheme for obtaining resonance assignments and structural constraints.

2.2.1 Backbone Assignment

Three pairs of triple-resonance experiments are normally sufficient to allow complete and unambiguous backbone assignments for most proteins. By relying exclusively upon through-bond correlations to connect spins along the backbone, these experiments eliminate the ambiguities inherent in earlier assignment approaches that relied on through-space correlations as well (30). An $^{15}N,^{13}C$-labeled sample with 70–90% ^2H-enrichment is used to record the experiments HNCA and HN(CO)CA (31–35), HNCO and HN(CA)CO (33,35–38), and CBCANH and CBCA(CO)NH (33,36,39) (Table 2). Each of these pairs of data sets gives information about intra-residue correlations and the corresponding interresidue correlations in the form of a three-dimensional spectrum with the amide proton (H^N) chemical shift on one axis, the amide nitrogen (N) on another, and the carbon chemical shift ($C\alpha$, $C\beta$, or C') on the third axis. By analyzing the HNCA and HN(CO)CA data together, for example, the H^N, N, and $C\alpha$ spins along the entire backbone (except for the prolines) can be correlated: The HNCA correlates each H^N and N with the intraresidue $C\alpha$, while the HN(CO)CA correlates each $C\alpha$ with the H^N and N of the following residue (Fig. 1). Similarly, the other two pairs of experiments correlate the carbonyl carbon (C') and $C\beta$ resonances with the amide H^N and N. Any ambiguities caused

Table 2 Triple-Resonance Experiments Used for Backbone Assignments

Experiment	Correlations observed	Magnetization transfer	Refs.
HNCA	H_i–N_i–$C\alpha_i$ H_i–N_i–$C\alpha_{i-1}$		31–34
HN(CO)CA	H_i–N_i–$C\alpha_{i-1}$		31–33, 35
HNCO	H_i–N_i–C_{i-1}		33, 35, 36
HN(CA)CO	H_i–N_i–C_i H_i–N_i–C_{i-1}		35, 37, 38

39

CBCANH $\qquad$ $C\beta_{i-1}/C\alpha_{i-1}-N_i-H_i$
$C\beta_i/C\alpha_i-N_i-H_i$

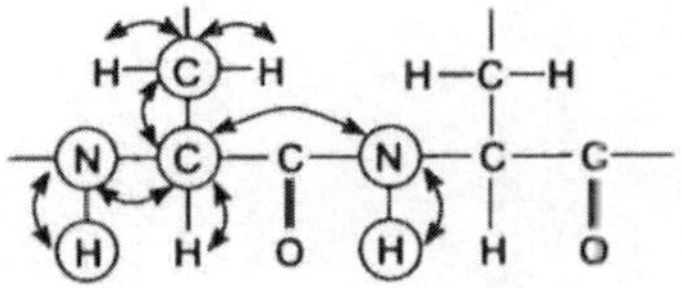

33, 36

CBCA(CO)NH $\qquad$ $C\beta_{i-1}/C\alpha_{i-1}-N_i-H_i$

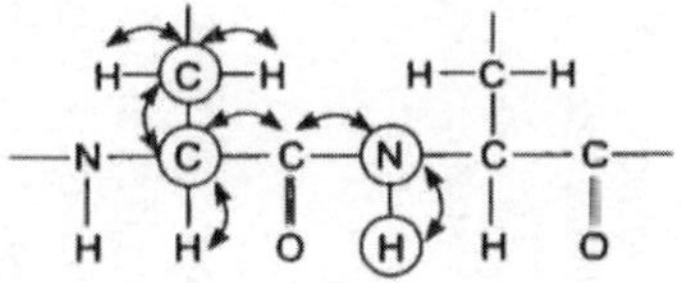

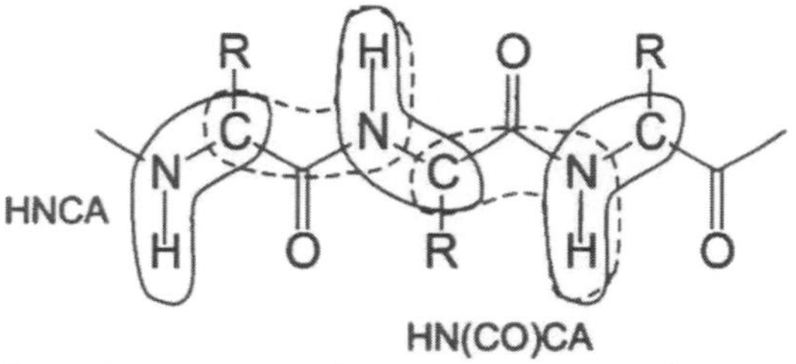

Figure 1 Schematic depiction of backbone assignment using the HNCA and HN(CO)CA spectra. Each H^N–N pair is correlated with the $C\alpha$ of the previous residue using the HN(CO)CA (dotted lines) and the $C\alpha$ of its own residue using the HNCA (solid line). To trace along the backbone, one searches for pairs of amides in which the $C\alpha$ chemical shift of one in the HNCA is identical to the $C\alpha$ chemical shift observed from the second in the HN(CO)CA. Two such amides belong to adjacent residues in the protein. Because of the requirement for amide protons, the correlations are interrupted at proline residues.

by degeneracies in $C\alpha$ chemical shifts can be resolved by examining the $C\beta$ or C' correlations. The $C\beta$ chemical shifts are particularly useful in this regard, since they are very well dispersed. Together the $C\alpha$ and $C\beta$ chemical shifts can be used to identify amino acid types and thus to map segments of connected spins onto the sequence of the protein. It is rare that any ambiguities remain in the backbone assignments after consideration of $C\alpha$, $C\beta$, and C' chemical shifts, and normally all residues except the terminal amino acids and some residues adjacent to prolines can be assigned. Use of these six experiments make data analysis so straightforward that the backbone can often be assigned within a few days using an interactive program like XEASY (39A). As ambiguities are further reduced by high-resolution experiments, the potential for automated data analysis increases.

Once the backbone assignments are complete, much useful information is already in hand. It has long been recognized that amino acids in beta strands and helices have characteristic chemical shifts. This information has been compiled into a "chemical shift index" for $C\alpha$, $H\alpha$, $C\beta$, and C' that can be used to predict the regions of secondary structure within a protein (40,41). Thus the $C\alpha$, $C\beta$, and C' chemical shifts determined during backbone assignment can be used immediately to identify regions of secondary structure.

Along the same lines, dihedral angles can be predicted on the basis of backbone chemical shifts. Some of these predictions contain the same information as the secondary structure predictions, while others provide new information about regions of the protein that do not have precise secondary structure. The TALOS method (torsion angle likelihood obtained from shift and sequence similarity) (42) uses a database of proteins for which both chemical shifts and high-resolution X-ray crystal structures are known. For each set of three consecutive amino acids in the target protein, the database is searched for the closest matches based on $C\alpha$, $C\beta$, C', $H\alpha$, and N chemical shifts and sequence similarity. If the central residues in the best ten matches have similar backbone ϕ and ψ angles, those values are taken as the predicted dihedral angles. Although about 3% of the predictions from TALOS may be wrong, mistakes can be identified during structure calculations by the inconsistency of a constraint with NOEs or other types of data.

2.2.2 Side-Chain Assignment

The determination of $C\alpha$ and $C\beta$ chemical shifts during backbone assignment provides a good starting point for the side-chain experiments. The H(CC-CO)NH-TOCSY and (H)C(C-CO)NH-TOCSY experiments (43,44) (Table 3) are particularly convenient for assigning the side chains of larger proteins (45). These experiments and their partner experiments, the H(CC)NH TOCSY and (H)C(C)NH TOCSY (46), correlate proton or carbon resonances within a side chain to one another and to the amide resonances in the backbone. Thus they are three-dimensional experiments in which the axes are the chemical shifts of H^N, N, and the side-chain protons or nitrogens. The amide correlations in these experiments make the spectra easy to interpret, since they contain much less ambiguity than an HCCH-TOCSY spectrum (47), for example. Ambiguities may remain as to which proton is attached to which carbon, but these can usually be resolved by the ^{13}C-NOESY-HSQC spectrum (48), since each H–C pair must show at least some NOESY cross-peaks. Complete assignment of the methyl groups is usually possible from the HC(C-CO)NH-TOCSY experiments, but other resonances may be missing. These can usually be supplied by either the ^{13}C-NOESY-HSQC or the HCCH-TOCSY, which becomes relatively easy to interpret once some resonances in each side chain have been assigned. Methyl group resonances are particularly useful entries into these spectra, since correlations of entire spin systems to the methyl groups are usually visible. In a streamlined structure determination, completing the assignments of the side chains may not even be necessary. So long as the methyl groups are assigned, most of the NOEs important for folding the protein can be obtained (see Sec. 3.3).

2.2.3 Structural Constraints

NOE-Based Distance Constraints. The compilation of distance constraints for structure calculations is based on the ^{13}C-NOESY-HSQC

Table 3 Heteronuclear Experiments Used for Side-Chain Assignments

Experiment	Correlations observed	Magnetization transfer	Refs.
(H)C(C)NH-TOCSY	$C_{x_i}/C\alpha_i\text{--}N_i\text{--}H_i$		46
H(CC)NH-TOCSY	$H_{x_i}/H\alpha_i\text{--}N_i\text{--}H_i$		46
(H)C(C-CO)NH-TOCSY	$C_{x_{i-1}}/C\alpha_{i-1}\text{--}N_i\text{--}H_i$		43, 34, 46

H(CC-CO)NH-TOCSY $H_{sc_{i-1}}/H\alpha_{i-1}-N_i-H_i$

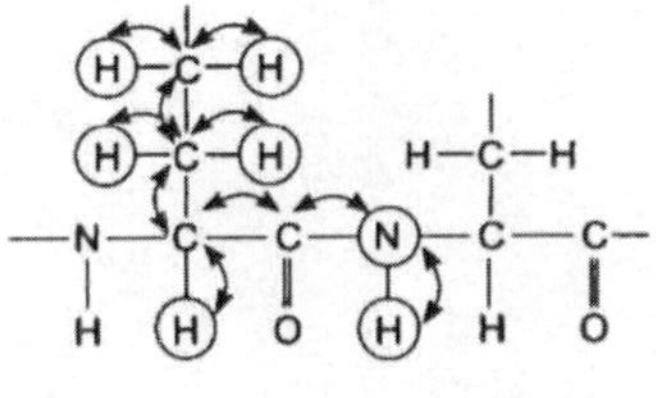

44, 46

HCCH-TOCSY $H_{sc_i}/H\alpha_i-H_{sc_i}/H\alpha_i-C_{sc_i}/C\alpha_i$

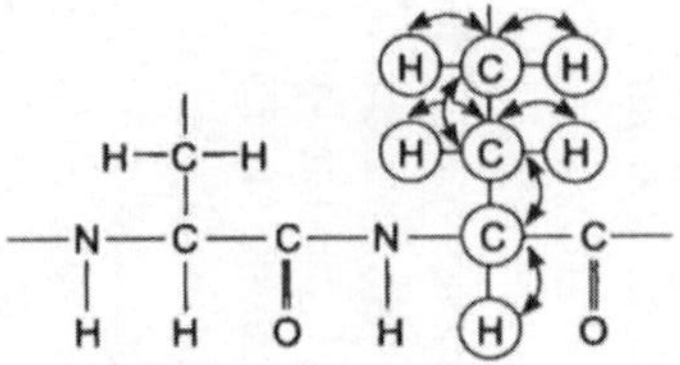

47

C_{sc} and H_{sc} are side-chain carbons and protons, respectively.

and ^{15}N-NOESY-HSQC spectra (49–52) and is the most time-consuming part of spectral analysis. In these experiments, the NOESY component is used to detect NOEs (through-space correlations) from ^{13}C- or ^{15}N-attached protons to other protons throughout the protein, while the HSQC component correlates each proton with the attached ^{13}C or ^{15}N. The resulting three-dimensional spectra have two ^{1}H axes and one heteronuclear axis. These spectra tend to be very dense, containing many thousands of cross-peaks, even for a small protein. Assignment typically begins with manual analysis to identify unambiguous NOEs. The most critical part of structure determination is obtaining correct assignments for a starting set of long-range NOEs that define the global fold of the protein. After unambiguous NOEs have been identified, additional NOEs are assigned that are consistent with the unambiguous ones. This is the stage at which specific labeling of the methyl groups and/or aromatic side chains in a protein is most useful. By having only the amides and methyl groups protonated in an ^{2}H,^{15}N-labeled sample, for example, the complexity of the ^{15}N-NOESY-HSQC spectrum would be greatly reduced. Only correlations from amide protons to the protonated methyls would be observed. The ^{13}C-NOESY-HSQC of a sample in which the methyls alone are ^{13}C labeled would contain only cross-peaks for NOEs between methyl groups, rather than all side chain–side chain NOEs as would be observed if the sample were fully ^{13}C labeled. Greatly reducing the number of intraresidue NOEs, which tend to be strong and of limited use in structure calculations, vastly simplifies data interpretation and allows for more unambiguous NOEs to be assigned in the initial stage of spectral analysis.

Once the global fold of a protein is identified, more NOEs can be assigned in an iterative process using automated or semiautomated methods. One such method is the NOAH/DYANA approach (53,54). Ambiguous NOESY cross-peaks are assigned to the proton pair predicted to cause the fewest violations, based on the preliminary family of structures. New distance restraints generated in this way are used to calculate a new set of structures. Consistent violations of restraints in these structures point to incorrect assignments, which are used to refine the NOE list. The process of assigning additional NOEs is repeated until finally an expanded distance restraint list and family of structures are derived simultaneously. This strategy currently requires some manual intervention to achieve good results and relies upon the initial accurate assignment of long-range NOEs to generate the preliminary structure. When NOAH is run in the absence of such initial assignments, the resulting distance constraint list is not as reliable.

The ARIA program exemplifies another approach to automated NOE assignment (55). In this method, all possible assignments of ambiguous

NOEs are considered at once during structure calculations using X-PLOR, so any pair of protons with the correct chemical shifts can satisfy the constraints. Ambiguities are resolved by determining which pairs of protons are actually satisfying which constraints in the resulting structures. As is the case for NOAH, having a good preliminary structure is important for success, but because the idea is to consider all possibilities, complete side-chain assignments play a more important role. This can be particularly problematic for large proteins, which are more difficult to assign completely. In order to address this limitation, ARIA has been combined with chemical-shift prediction methods to assign side-chain protons and NOEs simultaneously (56). In this way more than 40 side-chain protons and 400 new unambiguous NOEs were assigned in a 28-kDa single-chain T-cell receptor (56). As experiments for side-chain assignment improve, these automated NOE assignment methods will become more accurate and will come to play a more central role in structure determination strategies.

Dihedral Angle Constraints. In classical NMR-based protein structure determinations, dihedral angle constraints based on three-bond scalar couplings (57) were the traditional companion of distance constraints. With the ability to predict many of the backbone angles from chemical shifts using TALOS (see earlier), the determination of $^3J_{H^NH_\alpha}$ couplings (and the associated ϕ angles) from the HNHA (58) or HNCA (59) spectrum is in many cases superfluous. Dihedral angle constraints for the side chains can still be useful, though. The $\chi 1$ angle is most commonly determined using an HNHB experiment that allows measurement of the coupling between the backbone amide nitrogen and $H\beta$ (59,60). But this is a low-sensitivity experiment that does not work well on larger proteins, and the information gained would be useful only for high-resolution structures. Thus, it would be of little value for a streamlined structure determination process whose goal might be to produce large numbers of lower-resolution structures. New types of structural constraints are proving to be easier to obtain and more useful in this regard.

Residual Dipolar Couplings. Within the past few years methods have been developed that use residual dipolar couplings to obtain the orientations of bond vectors within a protein. This is a very exciting development because such a measurement provides a completely new type of structural constraint that is unrelated to interproton distances or dihedral angles. Moreover, this is the only type of constraint that can define the relative orientations of distant parts of a protein. Residual dipolar couplings are observed when a protein adopts a small degree of orientation in solution. Such a sample is anisotropic, so the residual dipolar couplings in its spectra do not average to zero as they would for an isotropic sample. Orientation can be induced by dissolving a protein in a dilute mixture of phospholipid bicelles in water (61). Above a critical temperature, which depends upon the lipids used, their ratio, and their concentration, the bicelles orient in the magnetic field and in turn confer a small degree of orientation on the protein. Below this temperature, the mixture is isotropic and the residual dipolar couplings average to zero. Thus, differences in couplings observed below and above the critical temperature reveal the residual dipolar coupling. One difficulty in applying this method is the instability of many bicelle-based samples. To overcome this problem, alternate bicelle mixtures have been developed and solutions of filamentous phage have been used to orient samples (62,63).

Once a stable sample has been obtained, the residual dipolar couplings for many bond vectors can be measured. Early efforts focused on obtaining couplings for $N-H^N$, $C\alpha-H\alpha$, and $C\alpha-C'$ bond pairs and developing methods for utilizing the resulting bond vector orientations in structure calculations (64). Since then, many other bond pairs have been added to the list, including $N-C'$, H^N-C', $H^N-C\alpha$, $N-C\alpha$, $H^N-C'_{(i-1)}$, $N-C'_{(i-1)}$, and $C\alpha-C\beta$ (65–68). $N-H^N$ dipolar couplings are the simplest to measure, being derived from the ^{15}N-HSQC spectrum or the IPAP ^{15}N-HSQC, in which the multiplet components are separated (69). Measurements of other couplings require the use of modified triple-resonance experiments: $C\alpha-H\alpha$ and $C\alpha-C'$ couplings are detected in the 3D (HA)CA(CO)NH and 2D H(N)CO, respectively (65), while HNCO-based experiments have been used to measure $C\alpha-H\alpha$, $N-C'$, H^N-C' $H^N-C\alpha$, $N-C\alpha$, $H^N-C'_{(i-1)}$, $N-C'_{(i-1)}$, and $C\alpha-C\beta$ couplings (66–68,70).

Bond vector orientations may be most valuable as supplementary restraints in systems where the long-range NOEs are insufficient to determine some aspect of the structure. In particular, structures of multidomain proteins or those in which distance restraints fail to determine the relative orientation of subdomains can benefit from the use of residual dipolar coupling data (71–73). There have been recent reports of structure determinations in the complete absence of NOE-derived distance restraints, but these calculations either depend upon some degree of homology modeling (74,75) or require the presence of a paramagnetic center in the protein (76). Residual dipolar couplings will likely take their place beside NOEs and dihedral angle constraints as the third main type of constraint used in structure determinations. Since couplings are derived from spectra that have already been analyzed during the backbone-assignment phase of structure determination, spectral analysis is relatively straightforward. When added to a minimal number of NOEs, such as sets of methyl and aromatic NOEs, these additional constraints are expected to facilitate structure determination of larger proteins (15,77). Methods for incorporating residual dipolar coupling data into structure calculations are still evolving (73,78); as they become more refined, the use of bond vector orientations will become a standard part of protein NMR spectroscopy.

Direct Detection of Hydrogen Bonds. J couplings across hydrogen bonds were first discovered in nucleic acids and provided the first direct way to detect these bonds using NMR spectroscopy (79). Reliable methods for detecting hydrogen bonds in proteins would provide important additional constraints for structure calculations. The major obstacle is that the scalar couplings through hydrogen bonds in proteins are so small, but $^{3h}J_{NC'}$ couplings have been detected in HNCO experiments modified to detect small couplings (0.25–0.9 Hz) (80–82). Moreover, anticorrelation has been observed between the length of a hydrogen bond and the magnitude of its $^{3h}J_{NC'}$ coupling, leading to measurement of hydrogen bond lengths by quantitative treatment of the coupling constants (83). $^{2h}J_{HC'}$ and $^{3h}J_{HC_\alpha}$ couplings through hydrogen bonds have also been observed, but they tend to be even smaller and more difficult to measure than $^{3h}J_{NC'}$ couplings (84,85).

These techniques are all inherently low in sensitivity due to the small magnitude of the couplings used for coherence transfer, and sensitivity decreases further in larger proteins. While deuteration is generally helpful for large proteins, it can be problematic for these experiments. since deuterons in strong hydrogen bonds cannot always be exchanged for protons. In one case almost 40% of the expected $^{3h}J_{NC'}$ couplings in a 30-kDa protein could not be detected because tightly hydrogen-bonded amide protons were missing (86). Thus the strongest hydrogen bonds are the ones least likely to be observed. In cases where hydrogen bonds can be observed, though, they would provide valuable constraints that could expedite structure determination substantially.

Spin Labeling. Distance-dependent line broadening of resonances in NMR spectra of proteins containing paramagnetic electrons (e.g., metals or nitroxide spin labels) was first observed as long ago as 1976 (87). Yet there have been few attempts at translating this broadening into distance information for structure calculations (88,89). Nitroxide spin labels are convenient for such studies because (1) they react only with cysteine residues and can thus be incorporated specifically at the site of a single cysteine within a protein, and (2) the paramagnetic (oxidized) label can be conveniently reduced to provide a comparison between spectra of labeled and unlabeled samples. In the first demonstration of the usefulness of such a label, single-cysteine versions of staphococcal nuclease were engineered to which nitroxide spin labels were attached (89,90). ^{15}N-HSQC spectra were acquired before and after reduction of the spin label. Comparing the relaxation properties of the HN spins in the oxidized and reduced proteins allowed direct measurement of the effects of the paramagnetic label on the spectra and yielded information on distances between the amide protons and the spin label (89).

More recently, the global fold of perdeuterated eIF4E has been determined largely on the basis of distance restraints derived from paramagnetic broadening of ^{15}N-HSQC resonances in a set of five samples of the protein, each with a nitroxide spin label at a different position (91). Relaxation rates were derived from the ^{1}H,^{15}N-HSQC by taking the ratios of cross-peak heights in the spectra of oxidized and reduced protein (I_{ox}/I_{red}). Three categories of distance constraints were defined: peaks undetectable in the HSQC spectrum of the oxidized protein correspond to protons less than ~ 14 Å from the spin label, those with I_{ox}/I_{red} less than 0.85 are ~ 14–23 Å from the label, and those for which I_{ox}/I_{red} is > 0.90 are greater than ~ 23 Å from the label. In this way, ~ 500 semiquantitative restraints were obtained that supplemented H^N–H^N distance constraints obtained from ^{15}N-edited NOESY spectra. Along with loose backbone angle restraints for secondary structure elements derived from the chemical shift index, these constraints were sufficient to determine correctly the global fold of eIF4E with a backbone precision of 2.3 Å (91). Since eIF4E samples are made up in CHAPS micelles having a molecular weight of ~ 45–50 kDa, it is expected that this methods will be useful for proteins at least that large.

There are some drawbacks to this approach for deriving long-distance restraints. First is the concern that the spin label will perturb the structure of the protein being studied. But the nitroxide spin label has been shown by electron paramagnetic resonance (EPR) to be readily incorporated into secondary structure elements (particularly helices) and to leave protein structures unperturbed (92). Moreover, even with no prior knowledge of a structure, spin labels could be positioned at the predicted surface of a protein on the basis of the protein's secondary structure and the hydrophilicity patterns in the sequence. The second, and more serious, drawback is the need for site-directed mutagenesis and the preparation of multiple samples. The approach is also unsuitable for proteins containing many cysteine residues. Despite the additional investment in sample preparation, spin-labeling may ultimately save time when solving the structures of systems too large for many unambiguous NOEs to be identified. Acquisition and analysis of the data are straightforward, and the information gained is easily combined with other restraints that rely only on the backbone assignments, such as H^N–H^N NOEs or orientational constraints for H^N–N bonds. When used in this way, paramagnetic broadening restraints could provide extremely valuable information for determining the folds of large proteins.

2.3 Structure Calculations

After compilation of distance and dihedral angle constraints, along with any constraints for hydrogen bonds, long-distance spin-labeling constraints, or bond vector orientation constraints from residual dipolar couplings, the data must be assembled to derive a picture of the three-dimensional structure of the protein under study. This is an iterative process, as mentioned earlier, that involves deriving a preliminary model of the protein from an initial set of constraints and subsequent addition of further constraints based upon that model. There are a variety of approaches for doing this that can be implemented using different software packages. The most widely used programs include X-PLOR (93), CNS (the successor of X-PLOR) (94), DYANA (95), and CONGEN (96).

All methods share some basic features: They allow for input of various types of structural constraints and sampling of a wide range of possible conformations for the protein, and all provide a means of assessing whether the resulting structure violates the constraints and of optimizing the "good" structures. How constraints are described and how conformational space is sampled differ in the various approaches. Distance geometry methods use internal distances [DG-II (10), DISGEO, DIAMOND (97)] or torsion angles [DIANA (98,99)] to build structures that are then converted into Cartesian coordinates for optimization. Restrained molecular dynamics (X-PLOR, CNS) starts from an initial conformation (typically an extended chain with randomized dihedral angles) that is allowed to evolve over time in the presence of a force field. The force fields used by different programs differ slightly from each other, but all describe the potential energy of a protein conformation in terms of the sum of the potential energies for bonds, angles, dihedral angles, improper angles, van der Waals interactions, electrostatic terms, and hydrogen bonding, to which the constraints from NMR data are added. Evolution of the coordinates is accomplished by assigning velocities to the atoms based on a temperature defined by the user. Simulated annealing (X-PLOR, CONGEN) is molecular dynamics carried out at a high temperature initially (for best sampling of conformational space), followed by a gradual lowering of the temperature that allows the structure to anneal in the presence of the experimental constraints and force field. A version of simulated annealing using molecular dynamics in torsion angle space is available using the DYANA program at a great savings in computational time due to the use of internal rather than Cartesian coordinates. CNS (Crystallography and NMR System) is the most versatile package to date, allowing implementation of both distance geometry and simulated annealing using molecular dynamics in either Cartesian or torsion angle space (94). More detailed reviews of methods for structure refinement can be found elsewhere (100,101).

The challenge for automation of this phase of structure determination is that there is no single best protocol for calculating the structures of proteins. Currently, the user adjusts the weight of various constraints and the magnitude of the penalties encountered when a given constraint is violated. Constraints are described as functions having specified upper and lower bounds, outside of which an error is incurred in proportion to the magnitude of the constraint violation. A user may also exploit different methods at different stages of the structure calculations. For example, DIANA can be quite useful in the early stages of a project for finding errors in the initial NOE list. Later, a combination of distance geometry followed by simulated annealing may provide the best sampling of conformational space. But the temperatures for annealing, the rate at which the temperature is lowered, and the length of time at a given temperature are all parameters set by the user. Automated methods will need to standardize the entire process from which data sets are acquired through what protocol is used for structure determination. Ideally, a completely unambiguous set of constraints will be used to determine initial structures that are then refined by iterative analysis of NMR data to derive more structural constraints with minimal human intervention (see Sec. 3.3).

2.4 Structures of Large Proteins

An ongoing goal of NMR technique development is to facilitate studies of larger systems. Several recent technological developments can now be combined so that structures of proteins over ~ 25 kDa are well within the reach of NMR spectroscopy. Using deuterium-labeled samples, pulse-field gradients, cryogenics probes, and transverse relaxation-optimized spectroscopy (TROSY), triple-resonance experiments have been refined to allow for assignment of systems as large as 110 kDa (3) and determination of the tertiary structure of a 42-kDa protein (73). The substitution of deuterons for protons lengthens the relaxation times of the attached nuclei, which means that samples deuterated at Hα and Hβ give substantially greater signal than protonated samples in triple-resonance experiments such as the HNCA and HNCACB. This difference becomes particularly critical for obtaining good data on systems larger than ~ 25 kDa.

For even larger proteins, the increased sensitivity of cryogenic probes has proven extremely valuable, as are new TROSY-based pulse sequences (102). TROSY, like deuteration, seeks to address the problem of the fast relaxation of larger systems. Instead of altering the relaxation properties of heteronuclei, though, TROSY dissects the various relaxation pathways in large proteins in order to select for the slowest one. In a two-spin system (e.g., $^1H-^{15}N$ or $^1H-^{13}C$), both dipole–dipole coupling and chemical shift anisotropy contribute to fast transverse relaxation. If the spins are not decoupled, as they normally would be, four peaks are observed for each $^1H-^{15}N$ pair in a $^1H-^{15}N$ correlation experiment instead of one peak. TROSY selects for only the most slowly relaxing of these components (i.e., the sharpest peak), which can result in as much as a 10-fold increase in signal-to-noise ratio in a two-dimensional spectrum. In combination with deuteration and cryogenic probe technology, TROSY versions of triple-resonance experiments provide the way to obtain the maximum possible signal for very large systems (103,104).

These optimized triple-resonance experiments vastly simplify the assignment of large proteins and often lead to complete proton and carbon assignments. This in turn means that unambiguous NOEs can be assigned more easily from the ^{15}N- and ^{13}C-NOESY-HSQC spectra. As systems become larger, though, obtaining complete assignments for the side chains becomes more laborious. In these cases, the methyl-labeled samples discussed in Section 2.1.3 can be used to obtain partial assignments for the side chains and simplified ^{13}C-NOESY spectra, which facilitate the assignment of unambiguous long-range NOEs (15,105). Even with these methods, the number of unambiguous NOEs may not be sufficient to define the fold of a very large protein. The use of new types of structural constraints then comes into play. In the case of the 42-kDa maltose-binding protein, residual dipolar couplings were successfully combined with a relatively low density of NOEs (five per residue) to obtain the global fold of the protein (73).

One other approach being explored for studying large systems is to label only one part of a protein at a time by ligating labeled and unlabeled polypeptides together. "Segmental labeling" dramatically reduces spectral complexity, enabling one to focus on a single region of interest within a larger protein. The labeled and unlabeled segments can be joined using intein-based enzymatic ligation (106) or chemical ligation (107). In nature, inteins are excised from the middle of polypeptide chains, resulting in splicing together of the surrounding sequences (the exteins). This reaction can be used in vitro to label a segment of a protein by mixing together a fusion protein containing the N-terminus of the protein and the N-terminal half of the intein with another fusion containing the C-terminus of the intein along with the C-terminus of the protein. Labeling these two fusion proteins differently will result in different labeling patterns in the two halves of the protein. When the two fusion proteins are mixed together, they refold, producing an active intein. The fusion proteins are spliced together, reconstituting the segmentally labeled target protein. Using two different inteins to mediate two splicing reactions, the central region of a protein can be labeled while the ends remain unlabeled (108). The major drawbacks of this method are that splicing introduces extra amino acids at the junctions between segments and that refolding and splicing conditions need to be optimized for each protein individually (109). In the chemical ligation approach, extra amino acids are not introduced between the segments, but the C-terminal fragment must begin with a cysteine. Meanwhile, the N-terminal fragment contains a C-terminal α-thioester that can react with the cysteine to form a peptide bond. This α-thioester is produced by expressing the N-terminus of the target protein as a fusion with a C-terminal intein and treating this hybrid with ethanethiol (107). The reaction of the α-thioester with cysteine is not quantitative, but yields up to 70% have been reported (107). If a method for segmental labeling could be made more reliable, it would be a very useful tool for simplifying structural studies of very large systems and might come into wider use.

2.5 Studies of Protein Complexes

Despite the recent advances that now enable NMR spectroscopic studies of large systems, protein complexes continue to present their unique challenges. Difficulties include sample preparation and the analysis of data that include signals from more than one protein, in particular the assignment of NOESY spectra containing and both intraprotein and interprotein NOEs. Studies of multimeric proteins or heterodimers of two closely related proteins are particularly plagued by the latter problem. The general strategy for coping with this challenge is to label the two sides of the dimer or complex differently and then to use experiments that select for NOEs between the differently labeled segments. The original versions of this strategy involved using filtered NOESY experiments on complexes containing ^{15}N- or ^{13}C-labeled protein plus unlabeled protein (110–115). These half-filter experiments tend to be quite insensitive, though, and if a homodimeric protein is being studied, the sample contains only 50% of the labeled-unlabeled heterodimer.

Deuteration has provided a much more sensitive method for identifying intermonomer NOEs in dimeric proteins. A simple ^{15}N-NOESY-HSQC on a mixture of 100% ^{2}H, ^{15}N-labeled protein and unlabeled protein selects for NOEs from amide protons attached to ^{15}N to side-chain protons, which are in the unlabeled monomer (116). This experiment is limited to detection of only NOEs from the backbone of one monomer to the side chains of the other. But this limitation has its advantage in that identification of the dimerization interface depends only upon backbone assignments that are acquired early in the structure determination process. In studies of the UmuD' dimer, the rapid identification of the dimerization interface in solution (117) resolved a question left open by the crystal structure as to which of two possible interfaces observed in the crystal was the interface in solution (Fig. 2) (118,119). A complete discussion of the issues involved in solving the structures of oligomeric proteins can be found elsewhere (120).

A major issue in studying multiprotein complexes is how to reliably produce uniform samples containing the desired components in the correct ratios. One approach is to use flexible linkers to join together the modules in the complex. This method was inspired by the single-chain antibodies that have long been used in studies of antibody–antigen binding in the immune system. The finding that the structures of the variable domain (F_v) of the McPC603 antibody and an F_v single-chain construct are virtually identical means that such linkers do not alter the structure of the complex being studied (121). In addition to ensuring a one-to-one ratio of the modules of a complex, covalently linking them together also reduces the entropic penalty for complex formation. The single-chain strategy may thus be particularly valuable for weakly associated complexes or those containing components that express poorly or suffer from solubility problems when expressed individually. One drawback of this approach is the resulting difficulty of identifying interdomain NOEs, since it is not straightforward to label each half of the complex separately. Combining this method with segmental labeling could solve this problem. The single-chain approach has been used recently to solve the structure of the variable domains from a major histocompatibility complex (MHC) class II T-cell receptor (122). This solution structure was helpful in the subsequent determination of the crystal structure of a complex of this receptor with an MHC class II molecule and a foreign peptide (123). Such a combination of NMR spectroscopy and crystallography can provide a very powerful approach for solving structures of large multiprotein complexes that present difficulties for either method alone (see Sec. 3.4).

2.6 Novel Methods for Drug Discovery

Nuclear magnetic resonance is well suited to drug discovery because of its unique ability to identify ligands that interact weakly with a target protein. A novel drug discovery technique called SAR (structure–activity relationships) by NMR takes advantage of this capability (124). Binding of a test compound to the target protein is assayed rapidly by monitoring chemical shift perturbations in the ^{15}N-HSQC spectrum of the protein, an assay that allows detection of binding as low as 10 mM. The

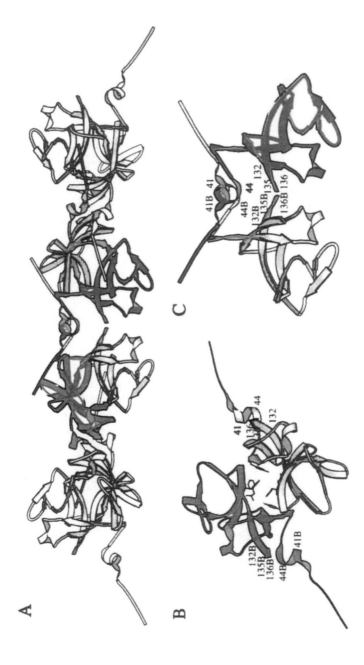

Figure 2 (a) The UmuD′ filament observed in X-ray crystallographic studies. (From Ref. 118.) (b) The originally reported dimer of UmuD′. Residues that showed intermonomer NOEs in solution are labeled. (c) The same residues mapped onto the "filament dimer" of UmuD′. This dimer was concluded to be the dimer in solution. (From Ref. 117.).

resulting "hit" rate is relatively high, which means that it is easy to identify lead compounds that can then be optimized for binding by screening analogs. Once the ^{15}N-HSQC spectrum has been assigned, the binding sites of the lead compounds can be determined simply by noting which peaks are perturbed upon addition of each compound. Two ligands are then identified that bind to adjacent sites in the protein, the structure of the ternary complex is determined by NMR or X-ray crystallography, and a linker is designed to connect the two ligands. The resulting compound will have a binding constant that is the product of the binding constants of the two separate ligands (i.e., a nanomolar binder can be derived from a pair of micromolar binders). This approach has been used to design molecules with nanomolar binding affinities for the FK506 binding protein (124) and nanomolar inhibitors of stromelysin (125,126). ^{13}C-HSQC spectra can also be used to screen for binding to a target protein and are particularly powerful when combined with ^{13}C-methyl labeling techniques that simplify the spectra (14). The resulting assay has an increased sensitivity because the three protons attached to ^{13}C-labeled methyl groups are observed rather than the single amide proton in the ^{15}N-HSQC. When combined with deuteration, this method has also proved useful for screening higher-molecular-weight targets, including the 110-kDa dihydroneopterin aldolase (14).

A recent drug discovery tool that does not require isotopic labeling or even assignment of the target protein is the SHAPES strategy (127). Lead compounds are generated by screening for binding of any of the 132 molecules in the "SHAPES library" to the target protein. These compounds represent the full range of molecular frameworks found in known drugs and are both soluble and easy to synthesize. Nuclear magnetic resonance screening involves observation of line broadening and transferred NOEs in the spectrum of the library molecule. For large targets (> 60 kDa), binding can be discerned from changes in the 1D tNOE NMR spectrum, while smaller targets (10–60 kDa) require additional 2D NOE spectra to detect weak μM–mM) binding. Thus this method requires only a single screen of a relatively small library, which means that relatively small amounts of protein are required. The results from the initial screen can be used to direct high-throughput screens, a process that typically results in a 10-fold increase in hits relative to screening random compounds.

3 PROSPECTS FOR HIGH-THROUGHPUT NMR

The technological advances of the past few years have dramatically increased the efficiency of NMR spectroscopy as a tool for solving protein structures. Innovations in spectrometer hardware, pulse programming, and isotopic labeling are now being combined to broaden the range of systems accessible to NMR while decreasing the amount of instrument time required to solve a structure. Both of these capabilities will be very important for high-throughput structure determination endeavors that seek to solve the structures of proteins on a genome-wide scale. An early challenge to such efforts will be to express thousands of proteins in quantities sufficient for structural studies. The abilities of NMR to rapidly assess protein folding, to work with samples at low concentrations, and to determine the structures of smaller proteins in a matter of weeks will all come into play as structural genomics develops.

3.1 High-Throughput Protein Expression

The most unreliable step in structure determination is expressing large quantities of soluble, isotopically labeled protein. Once a suitable sample is obtained, the technical parts of the process are relatively routine. Innovations in protein expression systems are therefore expected to have a substantial impact on the efficiency with which protein structures can be determined. Recent developments in bacterial expression will facilitate the process of testing a variety of expression vectors and protein constructs, thus streamlining the production of soluble samples. Recombinational cloning systems enable genes to be rapidly transferred into many different expression vectors with a variety of purification tags (128,129). A high-throughput approach to protein expression will involve the production of many expression vectors for many clones in parallel along with a highly parallel process for screening for the vectors for production of soluble protein (130). The process will involve testing expression with several tags (e.g., His_6, MBP, GST) in several expression hosts (e.g., various strains of *E. coli*, yeast, insect cells) in order to optimize the production of soluble samples. It is quite likely that as cell-free expression systems develop, they will become widely used for high-throughput protein production.

The major roadblock for high-throughput production of protein samples for structural studies is solubility. Proteins containing disulfide bonds, those requiring post-translational modifications, and membrane proteins present particular challenges at the present time. Since so many important proteins fall into these categories, it will be important for structural genomics endeavors to overcome these sample-production problems. Ideally, bacterial expression systems would be modified to allow for expression of these proteins, since *E. coli* provides the most convenient system for expressing large amounts of labeled protein. It is now possible to produce proteins with disulfide bonds in bacterial cells, thanks to the development of *E. coli* strains having an oxidizing cytoplasm instead of the normal reducing environment (131). The yeast *Picchia pastoris* can be also used to express disulfide-containing proteins, but yeast requires richer growth medium than bacteria and yields can be variable.

Post-translationally modified proteins cannot generally be expressed in bacteria, since glycosylation, myristoylation, phosphorylation, and sulfonation do not take place in *E coli*. Instead, they are typically expressed in yeast, insect cells, or mammalian cells, but isotopic labeling in these systems is only beginning to be developed. *P. pastoris* is to date the most successful eukaryotic system for producing isotopically labeled proteins with post-translational modifications (132). Despite the differences between the glycosylation patterns in *P. pastoris* and mammalian systems, the presence of any glycans helps mammalian proteins' folding and solubility. Alternatively, coexpression strategies can allow post-translationally modified proteins to be expressed in *E. coli*: The myristoylated protein recoverin has been successfully expressed alongside N-myristoyl CoA transferase (133). It is likely that more strategies like these will be developed so that other types of post-translationally modified proteins can be expressed in bacteria.

Membrane proteins are another type of system that is especially challenging at this time. It is possible for membrane proteins to be expressed in *E. coli* and then transferred to micelles after purification (134), but more frequently membrane proteins are expressed in yeast or mammalian cells (135). There are currently no reliable systems for producing correctly folded membrane proteins, so the efficient production of these proteins must await further development of both expression systems and labeling strategies.

In trying to produce soluble samples of thousands of proteins in parallel, it will be necessary to develop sets of standard expression conditions that are most likely to work for unknown proteins. This will involve a process of initial automatic sequence analysis to categorize each protein as, e.g., a membrane protein or one containing multiple disulfide bonds, followed by testing of a limited number of expression conditions that have been determined to be most promising for that type of protein. As more proteins are successfully expressed, the ability to predict expression conditions for new proteins will increase and the entire process will become more efficient. The classification of such data into successful and unsuccessful expression conditions for a wide range of proteins will be essential for structural genomics and useful to the greater biological community.

3.2 Nuclear Magnetic Resonance Spectroscopy as a Screening Tool for Structural Genomics

Once soluble protein has been produced, expression can be scaled up to produce NMR samples very quickly. A simple 1D NMR spectrum or a 2D ^{1}H,^{15}N-HSQC (Fig. 3) that can be acquired in approximately 10 minutes on a 50 μM sample provides a rapid assessment of the quality of a sample. Each protein can be tested under a few conditions (e.g., low salt and high salt at a few different pHs), and data collection can be automated by using a sample changer. Examining the spectral dispersion in the 1D or ^{15}N-HSQC spectrum serves as a rapid screen for whether a protein is folded or not (Fig. 3). Further information on the solubility and aggregation state of a sample can be obtained by examining the spectral linewidths and comparing the signal-to-noise ratio observed to that expected for a 50 μM sample. Sample impurities or other inhomogeneities are indicated by extra peaks in the ^{15}N-HSQC spectrum. The spectra can thus be used to guide decisions as to whether a protein is suitable for structural studies and whether NMR spectroscopy or X-ray crystallography would be more suitable for solving the

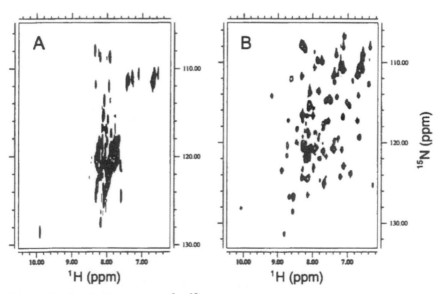

Figure 3 Comparison of the ^{1}H,^{15}N-HSQC spectra of a protein domain that is unfolded (A) vs. folded (B). The lack of dispersion and sharpness of the peaks in (A) are typical of unfolded proteins, while folded regions have the broader, well-dispersed peaks seen in (B). Thus the appearance of the ^{1}H,^{15}N-HSQC can be used to assess the folding state of a protein. (Figure courtesy of John D. Gross.)

structure. Since the position of peaks in an HSQC spectrum reveals whether there are disordered regions in a protein, NMR can also be used to guide truncation of a protein to its structured region.

3.3 Rapid Structure Determination by Nuclear Magnetic Resonance Spectroscopy

The structures of proteins up to 25 kDa can now be routinely solved by common NMR methods within two months. By using state-of-the-art technologies and optimizing all phases of structure determination, the fold of a protein of this size has been determined from only four days of data acquired on three samples, with an additional three days of data collection being required for a refined structure (15). Such a streamlined approach to structure determination will be an essential component of high-throughput strategies. By integrating labeling schemes and data collection protocols, the spectra are simplified. This facilitates data analysis and makes it more amenable to automation. The amount of time required for data collection is dramatically reduced by the use of cryogenic probes, which triple the sensitivity of NMR experiments, resulting in a ninefold reduction in acquisition times for samples that give strong signals (136). Only essential experiments are recorded, always with the goal of obtaining unambiguous NOEs with which to calculate the global fold of the protein. The Fesik group has shown that the six triple-resonance experiments used to assign the backbone can be acquired in ~ 1.5 days using an $^{15}N,^{13}C,^{2}H$ sample in which the methyl groups of valine, leucine, and isoleucine ($\delta 1$) are protonated (15). The same sample can then be used to record (H)C(CO)HN-TOCSY and H(CCO)NH-TOCSY spectra to assign the methyl groups, and to obtain residual dipolar coupling data. Aromatic side chains are assigned from TOCSY spectra of a second sample, in which phenylalanine and tyrosine are protonated. The second sample also contains $^{13}C,^{1}H$-methyl–labeled valine, leucine, and isoleucine in an otherwise deuterated ^{15}N-labeled background, so it can be used to acquire ^{15}N- and ^{13}C-NOESY spectra that contain only cross-peaks involving the labeled methyl groups and aromatic side chains and the amide protons. These NOEs are sufficient to determine the global fold of a protein, which can then be refined by automated methods using more NOEs and residual dipolar couplings (15). If experiments for direct detection of hydrogen bonds could be made more sensitive, they would provide a valuable addition to this scheme, since hydrogen bond constraints, along with the chemical shift index, can define the tertiary structure of a protein at an even earlier stage of data analysis.

High-throughput structure determination will necessarily involve automation of spectral analysis. Currently an experienced spectroscopist can spend two months solving the structure of a 25-kDa protein using semiautomated tools. This process is far too labor intensive and time consuming for high-throughput endeavors and requires constant decision making by the researcher. Automation of data analysis and structure calculations will relieve the spectroscopist of all but the most complex decisions. Automated analysis of spectra necessarily requires the following steps: (1) peak picking, (2) grouping of peaks into spin systems, (3) typing spin systems according to amino acid type, (4) linking spins systems together into segments, and (5) mapping these segments onto the sequence of the protein (101). One issue in automating the assignment process is that peaks in different spectra must align perfectly in order to be recognized by the program. The ability to obtain all the required data in a short time using very few samples means that differences in chemical shifts between spectra will be minimized, which is expected to alleviate this problem. Overlapping peaks are another particular challenge for automatic analysis. Because of this, simplifying the data used to assign proteins and obtain structural constraints will greatly assist in automating spectral analysis. There are a number of available programs that use this strategy (recently reviewed in Ref. 101), but the package one uses must be tailored to the specific experiments being analyzed. Thus one of the goals of high-throughput NMR might be to develop a very flexible program that could be adapted to use many different sets of experiments, including those that have not yet been devised.

3.4 Synergy of Nuclear Magnetic Resonance Spectroscopy and X-Ray Crystallography

Nuclear magnetic resonance spectroscopy and X-ray crystallography are complementary techniques in many ways. The NMR technique provides a dynamic view of the structure of proteins in solution, while X-ray crystallography gives a high-resolution glimpse into a protein crystal. The method of choice for studies of smaller proteins is NMR, since they generally give high-quality spectra with few ambiguities, making for rapid spectral analysis and structure determination. Crystallography may be the better approach for larger systems, although recent advances in NMR spectroscopy mean that it can be applied to larger systems than ever before. Crystallographers are experts at screening conditions for crystallization, and NMR spectroscopists might do well to adapt such sparse-matrix approaches to the screening of conditions for NMR samples (137). Meanwhile NMR spectroscopists are able to use simple spectra that can be acquired in a matter of minutes to assess the quality of a protein sample. Such information can be immensely helpful to crystallographers in terms of assessing whether a sample is homogeneous and whether a protein has unstructured regions that would require truncation prior to successful crystallization. These sorts of simple, rapid, and semiautomatic decision-making processes will doubtless play an important role as structure determination expands to genomic-scale efforts.

The ability of NMR to determine rapidly the secondary structure elements of a protein could also be useful for crystallographers. Using data acquired in just 1.5 days (15), the backbone of a protein could be assigned (automatically) and the regions of secondary structure determined from the chemical shifts using TALOS. Even if unambiguous NOEs could not be readily assigned, this information could guide crystallographers in interpreting their data. This type of synergy has already been used in solving the structure of the antiapoptotic protein Bcl-xL, which contains a long unstructured internal loop that hampered crystallographic structure determination. However, when secondary structure information from NMR spectra was combined with the crystallographic data, the structure could be solved (138).

Another illustration of the power of combining NMR spectroscopy and X-ray crystallography is in the area of T-cell receptors. After the NMR structure of human CD2 with the N-linker high-mannose glycan was solved (139), a mutant was designed that could function even without the carbohydrate. Next a mutant of the counter-receptor CD58 was devised that is folded and functional in the absence of its glycan, even though the glycan comprises two-thirds of the molecular weight of the wild-type protein (140). And NMR spectroscopy was used to show that the carbohydrate-free mutants of CD2 and CD58 provide good samples for structural studies and form a tight complex. With this knowledge, the complex was crystallized and the structure solved (141). It would have taken much longer to solve this structure by either technique alone. Only by taking advantage of the ability of NMR to screen for mutants that are well behaved and form a complex and of the ability of crystallography to solve the structures of large complexes could the structure be determined efficiently.

4 CONCLUSION

Nuclear magnetic resonance spectroscopy is an extremely powerful tool in structural biology that is capable of providing structural information on proteins larger than 100 kDa. Although data acquisition and analysis for complete protein structure determination are not as rapid as they are for X-ray crystallography, the relative ease of sample preparation means that many protein structures can be solved as quickly using NMR techniques as they can by crystallography. High-throughput structure determination endeavors will take advantage of both streamlined methods for solution structure determination by NMR and the ability of NMR to screen for samples that are amenable to structure determination by either NMR or crystallography. As NMR spectroscopy and X-ray crystallography become more synergic, a wider range of proteins and complexes will be more easily accessible to structural studies, and structures will be solved more and more efficiently.

REFERENCES

1. V Dötsch, G Wagner. New approaches to structure determination by NMR. Curr Opin Struct Biol 8:619–623, 1998.
2. G Wagner. An account of NMR in structural biology. Nature Struct Biol 4:841–844, 1997.
3. M Salzmann, K Pervushin, G Wider, H Senn, K Wüthrich. NMR assignment and secondary structure determination of an octameric 110-kDa protein using TROSY in triple resonance experiments. J Am Chem Soc 122:7543–7548, 2000.
4. HM Berman, J Westbrook, Z Feng, G Gilliland, TN Bhat, H Weissig, IN Shindyalov, PE Bourne. The protein data bank. Nucleic Acids Research 28:235–242, 2000.
5. GT Montelione, D Zheng, YJ Huang, KC Gunsalus, T Szyperski. Protein NMR spectroscopy in structural genomics. Nature Struct Biol 7:982–985, 2000.
6. S Yokoyama, H Hirota, T Kigawa, T Yabuki, M Shirouzu, T Terada, Y Ito, Y Matsuo, Y Kuroda, Y Nishimura, Y Kyogoku, K Miki, R Masui, S Kuramitsu. Structural genomics projects in Japan. Nature Struct Biol 7:943–945, 2000.
7. U Heinemann. Structural genomics in Europe: slow start, strong finish? Nature Struct Biol 7:940–942, 2000.
8. MP Williamson, TF Havel, K Wüthrich. Solution conformation and proteinase inhibitor IIA from bull seminal plasma by proton NMR and distance geometry. J Mol Biol 182:295–315, 1985.
9. G Wagner, K Wüthrich. Truncated driven nuclear Overhauser effect (TOE). A new technique for studies of selective ^{1}H-^{1}H Overhauser effects in the presence of spin diffusion. J Magn Reson 33:675–680, 1979.
10. TF Havel, K Wüthrich. A distance geometry program for determining the structure of small proteins and other macromolecules from nuclear magnetc resonance measurements of intramolecular ^{1}H-^{1}H proximities in solution. Bull Math Biol 46:673–698, 1984.
11. KH Gardner, LE Kay. The use of ^{2}H,^{13}C,^{15}N multidimensional NMR to study the structure and dynamics of proteins. Annu Rev Biophys Biomol Struct 27:357–406, 1998.
12. N Goto, K Gardner, G Mueller, R Willis, L Kay. A robust and cost-effective method for the production of Val, Leu, Ile (δ1) methyl-protonated ^{15}N-, ^{13}C-, ^{2}H-labeled proteins. J Biomol NMR 13:369–374, 1999.

13. K Gardner, L Kay. Production and incorporation of ^{15}N, ^{13}C, ^{2}H (^{1}H-δ1-methyl) isoleucine into proteins for multidimensional NMR studies. J Am Chem Soc 119:7599–7600, 1997.

14. P Hajduk, D Augeri, J Mack, R Mendoza, J Yang, S Betz, S Fesik. NMR-based screening of proteins containing ^{13}C-labeled methyl groups. J Am Chem Soc 122:7898–7904, 2000.

15. A Medek, E Olejniczak, R Meadows, S Fesik. An approach for high-throughput structure determination of proteins by NMR spectroscopy. J Biomol NMR 18:229–238, 2000.

16. G Vuister, S Kim, W C, B A. 2D and 3D NMR-study of phenylalanine residues in proteins by reverse isotopic labeling. J Am Chem Soc 116:9206–9210, 1994.

17. B Aghazadeh, K Zhu, T Kubiseski, G Liu, T Pawson, Y Zheng, M Rosen. NMR structure and mutagenesis of the Dbl homology domain. Nat Struct Biol 5:1098–1107, 1998.

18. M Kelly, C Krieger, L Ball, Y Yu, G Richter, P Schmeider, A Bacher, H Oschkinat. Application of amino acid type-specific ^{1}H- and ^{14}N-labeling in a ^{2}H-,^{15}N-lableled background to a 47-kDa homodimer: potential for NMR structure determination of large proteins. J Biomol NMR 14:79–83, 1999.

19. H Wang, D Janowick, J Schkeryantz, X Liu, F SW. A method for assigning phenyalanines in proteins. J Am Chem Soc 121:1611–1612, 1999.

20. J Cereghino, J Cregg. Heterologous protein expression in the methylotrophic yeast *Pichia pastoris*. FEMS Microbiol Rev 24:45–66, 2000.

21. J Cregg, T Vedvick, W Raschke. Recent advances in the expression of foreign genes in *Pichia pastoris*. Bio/Technology 11:905–910, 1993.

22. C Scorer, R Buckholz, J Clare, M Romanos. The intracellular production and secretion of HIV-1 envelope protein in the methylotrophic yeast *Pichia pastoris*. Gene 136:111–119, 1993.

23. M Wood, E Komives. Production of large quantities of isotopically labeled protein in *Pichia pastoris* by fermentation. J Biomol NMR 13:149–159, 1999.

24. S Massou, V Puech, F Talmont, P Demange, N Lindley, M Tropis, A Milon. Heterologous expression of a deuterated membrane-integrated receptor and partial deuteration in methylotrophic yeasts. J Biomol NMR 14:231–239, 1999.

25. L Jermutus, L Ryabova, A Pluchthun. Recent advances in producing and selecting functional proteins by using cell-free translation. Curr Opin Biotech 9:534–548, 1998.

26. T Kigawa, T Yabuki, Y Yoshida, M Tsutsui, Y Ito, T Shibata, S Yokoyama. Cell-free production and stable-isotope labeling of milligram quantities of proteins. FEBS Letters 442:15–19, 1999.

27. K Madin, T Sawasaki, T Ogasawara, Y Endo. A highly efficient and robust cell-free protein synthesis system prepared from wheat embryos: plants apparently contain a suicide system directed at ribosomes. Proc Natl Acad Sci USA 97:559–564, 2000.

28. J Huppa, H Ploegh. In vitro translation and assembly of a complete T cell receptor–CD3 complex. J Exp Med 186:393–403, 1997.

29. L Ryabova, D Desplancq, A Spirin, A Pluckthun. Functional antibody production using cell-free translation: Effects of protein disulfide isomerase and chaperones. Nature Biotechnology 15:79–84, 1997.

30. K Wüthrich. NMR of Proteins and Nucleic Acids. New York: Wiley, 1986.

31. M Ikura, LE Kay, A Bax. A novel approach for sequential assignment of ^{1}H, ^{13}C and ^{15}N spectra of larger proteins: heteronuclear triple-resonance three-dimensional NMR spectroscopy. Application to calmodulin. Biochemistry 29:4659–4667, 1990.

32. M Ikura, D Marion, LE Kay, H Shih, M Krinks, CB Klee, A Bax. Heteronuclear 3D NMR and isotopic labeling of calmodulin. Towards the complete assignment of the ^{1}H NMR spectrum. Biochem Pharmacol 40:153–160, 1990.

33. S Grzesiek, A Bax. Improved 3D triple-resonance NMR techniques applied to a 31-kDa protein. J Magn Res 96:432–440, 1992.

34. T Yamazaki, W Lee, M Revingtom, DL Mattiello, FW Dahlquist, CH Arrowsmith, LE Kay. An HNCA pulse scheme for the backbone assignmnet of ^{15}N-,^{13}C,- ^{2}H-labeled proteins: applicaton to a 37-KDa Trp repressor-DNA complex. J Am Chem Soc 116:6464–6465, 1994.

35. T Yamazaki, W Lee, CH Arrowsmith, DR Muhandiram, LE Kay. A suite of triple resonance NMR experiments for the backbone assignment of ^{15}N-, ^{13}C-, ^{2}H-labeled proteins with high sensitivity. J Am Chem Soc 116:11655–11666, 1994.

36. DR Muhandiram, LE Kay. Gradient-enhanced triple-resonance three-dimensional NMR experiments with improved sensitivity. J Magn Res B 103:203–216, 1994.

37. LE Kay, GY Xu, T Yamazaki. Enhanced-sensitivity triple-resonance spectroscopy with minimal H_2O saturation. J Magn Reson, Ser A 109:129–133, 1994.

38. H Matsuo, H Li, G Wagner. A sensitive HN(CA)CO experiment for deuterated proteins. J Magn Res B110:112–115, 1996.

39. S Grzesiek, A Bax. An efficient experiment for sequential backbone assignment of medium-sized isotopically enriched proteins. J Magn Res 99:201–207, 1992.

39A. C Bartels, T Xia, M Billeter, P Güntert, K Wüthrich. The program XEASY for computer-supported NMR spectral analysis of biological molecules. J Biomol NMR 6:1–10, 1995.

40. D Wishart, B Sykes, F Richards. The chemical shift index: a fast and simple method for the assignment of protein secondary structure. Biochemistry 31:1647–1651, 1992.

41. DS Wishart, BD Sykes. The ^{13}C chemical-shift index: a simple method for the identification of protein secondary structure using ^{13}C chemical-shift data. J Biomol NMR 4:171–180, 1994.

42. G Cornilescu, F Delaglio, A Bax. Protein backbone angle restraints from searching a database for chemical shift and sequence homology. J Biomol NMR 13:289–302, 1999.

43. S Grzesiek, J Anglister, A Bax. Correlation of backbone amide and aliphatic side-chain resonances in ^{13}C-/^{15}N-enriched proteins by isotropic mixing of 13C magnetization. J Magn Res B 101:114–119, 1993.
44. TM Logan, ET Olejniczak, RX Xu, SW Fesik. A general method for assigning NMR spectra of denatured proteins using 3D HC(CO)NH-TOCSY triple resonance experiments. J Biomol NMR 3:225–231, 1993.
45. Y Lin, CM Fletcher, J Zhou, CD Allis, G Wagner. Solution structure of the catalytic domain of GCN5 histone acetyltransferase bound to coenzyme A. Nature 400:86–89, 1999.
46. Y Lin, G Wagner. Efficient side-chain and backbone assignment in large proteins: application to tGCN5. J Biomol NMR 15:227–239, 1999.
47. LE Kay, G-Y Xu, AU Singer, DR Muhandiram, JD Forman-Kay. A gradient-enhanced HCCH-TOCSY experiment for recording side-chain ^1H and ^{13}C correlations in H_2O samples of proteins. J Magn Res B 101:333–337, 1993.
48. DR Muhandiram, NA Farrow, G-Y Xu, SH Smallcombe, LE Kay. A gradient ^{13}C NOESY-HSQC experiment for recording NOESY spectra of ^{13}C-labeled proteins dissolved in H_2O. J Magn Res B 102:317–321, 1993.
49. SW Fesik, ERP Zuiderweg. Heteronuclear three-dimensional NMR spectroscopy. A strategy for the simplification of homonuclear two-dimensional NMR spectra. J Magn Reson 78:588–593, 1988.
50. ERP Zuiderweg, SW Fesik. Heteronuclear three-dimensional NMR spectroscopy of the inflammatory protein C5a. Biochemistry 28:2387–2391, 1989.
51. D Marion, PC Driscoll, LE Kay, PT Wingfield, A Bax, AM Gronenborn, GM Clore. Overcoming the overlap problem in the assignment of ^1H NMR spectra of larger proteins by use of three-dimensional heteronuclear ^1H-^{15}N Hartmann–Hahn–multiple quantum coherence and nuclear Overhauser–multiple quantum coherence spectroscopy: application to interleukin 1β. Biochemistry 28:6150–6156, 1989.
52. GW Vuister, R Boelens, R Kaptein, M Burgering, PCM van Zijl. Gradient-enhanced 3D NOESY-HMQC spectroscopy. J Biomol NMR 2:301–305, 1992.
53. C Mumenthaler, P Güntert, W Braun, K Wüthrich. Automated combined assignment of NOESY spectra and three-dimensional protein structure determination. J Biomol NMR 10:351–362, 1997.
54. Y Xu, J Wu, D Gorenstein, W Braun. Automated 2D NOESY assignment and structure calculation of crambin (S22/I25) with the self-correcting distance geometry–based NOAH/DIAMOD programs. J Magn Res 136:76–85, 1999.
55. M Nilges, MJ Macias, SI O'Donoghue, H Oschkinat. Automated NOESY interpretation with ambiguous distance restraints: the refined NMR solution structure of the pleckstrin homology domain from β-spectrin. J Mol Biol 269:408–422, 1997.
56. BJ Hare, G Wagner. Application of automated NOE assignment to three-dimensional structure refinement of a 28-kDa single-chain T cell receptor. J Biomol NMR 15103–113 15:103–113, 1999.

57. M Karplus. J Phys Chem 30:11–15, 1959.
58. GW Vuister, A Bax. Quantitative J correlations: a new approach for measuring homonuclear three-bond $J(H^N H\alpha)$ coupling constants in ^{15}N-enriched proteins. J Am Chem Soc 115:7772–7777, 1993.
59. J Madsen, O Sorensen, P Sorensen, F Poulsen. Improved pulse sequences for measuring coupling constants in ^{13}C-, ^{15}N-labeled proteins. J Biomol NMR 3:239–244, 1993.
60. SJ Archer, M Ikura, DA Torchia, A Bax. J Magn Res 95:636–641, 1991.
61. N Tjandra, A Bax. Direct measurement of distances and angles in biomolecules by NMR in a dilute liquid crystalline medium. Science 278:1111–1114, 1997.
62. GM Clore, MR Starich, AM Gronenborn. Measurement of residual dipolar couplings of macromolecules aligned in the nematic phase of a colloidal suspension of rod-shaped viruses. J Am Chem Soc 120:10571–10572, 1998.
63. MR Hansen, L Mueller, A Pardi. Tunable alignment of macromolecules by filamentous phage yields dipolar coupling interactions. Nature Struct Biol 5:1065–1074, 1998.
64. N Tjandra, J Omichinski, A Gronenborn, G Clore, A Bax. Use of dipolar ^{1}H-^{15}N and ^{1}H-^{13}C couplings in the structure determination of magnetically oriented macromolecules in solution. Nature Struct Biol 4:732–738, 1997.
65. M Ottiger, A Bax. Determination of relative N-H^N, N-C′, Cα-C′, and Cα-Hα effective bond lengths in a protein by NMR in a dilute liquid crystalline phase. J Am Chem Soc 120:12334–12341, 1998.
66. D Yang, J Tolman, N Goto, L Kay. An HNCO-based pulse scheme for the measurement of ^{13}Cα-^{1}Hα one-bond dipolar couplings in ^{15}N-, ^{13}C-labeled proteins. J Biomol NMR 12:325–332, 1998.
67. P Permi, A Annila. Transverse relaxation–optimized spin-state selective NMR experiments for measurement of residual dipolar couplings. J Biomol NMR 16:221–227, 2000.
68. P Permi, P Rosevear, A Annila. A set of HNCO-based experiments for measurement of residual dipolar couplings in ^{15}N-, ^{13}C-, (^{2}H)-labeled proteins. J Biomol NMR 17:43–54, 2000.
69. M Ottiger, F Delaglio, A Bax. Measurement of J and dipolar couplings from simplified two-dimensional NMR spectra. J Magn Res 131:373–378, 1998.
70. J Chou, F Delaglio, A Bax. Measurement of one-bond N-15-C-13′ dipolar couplings in medium-sized proteins. J Biomol NMR 18:101–105, 2000.
71. MA Markus, RB Gerstner, DE Draper, DA Torchia. Refining the overall structure and subdomain orientation of ribosomal protein S4 Δ41 with dipolar couplings measured by NMR in uniaxial liquid crystalline phases. J Mol Biol 292:375–387, 1999.
72. MW Fischer, JA Losonczi, JL Weaver, JH Prestegard. Domain orientation and dynamics in multidomain proteins from residual dipolar couplings. Biochemistry 38:9013–9022, 1999.
73. G Mueller, W Choy, D Yang, F-K JD, R Venters, L Kay. Global folds of proteins with low densities of NOEs using residual dipolar couplings: applica-

tions to the 370-residue maltodextrin-binding protein. J Mol Biol 300:197–212, 2000.

74. F Delaglio, G Kontaxis, A Bax. Protein structure determination using molecular fragment replacement and NMR dipolar couplings. J Am Chem Soc 122:2142–2143, 2000.

75. J Chou, S Li, A Bax. Study of conformational rearrangement and refinement of structural homology models by the use of heteronuclear dipolar couplings. J Biomol NMR 18:217–227, 2000.

76. J-C Hus, D Marion, M Blackledge. De novo determination of protein structure by NMR using orientational and long-range order restraints. J Mol Biol 298:927–936, 2000.

77. G Clore, M Starich, C Bewley, M Cai, J Kuszewski. Impact of residual dipolar couplings on the accuracy of NMR structures determined from a minimal number of NOE restraints. J Am Chem Soc 121:6513–6514, 1999.

78. J Meiler, N Blomberg, M Nilges, C Griesinger. A new approach for applying residual dipolar couplings as restraints in structure elucidation. J Biomol NMR 16:245–252, 2000.

79. AJ Dingley, S Grzesiek. Direct observation of hydrogen bonds in nucleic acid base pairs by internucleotide $^2J_{NN}$ couplings. J Am Chem Soc 120:8293–8297, 1998.

80. G Cordier, S Grzesiek. Direct observation of hydrogen bonds in proteins by interresidue $^{3h}J_{NC'}$ scalar couplings. J Am Chem Soc 121:1601–1602, 1999.

81. G Cornilescu, J-S Hu, A Bax. Identification of the hydrogen bonding network in a protein by scalar coupling. J Am Chem Soc 121:2949–2950, 1999.

82. A Meissner, O Sorensen. New techniques for the measurement of C'N and $C'H^N$ J coupling constants across hydrogen bonds in proteins. J Magn Res 143:387–390, 2000.

83. G Cornilescu, BE Ramirez, MK Frank, GM Clore, AM Gronenborn, A Bax. Correlation between $^{3h}J_{NC'}$ and hydrogen bond length in proteins. J Am Chem Soc 121:6275–6279, 1999.

84. F Cordier, M Rogowski, S Grzesiek, A Bax. Observation of through-hydrogen-bond $^{2h}J_{HN'}$ in a perdeuterated protein. J Magn Res 140:510–512, 1999.

85. A Meissner, O Sorensen. ^{3h}J coupling between C^α and H^N across hydrogen bonds in proteins. J Magn Res 143:431–434, 2000.

86. Y-X Wang, J Jacob, F Cordier, P Wingfield, SJ Stahl, S Lee-Huang, D Torchia, S Grzesiek, A Bax. Measurement of $^{3h}J_{NC'}$ connectivities across hydrogen bonds in a 30-kDa protein. J Biomol NMR 14: 181-184, 1999.

87. TR Krugh. In: LJ Berliner, ed. Spin-Labeling Theory and Applications. New York: Academic Press, 1976, pp 339–372.

88. ME Girvin, RH Fillingame. Determination of local protein structure by spin label difference 2D NMR: the region neighboring Asp61 of subunit c of the F_1F_0 ATP synthase. Biochemistry 34:1635–1645, 1995.

89. JR Gillespie, D Shortle. Characterization of long-range structure in the denatured state of staphylococcal nuclease. II. Distance restraints from paramag-

netic relaxation and calculation of an ensemble of structures. J Mol Bio 268:170–184, 1997.

90. JR Gillespie, D Shortle. Characterization of long-range structure in the denatured state of staphylococcal nuclease. I. Paramagnetic relaxation enhancement by nitroxide spin labels. J Mol Biol 268:158–169, 1997.

91. JL Battiste, G Wagner. Utilization of site-directed spin lableing and high resolution heteronuclear NMR for global fold determination of large proteins with limited NOE data. Biochemistry 39:5355–5365, 2000.

92. HS Mchaourab, MA Lietzow, K Hideg, WL Hubbell. Motion of spin-labeled side chains in T4 lysozyme. Correlation with protein structure and dynamics. Biochemistry 35:7692–7704, 1996.

93. A Brünger. X-PLOR version 3.1 a system for X-ray crystallography and NMR. New Haven, CT: Yale University Press, 1987.

94. A Brünger, P Adams, C GM, W DeLano, P Gros, R Grosse-Kunstleve, J-S Jiang, J Kuszewski, M Nilges, N Pannu, R Read, L Rice, T Simonson, G Warren. Crystallography & NMR System: a new software suite for macromolecular structure determination. Acta Cryst D54:905–921, 1998.

95. P Güntert, C Mumenthaler, K Wüthrich. Torsion angle dynamics for NMR structure calculation with the new program DYANA. J Mol Biol 273:1997.

96. D Bassolino-Klimas, R Tejero, S Krystek, W Metzler, G Montelione, R Bruccoleri. Simulated annealing with restrained molecular dynamics using a flexible restraint potential: theory and evaluation with simulated NMR constraints. Protein Sci 5:593–603, 1996.

97. Y Xu, J Wu, D Gorenstein, W Braun. Automated 2D NOESY assignment and structure calculation of crambin (S22/I25) with the self-correcting distance geometry–based NOAH/DIAMOD programs. J Magn Res 136:76–85, 1999.

98. P Güntert, W Braun, K Wüthrich. Efficient computation of three-dimensional protein structures in solution from nuclear magnetic resonance data using the program DIANA and the supporting programs CALIBA, HABAS and GLOMSA. J Mol Biol 217:517–530, 1991.

99. P Güntert, W K. Improved efficiency of protein structure calculations from NMR data using the program DIANA with redundant dihedral angle constraints. J Biomol NMR 1: 446–456, 1991.

100. P Güntert. Structure calculations of biological macromolecules from NMR data. Q Rev Biophys 31:145–237, 1998.

101. HNB Moseley, GT Montelione. Automated analysis of NMR assignments and structures for proteins. Current Opin Struct Biol 9:635–642, 1999.

102. K Pervushin, R Riek, G Wider, K Wüthrich. Attenuating T_2 relaxation by mutual cancellation of dipole–dipole coupling and chemical shift anisotropy indicates an avenue to NMR structures of very large biological macromolecules in solution. Proc Natl Acad Sci USA 94:12366–12371, 1997.

103. M Saltzmann, K Pervushin, G Wider, H Senn, K Wüthrich. TROSY in triple-resonance experiments: new perspectives for sequential NMR assignment of large proteins. Proc Natl Acad Sci USA 95:13585–13590, 1998.

104. JP Loria, M Rance, AG Palmer. Transverse-relaxation-optimized (TROSY) gradient-enhanced triple-resonance NMR spectroscopy. J Magn Res 141:180–184, 1999.
105. G Kelly, S Prasannan, S Daniell, K Fleming, G Frankel, G Dougan, I Connerton, S Matthews. Structure of the cell-adhesion fragment of intimin from enteropathogenic *Escherichia coli*. Nat Struct Biol 6:313–318, 1999.
106. T Yamazaki, T Otomo, N Oda, Y Kyogoku, K Uegaki, N Ito, Y Ishino, H Nakamura. Segmental isotope labeling for protein NMR using peptide splicing. J Am Chem Soc 120:5591–5592, 1998.
107. R Xu, B Ayers, D Cowburn, TW Muir. Chemical ligation of folded recombinant proteins: segmental isotopic labeling of domains for NMR studies. Proc Natl Acad Sci USA 96:388–393, 1999.
108. T Otomo, N Ito, Y Kyogoku, T Yamazaki. NMR observation of selected segments in a larger protein: central-segment isotope labeling through intein-mediated ligation. Biochemistry 38:16040–16044, 1999.
109. T Otomo, K Teruya, K Uegaki, T Yamazaki, Y Kyogoku. Improved segmental labeling of proteins and application to a larger protein. J Biomol NMR 14:105–114, 1999.
110. G Wider, C Weber, R Traber, H Widmer, K Wüthrich. Use of a double-half filter in two-dimensional ^{1}H nuclear magnetic resonance studies of receptor-bound cyclosporin. J Am Chem Soc 112:9015–9016, 1990.
111. PJM Folkers, RHA Folmer, RNH Konings, CW Hilbers. Overcoming the ambiguity problem encountered in the analysis of nuclear Overhauser magnetic resonance spectra of symmetric dimer proteins. J Am Chem Soc 115:3798–3799, 1993.
112. H Matsuo, M Shirakawa, Y Kyogoku. Three-dimensional dimer structure of the λ-Cro repressor in solution as determined by heteronuclear multidimensional NMR. J Mol Biol 254:668–680, 1995.
113. M Ikura, A Bax. Isotope-filtered 2D NMR of a protein–peptide complex: study of a skeletal muscle myosin light chain kinase fragment bound to calmodulin. J Am Chem Soc 114:2433–2440, 1992.
114. M Burgering, R Boelens, R Kaptein. Observation of intersubunit NOEs in a dimeric P22 Mnt repressor mutant by a time-shared [^{15}N,^{13}C] double half-filter technique. J Biomol NMR 3:709–714, 1993.
115. MJM Burgering, R Boelens, DE Gilbert, JN Breg, KL Knight, RT Sauer, R Kaptein. Solution structure of dimeric Mnt repressor (1-76). Biochemistry 33:15036–15045, 1994.
116. KJ Walters, H Matsuo, G Wagner. Use of deuteration to distinguish inter-monomer NOEs in homodimeric proteins with C_2 symmetry. J Am Chem Soc 119:5958–5959, 1996.
117. A Ferentz, T Opperman, G Walker, G Wagner. Dimerization of the UmuD′ protein in solution and its implications for regulation of SOS mutagenesis. Nature Struct Biol 4:979–983, 1997.
118. TS Peat, EG Frank, JP McDonald, AS Levine, R Woodgate, WA Hendrickson. Structure of the UmuD′ protein and its regulation in response to DNA damage. Nature 380:727–730, 1996.

119. TS Peat, EG Frank, JP McDonald, AS Levine, R Woodgate, WA Hendrickson. The UmuD' protein filament and its role in damage induced mutagenesis. Structure 4:1401–1412, 1996.

120. K Walters, A Ferentz, B Hare, P Hidalgo, A Jasanoff, H Matsuo, G Wanger. Experimental approaches for characterizing protein–protein complexes and oligomers by NMR spectroscopy. Methods in Enzymology. Vol. 339B, 238–258, 2001.

121. C Freund, A Ross, A Pluckthun, TA Holak. Structural and dynamics properties of the Fv fragment and the single-chain F_v fragment of an antibody in solution investigated by heteronuclear three-dimensional NMR spectroscopy. Biochemistry 33:3296–3303, 1994.

122. BJ Hare, DF Wyss, MS Osburne, PS Kern, EL Reinherz, G Wagner. Structure, specificity and CDR mobility of a class II restricted single-chain T-cell receptor. Nature Struct Biol 6:574–581, 1999.

123. EL Reinherz, K Tan, L Tang, P Kern, J-h Liu, Y Xiong, RE Hussey, A Smolyar, B Hare, R Zhang, A Joachimiak, H-C Chang, G Wagner, J-h Wang. The crystal structure of a T cell receptor in complex with peptide and MHC class II. Science 286:1913–1921, 1999.

124. SB Shuker, PJ Hajduk, RP Meadows, SW Fesik. Discovering high-affinity ligands for proteins: SAR by NMR. Science 274:1531–1534, 1996.

125. ET Olejniczak, PJ Hajduk, PA Marcotte, DG Nettesheim, RP Meadows, R Edalji, TF Holtzman, SW Fesik. Stromelysin inhibitors designed from weakly bound fragments: effects of linking and cooperativity. J Am Chem Soc 119:5828–5832, 1997.

126. PJ Hajduk, G Sheppard, DG Nettesheim, ET Olejniczak, SB Shuker, RP Meadows, DH Steinman, GM Carrera, Jr., PA Marcotte, J Severin, K Walter, J Smith, E Gubbins, R Simmer, TF Holtzman, DW Morgan, SK Davidsen, JB Summers, SW Fesik. Discovery of potent nonpeptide inhibitors of stromelysin using SAR by NMR. J Am Chem Soc 119:5818–5827, 1997.

127. J Fejzo, CA Lepre, JW Peng, GW Bemis, Ajay, MA Murcko, JM Moore. The SHAPES strategy: an NMR-based approach for lead generation in drug discovery. Chemistry Biology 6:755–769, 1999.

128. Q Liu, MZ Li, D Leibham, D Cortez, SJ Elledge. The univector plasmid-fusion system, a method for rapid construction of recombinant DNA without restriction enzymes. Curr Biol 8:1300–1309, 1998.

129. AJ Walhout, R Sordella, X Lu, JL Hartley, GF Temple, MA Brasch, N Thierry-Mieg, M Vidal. Protein interaction mapping in *C. elegans* using proteins involved in vulval development. Science 287:116–122, 2000.

130. R Stevens. Design of high-throughput methods of protein production for structural biology. Structure 8:R177–R185, 2000.

131. PH Bessette, F Aslund, J Beckwith, G Georgiou. Efficient folding of proteins with multiple disulfide bonds in the *Escherichia coli* cytoplasm. Proc Natl Acad Sci USA 96:13703–13708, 1999.

132. H Denton, M Smith, H Husi, D Uhrin, PN Barlow, CA Batt, L Sawyer. Isotopically labeled bovine beta-lactoglobulin for NMR studies expressed in *Pichia pastoris*. Protein Expr Purif 14:97–103, 1998.

133. JB Ames, T Tanaka, L Stryer, M Ikura. Secondary structure of myristoylated recoverin determined by three-dimensional heteronuclear NMR: implications for the calcium-myristoyl switch. Biochemistry 33:10743–10753, 1994.

134. KR MacKenzie, JH Prestegard, DM Engelman. A transmembrane helix dimer: structure and implications. Science 276:131–133, 1997.

135. M Eilers, PJ Reeves, W Ying, HG Khorana, SO Smith. Magic angle spinning NMR of the protonated retinylidene Schiff base nitrogen in rhodopsin: expression of 15N-lysine- and 13C-glycine-labeled opsin in a stable cell line. Proc Natl Acad Sci USA 96:487–492, 1999.

136. P Hajduk, T Gerfin, J Boehlen , M Haberli, D Marek, F SW. High-through-put nuclear magnetic resonance–based screening. J Med Chem 42:2315–2317, 1999.

137. C Lepre, J Moore. Microdrop screening: a rapid method to optimize solvent conditions for NMR spectroscopy of proteins. J Biomol NMR 12:493–499, 1998.

138. SW Muchmore, M Sattler, H Liang, RP Meadows, JE Harlan, HS Yoon, D Nettesheim, BS Chang, CB Thompson, SL Wong, SL Ng, SW Fesik. X-ray and NMR structure of human Bcl-xL, an inhibitor of programmed cell death. Nature 381:335–341, 1996.

139. DF Wyss, JS Choi, J Li, MH Knoppers, KJ Willis, AR Arulanandam, A Smolyar, EL Reinherz, G Wagner. Conformation and function of the N-linked glycan in the adhesion domain of human CD2. Science 269:1273–1278, 1995.

140. ZY Sun, V Dotsch, M Kim, J Li, EL Reinherz, G Wagner. Functional glycan-free adhesion domain of human cell surface receptor CD58: design, production and NMR studies. EMBO J 18:2941–2949, 1999.

141. JH Wang, A Smolyar, K Tan, JH Liu, M Kim, ZY Sun, G Wagner, EL Reinherz. Structure of a heterophilic adhesion complex between the human CD2 and CD58 (LFA-3) counterreceptors. Cell 97:791–803, 1999.

6

Automated Molecular Replacement

Jorge Navaza
Centre National de la Recherche Scientifique, Gif-sur-Yvette, France

Pedro M. Alzari
Institut Pasteur, Paris, France

1 INTRODUCTION

The ultimate goal of a crystallographic study is to obtain a molecular model of the crystal electron density, starting from the measured moduli of its Fourier coefficients. Two major approaches are employed to obtain the final model. The first one relies on experimental methods such as multi-wavelength isomorphous replacement (MIR) and multiwavelength anomalous dispersion (MAD) which provide the phases of the Fourier coefficients, in which case the electron density can be directly calculated and interpreted in terms of molecular models. The second approach—the molecular replacement (MR) methods—exploits the structural similarity between the molecule(s) in the crystal with other molecules or fragments of known 3D structure. In this case, the crystal is assembled from the known molecular models so that the calculated diffraction pattern fits the observed data. In both approaches, due to experimental errors in the phases or inaccuracies in the model used for MR calculations, the final molecular model of the crystal is obtained after model rebuilding and refinement.

The basic ideas and techniques of MR originated in the early days of protein crystallography, from the interest in exploiting the so-called non-crystallographic symmetry (NCS) that occurs fairly often in protein crystals (1). Nowadays, the purpose of MR methods is different: It usually involves relating a search model, derived from a known crystal structure, to the molecule (or molecules) in an unknown crystal. When an appropriate search model is available, MR can directly provide the structure solution without the need for tedious preparations of heavy-atom or selenomethionine derivatives. The MR methods can thus be expected to play a central role in this new era of protein crystallography, when the number of known macromolecular structures will increase dramatically, fueled by structure-based biopharmaceutical discovery and ongoing structural genomics initiatives.

We will first describe the MR method and its implementation in the program AMoRe (2). Then we will present some selected examples to illustrate specific aspects of the method and conclude with a discussion of perspectives.

2 THE MOLECULAR REPLACEMENT METHOD

The aim of MR methods is to assemble a tentative crystal structure using known molecular models, similar to the molecules that constitute the actual crystal, in order to start the crystallographic refinement. In practice, this implies determining the position of the different independent molecules within the crystal unit cell. The search model (a whole molecule or a fragment) is treated as a rigid body, whose position is specified by six parameters: three angles that define its orientation with respect to the crystal axes and three translations. As a consequence, building a crystal structure composed of N independent molecules or fragments amounts to determining $6N$ parameters. The exhaustive exploration of a $6N$-dimensional domain would involve extremely long calculations, although 6D searches are now feasible (3). Furthermore, nonexhaustive 6D search methods using either stochastic approaches (4) or genetic algorithms (5,6) have recently been proposed and applied with success.

Fortunately enough, less time-consuming procedures can be successfully used following the "classical" MR approach. This approach, which is implemented in most currently available software, is based on the possibility of determining the orientational parameters of each individual molecule, independent of all other parameters. For each independent molecule, the orientation is first determined, and the translation of the orientated model is then searched in a second stage. This is done using appropriate rotation and translation functions, whose optimal values hopefully correspond to the correct values of the parameters. In this way the original $6N$-dimensional search is split into at most $2N$ three-dimensional searches.

The accuracy and size of the search model are critical for the success of the MR method. Standard models used in MR calculations are the atomic coordinates of known crystal structures, but other type of probes can also be used, such as NMR ensembles, theoretical homology models, or even electron density maps issued from electron microscopy or heavy-atom/MAD data. It is always difficult to estimate quantitatively how similar the search and the target molecules must be in order to ensure the successful application of MR. For reasonable-sized models, rmsd values in main-chain atomic coordinates higher than 2 Å often (but not always) render the structure determination uncertain. Indeed, the optimal values of the rotation or translation functions may not correspond to the correct solution when using poor models.

In recent decades, great effort was devoted to developing new functions and concocting a number of more or less successful recipes to enhance the signal of the right solution. This collective effort converted MR into an effective means for solving macromolecular crystal structures. However, the ultimate success or failure of MR remained unpredictable to a considerable extent, and the technique required a good deal of user intervention. The introduction of fast and accurate algorithms for screening possible solutions helped to improve this situation and opened the way for automation, thus putting MR methods within the realm of high-throughput structure determination.

3 IMPLEMENTATION OF THE MOLECULAR REPLACEMENT METHOD IN AUTOMATED MOLECULAR REPLACEMENT

The central idea in automated molecular replacement (AMoRe) is to use fast rotation and translation functions to sample many crystal configurations, i.e., tentative crystal structures built from molecular models. The actual values of these functions are not taken as figures of merit per se, but simply as a means to select a large number of potential solutions. The tentative crystal configurations thus selected are eventually assessed by using more robust criteria involving the comparison between observed and calculated structure factor amplitudes. Eventually crystal packing analysis may be used to exclude unrealistic configurations. Many structures have been solved where the correct solutions were ranked very low in terms of the values of fast functions.

The primary agreement criterion to assess crystal configurations in AMoRe is the (linear) correlation coefficient:

$$CC_F = \frac{\sum_H \left(\left| F_H^{obs} \right| - \left\langle \left| F_H^{obs} \right| \right\rangle \right) \times \left(\left| F_H^{cal} \right| - \left\langle \left| F_H^{cal} \right| \right\rangle \right)}{\sqrt{\sum_H \left(\left| F_H^{obs} \right| - \left\langle \left| F_H^{obs} \right| \right\rangle \right)^2} \times \sqrt{\sum_H \left(\left| F_H^{cal} \right| - \left\langle \left| F_H^{cal} \right| \right\rangle \right)^2}}$$

where $\langle \ldots \rangle$ means "average over reflections". The values of CC_F fall in the interval $[-1,1]$. Additional useful criteria involve other functions derived from the observed and calculated data, such as the linear correlation coefficient in intensities and the crystallographic R-factor. As a general rule, it is the contrast in the values of these criteria—not their absolute values—that gives us confidence in the assessment.

In this section we will first define the variables that specify the position of a molecule and their relationship with the molecular scattering factors, which are a cornerstone of the package. Then we will describe the fast rotation and translation functions used to sample crystal configurations and the rigid-body refinement program used to optimize the values of the positional variables. Finally, we will outline the overall strategy that is usually employed for crystal structure determination using AMoRe.

3.1 Positional Variables and Crystal Configurations

The position of one molecule or fragment within the crystal is determined by the rotation R and the translation T that move the search model from the reference initial position r° to the current position r:

$$r = Rr^\circ + T$$

The translation T is usually expressed in fractional coordinates (x, y, z) within the crystal cell. The rotation R is parameterized with the Euler angles (α, β, γ), associated with an orthonormal frame (X, Y, Z). A good choice for the orthonormal frame is Z parallel to the highest crystal symmetry axis, since it reduces the search volume in the orientational space. Several conventions exist for the names of angles and definitions of the axes involved in this parameterization. We will follow the convention illustrated in Figure 1: $(\alpha, \beta,)\gamma$ denotes a rotation of α_about the Z-axis, followed by a rotation of β about the new Y-axis, and finally a rotation of γ about the new Z-axis. The angles (in degrees) take values within the parallelepiped $\{0 \leq \alpha < 360;$ $0 \leq \beta \leq 180; 0 \leq \gamma < 360\}$. For $\theta = 0$ or 180, only the $(\alpha + \gamma)$ or $(\alpha - \gamma)$ are independent, respectively.

Another useful parameterization to represent the rotation R is the use of polar angles (θ, ϕ, κ), for it facilitates the detection of local NCS. In this representation, κ specifies the rotation angle about an axis whose orientation is defined by the colatitude and longitude (θ, ϕ), as shown in Figure 1. In this case, the angles can take values within the parallelepiped $\{0 \leq \theta \leq 180;$ $0 \leq \phi < 360; 0 \leq \kappa \leq 180\}$.

Given the initial positions of the search models, the crystal cell parameters, the space group symmetry, and the orientation of the orthonormal frame, a particular crystal configuration is uniquely determined by specify-

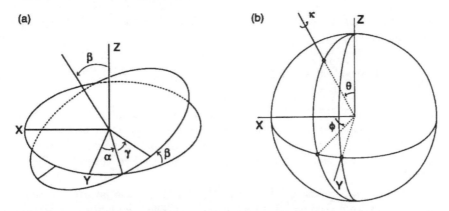

Figure 1 (a) Eulerian angles (α, β, γ) and (b) polar angles (θ, ϕ, κ).

ing the positions of the independent molecules within the unit cell, expressed in terms of the positional variables $(\alpha_m, \beta_m, \gamma_m, x_m, y_m, z_m)$, where the label m identifies each independent molecule within the crystal.

3.2 The Molecular Scattering Factor

Structure factor calculation recurs very often in MR. A central feature of AMoRe is to perform these calculations not in terms of atomic coordinates but in terms of the molecular scattering factor $f(\mathbf{h})$. This form factor corresponds to the Fourier transform of the electron density of the molecule placed at an initial reference position. Usually, the center of mass of the model is placed at the origin, and its principal axes of inertia are aligned with the orthonormal frame $(\mathbf{X}, \mathbf{Y}, \mathbf{Z})$, because this leads to an efficient sampling of configurations. In some cases it may be useful to maintain a predefined orientation for the initial position, for instance, if one wishes to compare the results obtained with different search models prearranged in a similar orientation. To calculate molecular scattering factors, each search model is placed within a cell (model box) large enough to allow for a fine sampling in reciprocal space, typically four times the molecular dimensions in each direction. The corresponding electron density map is then constructed and eventually transformed by Fast Fourier techniques.

If $\mathbf{R}$ and $\mathbf{T}$ denote, respectively, the rotation and translation that define the current position of an independent molecule, $\mathbf{M}_g$ and $\mathbf{t}_g$ denote the space group transformation matrix and translation vector of the gth symmetry operation, and $\mathbf{H}$ denotes the coordinates of a crystal reciprocal vector, then the contribution of the molecule to the calculated crystal structure factor is

$$F_H^{cal}(\mathbf{R}, \mathbf{T}) = \sum_{g=1}^{G} f(\mathbf{HM}_g\mathbf{DRO})e^{2\pi i\mathbf{H}(\mathbf{M}_g\mathbf{T}+\mathbf{t}_g)}$$

In this expression, **DRO** is the rotation matrix **R** expressed on a mixed basis, where **D** and **O** are orthogonalizing and deorthogonalizing matrices, in the unit cell and the model box, respectively. The calculated structure factor will contain as many such terms as these are independent molecules in the crystal.

The molecular scattering factor $f(\mathbf{h})$ carries all the information concerning the search model and is well suited for MR calculations. Instead of calculating structure factors from the rotated model coordinates, the evaluation of F_H^{cal} is now obtained by interpolation of the molecular scattering factors $f(\mathbf{h})$ at the rotated crystal reciprocal vectors. One feature of AMoRe is that the search model may be input as atomic coordinates as well as electron density maps, for they are only used to produce $f(\mathbf{h})$.

3.3 The Rotation Function

The rotations **R** that superimpose a search molecule upon the homologous ones within the target crystal may be determined by calculating the overlap, within a conveniently chosen region Ω of volume v (usually chosen as a spherical domain), of the observed Patterson function (the target function P_t) and a rotated version of the Patterson function corresponding to the isolated search molecule (the search function P_s), as defined by Rossmann and Blow (1):

$$R(\mathbf{R}) = \frac{1}{v}\int_{\Omega} P_t(\mathbf{r})P_s(\mathbf{R}^{-1}\mathbf{r})d^3\mathbf{r}$$

This function is usually referred to as the *cross-rotation function*, to emphasize the fact that it relates two different Patterson functions. When the target and search Patterson functions are the same, the overlap function is called the *self-rotation function*.

The rotation function R should display a local maximum for the sought rotations **R**. To compare rotation function values obtained under different conditions, we can define a normalized function R_N having the form of a correlation coefficient,

$$R_N(\mathbf{R}) = \frac{\int_{\Omega} P_t(\mathbf{r})P_s(\mathbf{R}^{-1}\mathbf{r})d^3\mathbf{r}}{\sqrt{\int_{\Omega} P_t^2(\mathbf{r})d^3\mathbf{r} \int_{\Omega} P_s^2(\mathbf{r})d^3\mathbf{r}}}$$

The reciprocal space formulation of the rotation function is obtained by substituting the Patterson functions with their Fourier summations,

$$P_{t,s}(\mathbf{r}) = \frac{1}{V} \sum_{\mathbf{h}} I_{t,s}(\mathbf{h}) e^{-2\pi i \mathbf{h} \mathbf{r}}$$

The resulting expression for the rotation function has the disadvantage of containing entangled contributions from the target and search functions, which renders its computation time consuming if the whole domain of rotations has to be explored. This difficulty may be overcome by expanding the Patterson functions in the preceding equation in terms of spherical harmonics, $Y_{l,m}$ (7). Taking advantage of the transformation of the $Y_{l,m}$ under rotations, and using recurrence relationships between spherical Bessel functions j_ℓ, it can be shown that

$$R(\mathbf{R}) = \frac{1}{V_s V_t} \sum_{\mathbf{h}} I_t(\mathbf{h}) \sum_{\mathbf{k}} I_s(\mathbf{k}) \sum_{\ell=0}^{\infty} \left\{ \sum_{n=1}^{\infty} 12\pi(2(\ell + 2n) - 1) \right.$$

$$\left. \frac{j_{\ell+2n-1}(2\pi hb) j_{\ell+2n-1}(2\pi kb)}{2\pi hb \quad\quad 2\pi kb} \right\}$$

$$\times \sum_{m,m'=-\ell}^{\ell} \overline{Y_{\ell,m}(\mathbf{h}/h)} Y_{\ell,m'}(\mathbf{k}/k) D_{m,m'}^{\ell}(\mathbf{R})$$

w $D_{m,m'}^{\ell}$ are the matrices of the irreducible representations of the rotation group (8).

The preceding equation has several advantages:

The angular variables are separated from the crystal-dependent ones. It also separates the contributions from target and search Patterson functions.

The equation is accurate, even when truncating the summations on ℓ and n to reasonable values. The upper limit for ℓ is of the order of the highest argument of the spherical Bessel functions, $\ell_{max} \approx 2\pi b/d_{min}$, where d_{min} i the resolution of the data.

When the rotations are parameterized in terms of the Euler angles (α, β, γ), the matrices $D_{m,m'}^{\ell}$ take the form

$$D_{m,m'}^{\ell}(\alpha, \beta, \gamma) = d_{m,m'}^{\ell}(\beta) e^{i(m\alpha + m'\gamma)}$$

which enables the computation of R or R_N, for each given value of β, by means of 2-dimensional fast Fourier transforms (FFTs). This fast rotation function is implemented in the program ROTING of AMoRe.

3.4 The Translation Function

Different types of translation functions have been proposed and are used in MR to position a correctly oriented model in the unknown unit cell. These functions may compare the target and search Patterson functions (9,10), the observed and calculated structure factor amplitudes or intensities (the so-called R-factor or correlation searches) (11–13) or even the target and search electron density maps (i.e., the phased translation function) (14–17).

In AMoRe, the sampling of the positional (translation) space is carried out with the TRAING program. The program includes the option to compute several fast translation functions, all of which comprise and generalize most previous propositions and are computed by FFT techniques.

If we write the contribution to the Fourier coefficient of the oriented model, rotated by a given **R** and placed at position **T**, as

$$\sum_{g=1}^{G} \left[f(\mathbf{HM}_g\mathbf{DRO})e^{2\pi i \mathbf{H}t_s} \right] e^{2\pi i \mathbf{HM}_s \mathbf{T}} = \sum_{g=1}^{G} u_g(\mathbf{H})e^{2\pi i \mathbf{HM}_s \mathbf{T}}$$

then the options for one-body search (i.e., no contribution from the previously positioned models) fast translation functions are the following (the overbar denotes complex conjugate):

Centered overlap:

$$\mathrm{CO(T)} = \sum_{\mathbf{H}} \left(I_{\mathbf{H}}^{\mathrm{obs}} - \left\langle I_{\mathbf{H}}^{\mathrm{obs}} \right\rangle \right) \times \left(I_{\mathbf{H}}^{\mathrm{cal}}(\mathbf{T}) - \left\langle I_{\mathbf{H}}^{\mathrm{cal}}(\mathbf{T}) \right\rangle \right)$$

$$\propto \sum_{\mathbf{H}} \left(I_{\mathbf{H}}^{\mathrm{obs}} - \left\langle I_{\mathbf{H}}^{\mathrm{obs}} \right\rangle \right) \overline{u_g(\mathbf{H})} u_{g'}(\mathbf{H}) e^{-2\pi i \mathbf{H}(\mathbf{M}_s 0 \mathbf{M}_{s'})\mathbf{T}}$$

Harada–Lifchitz:

$$\mathrm{HL(T)} = \left(\sum_{\mathbf{H}} \left(I_{\mathbf{H}}^{\mathrm{obs}} - \left\langle I_{\mathbf{H}}^{\mathrm{obs}} \right\rangle \right) \times \left(I_{\mathbf{H}}^{\mathrm{cal}}(\mathbf{T}) - \left\langle I_{\mathbf{H}}^{\mathrm{cal}}(\mathbf{T}) \right\rangle \right) \right) \bigg/ \sum_{\mathbf{H}} I_{\mathbf{H}}^{\mathrm{cal}}(\mathbf{T})$$

Correlation coefficient:

$$\mathrm{CC(T)} = \frac{\sum_{\mathbf{H}} \left(I_{\mathbf{H}}^{\mathrm{obs}} - \left\langle I_{\mathbf{H}}^{\mathrm{obs}} \right\rangle \right) \times \left(I_{\mathbf{H}}^{\mathrm{cal}}(\mathbf{T}) - \left\langle I_{\mathbf{H}}^{\mathrm{cal}}(\mathbf{T}) \right\rangle \right)}{\sqrt{\sum_{\mathbf{H}} \left(I_{\mathbf{H}}^{\mathrm{obs}} - \left\langle I_{\mathbf{H}}^{\mathrm{obs}} \right\rangle \right)^2 \sum_{\mathbf{H}} \left(I_{\mathbf{H}}^{\mathrm{cal}}(\mathbf{T}) - \left\langle I_{\mathbf{H}}^{\mathrm{cal}}(\mathbf{T}) \right\rangle \right)^2}}$$

Phased translation with external phases ϕ_H^{ext} (i.e., map correlation):

$$PTF(T) = \sum_H F_H^{obs} e^{i\phi_H^{ext}} \times \overline{F_H^{cal}(T)}$$

Full-symmetry phased translation (without external phases):

$$PT(T) = \sum_{g,g'=1}^{G} \sum_H \left(\left| \frac{F_H^{obs}}{u_g(H)} \right| + \left| \frac{F_H^{obs}}{u_{g'}(H)} \right| - 2K \right)$$
$$\times \overline{u_g(H)} u_{g'}(H) e^{-2\pi i H(M_g - M_{g'})T}$$

where K is a scale factor to substract the contribution of the phasing position.

For the n-body search, the phased translation function with a partial phasing model is given by

$$PTN(T) = \sum_{g,g'=1}^{G} \sum_H \left(\left| \frac{F_H^{obs}}{F_H^{fix}} \right| - K \right) F_H^{fix} \times \overline{F_H^{cal}}$$

Here, F_H^{fix} denotes the contribution to the calculated structure factor from one or more previously positioned molecules. In the many-body versions of CO(T), HL(T), and CC(T), the value of f_H^{cal} is substituted with $F_H^{cal} + F_H^{fix}$.

3.5 The FITING Program

Crystal configurations, either partially or fully defined, are optimized using a rigid-body least squares refinement program, called FITING (18), that takes advantage of a fast technique first proposed by Huber and Schneider (19). The quadratic misfit

$$R_F = \sum_H \left(\left| F_H^{obs} \right| - \lambda e^{BH^2/4} \left| F_H^{cal}(\{R_m, T_m\}) \right| \right)^2$$

is minimized with respect to the positional variables $\{R_m, T_m\}$ the overall scale factor λ, and the overall temperature factor B.

3.6 The Overall Strategy

The "classical" MR approach as implemented in AMoRe consists of three major steps. First, the rotation search aims at sampling the orientational space for all search models within the unknown crystal. The ROTING program based on the fast rotation function, whose mathematical structure was described earlier, is used to determine the possible orientations of the search models. Alternatively, if the calculated intensities are approximated by

$$I_H^{cal} \approx \sum_{g=1}^{G} |f(HM_g DRO)|^2$$

then the highest peaks of CC_I—as a function of $\mathbf{R}$—are selected. This function is essentially the direct rotation function (20). Even though CC_I with I_H^{cal} given by the preceding equation, cannot be calculated by standard fast techniques, then available computing resources allow for a point-by-point evaluation of CC_I at reasonable speed.

Second, a one-body translation search is carried out for each molecule and for each selected orientation, to sample the possible translations. The calculated intensities are approximated by

$$I_H^{cal} \approx \sum_{g',g=1}^{G} f(HM_g DRO)\overline{f(HM_{g'} DRO)} \times e^{2\pi i H((M_s - M_{s'})T + t_s - t_{s'})}$$

and CC_I—as a function of $\mathbf{T}$—is evaluated by FFT (13). Alternatively, other fast translation functions based on FFT techniques can also be used. The positions corresponding to the top partial (one independent molecule) crystal configurations are then refined by fast rigid-body least squares, and that with the highest CC_F value is assumed to be the correct position for the first molecule.

When there is more than one independent molecule in the crystal, the last stage of the method is the n-body translation search. In this case, the contribution of already placed models dramatically increases the chances of success of the method. If $M' < M$ molecules are already positioned, then the possible translations are determined for the top orientations of the remaining molecules. As before, the top positions are refined and that with the highest CC_F value corresponding to the partial $(M' + 1)$-body configuration is assumed to be the correct solution.

The fast algorithms used for structure factor calculations, the precision of the fast rotation function, and the facility of multiple inputs to translation searches and rigid-body refinement allow for a fast multiple exploration of the crystal configuration space with a high level of automation. Indeed, a situation where the foregoing protocol fails is often one in which a full six-dimensional search would fail too. As a rule, this corresponds to a poor quality of the search model or a small size of the search fragment with respect to the asymmetric unit content.

4 SOME APPLICATIONS OF MOLECULAR REPLACEMENT STRUCTURE DETERMINATIONS WITH AUTOMATED MOLECULAR REPLACEMENT

Two simple examples in which there is a high structural similarity between the target and search molecules illustrate the standard use of AMoRe. The crystal structure of fasciculin 2 from Green Mamba snake venom has been determined using as probe the atomic coordinates of fasciculin 1, which differ by only one out of 61 residues (21). There is a single molecule in the asymmetric unit, and the correct crystal configuration corresponds to the top peaks in both the rotation and translation functions calculated with data in the 15-Å to 3-Å resolution range (Table 1). Note the high contrast in the values of different criteria (CC_F, R_F, CC_I) after the final rigid-body least squares refinement. In this example any translation function could have been used to sample the translational space, as shown in Table 2.

The crystal structure of *C. thermocellum* cellobiohydrolase CelS (B. Gomes Guimaraes & PMA, unpublished results) has been determined using the coordinates of *C. cellulolyticum* cellobiohydrolase CelF (22). CelS crystals (space group $P2_12_12_1$) contain six independent molecules in the asymmetric unit and additional translation steps (*n*-body searches) are therefore required to obtain the complete crystal configuration. As in the previous example, the correct solution can be assembled directly from the top peaks in the rotation and subsequent translation functions (Tables 3 and 4 and Fig. 2). A significant increase in contrast in the translation function is observed after a partial configuration (one or more molecules) has been correctly determined. Indeed, the whole crystal structure could have been assembled from the output of the 2-body translation search (Table 4).

The structure determination of the complex between β-lactamase and the inhibitor Blip (23) represented a more complicated challenge for MR methods. There is only one complex in the asymmetric unit. β-Lactamase accounts for 60% of the independent scattering matter; its correct position corresponds to the top of the rotation and translation functions. For Blip, the fast rotation function is highly contrasted, but the correct orientation is one of the last positive peaks (Fig. 3). Moreover, the orientation is easily lost when slightly varying some of the parameters that define the function. The structure was originally solved by splitting Blip into two domains and test-ing several orientations calculated under different conditions (23). This example illustrates the importance of sampling and the inadequacy of the values of fast functions to assess putative solutions.

A common difficulty often encountered in MR is typified by low sequence (and therefore structural) similarities between the target and search

Table 1 Structure Determination of Fasciculin 2

(a)

α	β	γ	CF$_1$	RF$_1$	Cl$_1$	R$_N$
65.0	**69.7**	**34.9**	**17.8**	**53.0**	**29.3**	**19.7**
47.8	70.3	262.2	16.0	53.3	25.5	11.9
44.4	69.3	264.0	15.3	53.4	23.5	11.8
28.5	78.9	265.2	14.3	53.7	22.7	9.9
8.7	85.7	127.9	12.7	54.4	20.2	9.8
52.2	62.9	341.7	11.3	54.6	18.3	9.6

(b)

α	β	γ	x	y	z	CCF$_F$	R$_F$	CC$_I$	PT
65.0	**69.7**	**34.9**	**0.1066**	**0.4400**	**0.4916**	**49.6**	**43.0**	**49.1**	**100.0**
65.0	69.7	34.9	0.1066	0.4373	0.4704	38.4	47.6	41.3	80.8
65.0	69.7	34.9	0.1064	0.4372	0.3592	36.9	47.5	38.8	75.6
65.0	69.7	34.9	0.1064	0.4405	0.1127	35.8	48.1	35.8	66.1
65.0	69.7	34.9	0.1045	0.4405	0.1612	35.4	48.4	38.6	63.7
47.8	70.3	262.2	0.8253	0.5174	0.2836	23.3	52.2	23.9	86.9
47.8	70.3	262.2	0.8814	0.2208	0.4496	23.0	52.0	21.9	71.1
47.8	70.3	262.2	0.0557	0.5424	0.2896	22.7	52.7	21.7	78.2
47.8	70.3	262.2	0.8380	0.5124	0.1457	22.7	53.0	22.0	100.0
47.8	70.3	262.2	0.8811	0.2170	0.2117	22.4	52.3	19.5	80.9
44.4	69.3	264.0	0.0575	0.0589	0.4965	23.4	53.5	22.5	67.2
44.4	69.3	264.0	0.0555	0.5383	0.3164	23.1	52.6	20.9	78.9
44.4	69.3	264.0	0.0530	0.5430	0.2868	22.9	53.1	21.1	76.8

| 44.4 | 69.3 | 264.0 | 0.8897 | 0.2069 | 0.0237 | 22.8 | 52.5 | 20.1 | 66.8 |
| 44.4 | 69.3 | 264.0 | 0.9997 | 0.5107 | 0.0661 | 22.8 | 53.5 | 22.4 | 100.0 |

(c)

α	β	γ	x	y	z	CC_F	R_F	CC_I
63.7	**71.4**	**33.9**	**0.1065**	**0.4400**	**0.4881**	**55.8**	**40.5**	**56.0**
66.2	69.6	33.5	0.1080	0.4390	0.4097	39.6	47.0	41.4
63.6	70.9	33.8	0.1069	0.4374	0.3575	39.0	46.8	39.5

(a) The top six peaks of the rotation function (program ROTING) are shown. (b) Five optimal values of the full-symmetry-phased translation function for each of the top three orientations (program TRAING). (c) Rigid-body least squares refinement for the three optimal translations (program FITING). In each case, values for the right solution are shown in bold.

All descriptions are expressed in percentages. The meaning of descriptors for the rotation function output is: CF_1, correlation of amplitudes in P1; RF_1, crystallographic R-factor in P1; CI_1, correlation of intensities including all symmetry-related intensities. The fast translation function values (PT in this case) are rescaled to a maximum of 100.

Table 2 Translation Fuctions – Fasciculin 2

α	β	γ	x	y	z	CC_F	R_F	CC_I	CO
65.0	69.7	34.9	0.1044	0.4435	0.4910	49.5	43.1	49.4	100.0
65.0	69.7	34.9	0.1109	0.4363	0.4075	38.3	47.8	41.1	77.7
65.0	69.7	34.9	0.1054	0.4364	0.3565	36.6	47.4	38.8	66.1
65.0	69.7	34.9	0.1031	0.4442	0.1094	34.9	49.0	37.0	64.1
65.0	69.7	34.9	0.1073	0.4370	0.4321	34.8	48.7	38.4	67.1

α	β	γ	x	y	z	CC_F	R_F	CC_I	PT
65.0	69.7	34.9	0.1066	0.4400	0.4916	49.6	43.0	49.1	100.0
65.0	69.7	34.9	0.1066	0.4373	0.4074	38.4	47.6	41.3	80.8
65.0	69.7	34.9	0.1064	0.4372	0.3592	36.9	47.5	38.8	75.6
65.0	69.7	34.9	0.1064	0.4405	0.1127	35.8	48.1	35.8	66.1
65.0	69.7	34.9	0.1045	0.4405	0.1612	35.4	48.4	38.6	63.7

α	β	γ	x	y	z	CC_F	R_F	CC_I	HL
65.0	69.7	34.9	0.1031	0.4436	0.4909	49.1	43.3	49.2	100.0
65.0	69.7	34.9	0.1105	0.4358	0.4083	38.5	47.8	41.3	83.8
65.0	69.7	34.9	0.1050	0.4360	0.3570	36.6	47.5	38.9	78.0
65.0	69.7	34.9	0.1063	0.4376	0.4320	34.8	48.8	38.4	79.1
65.0	69.7	34.9	0.1024	0.4451	0.1096	34.6	49.2	36.7	76.3

α	β	γ	x	y	z	CC_F	R_F	CC_I	CC
65.0	69.7	34.9	0.1073	0.4433	0.4875	52.0	42.0	53.2	100.0
65.0	69.7	34.9	0.1062	0.4394	0.4082	38.3	47.4	41.2	77.2
65.0	69.7	34.9	0.1052	0.4361	0.3576	36.7	47.5	39.0	73.5
65.0	69.7	34.9	0.1069	0.4363	0.0550	35.4	48.4	34.0	64.1
65.0	69.7	34.9	0.1100	0.4386	0.4322	35.2	48.7	38.2	72.1

The optimal value corresponds to the correct solution for fasciculin 2 in all translation functions implemented in TRAING (CO, centered overlap; PT, full symmetry-phased translation; HL, Harada–Lifshitz; CC, correlation coefficient in intensities).

Table 3 Structure Determination of CelS, One-Body Calculations

(a)

α	β	γ	CF_1	RF_1	CI_1	R_N
70.8	64.0	81.3	4.6	53.3	7.1	8.1
123.4	62.5	78.3	4.3	53.4	6.9	7.2
40.0	15.8	170.0	4.3	53.3	6.6	6.8
166.6	45.1	37.7	4.1	53.4	6.4	6.9
58.7	89.1	132.7	4.1	53.4	6.6	7.6
80.5	49.7	144.5	3.4	53.7	5.6	6.6
51.2	57.4	240.2	2.9	53.8	4.9	5.0
66.6	23.6	104.7	3.2	53.7	5.3	4.8
83.8	59.7	53.8	2.9	53.8	5.1	4.7
104.7	16.8	277.0	2.9	53.8	5.1	4.7

(b)

α	β	γ	x	y	z	CC_F	R_F	CC_I	PT
70.8	64.0	81.3	0.2151	0.0433	0.0814	9.3	53.2	9.1	100.0
70.8	64.0	81.3	0.4840	0.2219	0.3298	8.2	53.5	7.5	53.4
70.8	64.0	81.3	0.1906	0.0439	0.0822	8.0	53.6	7.7	53.3
70.8	64.0	81.3	0.0031	0.1213	0.0878	7.9	53.4	7.8	55.1
70.8	64.0	81.3	0.3746	0.0437	0.0807	7.8	53.4	7.4	51.7
123.4	62.5	78.3	0.3254	0.0627	0.1531	11.1	52.5	10.8	100.0
123.4	62.5	78.3	0.3278	0.0629	0.3417	8.8	53.1	8.7	55.3
123.4	62.5	78.3	0.3241	0.1044	0.1545	8.8	53.1	8.8	60.5
123.4	62.5	78.3	0.2821	0.1817	0.0164	8.7	53.4	8.4	51.8
123.4	62.5	78.3	0.0323	0.0611	0.1531	8.7	53.0	8.4	48.8
40.0	15.8	170.0	0.2327	0.1721	0.2269	9.8	53.1	9.7	100.0
40.0	15.8	170.0	0.2363	0.3742	0.2277	8.7	53.3	8.7	65.5

α	β	γ	x	y	z	CC_F	R_F	CC_I	
40.0	15.8	170.0	0.1236	0.4133	0.3550	8.4	53.3	8.2	55.4
40.0	15.8	170.0	0.2314	0.1738	0.2721	8.3	53.4	8.5	53.3
40.0	15.8	170.0	0.2344	0.0817	0.2279	8.3	53.4	8.4	50.9
166.6	45.1	37.7	0.1611	0.0226	0.3694	10.3	52.7	10.0	100.0
166.6	45.1	37.7	0.1165	0.4381	0.3496	8.8	53.1	8.3	50.2
166.6	45.1	37.7	0.1620	0.4875	0.3724	8.6	53.2	8.1	60.4
166.6	45.1	37.7	0.1609	0.4049	0.3688	8.6	53.1	8.1	51.5
166.6	45.1	37.7	0.4695	0.1184	0.2885	8.5	53.4	7.9	58.9
58.7	89.1	132.7	0.4220	0.1897	0.0319	10.8	52.7	11.0	100.0
58.7	89.1	132.7	0.4229	0.1117	0.0300	8.9	53.1	8.6	55.4
58.7	89.1	132.7	0.4228	0.4181	0.0328	8.7	53.3	8.8	61.0
58.7	89.1	132.7	0.4213	0.3230	0.0309	8.4	53.2	8.5	46.9
58.7	89.1	132.7	0.2685	0.1925	0.0329	8.4	53.2	8.5	51.1
80.5	49.7	144.5	0.2883	0.2102	0.2942	9.5	53.2	9.5	100.0
80.5	49.7	144.5	0.2829	0.4596	0.2936	7.9	53.5	7.9	62.1
80.5	49.7	144.5	0.2859	0.4149	0.2962	7.9	53.4	8.0	59.2
80.5	49.7	144.5	0.2857	0.1027	0.2942	7.8	53.4	7.8	51.2
80.5	49.7	144.5	0.2843	0.2789	0.2929	7.7	53.4	7.5	54.3

(c)

α	β	γ	x	y	z	CC_F	R_F	CC_I
59.5	89.8	132.7	0.4225	0.1932	0.0319	12.0	52.2	11.7
123.1	62.4	78.4	0.3268	0.0628	0.1544	11.2	52.4	11.0
81.0	49.2	146.2	0.2863	0.2101	0.2935	10.9	52.6	10.6
167.6	45.2	37.7	0.1629	0.0230	0.3693	10.8	52.6	10.4
39.4	15.3	171.3	0.2319	0.1722	0.2263	10.0	53.0	9.9
71.6	63.4	81.5	0.2115	0.0439	0.0812	9.7	52.9	9.4

(a) The top six orientations of the fast rotation function correspond to the correct orientations of the independent molecules within the crystal. (b) Output of the one-molecule translation function to the six top orientations. (c) Six top solutions after translation output, sorted by their CC_F values.

Table 4   Structure Determination of CelS

α	β	γ	x	y	z	CC_F	R_F	CC_I	PTN
59.5	89.8	132.7	0.4225	0.1932	0.0319	Fixed molecule ←			
123.4	62.5	78.3	0.8268	0.5578	0.6512	16.0	51.0	15.3	100.0
123.4	62.5	78.3	0.3784	0.1286	0.0396	10.7	52.4	10.5	69.4
123.4	62.5	78.3	0.8588	0.8913	0.3392	10.6	52.4	10.2	61.6
59.5	89.8	132.7	0.4225	0.1932	0.0319	Fixed molecule ←			
166.6	45.1	37.7	0.1703	0.5242	0.8719	16.0	51.1	15.8	100.0
166.6	45.1	37.7	0.1423	0.3310	0.8851	11.0	52.3	10.8	50.4
166.6	45.1	37.7	0.4646	0.1971	0.1318	10.8	52.5	10.6	50.6
59.5	**89.8**	**132.7**	**0.4225**	**0.1932**	**0.0319**	**Fixed molecule ←**			
80.5	**49.7**	**144.5**	**0.2902**	**0.7133**	**0.2928**	**16.4**	**51.1**	**16.5**	**100.0**
80.5	49.7	144.5	0.2900	0.2136	0.1171	10.4	52.8	10.7	44.5
80.5	49.7	144.5	0.4549	0.6331	0.4808	10.3	52.6	10.1	59.4
59.5	89.8	132.7	0.42225	0.1932	0.0319	Fixed molecule ←			
40.0	15.8	170.0	0.7272	0.6762	0.2319	13.6	51.6	13.6	100.0
40.0	15.8	170.0	0.6549	0.2943	0.9953	10.6	52.5	9.9	64.1
40.0	15.8	170.0	0.6679	0.1774	0.9937	10.6	52.5	10.3	85.8
59.5	89.8	132.7	0.4225	0.1932	0.0319	Fixed molecule ←			
70.8	64.0	81.3	0.2104	0.0436	0.5841	16.1	51.0	15.7	100.0
70.8	64.0	81.3	0.4144	0.8533	0.3178	10.6	52.6	10.7	55.0
70.8	64.0	81.3	0.6121	0.0742	0.9240	10.5	52.6	10.1	60.2

Two-molecule search, having fixed the position of the molecule with the highest CC_F in the one-molecule search (see Table 3). Only the three top peaks for each of five optimal orientations are shown. The procedure would now follow by selecting the crystal configuration with the highest CC_F value (shown in bold) and carrying out successive samplings of the translational space with n-body searches (n = 3, 4, 5, 6) until all independent molecules have been placed within the unit cell.

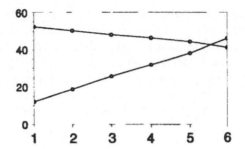

Figure 2 Cellobiohydrolase CelS. Progress of the assessment criteria CC_F and R_F during the *n*-body search as a function of n. The values of CC_I (not shown) are quite similar to those of CC_F.

molecules, a situation that will acquire greater relevance with the rapid increase of structural and genomic databases. The crystal structure of the *Ascaris* hemoglobin domain I (AhdI), which has been solved using heavy-atom methods, constitutes a representative example. When compared to other globins, the degree of sequence identity ranges from 10% to 20%, a

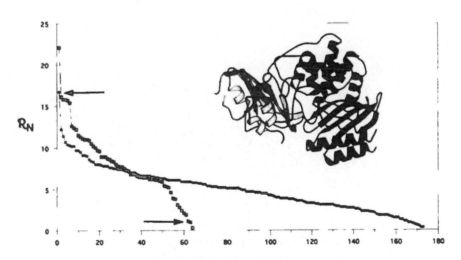

Positive Peaks in Rotation Function

Figure 3 β-Lactamase–Blip complex. List of all positive peaks in the rotation function R_N for the two partners, β-lactamase (circles) and Blip (squares). The insert shows the 3D structure of the complex in ribbon representation; β-lactamase is depicted in light gray, Blip in dark gray.

limit case for its use as a search probe in MR. However, the AdhI structure can indeed be determined using as a template the coordinates of sperm whale myoglobin (24). The two proteins share only 19 identical residues (14%), with five small insertions or deletions in helix-connecting loops. The correct crystal configuration can be found automatically with good contrast at low resolution (15–7 Å), but it is lost when using data in the 10-Å to 4-Å resolution range (Fig. 4). The root mean square (rms) deviation

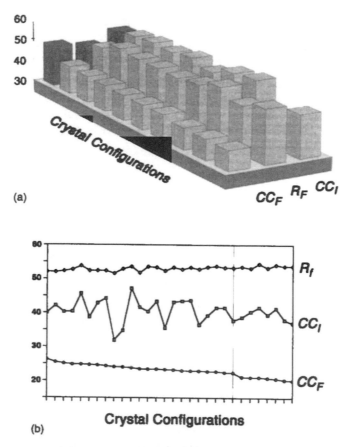

Figure 4 Hemoglobin domain. Sampling of crystal configurations assessed using different criteria (CC_F, R_F, CC_I). (a) Calculations in the 15-Å to 7-Å resolution range. CC_F correctly identifies the solution (shown in dark gray). (b) Calculations carried out using data between 10- and 4-Å resolution. Due to model inaccuracy, the solution (vertical line) cannot be identified by standard criteria.

between the target and search models is 1.97 Å for 133 equivalent C_α positions and increases to 2.3 Å when the overlap between the complete models is optimized in reciprocal space. A structural comparison (Fig. 5) indicates that the differences in amino acid sequences promote significant variations of the á-helical arrangement within the globular core, thus accounting for the better signal-to-noise ratio at low resolution.

The introduction of NCS in MR reduces the number of molecules to be placed and considerably increases the chances of success in many-body searches. Although easily detectable, translational NCS is neither systematically tested for nor employed in MR. An interesting example is provided by the crystal structure of a Fab fragment, Fab CC49, with four molecules in the asymmetric unit (E. Padlan, and C. Abergel, personnal communication). The four independent Fab molecules are associated in pairs, each pair being linked by a translational NCS. In a single-molecule rotation and translation search, the configuration with the highest, well-contrasted CC_F value is wrong. Starting from it, up to three molecules can be positioned in the unit cell with a plausible packing and R-factor. This is indeed a case where a full six-dimensional search with classical target functions would also fail. However, the use of translational NCS in MR avoids the traps often encountered in many-body searches and leads to the correct four-molecule solution.

The capability of using electron density maps as search probes opens new and interesting perspectives in MR, extending the possible field of applications of the method to address docking problems in electron micro-

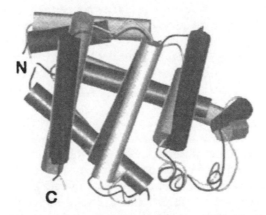

Figure 5 Hemoglobin domain. Structural superposition between the target molecule, *Ascaris* hemoglobin domain I (PDB code 1ash, shown in light gray), and the search probe, sperm whale myoglobin (PDB code 2mgm, shown in dark gray).

scopy (25) and to exploit weak phase information from MIR or MAD experiments in MR calculations. As an example, the 3D structure of endoglucanase CelC (26), for which no homology model was available, was determined using a combination of heavy-atom and MR methods. An uninterpretable electron density map calculated with heavy-atom phases within a molecular envelope was employed as a search probe to solve a second crystal form. Eventually, density-averaging techniques led to an interpretable map. A similar example is afforded by the crystallographic study of carbamate kinase (27), in which a portion of the electron density was used to identify NCS mates in a single-crystal form.

5   CONCLUSIONS AND PERSPECTIVES

Molecular replacement is an efficient technique for solving crystal structures. It is the method of choice for crystallographic studies of protein–ligand complexes in drug design and protein engineering. In these cases the solutions can be obtained almost automatically given the performance of available software. But MR has also proved to be useful when the target and search molecules have weak structural or sequence similarities. Indeed, models successfully used as templates in MR may not be accurate enough to start crystallographic refinement, as is the case with NMR ensembles. It is not unlikely that further improvements in MR will increase the efficiency of the method (i.e., find the correct crystal configuration) without necessarily solving the phase problem.

The most common reasons for MR failures involve model inaccuracies stemming from the low structural similarity between the search and target molecules (low sequence identity, NMR ensembles) or internal flexibility in the template. While this is undoubtedly the major limitation of the MR method, sampling size is another critical factor, as illustrated earlier by the β-lactamase–Blip complex case. Sometimes, unsuccessful applications of the method can actually be attributed to a scare sampling of positional space.

The rapid growth of NMR and X-ray structural databases will certainly make MR methods an important tool for high-throughput structure determination in genomic programs. This task will require highly automated computational methods. At present, albeit over half of the structures are solved straightforwardly, a dialog between numerical computation and human decision is part of the process of crystal structure determination. Automation will not only speed up the process but will also allow us to pursue challenging structural problems abondoned unnecessarily. This will require clear diagnostics and sensible guidance.

BIBLIOGRAPHY

Many topics of MR have not been discussed, because they are beyond the scope of the presentation. For good compilations of MR-related articles, the reader is referred to the seminal book on molecular replacement edited by M.G. Rossmann (28), the Proceedings from the CCP4 study weekends dedicated to molecular replacement in 1985 (29), 1992 (30), and 2001 (which will be published as a special issue in *Acta Crystallogr.* D), and the MR section in the new volume F of the *International Tables of Crystallography: Crystallography of Biological Macromolecules*.

Without pretending to be exhaustive, we quote here some important contributions in relation to rotation and translation functions, for they are the essential tools in the classical formulation of the MR method. Besides the classical article by Rossmann and Blow (1), other formulations of the rotation function are discussed by Nordman (31), Steigemann (32), and DeLano and Brünger (20). The problems of sampling and symmetry of the rotation function have been considered by Lattman (33), Moss (34), and Burdina (35). The use of NCS in self- and cross-rotation functions was first introduced by Rossmann and coworkers (36,37). The computation of the fast rotation function is discussed in Refs. 7, 38, and 39. The use of molecular scattering factors to speed up calculations was introduced by Lattman and Love (40), and in particular for fast rigid-body refinement by Huber and Schneider (19) and Navaza and coworkers (18).

Following the pioneering work of Crowther and Blow (9), many authors have contributed to the improvement of translation functions. Some of them were quoted earlier (9–17), and good reviews of classical formulations have been presented by Tickle (41,42). The symmetry of one-body translation functions is a special topic seldom discussed in the literature; the seminal reference for this is undoubtly Hirshfeld (43). Finally, a number of MR software packages are currently employed in protein crystallography. These include AMoRe (2) (both as a stand-alone program and as part of the CCP4 package), CNS (44), MOLREP (45), MERLOT (46), REPLACE (47), and EPMR (6).

REFERENCES

1. Rossmann, M.G., Blow, D.M. The detection of subunits within the crystallographic asymmetric unit. Acta Crystallogr. 15:24–31, 1962.
2. Navaza, J. AMoRe: an automated package for molecular replacement. Acta Crystallogr. A50:157–163, 1994.
3. Sheriff, S., Klei, H.E., Davis, M.E. Implementation of a six-dimensional search using the AMoRe translation function for difficult molecular-replacement problems. J. Appl. Crystallogr. 32:98–101, 1999.

4. Glykos, N.M., Kokkinidis, M. A stochastic approach to molecular replacement. Acta Crystallogr. D 56:169–174, 2000.
5. Chang, G., Lewis, M. Molecular replacement using genetic algorithms. Acta Crystallogr. D 53:279–289, 1997.
6. Kissinger, C.R., Gehlhaar, D.K., Fogel, D.B. Rapid automated molecular replacement by evolutionary search. Acta Crystallogr. D 55:484–491, 1999.
7. Crowther, R.A. The fast rotation function. In: Rossmann, M.G., ed. The molecular replacement method. A collection of papers on the use of non-crystallographic symmetry. Gordon & Breach: New York, 1972, pp. 173–178.
8. Navaza, J. Rotation function. In: Rossmann, M.G. & Arnold, E., eds. International Tables for X-ray Crystallography. Vol. F: Crystallography of biological macromolecules. International Union of Crystallography, 2001.
9. Crowther, R.A., Blow, D.M. A method of positioning a known molecule in an unknown crystal structure. Acta Crystallogr. 23:544–548, 1967.
10. Harada, Y., Lifchitz, A., Berthou, J., Jolles, P. A translation function combining packing and diffraction information: an application to lysozyme (high-temperature form). Acta Crystallogr. A37:398–406, 1981.
11. Taylor, C.A., Morley, K.A. An improved method for determining the relative positions of molecules. Acta Crystallogr. 12:101–105, 1959.
12. Fujinaga, M., Read, R.J. Experiences with a new translation function program. J. Appl. Crystallogr. 20:517, 1987.
13. Navaza, J., Vernoslova, E. On the fast translation functions for molecular replacement. Acta Crystallogr. A51:44–449, 1995.
14. Read, R.J., Schierbeek, A.J. A phased translation function. J. Appl. Crystallogr. 21: 490–495, 1988.
15. Colman, P.M., Fehlhammer, H., Bartels, K. In: Ahmed, F.R.T., Huml, K., & Sedlacek, B., eds. Crystallographic computing techniques. Munksgaard: Copenhagen, 1976, p. 248.
16. Cygler, M., Desrochers, M. A full-symmetry translation function based on electron density. Acta Crystallogr. A45:563–572, 1989.
17. Bentley, G.A., Houdusse, A. Some applications of the phased translation function in macromolecular structure determination. Acta Crystallogr. A48:312–322, 1992.
18. Castellano, E.E., Oliva, G., Navaza, J. Fast rigid-body refinement for molecular replacement techniques. J. Appl. Crystallogr. 25:281–284, 1992.
19. Huber, R., Schneider, M. A group refinement procedure in protein crystallography using Fourier transforms. J. Appl. Crystallogr. 18:165–169, 1985.
20. DeLano, W.L., Brünger, A.T. The direct rotation function: Patterson correlation search applied to molecular replacement. Acta Crystallogr. D51:740–748, 1995.
21. Le Du, M.H., Housset, D., Marchot, P., Bougis, P. E., Navaza, J., Fontecilla-Camps, J.C. Structure of fasciculin 2 from green mamba snake venom: evidence for unusual loop flexibility. Acta Crystallogr. D52:87–92, 1996.
22. Parsiegla, G., Juy, M., Reverbel-Leroy, C., Tardif, C., Belaich, J. P., Driguez, H., Haser, R. The crystal structure of the processive endocellulase CelF of

Clostridium cellulolyticum in complex with a thiooligosaccharide inhibitor at 2.0-Å resolution. EMBO J. 17:5551–5562, 1998.

23. Strynadka, N.C., Jensen, S.E., Alzari, P.M., James, M.N. A potent new mode of beta-lactamase inhibition revealed by the 1.7-Å X-ray crystallographic structure of the TEM-1-BLIP complex. Nature Struct. Biol. 3:290–297, 1996.

24. Phillips, G.N., Arduini, R.M., Springer, B.A., Sligar, S.G. Crystal structure of myoglobin from a synthetic gene. Proteins: Struct, Funct, & Genet. 7:358–365, 1990.

25. Lepault, J., Petitpas, I., Erk, I., Navaza, J., Bigot, D., Dona, M., Vachette, P., Cohen, J., Rey, F.A. Structural polymorphism of the major capsid protein of rotavirus. EMBO J. 2:1498–1507, 2001.

26. Dominguez, R., Souchon, H., Spinelli, S., Dauter, Z., Wilson, K. S., Chauvaux, S., Béguin, P., Alzari, P.M. A common protein fold and similar active site in two distinct families of beta-glycanases. Nature Struct. Biol. 2:569–576, 1995.

27. Marina, A., Alzari, P. M., Bravo, J., Uriarte, M.,Barcelona, B., Fita, I., Rubio, V. Carbamate kinase: new structural machinery for making carbamoyl phosphate, the common precursor of pyrimidines and arginine. Protein Sci. 8:934–940, 1999.

28. Rossmann, M.G., ed. The Molecular Replacement Method. Gordon and Breach: New York, 1972.

29. Machin, P.A., ed. Molecular Replacement. Proceedings of the Daresbury study weekend. SERC: Daresbury Laboratory, 1985.

30. Dodson, E.J., Gover, S., Wolf, W., eds. Molecular Replacement. Proceedings of the CCP4 study weekend. SERC: Daresbury Laboratory, 1992.

31. Nordman, C.E. Vector space search and refinement procedures. Transactions of the Am. Cryst. Assoc. 2: 29–38, 1966.

32. Steigemann, W. PhD dissertation, Technische Universitat, München, 1974.

33. Lattman, E.E. Optimal sampling of the rotation function. Acta Crystallogr. B28:1065–1068, 1972.

34. Moss, D.S. The symmetry of the rotation function. Acta Crystallogr. A41:470–475, 1985.

35. Burdina, V.I. Symmetry of the rotation function. Soviet Phys. Crystallogr. 15:545–550, 1971.

36. Rossmann, M.G., Ford, G.C., Watson, H.C., Banaszak, L.J. Molecular symmetry of glyceraldehyde-3-phosphate dehydrogenase. J. Mol. Biol. 64:237–245, 1972.

37. Tong, L., Rossmann, M.G. The locked rotation function. Acta Crystallogr. A46:783–792, 1990.

38. Dodson, E.J. Molecular replacement: the method and its problems. In: Machin, P.A., ed. Molecular Replacement. Proceedings of the Daresbury study weekend. SERC: Daresbury Laboratory, 1985, pp. 33–45.

39. Navaza, J. On the computation of the fast rotation function. Acta Crystallogr. D49:588–591, 1993.

40. Lattman, E.E., Love, W.E. A rotational search procedure for detecting a known molecule in a crystal. Acta Crystallogr. B26:1854–1857, 1970.

41. Tickle, I.J. Review of space group general translation functions that make use of known structure information and can be expanded as Fourier series. In: Machin, P.A., ed. Molecular Replacement. Proceedings of the Daresbury study weekend. SERC: Daresbury Laboratory, 1985, pp. 22–26.

42. Tickle, I.J. Fast Fourier transform functions. In: Dodson, E.J., Gover, S., & Wolf, W., eds. Molecular Replacement. Proceedings of the CCP4 study weekend. SERC: Daresbury Laboratory, 1992, pp. 20–31.

43. Hirshfeld, D. Symmetry in the generation of trial structures. Acta Crystallogr. 24:301–311, 1968.

44. Brünger, A.T. Patterson correlation searches and refinement. Methods Enzymol. 276:558–580, 1997.

45. Vagin, A., Teplyakov, A. MOLREP: an automated program for molecular replacement. J. Appl. Crystallogr. 30:1022–1025, 1997.

46. Fitzgerald, P.M.D. MERLOT, an integrated package of computer programs for the determination of crystal structures by molecular replacement. J. Appl. Crystallogr. 21:273–278, 1988.

47. Tong, L. REPLACE, a suite of computer programs for molecular replacement. J. Appl. Crystallogr. 26:48–751, 1993.

7

Comparative Protein Structure Modeling

András Fiser and Andrej Sali
The Rockefeller University, New York, New York, U.S.A.

1 INTRODUCTION

Functional characterization of a protein sequence is one of the most frequent problems in biology. This task is usually facilitated by an accurate three-dimensional (3D) structure of the studied protein. A three-dimensional structure of natural proteins is guided by two distinct sets of principles operating on vastly different time scales: the laws of physics and the theory of evolution. Each of the two sets of principles that apply to the natural protein sequences gave rise to a class of protein structure prediction methods (Fig. 1) (Baker and Sali, 2001; Fiser et al., 2002).

The first approach, de novo or ab initio methods, predict the structure from sequence alone, without relying on similarity at the fold level between the modeled sequence and any of the known structures (Bonneau, Baker, 2001). The de novo methods assume that the native structure corresponds to the global free-energy minimum accessible during the lifespan of the protein and attempt to find this minimum by an exploration of many conceivable protein conformations. The two key components of de novo methods are the procedure for efficiently carrying out the conformational search and the free-energy function used for evaluating possible conformations.

The second class of methods, including threading (Domingues et al., 2000) and comparative modeling (Blundell et al., 1987; Marti-Renom et al.,

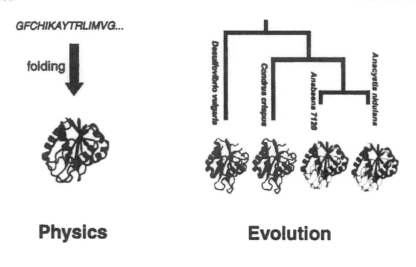

Figure 1 De novo structure prediction and comparative protein structure modeling. Proteins obey two distinct sets of principles, the laws of physics and the theory of evolution, each giving rise to the corresponding variety of protein structure prediction methods. (From Fiser et al., 2002.)

2000), rely on detectable similarity spanning most of the modeled sequence and at least one known structure. When the structure of one protein in the family has been determined by experiment, the other members of the family can be modeled based on their alignment to the known structure.

Comparative, or homology, protein structure modeling builds a three-dimensional model for a protein of unknown structure (the target) based on one or more related proteins of known structure (the templates) (Blundell et al., 1987; Greer, 1981; Johnson et al., 1994; Sali, Blundell, 1993; Sali, 1995; Sanchez, Sali, 1997a; Marti-Renom et al., 2000; Fiser et al., 2001; Fiser et al., 2002; Sanchez, Sali, 2000; Fiser, Sali, 2002). The necessary conditions for calculating a useful model are (1) detectable similarity between the target sequence and the template structures and (2) availability of a correct alignment between them. The comparative approach to protein structure prediction is possible because a small change in the protein sequence usually results in a small change in its 3D structure (Chothia, Lesk, 1986). It is also facilitated by the fact that 3D structure of proteins from the same family is more conserved than their primary sequences (Lesk, Chothia, 1980). Therefore, if similarity between two proteins is detectable at the sequence level, structural similarity can usually be assumed. Moreover, proteins that share low or even nondetectable sequence similarity many times also have similar structures. Despite progress in ab initio protein structure prediction (Bonneau, Baker, 2001), comparative modeling remains the only method that can reliably predict the 3D structure of a protein with an accuracy comparable to a low-resolution experimentally determined structure (Marti-Renom et al., 2000).

All current comparative modeling methods consist of five sequential steps (Fig. 2). The first step is to search for proteins with known 3D structures that are related to the target sequence. The second step is to pick those structures that will be used as templates. The third step is to align their sequences with the target sequence. The fourth step is to build the model for the target sequence given its alignment with the template structures. The last step is to evaluate the model using a variety of criteria. If necessary, template selection, alignment, and model building can be repeated until a satisfactory model is obtained.

Currently, the probability of finding related proteins of known structure for a sequence picked randomly from an organism's genome ranges approximately from 30% to 65%, depending on which genome is examined (Kelley et al., 2000; Sanchez, Sali, 1998; Teichmann et al., 1999; Pieper et al., 2002). Approximately 57% of all known sequences have at least one domain that is detectably related to at least one protein of known structure (Pieper et al., 2002). Since the number of known protein sequences is approximately 1,200,000 (Benson et al., 2002; Bairoch, Apweiler, 2000), comparative modeling can be applied to domains in approximately 600,000 proteins. This number is an order of magnitude larger than the number of experimentally determined protein structures deposited in the Protein Data Bank (PDB) ($\sim$ 15,000) (Westbrook et al., 2002). Furthermore, the usefulness of comparative modeling is steadily increasing because the number of different structural folds that proteins adopt is limited (Chothia, 1992; Lo et al., 2000; Holm, Sander, 1997; Bray et al., 2000) and because the number of experimentally determined novel structures is increasing. This trend is accentuated by the recently initiated structural genomics project that aims to determine at least one structure for most protein families (Burley et al., 1999). It is conceivable that this aim will be substantially achieved in less than 10 years, making comparative modeling applicable to most protein sequences (Vitkup et al., 2001).

There are several computer programs and Web servers that automate the comparative modeling process. The first Web server for automated comparative modeling was the Swiss-Model server (http://www.expasy.ch/swissmod/), followed by CPHModels (http://www.cbs.dtu.dk/services/CPHmodels/), SDSC1 (http://cl.sdsc.edu/hm.html), FAMS (http://physchem.pharm.kitasato-u.ac.jp/FAMS/fams.html), and ModWeb

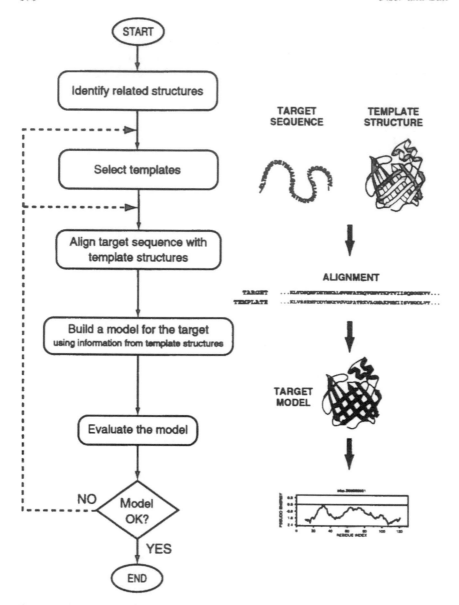

Figure 2 Steps in comparative protein structure modeling. See text for a description of each step. (From Fiser et al., 2001.)

(http://guitar.rockefeller.edu/modweb). These servers accept a sequence from a user and return an all-atom comparative model when possible. In addition to modeling a given sequence, ModWeb is capable of returning comparative models for all sequences in the TrEMBL database that are detectably related to an input, user-provided structure. While the Web servers are convenient and useful, the best results in the difficult or unusual modeling cases, such as problematic alignments, modeling of loops, existence of multiple conformational states, and modeling of ligand binding, are still obtained by nonautomated, expert use of the various modeling tools. A number of resources useful in comparative modeling are listed in Table 1.

This chapter begins with a description of all the steps in comparative modeling, fold assignment, template selection, sequence-structure alignment, model building, and model assessment. We conclude by describing errors in comparative models and sample applications of comparative modeling to individual proteins and to whole genomes. We emphasize our own work and experience, although we have profited greatly from the contributions of many others, cited in the list of references.

2   STEPS IN COMPARATIVE MODELING

2.1   Searching for Structures Related to the Target Sequence

Comparative modeling usually starts by searching the PDB (Westbrook et al., 2002) of known protein structures using the target sequence as the query. This search is generally done by comparing the target sequence with the sequence of each of the structures in the database.

There are three main classes of protein comparison methods that are useful in fold identification. The first class compares the target sequence with each of the database sequences independently, using pairwise sequence-sequence comparison (Apostolico, Giancarlo, 1998). The performance of these methods in sequence searching (Pearson, 2000; Pearson, 1995) and fold assignments has been evaluated exhaustively (Brenner et al., 1998). The most popular programs in the class include FASTA (Pearson, 2000) and BLAST (Altschul et al., 1997).

The second class of methods relies on multiple sequence comparisons to improve greatly the sensitivity of the search (Henikoff et al., 2000; Krogh et al., 1994; Gribskov, Veretnik, 1996; Altschul et al., 1997; Jaroszewski et al., 1998). The most well known program in this class is PSI-BLAST (Altschul et al., 1997). Another, similar approach that appears to perform even slightly better than PSI-BLAST has been implemented in the program PDB-BLAST (Jaroszewski et al., 1998). PDB-BLAST begins by finding all

Table 1 Programs and Servers Useful for Comparative Protein Structure Modeling

Databases
NCBI	www.ncbi.nlm.nih.gov/
PDB	www.rcsb.org/
MSD	www.rcsb.org/databases.html
CATH	www.biochem.ucl.ac.uk/bsm/cath/
TrEMBL	srs.ebi.ac.uk/
Scop	scop.mrc-lmb.cam.ac.uk/scop/
Presage	presage.stanford.edu
ModBase	guitar.rockefeller.edu/modbase/
GeneCensus	bioinfo.mbb.yale.edu/genome
GeneBank	www.ncbi.nlm.nih.gov.Genbank/GenbankSearch.html
PSI	www.structuralgenomics.org

Template Search, fold assignment
PDB-Blast	bioinformatics.burnham-inst.org/pdb_blast
BLAST	www.ncbi.nlm.nih.gov/BLAST/
FastA	www.ebi.ac.uk/fasta33
DALI	www2.ebi.ac.uk/dali/
PhD, TOPITS	www.embl-heidelberg.de/predictprotein/predictprotein/html
THREADER	bioinf.cs.ucl.ac.uk/threader/
123D	123d.ncifcrf.gov
UCLA-DOE	fold.doe-mbi.ucla.edu
PROFIT	lore.came.sbg.ac.at/
MATCHMAKER	www.tripos.com/software/mm.html
3D-PSSM	www.sbg.bio.ic.ac.uk/~3dppsm
BIOINBGU	www.cs.bgu.ac.il/~bioinbgu/
FUGUE	www.cryst.bioc.cam.ac.uk/~fugue
LOOPP	ser-loopp.tc.cornell.edu/loopp.html
FASS	bioinformatics.burnham-inst.org/FFAS/index.html
SAM-T99/T98	www.cse.ucsc.edu/research/compbio/sam.html

Comparative modeling
3D-JIGSAW	www.bmm.icnet.uk/servers/3djigsaw/
CPH-Models	www.cbs.dtu.dk/services/CPHmodels/
COMPOSER	www-cryst.bioc.cam.ac.uk/
FAMS	physchem.pharm.kitasato-u.ac.jp/FAMS/fams.html
Modeller	guitar.rockefeller.edu/modeller/modeller/html
PrISM	honiglab.cpmc.columbia.edu/
SWISS-MODEL	www.expasy.ch/swissmod/SWISS-MODEL.html
SDSC1	cl.sdsc.edu.hm.html
WHAT IF	www.combi.kun.nl/whatif/
ICM	www.molsoft.com/
SCWRL	www.fccc.edu/research/labs/dunbrack/scwrl/

Table 1 *Continued*

InsightII	www.accelrys.com
SYBYL	www.tripos.com
Model evaluation	
PROCHECK	www.biochem.ucl.ac.uk/~roman/procheck/procheck.html
WHATCHECK	www.cmbi.kun.nl/gv/servers/WIWWWI/
Prosall	www.came.sbg.ac.at
BIOTECH	biotech.embl-ebi.ac.uk:8400/
VERIFY3D	www.doe.mbi.ucla.edu/Services.Verify_3D/
ERRAT	www.doe-mbi.ucla.edu/Services/Errat.html
ANOLEA	guitar.rockefeller.edu/~fmelo/anolea/anolea.html
AQUA	urchin.bmrb.wisc.edu/~jurgen/Aqua/server/
SQUID	www.yorvic.york.ac.uk/~oldfield/squid
PROVE	www.ucmb.ulb.ac.be/UCMB/PROVE/

An up-to-date version of this table can be found on the Web at http://guitar.rockefeller.edu/bioinformatics_resources.shtml.

sequences in a sequence database that are clearly related to the target and easily aligned with it. The multiple alignment of these sequences is the target sequence profile. Similar profiles are also constructed for all potential template structures. The templates are then found by comparing the target sequence profile with each of the template sequence profiles, using a local dynamic programming method that relies on the common BLOSUM62 residue substitution matrix (Henikoff, Henikoff, 2000). These more sensitive fold identification techniques based on sequence profiles are especially useful for finding structural relationships when sequence identity between the target and the template drops below 25%.

The third class of methods relies on pairwise comparison of a protein sequence and a protein structure; that is, structural information is used for one of the two proteins that are being compared, and the target sequence is matched against a library of 3D profiles or threaded through a library of 3D folds. These methods are also called fold assignment, threading, or 3D template matching (Johnson, Overington, 1993; Bowie et al., 1991; D.T Jones et al., 1992; Godzik, 1996; Sippl, 1995). They are reviewed in D.T. Jones, 1997; Smith et al., 1997; and Torda, 1997, and evaluated in Domingues et al., 2000. These methods are especially useful when sequence profiles are not possible to construct because there are not enough known sequences that are clearly related to the target or potential templates.

What similarity between the target and template sequences is needed to have a chance of obtaining a useful comparative model? The answer depends on the question that is asked of a model. In general, the usefulness of a template should be assessed by evaluation of the corresponding 3D model based on a given template, using methods described later. This approach is optimal because the evaluation of a 3D model is generally more sensitive and robust than the evaluation of an alignment (Sanchez, Sali, 1998). A good starting point for template searches are the many database search servers on the Web (Table 1).

2.2 Selecting Templates

Once a list of potential templates is obtained using searching methods, it is necessary to select one or more templates that are appropriate for the particular modeling problem. Several factors need to be taken into account when selecting a template.

The quality of a template increases with its overall sequence similarity to the target and decreases with the number and length of gaps in the alignment. The simplest template selection rule is to select the structure with the highest sequence similarity to the modeled sequence.

The family of proteins that includes the target and the templates can frequently be organized into subfamilies. The construction of a multiple alignment and a phylogenetic tree (Retief, 2000; Felsenstein, 1981) can help in selecting the template from the subfamily that is closest to the target sequence.

The similarity between the "environment" of the template and the environment in which the target needs to be modeled should also be considered. The term *environment* is used here in a broad sense, including everything that is not the protein itself (e.g., solvent, pH, ligands, quaternary interactions). If possible, a template bound to the same or similar ligands as the modeled sequence should generally be used.

The quality of the experimentally determined structure is another important factor in template selection. The resolution and R-factor of a crystallographic structure and the number of restraints per residue for an NMR structure are indicative of the accuracy of the structure. For instance, if two templates have comparable sequence similarity to the target, the one determined at the highest resolution should generally be used.

The criteria for selecting templates also depend on the purpose of a comparative model. For example, if a protein–ligand model is to be constructed, the choice of the template that contains a similar ligand is probably more important than the resolution of the template. On the other hand, if the model is to be used to analyze the geometry of the active site of an enzyme, it may be preferable to use a high-resolution template structure.

It is not necessary to select only one template. In fact, the use of several templates generally increases the model accuracy. One strength of the comparative modeling program MODELLER (Sali, Blundell, 1993) is that it can combine information from multiple template structures, in two ways. First, multiple template structures may be aligned with different domains of the target, with little overlap between them, in which case the modeling procedure can construct a homology-based model of the whole target sequence. Second, the template structures may be aligned with the same part of the target, in which case the modeling procedure is likely to automatically build the model on the locally best template (Sanchez, Sali, 1997b; Sali et al., 1995). In general, it is frequently beneficial to include in the modeling process all the templates that differ substantially from each other, if they share approximately the same overall similarity to the target sequence.

An elaborate way to select suitable templates is to generate and evaluate models for each candidate template structure and/or their combinations. The optimized all-atom models are evaluated by an energy or scoring function, such as the Z-score of PROSA (Sippl, 1993). The PROSA Z-score of a model is a measure of compatibility between its sequence and its structure. Ideally, the Z-score of the model should be comparable to the Z-score of the template. The PROSA Z-score is frequently sufficiently accurate to identify one of the most accurate of the generated models (Wu et al., 2000). This trial-and-error approach can be viewed as limited threading (i.e., the target sequence is threaded through similar template structures).

2.3 Aligning the Target Sequence with One or More Structures

To build a model, all comparative modeling programs depend on a list of assumed structural equivalences between the target and template residues. This list is defined by an alignment of the target and template sequences. Although many template search methods will produce such an alignment, it is usually not the optimal target–template alignment in the more difficult alignment cases (e.g., at less than 30% sequence identity). Search methods tend to be tuned for the detection of remote relationships, not for optimal alignment. Therefore, once the templates are selected, an alignment method should be used to align them with the target sequence.

The alignment is relatively simple to obtain when the target–template sequence identity is above 40%. In most such cases, an accurate alignment can be calculated automatically using standard sequence–sequence alignment methods. If the target–template sequence identity is lower than 40%, the alignment generally has gaps and needs manual intervention to minimize the number of misaligned residues. In these low-sequence identity cases, the alignment accuracy is the most important factor affecting the quality of the resulting model. Alignments can be improved by including structural information from the template. For example, gaps should be avoided in secondary structure elements, in buried regions, or between two residues that are far apart in space. Some alignment methods take such criteria into account (Sanchez, Sali, 1998; Jennings et al., 2001; Blake, Cohen, 2001; Shi et al., 2001). It is important to inspect and edit the alignment in view of the template structure, especially if the target–template sequence identity is low. A misalignment by only one residue position will result in an error of approximately 4Å in the model because the current modeling methods generally cannot recover from errors in the alignment.

When multiple templates are selected, a good strategy is to superpose them with each other first, to obtain a multiple structure–based alignment. In the next step, the target sequence is aligned with this multiple structure–based alignment. Another improvement is to calculate the target and template sequence profiles, by aligning them with all sequences from a nonredundant sequence database that are sufficiently similar to the target and template sequences, respectively, so that they can be aligned without significant errors (e.g., better than 40% sequence identity). The final target–template alignment is then obtained by aligning the two profiles, not the template and target sequences alone. The use of multiple structures and multiple sequences benefits from the evolutionary and structural information about the templates as well as evolutionary information about the target sequence, and often produces a better alignment for modeling than the pairwise sequence alignment methods (Sauder et al., 2000; Jaroszewski et al., 2000).

2.4 Model Building

2.4.1 Modeling by Assembly of Rigid Bodies

The first and still widely used approach in comparative modeling is to assemble a model from a small number of rigid bodies obtained from the aligned protein structures (Greer, 1990; Blundell et al., 1987; Browne et al., 1969). The approach is based on the natural dissection of the protein structure into conserved core regions, variable loops that connect them, and side chains that decorate the backbone. For example, the following semiautomated procedure is implemented in the computer program COMPOSER (Sutcliffe et al., 1987). First, the template structures are selected and superposed. Second, the "framework" is calculated by averaging the coordinates of the C_α atoms of structurally conserved regions in the template structures. Third, the mainchain atoms of each core region in the target model are obtained by superposing on the framework the core segment from the template whose sequence is closest to the target. Fourth, the loops are generated by scanning a database of all known protein structures to identify the structurally variable regions that fit the anchor core regions and have a compatible sequence (Topham et al., 1993). Fifth, the side chains are modeled based on their intrinsic conformational preferences and on the conformation of the equivalent side chains in the template structures (Sutcliffe et al., 1987). And finally, the stereochemistry of the model is improved by either a restrained energy minimization or a molecular dynamics refinement. The accuracy of a model can be somewhat increased when more than one template structure is used to construct the framework and when the templates are averaged into the framework using weights corresponding to their sequence similarities to the target sequence (Srinivasan, Blundell, 1993). For example, differences between the model and X-ray structures may be slightly smaller than the differences between the X-ray structures of the modeled protein and the homologs used to build the model. Possible future improvements of modeling by rigid-body assembly include incorporation of rigid-body shifts, such as the relative shifts in the packing of α-helices and β-sheets (Reddy, Blundell, 1993; Nagarajaram et al., 1999).

2.4.2 Modeling by Segment Matching or Coordinate Reconstruction

The basis of modeling by coordinate reconstruction is the finding that most hexapeptide segments of protein structure can be clustered into only 100 structurally different classes (Unger et al., 1989; Bystroff, Baker, 1998). Thus, comparative models can be constructed by using a subset of atomic positions from template structures as "guiding" positions and by identifying and assembling short, all-atom segments that fit these guiding positions. The guiding positions usually correspond to the $C\alpha$ atoms of the segments that are conserved in the alignment between the template structure and the target sequence. The all-atom segments that fit the guiding positions can be obtained either by scanning all the known protein structures, including those that are not related to the sequence being modeled (Claessens et al., 1989; Holm, Sander, 1991), or by a conformational search restrained by an energy function (Bruccoleri, Karplus, 1990; van Gelder et al., 1994). For example, a general method for modeling by segment matching is guided by the positions of some atoms (usually $C\alpha$ atoms) to find the matching segments in the representative database of all known protein structures (Levitt, 1992). This method can construct both main-chain and side chain atoms and can also model gaps. It is implemented in the program SegMod. Even some side-chain modeling methods (Chinea et al., 1995) and the class of loop construction methods based on finding suitable fragments in the database of known structures

(Jones, Thirup, 1986) can be seen as segment matching or coordinate reconstruction methods.

2.4.3 Modeling by Satisfaction of Spatial Restraints

The methods in this class begin by generating many constraints or restraints on the structure of the target sequence, using its alignment to related protein structures as a guide. The procedure is conceptually similar to that used in determination of protein structures from NMR-derived restraints. The restraints are generally obtained by assuming that the corresponding distances between aligned residues in the template and the target structures are similar. These homology-derived restraints are usually supplemented by stereochemical restraints on bond lengths, bond angles, dihedral angles, and nonbonded atom–atom contacts that are obtained from a molecular mechanics force field. The model is then derived by minimizing the violations of all the restraints. This can be achieved by either distance geometry or real-space optimization. For example, an elegant distance geometry approach constructs all-atom models from lower and upper bounds on distances and dihedral angles (Havel, Snow, 1991). Lower and upper bounds on $C\alpha$–$C\alpha$ and main-chain–side-chain distances, hydrogen bonds, and conserved dihedral angles were derived for *E. coli* flavodoxin from four other flavodoxins; bounds were calculated for all distances and dihedral angles that had equivalent atoms in the template structures. The allowed range of values of a distance or a dihedral angle depended on the degree of structural variability at the corresponding position in the template structures. Distance geometry was used to obtain an ensemble of approximate 3D models, which were then exhaustively refined by restrained molecular dynamics with simulated annealing in water.

2.4.4 Modeling by Satisfaction of Spatial Restraints in the MODELLER Program

We now describe our own approach in more detail (Sali et al., 1990; Sali, Blundell, 1993; Fiser et al., 2000; Sali, Overington, 1994) (Fig. 3). The approach was developed to use as many different types of data about the target sequence as possible. It is implemented in the computer program MODELLER (Table 1). The comparative modeling procedure begins with an alignment of the target sequence with related known 3D structures. The output, obtained without any user intervention, is a 3D model for the target sequence containing all main-chain and side-chain non-hydrogen atoms.

In the first step of model building, distance and dihedral angle restraints on the target sequence are derived from its alignment with tem-

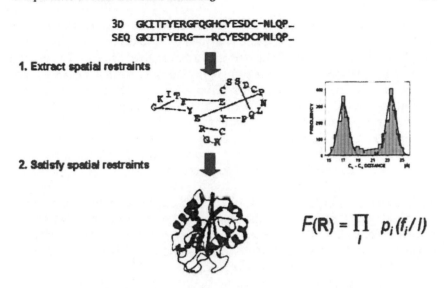

1. Extract spatial restraints

2. Satisfy spatial restraints

$$F(\mathbf{R}) = \prod_i p_i(f_i/I)$$

Figure 3 Comparative protein structure modeling by satisfaction of spatial restraints as implemented in MODELLER. First, spatial restraints are extracted from the input alignment, general spatial preferences found in known protein structures, and a molecular mechanics force field. Second, all the restraints are combined into an objective function that is optimized to obtain the final model.

plate 3D structures. The form of these restraints was obtained from a statistical analysis of the relationships between similar protein structures. The analysis relied on a database of 105 family alignments that included 416 proteins of known 3D structure (Sali, Overington, 1994). By scanning the database of alignments, tables quantifying various correlations were obtained, such as the correlations between two equivalent $C\alpha$–$C\alpha$ distances or between equivalent main-chain dihedral angles from two related proteins (Sali, Blundell, 1993). These relationships are expressed as conditional probability density functions (pdf's) and can be used directly as spatial restraints. For example, probabilities for different values of the main-chain dihedral angles are calculated from the type of a residue considered, from main-chain conformation of an equivalent residue, and from sequence similarity between the two proteins. Another example is the pdf for a certain $C\alpha$–$C\alpha$ distance given equivalent distances in two related protein structures. An important feature of the method is that the forms of spatial restraints were obtained empirically, from a database of protein structure alignments.

In the second step, the spatial restraints and the CHARMM22 force-field terms enforcing proper stereochemistry (MacKerell Jr. et al., 1998; Brooks III et al., 1983) are combined into an objective function. The general form of the objective function is similar to that in molecular dynamics programs, such as CHARMM22 (Brooks III et al., 1983). The objective function depends on the Cartesian coordinates of the atoms (3D points) that form the modeled molecules. For a 10,000-atom system, there can be on the order of 200,000 restraints. The functional form of each term is simple; it includes a quadratic function, harmonic lower and upper bounds, cosine, a weighted sum of a few Gaussian functions, Coulomb's law, Lennard–Jones potential, and cubic splines. The geometric features presently include a distance, an angle, a dihedral angle, a pair of dihedral angles between two, three, four, and eight atoms, respectively, the shortest distance in the set of distances, solvent accessibility in Å^2, and atom density, expressed as the number of atoms around the central atom. Some restraints can be used to restrain pseudo-atoms, such as the gravity center of several atoms.

Finally, the model is obtained by optimizing the objective function in Cartesian space. The optimization is carried out by the use of the variable target function method (Braun, Go, 1985), employing methods of conjugate gradients and molecular dynamics with simulated annealing (Clore et al., 1986). Several slightly different models can be calculated by varying the initial structure, and the variability among these models can be used to estimate the lower bound on the errors in the corresponding regions of the fold.

Because the modeling by satisfaction of spatial restraints can use many different types of information about the target sequence, it is perhaps the most promising of all comparative modeling techniques. One of the strengths of modeling by satisfaction of spatial restraints is that constraints or restraints derived from a number of different sources can easily be added to the homology-derived restraints. For example, restraints could be provided by rules for secondary structure packing (Cohen, Kuntz, 1989), analyses of hydrophobicity (Aszodi, Taylor, 1994) and correlated mutations (Taylor, Hatrick, 1994), empirical potentials of mean force (Sippl, 1990), nuclear magnetic resonance (NMR) experiments (Sutcliffe et al., 1992), cross-linking experiments, fluorescence spectroscopy, image reconstruction in electron microscopy, site-directed mutagenesis (Boissel et al., 1993), intuition, *etc.* In this way, a comparative model, especially in the difficult cases, could be improved by making it consistent with available experimental data and/or with more general knowledge about protein structure.

Accuracies of the various model building methods are relatively similar when used optimally (Marti-Renom et al., 2002). Other factors, such as template selection and alignment accuracy, usually have a larger impact on the model accuracy, especially for models based on less than 40% sequence identity to the templates. However, it is important that a modeling method allow a degree of flexibility and automation to obtain better models more easily and rapidly. For example, a method should allow for an easy recalculation of a model when a change is made in the alignment; it should be straightforward to calculate models based on several templates; and the method should provide tools for incorporation of prior knowledge about the target (e.g., cross-linking restraints, predicted secondary structure) and allow *ab initio* modeling of insertions (e.g., loops), which can be crucial for annotation of function. Loop modeling is an especially important aspect of comparative modeling in the range from 30% to 50% sequence identity. In this range of overall similarity, loops among the homologs vary, while the core regions are still relatively conserved and aligned accurately. Next, we review loop modeling.

2.4.5 Loop Modeling

In comparative modeling, target sequences often have inserted residues relative to the template structures or have regions that are structurally different from the corresponding regions in the templates. Thus, no structural information about these inserted segments can be extracted from the template structures. These regions frequently correspond to surface loops. Loops often play an important role in defining the functional specificity of a given protein framework, forming the active and binding sites. The accuracy of loop modeling is a major factor determining the usefulness of comparative models in applications such as ligand docking. Loop modeling can be seen as a mini-protein-folding problem because the correct conformation of a given segment of a polypeptide chain has to be calculated mainly from the sequence of the segment itself. However, loops are generally too short to provide sufficient information about their local fold. Even identical decapeptides in different proteins do not always have the same conformation (Kabsch, Sander, 1984; Mezei, 1998). Some additional restraints are provided by the core anchor regions that span the loop and by the structure of the rest of a protein that cradles the loop. Although many loop-modeling methods have been described, it is still not possible to model correctly and with high confidence loops longer than approximately eight residues (Fiser et al., 2000).

There are two main classes of loop-modeling methods: (1) the database search approaches, where a segment that fits on the anchor core regions is found in a database of all known protein structures (T.A. Jones, Thirup, 1986; Chothia, Lesk, 1987); (2) the conformational search approaches (Moult, James, 1986; Bruccoleri, Karplus, 1987; Shenkin et al., 1987).

There are also methods that combine these two approaches (van Vlijmen, Karplus, 1997; Deane, Blundell, 2001).

The database search approach to loop modeling is accurate and efficient when a database of specific loops is created to address the modeling of the same class of loops, such as β-hairpins (Sibanda et al., 1989), or loops on a specific fold, such as the hypervariable regions in the immunoglobulin fold (Chothia et al., 1989; Chothia, Lesk, 1987). For example, an analysis of the hypervariable immunoglobulin regions resulted in a series of rules that allowed a very high accuracy of loop prediction in other members of the family. These rules were based on the small number of conformations for each loop and on the dependence of the loop conformation on its length and certain key residues. There are attempts to classify loop conformations into more general categories, thus extending the applicability of the database search approach to more cases (Rufino et al., 1997; Oliva et al., 1997; Ring et al., 1992). However, the database methods are limited by the fact that the number of possible conformations increases exponentially with the length of a loop. As a result, only loops up to four to seven residues long have most of their conceivable conformations present in the database of known protein structures (Fidelis et al., 1994; Lessel, Schomburg, 1994). Even according to the more optimistic estimate, approximately 30% and 60% of all the possible eight- and nine-residue loop conformations, respectively, are missing from the database (Fidelis et al., 1994). This is made even worse by the requirement for an overlap of at least one residue between the database fragment and the anchor core regions, which means that the modeling of a five-residue insertion requires at least a seven-residue fragment from the database (Claessens et al., 1989). Despite the rapid growth of the database of known structures, there is no possibility to cover most of the conformations of a nine-residue segment in the foreseeable future. On the other hand, most of the insertions in a family of homologous proteins are shorter than 10–12 residues (Fiser et al., 2000).

To overcome the limitations of the database search methods, conformational search methods were developed (Moult, James, 1986; Bruccoleri, Karplus, 1987). There are many such methods, exploiting different protein representations, objective function terms, and optimization or enumeration algorithms. The search algorithms include the minimum perturbation method (Fine et al., 1986), molecular dynamics simulations (Bruccoleri, Karplus, 1990; van Vlijmen, Karplus, 1997), genetic algorithms (Ring, Cohen, 1993), Monte Carlo and simulated annealing (Abagyan, Totrov, 1994; Collura et al., 1993; Higo et al., 1992), multiple-copy simultaneous search (Zheng et al., 1993; Zheng et al., 1994), self-consistent field optimization (Koehl, Delarue, 1995), and an enumeration based on graph theory (Samudrala, Moult, 1998).

The loop-modeling module in MODELLER implements the optimization-based approach (Fiser et al., 2000; Fiser et al., 2002). The main reasons are the generality and conceptual simplicity of energy minimization, as well as the limitations on the database approach imposed by a relatively small number of known protein structures (Fidelis et al., 1994). Loop prediction by optimization is applicable to simultaneous modeling of several loops and loops interacting with ligands, which is not straightforward for the database search approaches. Loop optimization in MODELLER relies on conjugate gradients and molecular dynamics with simulated annealing. The pseudo-energy function is a sum of many terms, including some terms from the CHARMM-22 molecular mechanics force field (MacKerell Jr. et al., 1998) and spatial restraints based on distributions of distances (Sippl, 1990) and dihedral angles in known protein structures. The method was tested on a large number of loops of known structure, both in the native and near-native environments. In the case of five-residue loops in the correct environments, the average error was 0.6 Å, as measured by local superposition of the loop main-chain atoms alone. For eight-residue loops in the correct environments, 90% of the loops had less than 2-Å main-chain RMS error, with an average of less than 1.2 Å. Even 12-residue loops are modeled with useful accuracy in 30% of the cases. To simulate comparative modeling problems, the loop-modeling procedure was evaluated by predicting loops of known structure in only approximately correct environments. Such environments were obtained by distorting the anchor regions, corresponding to the three residues at either end of the loop, and all the atoms within 10 Å of the native loop conformation for up to 2–3 Å by molecular dynamics simulations. When the RMSD distortion of the environment atoms is 2.5 Å, the average loop prediction error increases by 180%, 25% and 3% for 4-, 8- and 12-residue loops, respectively. It is no longer too optimistic to expect useful models for loops as long as 12 residues, if the environment of the loop is at least approximately correct. It is possible to estimate whether or not a given loop prediction is correct, based on the structural variability of the independently derived lowest-energy loop conformations. Typically, the loop prediction corresponds to the lowest-energy conformation out of the 500 independent optimizations. The algorithm allows straightforward incorporation of additional spatial restraints, including those provided by template fragments, disulfide bonds, and ligand binding sites.

2.5 Evaluating a Model

After a model is built, it is important to check it for possible errors. The quality of a model can be predicted approximately from the sequence similarity between the target and the template (Figs. 2, 5, 7). Sequence identity above 30% is a relatively good predictor of the expected accuracy of a model. However, other factors, including the environment, can strongly influence the accuracy of a model. For instance, some calcium-binding proteins undergo large conformational changes when bound to calcium. If a calcium-free template is used to model the calcium-bound state of a target, it is likely that the model will be incorrect irrespective of the target–template similarity. This estimate also applies to determination of protein structure by experiment; a structure must be determined in the functionally meaningful environment. If the target–template sequence identity falls below 30%, the sequence identity becomes significantly less reliable as a measure of expected accuracy of a single model. The reason is that below 30% sequence identity, models are often obtained that deviate significantly, in both directions, from the average accuracy. It is in such cases that model evaluation methods are most informative.

Two types of evaluation can be carried out. "Internal" evaluation of self-consistency checks whether or not a model satisfies the restraints used to calculate it. "External" evaluation relies on information that was not used in the calculation of the model (Luthy et al., 1992; Sippl, 1993).

Assessment of a model's stereochemistry (e.g., bonds, bond angles, dihedral angles, and nonbonded atom–atom distances) with programs such as PROCHECK (Laskowski et al., 1993) and WHATCHECK (Hooft et al., 1996) is an example of internal evaluation. Although errors in stereochemistry are rare and less informative than errors detected by methods for external evaluation, a cluster of stereochemical errors may indicate that the corresponding region also contains other larger errors (e.g., alignment errors).

When the model is based on less than ≈30% sequence identity to the template, the first purpose of the external evaluation is to test whether or not a correct template was used. This test is especially important when the alignment is only marginally significant or several alternative templates with different folds are to be evaluated. A complication is that at low similarities the alignment generally contains many errors, making it difficult to distinguish between an incorrect template on one hand and an incorrect alignment with a correct template on the other hand. It is generally possible to recognize a correct template only if the alignment is at least approximately correct. This complication can sometimes be overcome by testing models from several alternative alignments for each template. One way to predict whether or not a template is correct is to compare the PROSA Z-score (Sippl, 1993) for the model and the template structure(s). Since the Z-score of a model is a measure of compatibility between its sequence and structure, the model Z-score should be comparable to that of the template.

However, this evaluation does not always work. For example, a well-modeled part of a domain is likely to have a bad Z-score because some interactions that stabilize the fold are not present in the model. Correct models for some membrane proteins and small disulfide-rich proteins also tend to be evaluated incorrectly, apparently because these structures have distributions of residue accessibility and residue–residue distances that are different from those for the larger globular domains, which were the source of the PROSA statistical potential function.

The second, more detailed kind of external evaluation is the prediction of unreliable regions in the model. One way to approach this problem is to calculate a "pseudo-energy" profile of a model, such as that produced by PROSA (Sippl, 1995). The profile reports the energy for each position in the model. Peaks in the profile frequently correspond to errors in the model. There are several pitfalls in the use of energy profiles for local error detection. For example, a region can be identified as unreliable only because it interacts with an incorrectly modeled region; there are also more fundamental problems (Fiser et al., 2000).

Finally, a model should be consistent with experimental observations, such as site-directed mutagenesis, cross-linking data, and ligand binding.

It is frequently difficult to select best templates or to calculate a good alignment. One way of improving a comparative model in such cases is to proceed with an iteration consisting of template selection, alignment, and model building, guided by model assessment. This iteration can be repeated until no improvement in the model is detected (Guenther et al., 1997; Sanchez, Sali, 1997b).

3 ERRORS IN COMPARATIVE MODELS

The overall accuracy of comparative models spans a wide range (Figs. 5, 7). At the low end of the spectrum are the low-resolution models, whose only essentially correct feature is their fold. At the high end of the spectrum are the models with an accuracy comparable to medium resolution crystallographic structures (Baker, Sali, 2001; Marti-Renom et al., 2000). Even low-resolution models are often useful for addressing biological questions, because function can many times be predicted from only coarse structural features of a model.

The errors in comparative models can be divided into five categories (Fig. 4): (1) errors in sidechain packing; (2) distortions or shifts of a region that is aligned correctly with the template structures; (3) distortions or shifts of a region that does not have an equivalent segment in any of the template structures; (4) distortions or shifts of a region that is aligned incorrectly with the template structures; (5) a misfolded structure resulting from using an

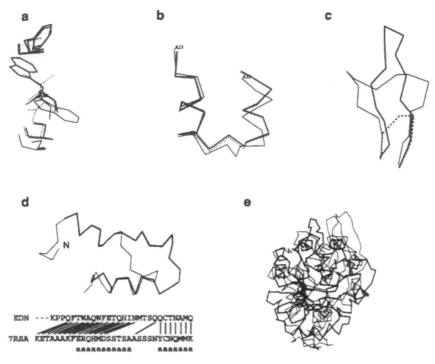

Figure 4 Errors in comparative protein structure modeling. (a) Errors in side-chain packing. The Trp 109 residue in the crystal structure of mouse cellular retinoic acid–binding protein I (thin line) is compared with its model (thick line) and with the template mouse adipocyte lipid–binding protein (broken line). (b) Distortions and shifts in correctly aligned regions. A region in the crystal structure of mouse cellular retinoic acid–binding protein I is compared with its model and with the template fatty acid–binding protein using the same representation as in panel a. (c) Errors in regions without a template. The Cα trace of the 112–117 loop is shown for the X-ray structure of human eosinophil neurotoxin (thin line), its model (thick line), and the template ribonuclease A structure (residues 111–117; broken line). (d) Errors due to misalignments. The N-terminal region in the crystal structure of human eosinophil neurotoxin (thin line) is compared with its model (thick line). The corresponding region of the alignment with the template ribonuclease A is shown. The black lines show correct equivalences, that is, residues whose Cα atoms are within 5 Å of each other in the optimal least squares superposition of the two X-ray structures. The "a" characters in the bottom line indicate helical residues. (e) Errors due to an incorrect template. The X-ray structure of α-trichosanthin (thin line) is compared with its model (thick line), which was calculated using indole-3-glycerophosphate synthase as the template. (From Fiser et al., 2001.)

incorrect template. Significant methodological improvements are needed to address all of these errors.

Errors 3–5 are relatively infrequent when sequences with more than 40% identity to the templates are modeled. For example, in such a case, approximately 90% of the main-chain atoms are likely to be modeled with an rms error of about 1 Å. In this range of sequence similarity, the alignment is mostly straightforward to construct, there are not many gaps, and structural differences between the proteins are usually limited to loops and side chains. When sequence identity is between 30% and 40%, the structural differences become larger, and the gaps in the alignment are more frequent and longer. As a result, the mainchain RMS error rises to about 1.5 Å for about 80% of residues. The rest of the residues are modeled with large errors because the methods generally fail to model structural distortions and rigid-body shifts and are unable to recover from misalignments. Below 40% sequence identity, misalignments and insertions in the target sequence become the major problems. When sequence identity drops below 30%, the main problem becomes the identification of related templates and their alignment with the sequence to be modeled (Figs. 5, 7). In general, it can be expected that about 20% of residues will be misaligned, and consequently incorrectly modeled with an error larger than 3 Å, at this level of sequence similarity (Johnson, Overington, 1993). These misalignments are a serious impediment to comparative modeling because it appears that presently at least one-half of all related protein pairs are related at less than 30% sequence identity (Rost, 1999; Sanchez, Sali, 1998).

It has been pointed out that a comparative model is frequently more distant from the actual target structure than the closest template structure used to calculate the model (Martin et al., 1997). However, at least for some modeling methods, this is only the case when there are errors in the template–target alignment used for modeling, and when the correct structure-based template–target alignment is used for comparing the template with the actual target structure (Sanchez, Sali, 1997b). In contrast, the model is generally closer to the target structure than any of the templates if the modeling target–template alignment is used in evaluating the similarity between the actual target structure and the template (Sanchez, Sali, 1997b). When more than one template is used for modeling, it is sometimes possible to obtain a model that is significantly closer to the target structure than any of the templates (Sanchez, Sali, 1997b). This improvement occurs because the model tends to inherit the best regions from each template. Therefore, using a model is generally better than using the template structure, even when the alignment is incorrect, because the actual target structure and, therefore, the correct template–target alignment are not available in practical modeling applications (Fig. 5).

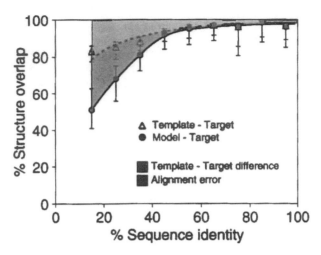

Figure 5 Average model accuracy as a function of sequence identity. As the sequence identity between the target sequence and the template structure decreases, the average structural similarity between the template and the target also decreases (dotted line, triangles). Structural overlap is defined as the fraction of equivalent $C\alpha$ atoms. For the comparison of the model with the actual structure (filled circles), two C_α atoms were considered equivalent if they belonged to the same residue and were within 3.5 Å of each other after least squares superposition of all $C\alpha$ atoms by the ALIGN3D command in MODELLER. For comparison of the template structure with the actual target structure (triangles), two $C\alpha$ atoms were considered equivalent if they were within 3.5 Å of each other after alignment and rigid-body superposition. At high sequence identities, the models are close to the templates and therefore also close to the experimental target structure (solid line, filled circles). At low sequence identities, errors in the target–template alignment become more frequent and the structural similarity of the model with the experimental target structure falls below the target–template structural similarity. The difference between the model and the actual target structure is a combination of the target–template differences (light area) and the alignment errors (dark area). The figure was constructed by calculating 3993 comparative models based on single templates of varying similarity to the targets. All targets had known (experimentally determined) structures, and therefore the comparison of the models and templates with the experimental structures was possible. (From Sanchez, Sali, 1998.)

    To put the errors in comparative models into perspective, we list the differences among structures of the same protein that have been determined experimentally (Fig. 6). The 1-Å accuracy of main-chain atom positions corresponds to X-ray structures defined at a low resolution of about 2.5 Å and with an R-factor of about 25% (Ohlendorf, 1994), as well as to medium-resolution NMR structures determined from

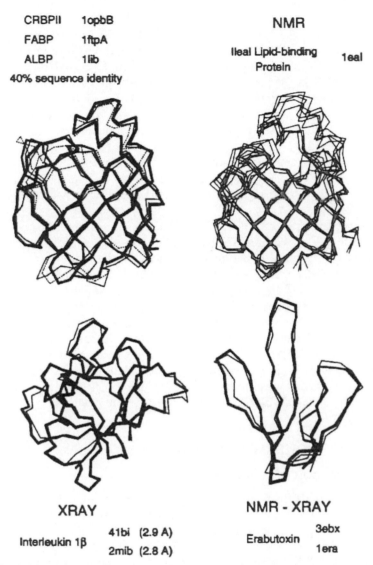

CRBPII 1opbB
FABP 1ftpA
ALBP 1lib
40% sequence identity

NMR

Ileal Lipid-binding Protein 1eal

XRAY

Interleukin 1β

41bi (2.9 A)
2mib (2.8 A)

NMR - XRAY

Erabutoxin

3ebx
1era

Figure 6 Accuracy of comparative models as compared to low-resolution crystallographic structure determination and medium-resolution NMR structure determination. *Upper left panel*: Comparison of homologous structures that share ~ 40% sequence identity. *Upper right panel*: 20 conformations of ileal lipid–binding protein that satisfy the NMR restraints equally well. *Lower left panel*: Comparison of two independently determined X-ray structures of interleukin 1β. *Lower right panel*: Comparison of the X-ray and NMR structures of erabutoxin. (From Fiser et al., 2001.)

10 interproton distance restraints per residue (Clore et al., 1993). Similarly, differences between the highly refined X-ray and NMR structures of the same protein also tend to be about 1 Å (Clore et al., 1993). Changes in the environment (e.g., oligomeric state, crystal packing, solvent, ligands) can also have a significant effect on the structure (Faber, Matthews, 1990). Overall, comparative models based on templates with more than 40% identity are almost as good as medium-resolution experimental structures, simply because the proteins at this level of similarity are likely to be as similar to each other as are the structures for the same protein determined by different experimental techniques under different conditions. However, the caveat in comparative protein modeling is that some regions, mainly loops and side chains, may have larger errors.

A way to test protein structure modeling methods, including comparative modeling, is provided by the biannual meetings on critical assessment of techniques for protein structure prediction (CASP) (Moult et al., 1995; Zemla et al., 2001; Marti-Renom et al., 2002). Protein modelers are challenged to model sequences with unknown 3D structure and to submit their models to the organizers before the meeting. At the same time, the 3D structures of the prediction targets are being determined by X-ray crystallography or NMR methods. They become available only after the models are calculated and submitted. Thus, a bona fide evaluation of protein structure modeling methods is possible. Large-scale, continuous, and automated complements to this experiment are implemented in two web servers, Live Bench (Bujnicki et al., 2001) and EVA (Eyrich et al., 2001).

4 APPLICATIONS OF COMPARATIVE MODELING

4.1 Modeling of Individual Proteins

Comparative modeling is often an efficient way to obtain useful information about the proteins of interest. For example, comparative models can be helpful in designing mutants to test hypotheses about the protein's function (Vernal et al., 2002; Wu et al., 1999a), identifying active and binding sites (Sheng et al., 1996), searching for, designing, and improving ligands for a given binding site (Ring et al., 1993), modeling substrate specificity (Xu et al., 1996), predicting antigenic epitopes (Sali et al., 1993), simulating protein–protein docking (Vakser, 1995), inferring function from calculated electrostatic potential around the protein (Matsumoto et al., 1995), facilitating molecular replacement in X-ray structure determination (Howell et al., 1992), refining models based on NMR constraints (Modi et al., 1996; Barrientos et al., 2001), testing and improving a sequence–structure alignment (Wolf et al., 1998), confirming a remote structural relationship (Guenther et al., 1997; Wu et al., 2000), and rationalizing known experimental observations (Fig. 7). For a lengthy review of comparative modeling applications see Johnson et al., 1994.

Fortunately, a 3D model does not have to be absolutely perfect to be helpful in biology, as demonstrated by the applications just listed. The type of a question that can be addressed with a particular model does depend on its accuracy.

At the low end of the accuracy spectrum, there are models that are based on less than 25% sequence identity and have sometimes less than 50% of their Cα atoms within 3.5 Å of their correct positions. However, such models still have the correct fold, and even knowing only the fold of a protein is frequently sufficient to predict its approximate biochemical function. More specifically, only nine out of 80 fold families known in 1994 contained proteins (domains) that were not in the same functional class, although 32% of all protein structures belonged to one of the nine superfolds (Orengo et al., 1997). Models in this low range of accuracy combined with model evaluation can be used for confirming or rejecting a match between remotely related proteins (Sanchez, Sali, 1997b; Sanchez, Sali, 1998).

In the middle of the accuracy spectrum are the models based on approximately 35% sequence identity, corresponding to 85% of the C atoms modeled within 3.5 Å of their correct positions. Fortunately, the active and binding sites are frequently more conserved than the rest of the fold and are thus modeled more accurately (Sanchez, Sali, 1998). In general, medium-resolution models frequently allow a refinement of the functional prediction based on sequence alone because ligand binding is most directly determined by the structure of the binding site rather than its sequence. It is frequently possible to correctly predict important features of the target protein that do not occur in the template structure. For example, the location of a binding site can be predicted from clusters of charged residues (Matsumoto et al., 1995), and the size of a ligand may be predicted from the volume of the binding site cleft (Xu et al., 1996). Medium-resolution models can also be used to construct site-directed mutants with altered or destroyed binding capacity, which in turn could test hypotheses about the sequence–structure–function relationships. Other problems that can be addressed with medium-resolution comparative models include designing proteins that have compact structures without long tails, loops, and exposed hydrophobic residues for better crystallization and designing proteins with added disulfide bonds for extra stability.

The high end of the accuracy spectrum corresponds to models based on 50% sequence identity or more. The average accuracy of these models approaches that of low-resolution X-ray structures (3Å resolution) or med-

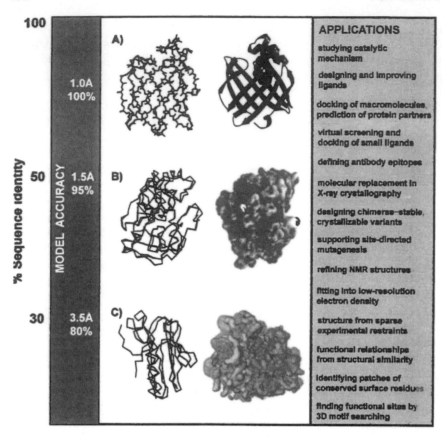

Figure 7 Accuracy of comparative models and their applications. The vertical axis indicates the different ranges of applicability of comparative protein structure modeling, the corresponding accuracy of protein structure models, and their sample applications. In panels A–C, typical overall accuracy of a comparative model (right) is indicated by a comparison of a model with an actual structure (left). (A) The complex between docosahexaenoic fatty acid (violet) and brain lipid–binding protein (right), modeled based on its 62% sequence identity to the crystallographic structure of adipocyte lipid–binding protein (PDB code 1ADL). (From Xu et al., 1996.) A number of fatty acids were ranked for their affinity to brain lipid–binding protein consistently with site-directed mutagenesis and affinity chromatography experiments, even though the ligand specificity profile of this protein is different from that of the template structure. (B) A putative proteoglycan–binding patch was identified on a medium-accuracy comparative model of mouse mast cell protease 7 (right), modeled based on its 39% sequence identity to the crystallographic structure of bovine pancreatic trypsin (2PTN) that does not bind proteoglycans. (From Matsumoto et al., 1995.) The prediction was confirmed by site-directed mutagenesis and heparin-affinity chromatography experiments. (C) A molecular model of the

ium-resolution NMR structures (10 distance restraints per residue) (Sanchez, Sali, 1997b). The alignments on which these models are based generally contain almost no errors. In addition to the already listed applications, high-quality models can be used for docking of small ligands (Ring et al., 1993) or whole proteins onto a given protein (Totrov, Abagyan, 1994; Vakser, 1995).

We now describe two applications of comparative modeling in more detail: (1) modeling of substrate specificity aided by a high-accuracy model and (2) substantiating a remote relationship between two proteins aided by a low-accuracy model.

Example 1: Modeling of Substrate Specificity. Brain lipid–binding protein (BLBP) is a member of the family of fatty acid–binding proteins that was isolated from brain (Xu et al., 1996). The problem was to find out which one of the many fatty acids known to bind to fatty acid–binding proteins in general is the likely physiological ligand of BLBP. To address this problem, comparative models of BLBP complexed with many fatty acids were calculated by relying on the structures of the adipocyte lipid–binding protein and muscle fatty acid–binding protein, in complex with their ligands. The models were evaluated by binding and site-directed mutagenesis experiments (Xu et al., 1996). The model of BLBP indicated that its binding cavity was just large enough to accommodate docosahexaenoic acid (DHA) (Fig. 8). Because DHA filled the BLBP–binding cavity completely, it was unlikely that BLBP would bind a larger ligand. Thus, DHA was the ligand predicted to have the highest affinity for BLBP. The prediction was confirmed by the measurement of binding affinities for many fatty acids. It turned out that the BLBP-DHA interaction was the strongest fatty acid–protein interaction known to date. The binding affinities of the ligands correlated with the surface areas buried by the protein–ligand interactions, as calculated from the corresponding models, and explained why DHA had the highest affinity. This case illustrates how a comparative model provides new information that cannot be deduced directly from the template structures despite their high, 60% sequence identity to BLBP. The two templates have smaller binding sites and consequently different patterns of binding affi-

---

whole yeast ribosome (right) was calculated by fitting atomic rRNA and protein models into the electron density of the 80S ribosomal particle, obtained by electron microscopy at 15-Å resolution. (From Spahn et al., 2001.) Most of the models for 40 out of the 75 ribosomal proteins were based on approximately 30% sequence identity to their template structures.

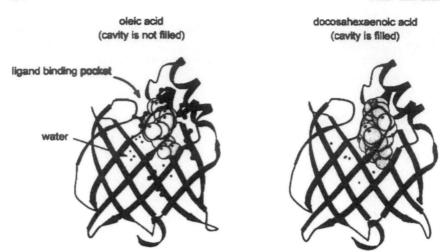

Figure 8 Modeling of the substrate specificity of the brain lipid–binding protein. The fatty acid ligand is shown in the CPK representation. The small spheres in the ligand–binding cavity are water molecules. *Left panel*, the model of the BLBP–oleic acid complex. *Right panel*, the model of the BLBP–docosahexaenoic acid complex. (From Xu et al., 1996.)

nities for the same set of ligands. The study also illustrated how new information is obtained relative to the target–template alignment even when the similarity between the target and the template sequences is high. The volumes and contact surfaces can be calculated only from a 3D model.

  Example 2: Detection of Remote Relationships. Genes coding for the core histones H2a, H2b, H3, and H4 of *Giardia lamblia* were sequenced (Wu et al., 1999b). The derived amino acid sequences of all four histones were similar to their homologs in other eukaryotes, although they were among the most divergent members of this protein family. Comparative protein structure modeling combined with energy evaluation (Sippl, 1993) of the resulting models indicated that the *G. lamblia* core histones individually and together can assume the same three-dimensional structures that were established by X-ray crystallography for *Xenopus laevis* histones and the nucleosome core particle (Wu et al., 2000) (Fig. 9). Since *G. lamblia* represents one of the earliest eukaryotes in many different molecular trees, the structure of its histones is potentially of relevance to understanding histone evolution. Our studies concluded that the *G. lamblia* histones do not represent an intermediate stage between archaeal and eukaryotic histones.

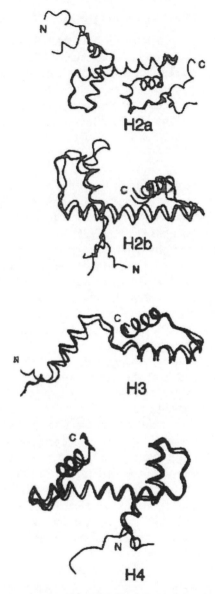

Figure 9 Substantiating the fold similarity of remotely related proteins by comparative modeling and assessment of the model energy. Comparative protein structure models of the *Giardia lamblia* core histones, based on the known structures of the *Xenopus histones*. The models and their evaluations indicate that the sequences of the *G. lamblia* histones are consistent with the structure of the corresponding *Xenopus* histones, with the exception of their terminal extension. (From Wu et al., 2000.)

4.2 Automated, Large-Scale Comparative Modeling

In a few years, the genome projects will have provided us with the amino acid sequences of millions of proteins—the catalysts, inhibitors, messengers, receptors, transporters, and building blocks of the living organisms. The full potential of the genome projects will be realized only once we assign and understand the function of these new proteins. This understanding will be facilitated by structural information for all or almost all proteins. Much of the structural information will be provided by structural genomics (Sali, 1998; Burley et al., 1999; Vitkup et al., 2001), a large-scale determination of protein structures by X-ray crystallography and nuclear magnetic resonance spectroscopy, combined efficiently with accurate, automated, and large-scale comparative protein structure modeling techniques (Sanchez et al., 2000a). Given limitations of the current modeling techniques, it seems reasonable to require models based on at least 30% sequence identity, corresponding to one experimentally determined structure per sequence family rather than fold family. It was estimated that the structures of representatives of approximately 16,000 sequence domain families need to be determined to provide comparative models based on at least 30% sequence identity for 90% of the protein sequences (Vitkup et al., 2001).

To enable large-scale comparative modeling needed for structural genomics, the steps of comparative modeling are being assembled into a completely automated pipeline (Sanchez, Sali, 1998). Since many computer programs for performing each of the operations in comparative modeling already exist, it may seem trivial to construct a pipeline that completely automates the whole process. In fact, it is not easy to do so in a robust manner. For a good reasons, most of the tasks in modeling of individual proteins, including template selection, alignment, and model evaluation, are typically performed with significant human intervention. This semiautomated modeling allows the use of the best tool for a particular problem at hand and consideration of many different sources of information that are difficult to take into account entirely automatically. Because large-scale modeling can be performed only in a completely automated manner, the main challenge is to build an automated and robust pipeline that approaches the performance of a human expert as much as possible.

Domains in approximately 57% of the 1,200,000 known protein sequences were modeled with MODELLER and deposited into a comprehensive database of comparative models, ModBase (http://guitar.rockefeller.edu/modbase/) (Sanchez et al., 2000b; Pieper et al., 2002; Sanchez, Sali, 1998). While the current number of modeled proteins may look impressive, usually only one domain per protein is modeled (on the average, proteins have slightly more than two domains), and two-thirds of the models are based on less than 30% sequence identity to the closest template. The Web interface to ModBase allows flexible querying for fold assignments, sequence–structure alignments, models, and model assessments of interest. An integrated sequence/structure viewer, ModView, allows inspection and analysis of the query results (Ilyin, Sali, 2002). ModBase will be increasingly interlinked with other applications and databases such that structures and other types of information can easily be used for functional annotation.

Large-scale comparative modeling opens new opportunities for tackling existing problems by virtue of providing many protein models from many genomes. One example is the selection of a target protein for which a drug needs to be developed. A good choice is a protein that is likely to have high ligand specificity; specificity is important because specific drugs are less likely to be toxic. Large-scale modeling facilitates imposing the specificity filter in target selection by enabling a structural comparison of the ligand binding sites of many proteins, either human or from other organisms. Such comparisons may make it possible to select rationally the target whose binding site is structurally most different from the binding sites of all the other proteins that may potentially react with the same drug. For example, when a human pathogenic organism needs to be inhibited, it may be possible to select as the target that pathogen's protein that is structurally most different from all the human homologs. Alternatively, when a human metabolic pathway needs to be regulated, the target identification could focus on that particular protein in the pathway that has the binding site most dissimilar from its human homologs.

ACKNOWLEDGEMENTS

We are grateful to the members of our group for many discussions about protein structure prediction. Research was supported by NIH/NIGMS R01 GM54762, NIH/NIGMS P50 GM62529, Merck Genome Research Award, and the Mathers Fund Award. András Fiser was a Burroughs Wellcome Fund Postdoctoral Fellow and is a Charles Revson Foundation Postdoctoral Fellow. Andrej Sali is an Irma T. Hirschl Trust Career Scientist. This perspective is based partly on previous papers (Fiser et al., 2001; Fiser, Sali, 2002; Fiser et al., 2002; Baker, Sali, 2001; Marti-Renom et al., 2000).

REFERENCES

Abagyan R, Totrov M. 1994. Biased probability Monte Carlo conformational searches and electrostatic calculations for peptides and proteins. J Mol Biol 235:983–1002.

Altschul SF, Madden TL, Schaffer AA, Zhang J, Zhang Z, Miller W, Lipman DJ. 1997. Gapped BLAST and PSI-BLAST: a new generation of protein database search programs. Nucleic Acids Res 25:3389–3402.

Apostolico A, Giancarlo R. 1998. Sequence alignment in molecular biology. J Comput Biol 5:173–196.

Aszodi A, Taylor WR. 1994. Secondary structure formation in model polypeptide chains. Protein Eng 7:633–644.

Bairoch A, Apweiler R. 2000. The SWISS-PROT protein sequence database and its supplement TrEMBL in 2000. Nucleic Acids Res 28:45–48.

Baker D, Sali A. 2001. Protein structure prediction and structural genomics. Science, in press.

Barrientos LG, Campos-Olivas R, Louis JM, Fiser A, Sali A, Gronenborn AM. 2001. 1H, 13C, 15N resonance assignments and fold verification of a circular permuted variant of the potent HIV-inactivating protein cyanovirin-N. J Biomol NMR 19:289–290.

Benson DA, Karsch-Mizrachi I, Lipman DJ, Ostell J, Rapp BA, Wheeler DL. 2002. GenBank. Nucleic Acids Res 30:17–20.

Blake JD, Cohen FE. 2001. Pairwise sequence alignment below the twilight zone. J Mol Biol 307:721–735.

Blundell TL, Sibanda BL, Sternberg MJ, Thornton JM. 1987. Knowledge-based prediction of protein structures and the design of novel molecules. Nature 326:347–352.

Boissel JP, Lee WR, Presnell SR, Cohen FE, Bunn HF. 1993. Erythropoietin structure–function relationships. Mutant proteins that test a model of tertiary structure. J Biol Chem 268:15983–15993.

Bonneau R, Baker D. 2001. Ab initio protein structure prediction: progress and prospects. Annu Rev Biophys Biomol Struct 30:173–189.

Bowie JU, Luthy R, Eisenberg D. 1991. A method to identify protein sequences that fold into a known three-dimensional structure. Science 253:164–170.

Braun W, Go N. 1985. Calculation of protein conformations by proton–proton distance constraints. A new efficient algorithm. J Mol Biol 186:611–626.

Bray JE, Todd AE, Pearl FM, Thornton JM, Orengo CA. 2000. The CATH Dictionary of Homologous Superfamilies (DHS): a consensus approach for identifying distant structural homologues. Protein Eng 13:153–165.

Brenner SE, Chothia C, Hubbard TJ. 1998. Assessing sequence comparison methods with reliable structurally identified distant evolutionary relationships. Proc Natl Acad Sci USA 95:6073–6078.

Brooks CL III, Bruccoleri RE, Olafson BD, States DJ, Swaminathan S, Karplus M. 1983. CHARMM: A program for macromolecular energy minimization and dynamics calculations. J Comp Chem 4:187–217.

Browne WJ, North ACT, Phillips DC, Brew K, Vanaman TC, Hill RC. 1969. A possible three-dimensional structure of bovine lactalbumin based on that of hen's egg-white lysozyme. J Mol Biol 42:65–86.

Bruccoleri RE, Karplus M. 1987. Prediction of the folding of short polypeptide segments by uniform conformational sampling. Biopolymers 26:137–168.

Bruccoleri RE, Karplus M. 1990. Conformational sampling using high-temperature molecular dynamics. Biopolymers 29:1847–1862.

Bujnicki JM, Elofsson, Fischer D, Rychlewski L. 2001. Livebench-1: Continuous benchmarking of protein structure prediction servers. Protein Sci 10:352–361.

Burley SK, Almo SC, Bonanno JB, Capel M, Chance MR, Gaasterland T, Lin D, Sali A, Studier FW, Swaminathan S. 1999. Structural genomics: beyond the human genome project. Nat Genet 23:151–157.

Bystroff C, Baker D. 1998. Prediction of local structure in proteins using a library of sequence–structure motifs. J Mol Biol 281:565–577.

Chinea G, Padron G, Hooft RW, Sander C, Vriend G. 1995. The use of position-specific rotamers in model building by homology. Proteins 23:415–421.

Chothia C. 1992. One thousand families for the molecular biologist. Nature 357:543–544.

Chothia C, Lesk AM. 1986. The relation between the divergence of sequence and structure in proteins. EMBO J 5:823–826.

Chothia C, Lesk AM. 1987. Canonical structures for the hypervariable regions of immunoglobulins. J Mol Biol 196:901–917.

Chothia C, Lesk AM, Tramontano A, Levitt M, Smith-Gill SJ, Air G, Sheriff S, Padlan EA, Davies D, Tulip WR. 1989. Conformations of immunoglobulin hypervariable regions. Nature 342:877–883.

Claessens M, Van Cutsem E, Lasters I, Wodak S. 1989. Modelling the polypeptide backbone with "spare parts" from known protein structures. Protein Eng 2:335–345.

Clore GM, Brunger AT, Karplus M, Gronenborn AM. 1986. Application of molecular dynamics with interproton distance restraints to three-dimensional protein structure determination. A model study of crambin. J Mol Biol 191:523–551.

Clore GM, Robien MA, Gronenborn AM. 1993. Exploring the limits of precision and accuracy of protein structures determined by nuclear magnetic resonance spectroscopy. J Mol Biol 231:82–102.

Cohen FE, Kuntz ID. 1989. Tertiary structure prediction. In: Fasman GD, ed. Prediction of Protein Structure and the Principles of Protein Conformations. New York: Plenum Press, pp 647–705.

Collura V, Higo J, Garnier J. 1993. Modeling of protein loops by simulated annealing. Protein Sci 2:1502–1510.

Deane CM, Blundell TL. 2001. CODA: a combined algorithm for predicting the structurally variable regions of protein models. Protein Sci 10:599–612.

Domingues FS, Lackner P, Andreeva A, Sippl MJ. 2000. Structure-based evaluation of sequence comparison and fold recognition alignment accuracy. J Mol Biol 297:1003–1013.

Eyrich V, Marti-Renom MA, Przybylski D, Fiser A, Pazos F, Valencia A, Sali A, Rost B. 2000. EVA: continuous automatic evaluation of protein structure prediction servers. Bioinformatics, 17:1242–1243.

Faber HR, Matthews BW. 1990. A mutant T4 lysozyme displays five different crystal conformations. Nature 348:263–266.

Felsenstein J. 1981. Evolutionary trees from DNA sequences: a maximum likelihood approach. J Mol Evol 17:368–376.

Fidelis K, Stern PS, Bacon D, Moult J. 1994. Comparison of systematic search and database methods for constructing segments of protein structure. Protein Eng 7:953–960.

Fine RM, Wang H, Shenkin PS, Yarmush DL, Levinthal C. 1986. Predicting antibody hypervariable loop conformations. II: Minimization and molecular dynamics studies of MCPC603 from many randomly generated loop conformations. Proteins 1:342–362.

Fiser A., Sali, A. Modeller: generation and refinement of homology models. Methods Enzymol, in press 2002.

Fiser A, Do RK, Sali A. 2000. Modeling of loops in protein structures. Protein Sci 9:1753–1773.

Fiser A, Sanchez R, Melo F, Sali A. 2001. Comparative protein structure modeling. In: Watanabe M, Roux B, MacKerell AD, Jr, Becker O, eds. Computational Biochemistry and Biophysics. New York: Marcel Dekker. pp 275–312.

Fiser A, Feig M, Brooks CL, III, Sali A. 2002. Evolution and Physics in Comparative Protein Structure Modeling. Acc Chem Res 35:413–421.

Godzik A. 1996. Knowledge-based potentials for protein folding: what can we learn from known protein structures? Structure 4:363–366.

Greer J. 1981. Comparative model-building of the mammalian serine proteases. J Mol Biol 153:1027–1042.

Greer J. 1990. Comparative modeling methods: application to the family of the mammalian serine proteases. Proteins 7:317–334.

Gribskov M, Veretnik S. 1996. Identification of sequence pattern with profile analysis. Methods Enzymol 266:198–212.

Guenther B, Onrust R, Sali A, O'Donnell M, Kuriyan J. 1997. Crystal structure of the δ-subunit of the clamp-loader complex of *E. coli* DNA polymerase III. Cell 91:335–345.

Havel TF, Snow ME. 1991. A new method for building protein conformations from sequence alignments with homologues of known structure. J Mol Biol 217:1–7.

Henikoff S, Henikoff JG. 2000. Amino acid substitution matrices. Adv Protein Chem 54:73–97.

Henikoff JG, Pietrokovski S, McCallum CM, Henikoff S. 2000. Blocks-based methods for detecting protein homology. Electrophoresis 21:1700–1706.

Higo J, Collura V, Garnier J. 1992. Development of an extended simulated annealing method: application to the modeling of complementary determining regions of immunoglobulins. Biopolymers 32:33–43.

Holm L, Sander C. 1991. Database algorithm for generating protein backbone and side-chain coordinates from a C alpha trace application to model building and detection of coordinate errors. J Mol Biol 218:183–194.

Holm L, Sander C. 1997. Dali/FSSP classification of three-dimensional protein folds. Nucleic Acids Res 25:231–234.

Hooft RW, Vriend G, Sander C, Abola EE. 1996. Errors in protein structures. Nature 381:272.

Howell PL, Almo SC, Parsons MR, Hajdu J, Petsko GA. 1992. Structure determination of turkey egg-white lysozyme using Laue diffraction data. Acta Crystallogr B 48 (Pt 2):200–207.

Ilyin V, Sali, A. Modview. Bioinformatics, in press, 2002.

Jaroszewski L, Rychlewski L, Zhang B, Godzik A. 1998. Fold prediction by a hierarchy of sequence, threading, and modeling methods. Protein Sci 7:1431–1440.

Jaroszewski L, Rychlewski L, Godzik A. 2000. Improving the quality of twilight-zone alignments. Protein Sci 9:1487–1496.

Jennings AJ, Edge CM, Sternberg MJ. 2001. An approach to improving multiple alignments of protein sequences using predicted secondary structure. Protein Eng 14:227–231.

Johnson MS, Overington JP. 1993. A structural basis for sequence comparisons. An evaluation of scoring methodologies. J Mol Biol 233:716–738.

Johnson MS, Srinivasan N, Sowdhamini R, Blundell TL. 1994. Knowledge-based protein modelling. CRC Crit Rev Biochem Mol Biol 29:1–68.

Jones DT. 1997. Progress in protein structure prediction. Curr Opin Struct Biol 7:377–387.

Jones DT, Taylor WR, Thornton JM. 1992. A new approach to protein fold recognition. Nature 358:86–89.

Jones TA, Thirup S. 1986. Using known substructures in protein model building and crystallography. EMBO J 5:819–822.

Kabsch W, Sander C. 1984. On the use of sequence homologies to predict protein structure: identical pentapeptides can have completely different conformations. Proc Natl Acad Sci USA 81:1075–1078.

Kelley LA, MacCallum RM, Sternberg MJ. 2000. Enhanced genome annotation using structural profiles in the program 3D-PSSM. J Mol Biol 299:499–520.

Koehl P, Delarue M. 1995. A self-consistent mean field approach to simultaneous gap closure and side-chain positioning in homology modeling. Nat Struct Biol 2:163–170.

Krogh A, Brown M, Mian IS, Sjolander K, Haussler D. 1994. Hidden Markov models in computational biology. Applications to protein modelling. J Mol Biol 235:1501–1531.

Laskowski RA, Moss DS, Thornton JM. 1993. Main-chain bond lengths and bond angles in protein structures. J Mol Biol 231:1049–1067.

Lesk AM, Chothia C. 1980. How different amino acid sequences determine similar protein structures: the structure and evolutionary dynamics of the globins. J Mol Biol 136:225–270.

Lessel U, Schomburg D. 1994. Similarities between protein 3-D structures. Protein Eng 7:1175–1187.

Levitt M. 1992. Accurate modeling of protein conformation by automatic segment matching. J Mol Biol 226:507–533.

Lo CL, Ailey B, Hubbard TJ, Brenner SE, Murzin AG, Chothia C. 2000. SCOP: a structural classification of proteins database. Nucleic Acids Res 28:257–259.

Luthy R, Bowie JU, Eisenberg D. 1992. Assessment of protein models with three-dimensional profiles. Nature 356:83–85.

MacKerell AD Jr., Bashford D, Bellott M, Dunbrack RL, Jr., Evanseck JD, Field MJ, Fischer S, Gao J, Guo H, Ha S, Joseph-McCarthy D, Kuchnir L, Muczera K, Lau FTK, Mattos C, Michnik S, Nguyen DT, Ngo T, Prodhom B, reiher WE, III, Roux B, Schlenkrich M, Smith JC, Stote R, Straub J, Watanabe M, Wiorkiewicz-Kuczera J, Yin D, Karplus M. 1998. All-atom empirical potential for molecular modleing and dynamics studies of proteins. J Phys Chem B 102:3586–3616.

Marti-Renom MA, Stuart AC, Fiser A, Sanchez R, Melo F, Sali A. 2000. Comparative protein structure modeling of genes and genomes. Annu Rev Biophys Biomol Struct 29:291–325.

Marti-Renom MA, Madhusudhan MS, Fiser A, Rost B, Sali A. 2002. Reliability of assessment of protein structure prediction methods. Structure 10:435–440.

Martin AC, MacArthur MW, Thornton JM. 1997. Assessment of comparative modeling in CASP2. *Proteins Suppl 1*:14-28.

Matsumoto R, Sali A, Ghildyal N, Karplus M, Stevens RL. 1995. Packaging of proteases and proteoglycans in the granules of mast cells and other hematopoietic cells. A cluster of histidines on mouse mast cell protease 7 regulates its binding to heparin serglycin proteoglycans. J Biol Chem 270:19524–19531.

Mezei M. 1998. Chameleon sequences in the PDB. Protein Eng 11:411–414.

Modi S, Paine MJ, Sutcliffe MJ, Lian LY, Primrose WU, Wolf CR, Roberts GC. 1996. A model for human cytochrome P450 2D6 based on homology modeling and NMR studies of substrate binding. Biochemistry 35:4540–4550.

Moult J, James MN. 1986. An algorithm for determining the conformation of polypeptide segments in proteins by systematic search. Proteins 1:146–163.

Moult J, Pedersen JT, Judson R, Fidelis K. 1995. A large-scale experiment to assess protein structure prediction methods. Proteins 23:ii–iv.

Nagarajaram HA, Reddy BV, Blundell TL. 1999. Analysis and prediction of inter-strand packing distances between beta-sheets of globular proteins. Protein Eng 12:1055–1062.

Ohlendorf DH. Accuracy of refined protein structures. Comparison of four independently refined models of human interleukin 1 beta. Acta Crystallogr D Biol Crystallogr D50:808–812. 1994.

Oliva B, Bates PA, Querol E, Aviles FX, Sternberg MJ. 1997. An automated classification of the structure of protein loops. J Mol Biol 266:814–830.

Orengo CA, Michie AD, Jones S, Jones DT, Swindells MB, Thornton JM. 1997. CATH—a hierarchic classification of protein domain structures. Structure 5:1093–1108.

Pearson WR. 1995. Comparison of methods for searching protein sequence databases. Protein Sci 4:1145–1160.

Pearson WR. 2000. Flexible sequence similarity searching with the FASTA3 program package. Methods Mol Biol 132:185–219.

Pieper U, Eswar N, Ilyin VA, Stuart A, Sali A. 2002. ModBase, a database of annotated comparative protein structure models. Nucleic Acids Res 30:255–259.

Reddy BV, Blundell TL. 1993. Packing of secondary structural elements in proteins. Analysis and prediction of interhelix distances. J Mol Biol 233:464–479.

Retief JD. 2000. Phylogenetic analysis using PHYLIP. Methods Mol Biol 132:243–258.

Ring CS, Cohen FE. 1993. Modeling protein structures: construction and their applications. FASEB J 7:783–790.

Ring CS, Kneller DG, Langridge R, Cohen FE. 1992. Taxonomy and conformational analysis of loops in proteins. J Mol Biol 224:685–699.

Ring CS, Sun E, McKerrow JH, Lee GK, Rosenthal PJ, Kuntz ID, Cohen FE. 1993. Structure-based inhibitor design by using protein models for the development of antiparasitic agents. Proc Natl Acad Sci USA 90:3583–3587.

Rost B. 1999. Twilight zone of protein sequence alignments. Protein Eng 12:85–94.

Rufino SD, Donate LE, Canard LH, Blundell TL. 1997. Predicting the conformational class of short and medium-size loops connecting regular secondary structures: application to comparative modelling. J Mol Biol 267:352–367.

Sali A. 1995. Modeling mutations and homologous proteins. Curr Opin Biotechnol 6:437–451.

Sali A. 1998. 100,000 protein structures for the biologist. Nat Struct Biol 5:1029–1032.

Sali A, Blundell TL. 1993. Comparative protein modeling by satisfaction of spatial restraints. J Mol Biol 234:779–815.

Sali A, Overington JP. 1994. Derivation of rules for comparative protein modeling from a database of protein structure alignments. Protein Sci 3:1582–1596.

Sali A, Overington JP, Johnson MS, Blundell TL. 1990. From comparisons of protein sequences and structures to protein modelling and design. Trends Biochem Sci 15:235–240.

Sali A, Matsumoto R, McNeil HP, Karplus M, Stevens RL. 1993. Three-dimensional models of four mouse mast cell chymases. Identification of proteoglycan binding regions and protease-specific antigenic epitopes. J Biol Chem 268:9023–9034.

Sali A, Potterton L, Yuan F, van Vlijmen H, Karplus M. 1995. Evaluation of comparative protein modeling by MODELLER. Proteins 23:318–326.

Samudrala R, Moult J. 1998. A graph-theoretic algorithm for comparative modeling of protein structure. J Mol Biol 279:287–302.

Sanchez R, Sali A. 1997a. Advances in comparative protein-structure modeling. Curr Opin Struct Biol 7:206–214.

Sanchez R, Sali A. 1997b. Evaluation of comparative protein structure modeling by MODELLER-3. Proteins Suppl 1:50–58.

Sanchez R, Sali A. 1998. Large-scale protein structure modeling of the *Saccharomyces cerevisiae* genome. Proc Natl Acad Sci USA 95:13597–13602.

Sanchez R, Sali A. 2000. Comparative protein structure modeling. Introduction and practical examples with modeller. Methods Mol Biol 143:97–129.

Sanchez R, Pieper U, Melo F, Eswar N, Marti-Renom MA, Madhusudhan MS, Mirkovic N, Sali A. 2000a. Protein structure modeling for structural genomics. Nat Struct Biol 7 Suppl:986–990.

Sanchez R, Pieper U, Mirkovic N, de Bakker PI, Wittenstein E, Sali A. 2000b. MODBASE, a database of annotated comparative protein structure models. Nucleic Acids Res 28:250–253.

Sauder JM, Arthur JW, Dunbrack RL, Jr. 2000. Large-scale comparison of protein sequence alignment algorithms with structure alignments. Proteins 40:6–22.

Sheng Y, Sali A, Herzog H, Lahnstein J, Krilis SA. 1996. Site-directed mutagenesis of recombinant human beta 2-glycoprotein I identifies a cluster of lysine residues that are critical for phospholipid binding and anti-cardiolipin antibody activity. J Immunol 157:3744–3751.

Shenkin PS, Yarmush DL, Fine RM, Wang HJ, Levinthal C. 1987. Predicting antibody hypervariable loop conformation. I. Ensembles of random conformations for ringlike structures. Biopolymers 26:2053–2085.

Shi J, Blundell TL, Mizuguchi K. 2001. FUGUE: sequence–structure homology recognition using environment-specific substitution tables and structure-dependent gap penalties. J Mol Biol 310:243–257.

Sibanda BL, Blundell TL, Thornton JM. 1989. Conformation of beta-hairpins in protein structures. A systematic classification with applications to modelling by homology, electron density fitting and protein engineering. J Mol Biol 206:759–777.

Sippl MJ. 1990. Calculation of conformational ensembles from potentials of mean force. An approach to the knowledge-based prediction of local structures in globular proteins. J Mol Biol 213:859–883.

Sippl MJ. 1993. Recognition of errors in three-dimensional structures of proteins. Proteins 17:355–362.

Sippl MJ. 1995. Knowledge-based potentials for proteins. Curr Opin Struct Biol 5:229–235.

Smith TF, Lo CL, Bienkowska J, Gaitatzes C, Rogers RG, Jr, Lathrop R. 1997. Current limitations to protein threading approaches. J Comput Biol 4:217–225.

Spahn CM, Beckmann R, Eswar N, Penczek PA, Sali A, Blobel G, Frank J. 2001. Structure of the 80S ribosome from *Saccharomyces cerevisiae*—tRNA-ribosome and subunit–subunit interactions. Cell 107:373–386.

Srinivasan N, Blundell TL. 1993. An evaluation of the performance of an automated procedure for comparative modeling of protein tertiary structure. Protein Eng 6:501–512.

Sutcliffe MJ, Haneef I, Carney D, Blundell TL. 1987. Knowledge-based modelling of homologous proteins. Part I: Three-dimensional frameworks derived from the simultaneous superposition of multiple structures. Protein Eng 1:377–384.

Sutcliffe MJ, Dobson CM, Oswald RE. 1992. Solution structure of neuronal bungarotoxin determined by two-dimensional NMR spectroscopy: calculation of tertiary structure using systematic homologous model building, dynamical simulated annealing, and restrained molecular dynamics. Biochemistry 31:2962–2970.

Taylor WR, Hatrick K. 1994. Compensating changes in protein multiple sequence alignments. Protein Eng 7:341–348.

Teichmann SA, Chothia C, Gerstein M. 1999. Advances in structural genomics. Curr Opin Struct Biol 9:390–399.

Topham CM, McLeod A, Eisenmenger F, Overington JP, Johnson MS, Blundell TL. 1993. Fragment ranking in modelling of protein structure. Conformationally constrained environmental amino acid substitution tables. J Mol Biol 229:194–220.

Torda AE. 1997. Perspectives in protein-fold recognition. Curr Opin Struct Biol 7:200–205.

Totrov M, Abagyan R. 1994. Detailed ab initio prediction of lysozyme–antibody complex with 1.6Å accuracy. Nat Struct Biol 1:259–263.

Unger R, Harel D, Wherland S, Sussman JL. 1989. A 3D building blocks approach to analyzing and predicting structure of proteins. Proteins 5:355–373.

Vakser IA. 1995. Protein docking for low-resolution structures. Protein Eng 8:371–377.

van Gelder CW, Leusen FJ, Leunissen JA, Noordik JH. 1994. A molecular dynamics approach for the generation of complete protein structures from limited coordinate data. Proteins 8:174–185.

van Vlijmen HW, Karplus M. 1997. PDB-based protein loop prediction: parameters for selection and methods for optimization. J Mol Biol 267:975–1001.

Vernal J, Fiser A, Sali A, Muller M, Jose CJ, Nowicki C. 2002. Probing the specificity of a trypanosomal aromatic alpha-hydroxy acid dehydrogenase by site-directed mutagenesis. Biochem Biophys Res Commun 293:633–639.

Vitkup D, Melamud E, Moult J, Sander C. 2001. Completeness in structural genomics. Nat Struct Biol 8:559–566.

Westbrook J, Feng Z, Jain S, Bhat TN, Thanki N, Ravichandran V, Gilliland GL, Bluhm W, Weissig H, Greer DS, Bourne PE, Berman HM. 2002. The Protein Data Bank: unifying the archive. Nucleic Acids Res 30:245–248.

Wolf E, Vassilev A, Makino Y, Sali A, Nakatani Y, Burley SK. 1998. Crystal structure of a GCN5-related *N*-acetyltransferase: *Serratia marcescens* aminoglycoside 3-*N*-acetyltransferase. Cell 94:439–449.

Wu G, Fiser A, ter Kuile B, Sali A, Muller M. 1999a. Convergent evolution of *Trichomonas vaginalis* lactate dehydrogenase from malate dehydrogenase. Proc Natl Acad Sci USA 96:6285–6290.

Wu G, Fiser A, ter Kuile B, Sali A, Muller M. 1999b. Convergent evolution of *Trichomonas vaginalis* lactate dehydrogenase from malate dehydrogenase. Proc Natl Acad Sci USA 96:6285–6290.

Wu G, McArthur AG, Fiser A, Sali A, Sogin ML, Müller M. 2000. Core histones of the amitochondriate protist, *Giardia lamblia*. Mol Biol Evol 17:1156–1163.

Xu LZ, Sanchez R, Sali A, Heintz N. 1996. Ligand specificity of brain lipid–binding protein. J Biol Chem 271:24711–24719.

Zemla A, Venclovas, Moult J, Fidelis K. 2001. Processing and evaluation of predictions in CASP4. Proteins 45 Suppl 5:13–21.

Zheng Q, Rosenfeld R, Vajda S, DeLisi C. 1993. Determining protein loop conformation using scaling-relaxation techniques. Protein Sci 2:1242–1248.

Zheng Q, Rosenfeld R, DeLisi C, Kyle DJ. 1994. Multiple copy sampling in protein loop modeling: computational efficiency and sensitivity to dihedral angle perturbations. Protein Sci 3:493–506.

8

Rising Accuracy of Protein Secondary Structure Prediction

Burkhard Rost
Columbia University, New York, New York, U.S.A.

1 INTRODUCTION

The Sequence–Structure Gap is Rapidly Increasing. Currently, databases for protein sequences (e.g., SWISS-PROT/TrEMBL* (14)) are expanding rapidly, largely due to large-scale genome sequencing projects: At

---

*Abbreviations used: *3D*, three-dimensional; *3D structure*, three-dimensional (coordinates of protein structure); *1D*, one-dimensional; *1D structure*, one-dimensional (e.g., sequence or string of secondary structure); *ASP*, method identifying regions of structure ambivalent in response to global changes (1); *DSSP*, database containing the secondary structure and solvent accessibility for proteins of known 3D structure; *HMMSTR*, hidden Markov model—based prediction of secondary structure (2); *HSSP*, database of protein structure–sequence alignments; *rmsd*, root mean square deviation; *JPred*, method combining other prediction methods (3,4); *JPred2*, divergent profile (PSI-BLAST) based neural network prediction (5); *MaxHom*, dynamic programming algorithm for conservation weight–based multiple sequence alignment; *PDB*, Protein Data Bank of experimentally determined 3D structures of proteins (6); *PHD*, Pairwise profile–based neural network prediction of secondary structure; *PHDpsi*, divergent profile (PSI-BLAST) based neural network prediction (7,8); *PROF*, divergent profile–based neural network prediction trained and tested with PSI-BLAST (9); *PSI-BLAST*, gapped and iterative specific profile-based, fast and accurate alignment method (10); *PSIPRED*, divergent profile (PSI-Blast) based neural network prediction (11); *SAM-T99sec*, neural network prediction using hidden Markov models as input (12)l *SSpro*, profile-based advanced neural network prediction method (13); *SWISS-PROT*, database of protein sequences (14); *U*, protein sequence of unknown 3D structure (e.g., protein to be predicted).

207

the beginning of 2001, we knew all sequences for more than 40 entire genomes (15–17). This implies that the gap between known structures and known sequences is rapidly increasing, despite significant improvements of structure determination techniques (PDB (6, 18)). The most successful theoretical approach to bridging this gap is comparative modeling. It effectively raises the number of "known" 3D structures from 10,000 to over 100,000 (19,20). In fact, our ability to find the appropriate template so that we can apply comparative modeling has risen continuously since the early 1990s. Now, we can predict 3D structure through comparative modeling for more than twice as many proteins as in 1993. However, after four decades of ardent research, we still cannot predict structure from sequence (21–23). Nevertheless, the field has had its success; Now the best methods can frequently get some features of the fold right (24).

Simplifying the Structure Prediction Problem. The rapidly growing sequence–structure gap has enticed theoreticians to solve simplified prediction problems (25). An extreme simplification is the prediction of protein structure in one dimension (1D), as represented by strings of, e.g., secondary structure, or residue solvent accessibility. Theoreticians are lucky in that simplified predictions in 1D (e.g., secondary structure or solvent accessibility (25–27))—even when only partially correct—are often useful, e.g., for predicting protein function or functional sites.

Topics Left Out Here. This chapter focuses on methods predicting secondary structure for globular proteins in general. In the infancy of analyzing the proteome of entirely sequenced organisms, the most useful structure prediction methods are those that focus on particular classes of proteins, such as proteins containing membrane helices and coiled-coil regions (28–31). For predicting the topology of helical membrane proteins, a number of new methods add interesting new facets (32–37). However, no method has really utilized the flood of recent experimental information about membrane proteins (38). Overall, membrane helices can be predicted much more accurately than globular helices. The current state of the art is to correctly predict all membrane helix topology for more than 80% of the proteins and to falsely predict membrane helices for less than 4% of all globular proteins. We have recently come across evidence suggesting that this figure overestimates performance (B. Rost, unpublished). Clearly, methods developed to predict helices in globular proteins go completely wrong for membrane helices! In contrast, porins appear to be predicted relatively accurately by methods developed for globular proteins (39,40). Few methods specifically predicting coiled-coil regions have recently been published (an older review is Ref. 41). Two interesting developments are the prediction of the dimeric state of coiled coils (42) and a method predicting 3D structure for coiled-coil regions (43). In fact, the latter is the only existing method predicting 3D structure below 2-Å main-chain deviation over more than 30 residues. Another example for successful specialized secondary structure prediction methods is the focus on beta-turns (44,45). The method from the Thornton group appears to be the most accurate current means of predicting turns. Successful methods specialized to predicting alpha-helix propensities have resulted from the experimental studies of short peptides in solution (46,47). Neither the turn nor the helix-in-solution methods have yet been combined with other secondary structure prediction methods.

2 MATERIALS

Secondary Structure Assigned by DSSP. Secondary structure is most often assigned automatically based on the hydrogen-bonding pattern between the backbone carbonyl and NH groups (e.g., by DSSP [48]). DSSP distinguishes eight secondary structure states that are often grouped into three classes: H = helix, E = strand, and L = nonregular structure. Typically the grouping is as follows: "H" (α-helix→ H, "G" (3_{10}-helix) → H, "T" (π-helix) → H, "E" (extended strand) → E, and "B" (residue in isolated β-bridge) → E, "T" (turn) → L, "S" (bend) → L, " " (blank = others) → L, with the "corrections": "B" → EE, but "B_B" → LLL. Note that some developers use different projections of the eight DSSP classes onto three predicted classes; most of these yield seemingly higher levels of prediction accuracy. For example, short helices are more difficult to predict ((49); see also Fig. 5). Hence, converting "GGG" to "LLL" lets authors report higher numbers.

Per-Residue Prediction Accuracy. The simplest and most widely used score for secondary structure prediction is the three-state per-residue accuracy, giving the percentage of correctly predicted residues predicted correctly in either of the three states: helix, strand, or other:

$$Q_3 = 100 \cdot \frac{\sum_{i=1}^{3} c_i}{N} \tag{1}$$

where c_i is the number of residues predicted correctly in state i (H, E, L) and N is the number of residues in the protein (or in a given data set). Because typical data sets contain about 32% H (helix), 21% E (strand), and 47% L (other), correct prediction of the nonregular class (L) tends to dominate the three-state accuracy. More fine-grained methods that avoid this shortcoming are defined in detail elsewhere (50,51).

Per-Segment Prediction Accuracy. Measures for single-residue accuracy do not completely reflect the quality of a prediction (51–56). Three simple measures assess the quality of predicting segments: (1) the number of correctly predicted segments, (2) the predicted vs. observed average segment length, and (3) the predicted vs. observed distributions of segments with length *L* (57). All these measures can, e.g., identify methods with fairly high per-residue accuracy yet an unrealistic distribution of segments. More elaborated scores are based on the overlap between predicted and observed segments (SOV: (51,58)).

Conditions for Evaluating Sustained Performance. A systematic testing of performance is a precondition for any prediction to become reliably useful. For example, the history of secondary structure prediction has partly been a hunt for highest-accuracy scores, with overoptimistic claims by predictors seeding the scepticism of potential users. Given a separation of a data set into a training set (used to derive the method) and a test set (or cross-validation set, used to evaluate performance), a proper evaluation (or cross-validation) of prediction methods needs to meet four requirements.

1. There is no significant pairwise sequence identity between proteins used for the training and test sets, i.e., < 25% (length-dependent cutoff (59)).
2. All available unique proteins should be used for testing, since proteins vary considerably in structural complexity; certain features are easier to predict, others harder.
3. No matter which data sets are used for a particular evaluation, a standard set should be used for which results are also always reported.
4. Methods should never be optimized with respect to the data set chosen for final evaluation. In other words, the test set should never be used before the method is set up.

Number of Cross-Validation Experiments Has No Meaning. Most methods are evaluated in *n*-fold cross-validation experiments (splitting the data set into *n* different training and test sets). How many separations should be used? That is, which value of *n* yields the best evaluation? A misunderstanding is often spread in the literature: the more separations (the larger the *n*) the better. However, the exact value of *n* is not important provided the test set is representative and comprehensive and the cross-validation results are *not* miss-used misused to readjust again change parameters. In other words, the choice of *n* has no meaning for the user.

3 METHODS

3.1 Dinosaurs of Secondary Structure Prediction Are Still Alive!

First Generation: Single-Residue Statistics. The first experimentally determined 3D structures of hemoglobin and myoglobin were published in 1960 (60,61). Almost a decade earlier, Pauling and Corey suggested an explanation for the formation of certain local conformational patterns like α-helices and β-strands (62,63). Shortly after (and still prior to the first experimental structure), the first attempt was made to correlate the content of a certain amino acids (e.g., Proline) with the content of the α-helix (64). The idea was expanded by correlating the content for all amino acids with that of the α-helix and the β-strand (65,66). The field of secondary structure prediction had been opened. Most early methods were first-generation methods, in that they were based on single-residue statistics. Preferences of particular amino acids for particular secondary structure states were extracted from the given small databases (67–75). By 1983, it became clear that the accuracy of these methods had been overestimated (76) (Fig. 1).

Second Generation: Segment Statistics. The principal improvement of the second generation profited from the growth of experimental information about protein structure. These data enabled the parameterization of the information contained in consecutive segments of residues. Typically 11–21 adjacent residues are taken from a protein and statistics are compiled to evaluate how likely the central residue in that segment is to be in a particular secondary structure state. Similar segments of adjacent residues were also used to base predictions on more elaborated algorithms, some of which were spun off from artificial intelligence. Since then, almost any algorithm has been applied to the problem of predicting secondary structure; all were limited to accuracy levels around 60% (Fig. 1). Reports of higher levels of accuracy were usually based on too small or nonrepresentative data sets (50,54,77,78). The main algorithms were based on: (1) statistical information (79–91); (2) physicochemical properties (92); (3) sequence patterns (93–95); (4) multilayered (or neural) networks (96–103); (5) graph theory (104,105); (6) multivariate statistics (106,107); (7) expert rules (105,108–112); and (8) nearest-neighbor algorithms (113–115).

Problems with First and Second Generation Methods. All methods from the first and second generation shared at least two of the following problems (most shared all three):

1. Three-state per-residue accuracy was below 70%.
2. β-strands were predicted at levels of 28–48%, i.e., only slightly better than random.
3. Predicted helices and strands were too short.

The first problem (< 100% accuracy) is commonly linked to two features. (1) Secondary structure formation is partially determined by long-range interactions, i.e., by contacts between residues that are not visible by any method based on segments of 11–21 adjacent residues. (2) Secondary structure assignments vary by 5–12% even between different crystals of the same protein. Hence, 100% identical assignments are an unrealistic and unreason-

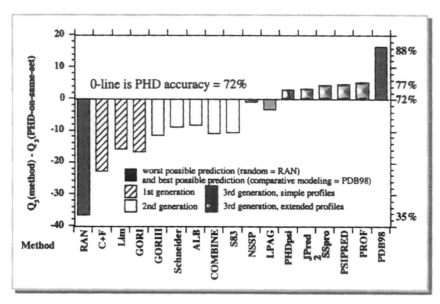

Figure 1 Three-state per-residue accuracy of various prediction methods: I included only methods for which I could run independent tests. Unfortunately, for most old methods this was not possible. However, for each method I had independent results from PHD (Refs. 7,50,78) available. I normalized the differences between data sets by simply compiling levels of accuracy with respect to PHD. For comparison, I added the worst possible prediction (random) and the best possible one (through comparative modeling of a close homolog). The methods were: $C+F$, Chou and Fasman (1st generation) (Refs. 73,242); *Lim* (1st) (Ref. 74); *GORI* (1st) (Ref. 83); *Schneider* (2nd) (Ref. 117); *ALB* (2nd) (Ref. 92); *GORIII* (2nd) (Ref. 84); *COMBINE* (2nd) (Ref. 243); *S83* (2nd) (Ref. 116); *LPAG* (3rd) (Ref. 159); *NSSP* (3rd) (Ref. 114); *PHDpsi* (3rd) (Ref. 8); JPred2 (3rd) (Ref. 5); SSpro (3rd) (Ref. 13); PSIPRED (3rd) (Ref. 11); PROF (3rd) (Ref. 244).

able aim. The second problem (β-strands are $< 50\%$ accurate) has been explained by the fact that β-sheet formation is determined by more nonlocal contacts than is α-helix formation. The third problem (too-short segments predicted) was basically overlooked by most developers (exceptions: Refs. 116 and 117). This problem makes predictions very difficult to use in practice (Fig. 2). Many of the recent third-generation prediction methods address all three problems simultaneously and are clearly superior to the old methods (Fig. 1). Nevertheless, many of the secondary structure prediction methods available today (e.g., in GCG (118) or from internet services (119)) are unfortunately still using the dinosaurs of secondary structure prediction.

3.2 Quantum Leap Through Using Pairwise Evolutionary Information

3.2.1 Evolutionary Odyssey Informative?

Variation in Sequence Space. The exchange of a few residues can already destabilize a protein (120). This implies that the majority of the 20^N possible sequences of length N form different structures. Has evolution really created such an immense variety? Random errors in the DNA sequence lead to a different translation of protein sequences. These "errors" are the basis for evolution. Mutations resulting in a structural change are not likely to survive, since the protein can no longer function appropriately. Furthermore, the universe of stable structures is not continuous: Minor changes on the level of the 3D structure may destabilize the structure. Thus, residue exchanges conserving structure are statistically extremely unlikely. However, the evolutionary pressure to conserve structure and function has led to a record of this unlikely event: Structure is more

SEQ	KELVLALYDYQEKSPREVTMKKGDILTLLNSTNKDWWKVEVNDRQGFVPAAYVKKLD
OBS	EEEE E--E EEEEEE EEEEE EEEEEEHHHHEEEE
TYP	EEHHH EE EEEE EE HHHEE EEEHH

Figure 2 Example of typical secondary structure prediction of the second generation: The protein sequence (*SEQ*) given was the SH3 structure. (From Ref. 184). The observed secondary structure (*OBS*) was assigned by DSSP. (From Ref. 48). (H = helix; E = strand; blank = nonregular structure; the dashes indicate the continuation of the second strand that was missed by DSSP). The typical prediction of too short segments (*TYP*) poses the following problems in practice: (1) Are the residues predicted to be strand in segments 1, 5, and 6 errors, or should the helices be elongated? (2) Should the second and third strands be joined, or should one of them be ignored, or does the prediction indicate two strands here? Note: The three-state per-residue accuracy is 60% for the prediction given.

conserved than sequence (121–123). Indeed, all naturally evolved protein pairs that have 35 of 100 pairwise identical residues have similar structures (59,124). However, the attractors of protein structures are even larger: the majority of protein pairs of similar structures has levels below 15% pairwise sequence identity (59,125,126).

Long-Range Information in Multiple Sequence Alignments. The residue substitution patterns observed between proteins of a particular structural family, i.e., changes that conserved structure, are highly specific for the structure of that family. Furthermore, multiple alignments of sequence families implicitly also contain information about long-range interactions. Suppose residues i and $i + 100$ are close in 3D, then the types of amino acids that can be exchanged (without changing structure) at position i are constrained by the need for their physicochemical characteristics to fit the amino acid types at position $i + 100$ (127,128).

3.2.2   Can Evolutionary Information Be Used?

Expert Predictions: Visual Use of Alignment Information. The first method that used information from family alignments was proposed in the 1970s (129). Since then, experts have based single-case predictions successfully on multiple alignments (129–146). In fact, analyzing the conservation patterns in sequence families is the first step when any expert wants to learn anything about a particular protein. Conversely, proteins without homologs constitute the dead-end road of sequence analysis.

Automatic Use of Pairwise Alignment Information. The simplest way to use alignment information automatically was first proposed by Maxfield and Scheraga and by Zvelebil et al. (147,148): Predictions were compiled for each protein in an alignment and then averaged over all proteins. A slightly more elaborated way of automatically using evolutionary information is to base prediction directly on a profile compiled from the multiple sequence alignment (7,50,78). The following steps are applied in particular for the *PHD* methods (7,149) (Fig. 3).

1. A sequence of unknown structure (U) is quickly (typically by *Blast* (150)) aligned against the database of known sequences (i.e., no information of structure required!).
2. Proteins with sufficient sequence identity to U to ensure structural similarity are extracted and realigned by a multiple alignment algorithm *MaxHom* (151).
3. For each position, the profile of residue exchanges in the final multiple alignment is compiled and used as input to a neural network.

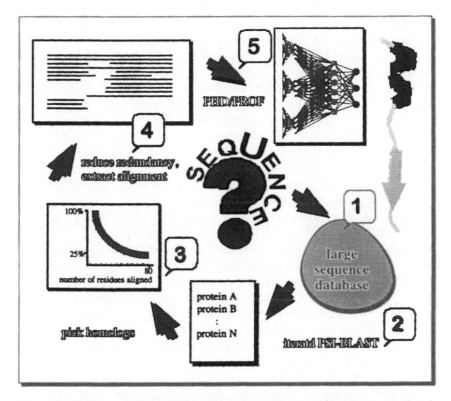

Figure 3 Using evolutionary information to predict secondary structure. Starting from a sequence of unknown structure (*SEQUENCE*), the following steps are required to finally feed evolutionary information into the *PHD* neural networks (upper right): (1) a database search for homologs through iterated *PSI-Blast* (Ref. 150), protocol from Ref. 8), (2) a decision for which proteins will be considered as homologs (BLAST score or length-dependent cutoff for pairwise sequence identity (Refs. 59,124)), (3) a reduction of redundancy (purge too many too-similar proteins), and (4) a final refinement and extraction of the resulting multiple alignment. Numbers 1–5 illustrated where users of the *PredictProtein* server (Refs. 7,119) can interfere to improve prediction accuracy without changes being made to the actual prediction method *PHD*.

3.2.3 Third Generation: Evolution to Better Predictions

Example Chosen: PHD. In the following, I illustrate the principal concepts of third-generation methods based on the particular neural network–based method *PHD* because it has been the most accurate method for many years and because most of these concepts were introduced by *PHD* (50,78). Meanwhile, several other methods have reported and/or achieved similar levels of performance (7,50,78,114,144,152–160). More recent methods will be discussed in more detail later.

Multiple Levels of Computations. PHD processes the input information on multiple levels (neural network in Fig. 3). The first level is a feed-forward neural network with three layers of units (input, hidden, and output). Input to this first-level sequence-to-structure network consists of two contributions: one from the local sequence, i.e., taken from a window of 13 adjacent residues, and another from the global sequence. Output of the first-level network is the 1D structural state of the residue at the center of the input window. The second level is a structure-to-structure network. The next level consists of an arithmetic average over independently trained networks (jury decision). The final level is a simple filter.

Balanced Predictions via Balanced Training. The distribution of the training examples (known structures) is rather uneven: About 32% of the residues are observed in helix, 21% in strand, and 47% in loop. Choosing the training examples proportional to the occurrence in the data set (unbalanced training) results in a prediction accuracy that mirrors this distribution; e.g., strands are predicted inferior to helix or loop (49,50,78). A simple way around the database bias is a balanced training: At each time step, one example is chosen from each class, i.e., one window with the central residue in a helix, one with the central residue in a strand, and one representing the loop class. This training results in a performance well balanced between the output states (Fig. 4).

Better Segment Prediction via Structure-to-Structure Networks. The first-level sequence-to-structure networks use as input the following information from 13 adjacent residues: (1) profile of amino acid substitutions for all 13 residues; (2) conservation weights compiled for each column of the multiple alignment; (3) number of insertions and deletions in each column; (4) position of the current segment of 13 residues with respect to the N- and C-term; (5) amino acid composition; and (6) length of the protein. The network output consists of three units for helix, strand, and nonregular structure. The second-level structure-to-structure networks use the same output. The major input for the second-level structure-to-structure networks are the output values of the first-level sequence-to-structure networks. The reason for introducing a second level is the following. Networks are trained by changing the connections between the units such that the error is reduced for each of the examples successively presented to the network during training. The examples are chosen at random. Therefore, the examples taken at time step t and at time step $t + 1$ are usually not adjacent in sequence. This implies that the network cannot learn that, e.g., helices contain at least three residues. The second-level structure-to-structure network introduces a correlation between adjacent residues, with the effect that predicted secondary

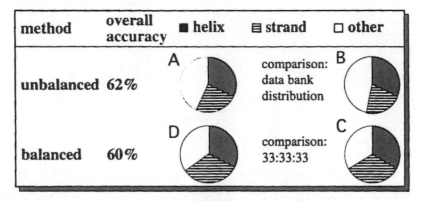

method	overall accuracy	■ helix	⊟ strand	□ other

Figure 4 Prediction balanced between three secondary structure states: The pies were valid for a simple neural network prediction not using evolutionary information (second generation). In their entirety, the pies represented 100% of (A + D) all correctly predicted residues, (B) all residues in a representative subset of PDB, and (C) all residues presented during balanced training. The basic message is that the prediction of strand is not inferior to the one for helix for second-generation methods (A) because strand formation is dominated more by long-range interactions (as previously argued), although the database distributions differ among the three states (B). Simply skewing the distribution (C) resulted in an equally accurate prediction for all three states (D).

structure segments have length distributions similar to the ones observed (57). The problem that remains after the second-level networks are is the underprediction of short segments (Fig. 5).

3.3 Continuous Advance Through Profile Searches in Growing Databases

Automatically Aligning Protein Families Based on Profiles: The PSI-BLAST Wonder. Just as experts have been using alignment information to predict aspects of structure and function, they have intruded into the twilight zone of sequence alignments (121) using profile-based alignment techniques. The idea of profile-based searches is simply to use the fact that profiles of evolutionary conservation are highly specific for every protein family. For example, glycines can often be mutated without major changes. However, in particular families, the conservation of some glycines may be crucial to maintain mobility. Many groups have successfully implemented semiautomatic profile-based databases searches (150,161–166). However, the breakthrough to large-scale routine searches was achieved via the development of PSI-BLAST (10) and hidden Markov models (12,167). In particular, the gapped, profile-based, and iterated

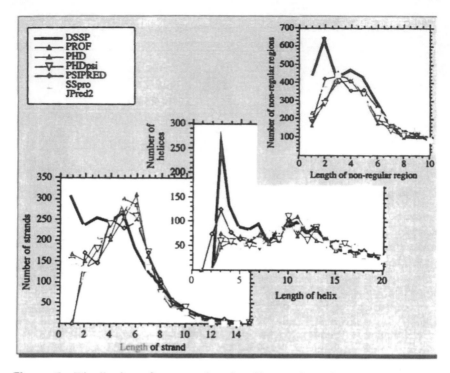

Figure 5 Distribution of segment lengths: The number of secondary structure segments observed (thick black line; according to DSSP (Ref. 48)) and predicted is plotted against their length. All methods miss short helices and strands. However, short regions lacking regular secondary structure were also underpredicted by all methods. Overall, most methods predict segments around the lengths of those observed. All results are based on a data set of 201 proteins taken from the EVA server (Refs. 180,181) that contained no protein used for training of any of the methods (also used for results in Table 1).

search tool PSI-BLAST continues to revolutionize the field of protein sequence analysis through its unique combination of speed and accuracy. More distant relationships are found through iteration, starting from the safe zone of comparisons and intruding deeply and reliably into the twilight zone (Fig. 6).

Jones Broke Through by Using PSI-BLAST Searches of Large Databases. David Jones pioneered using iterated PSI-BLAST searches automatically (11). The most important step reached by the resulting method, PSIPRED, has been the detailed strategy to avoid polluting the profile through unrelated proteins (Fig. 6). To avoid this trap, the database searched has to be filtered first (11). At the CASP meeting at which David

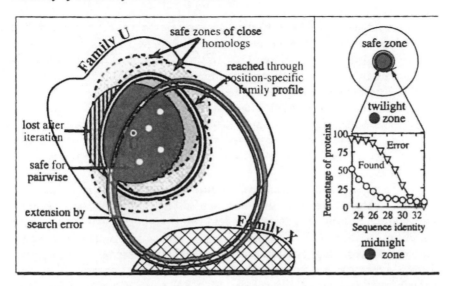

Figure 6 Profile-based searches extend evolutionary information: The cloud signifies a protein structural family for the query protein U, i.e., all proteins that have a similar 3D structure. A simple pairwise comparison of U with all other proteins covers the "safe zone" of sequence alignment (dark gray circle around U). This zone can be defined, e.g., by *BLAST* scores below 10^{-10} or by more than 35% pairwise identical residues over long alignments. Assume that there are only five other proteins (small white circles) in the safe zone, falling all on the same side of U. Now, *PSI-BLAST* starts the next iteration with the family-specific given by the proteins found in the safe zone. Searching the database again with this profile reaches safely into the twilight zone (zone marked by double-lined egg). However, no current method generally reaches all members of family U. Furthermore, in particular for *PSI-BLAST*, the new region may fall outside of the initial safe zone (vertically hatched crescent left of dark gray safe zone). Finally, the regions that could have been reached by sequence-space hopping or intermediate sequence searches (dashed light gray circles around five initial hits, (Refs. 59,245,246)) are not entirely covered by the profile-based search. The tricky bit is to avoid for the profile to pick unrelated proteins (transparent egg) and thus to connect two separate structural families (U and X). The three circles on the right-hand side signify the three zones: safe (no error), twilight (some to many errors), midnight (hardly any correct hit) of database searches. Their sizes are proportional to the "real" size of the regions they occupy. The graph shows that the number of false positives explodes in a brief region of the twilight zone (0 error at 33% sequence identity, > 90% error at 25%). At the same time, more than half the true homologs are found only in the midnight zone. Conclusions: (1) Iterated *PSI-BLAST* searches can safely identify fairly divergent family members. (2) Close homologs may be lost during the extension of the family. (3) The advanced search can lead one astray.

Jones introduced PSIPRED, Kevin Karplus and colleagues presented their prediction method (SAM-T99sec) for finding more diverged profiles through hidden Markov models (168,169). In 1999, Cuff and Barton et al. also successfully used PSI-BLAST alignments for JPred2 (170). Jennings et al. (171) explored an alternative to increasing divergence: They started with a safe zone alignment through ClustalW (166) and HMMer (167) and iteratively refined the alignment using the secondary structure prediction from DSC [160]. The resulting alignment is reported to be more accurate and to yield higher prediction accuracy than the initial ClustalW/HMMer alignments (171).

SSpro: Advanced Recursive Neural Network System. The only method published recently that appears to improve prediction accuracy significantly, not through more divergent profiles but through the particular algorithm, is SSpro (13). The major idea of the method aims at solving the problem of predicting too short segments. PHD addressed this problem by a second-level structure-to-structure network (50). Most authors have since implemented this idea (in particular PSIPRED and JPred2). Pierre Baldi and colleagues deviated substantially from this concept. Instead of using an additional network, they embedded the correlation into one single recursive neural network. In principle, the idea of a recursive network had been implemented before (172). However, the particular details of the algorithm implemented in SSpro are novel and—as Table 1 illustrates—prove highly successful. Interestingly, SSpro is less successful on improving the prediction of segments length than on improving overall accuracy (Fig. 5).

HMMSTR: Hidden Markov Models for Connecting the Library of Structure Fragments. Can we predict secondary structure for protein U by local sequence similarity to segments of known structures {S} even when overall U differs from any of the known structures {S}? Yes, as shown by many nearest-neighbor-based prediction methods, the most successful of which seems to be NSSP (158). A conceptually quite different realization of the same concept has been implemented in HMMSTR by Bystroff and colleagues (2). First, build a library of local stretches (3–19) of residues with "basic structural motifs" (I-sites). Second, assemble these local motifs through hidden Markov models, introducing structural context on the level of super secondary structure. Thus, the goal is to predict protein structure through identification of "grammatical units of protein structure formation." Although HMMSTR intrinsically aims at predicting higher-order aspects of 3D structure, a side result is the prediction of 1D secondary structure. I find two results surprising: (1) The authors do not find any significant effect of "overoptimizing" their method; i.e., HMMSTR appears as accurate in predicting secondary structure for proteins known today as it will be for those known next year. (2) Three-state per-residue accuracy is

Table 1 Accuracy of Secondary Structure Prediction Methods[a]

Method[b]	Q_3[c]	Q_3 claim[d]	BAD[e]	Info[f]	CorrH[g]	CorrE[h]	SOV[i]	Class[j]
PHD	71.7	71.6	4.1	0.25	0.59	0.60	68	78
JPred2	75.	76.4	2.4	0.34	0.64	0.63	70	77
PHDpsi	75.0		2.9	0.29	0.64	0.62	70	81
PROF	77.0		2.1	0.37	0.67	0.65	73	83
PSIPRED	76.7	76.5–78.3[k]	2.4	0.37	0.66	0.64	73	81
SSpro	76.2	76	2.6	0.36	0.67	0.65	71	83
EVA-4	77.8	2.0	0.38	0.69	0.67	0.67	83	

[a] Data set and sorting: The results are compiled via EVA (Ref. 248). All methods for which details are listed have been tested on 201 different new protein structures (EVA version Feb. 2001). None of these proteins was similar to any protein used to develop the respective method. This set comprised the largest such set by Feb. 7, 2001, for which we had results. Sorting and grouping reflects the following concept: If the data set is too small to distinguish between methods, these two are grouped. For the given set of 195 proteins, this yielded four groups. Inside each group, results are sorted alphabetically. Due to a lack of data, I could not add the performance of SAM-T99sec (Ref. 169); on a set of 105 proteins SAM-T99sec appears comparable to the best three: PSIPRED, Spro, and PROF. Another method that appeared at least as accurate when tested on an earlier EVA set is missing since it is not publicly available (Ref. 175).
[b] Method: See abbreviations in footnote at chapter opening; EVA-4 refers to a simple average over the binary prediction output from PHDpsi, PSIPRED, SSpro, and PROF.
[c] Q_3: three-state per-residue accuracy [Eq. (1)].
[d] Q_3 claim: three-state per-residue accuracy published in original publication of method: PSIPRED (Ref. 11), SSpro (Ref. 13), JPred2 (Ref. 5), PHD (Ref. 78).
[e] BAD: Percentage of helical residues predicted as strand and of strand residues predicted as helix (Ref. 56).
[f] Info: per-residue information content (Ref. 50)
[g] CorrH: Matthew's correlation coefficient for state helix (Ref. 249).
[h] CorrE: Matthew's correlation for state strand (Ref. 249).
[i] SOV: three-state per-segment score averaged over the three=state segment overlap between predicted and observed segments (Refs. 51,58).
[j] Class: percentage of proteins correctly sorted into one of the four classes: all-alpha (length > 60, helix > 45%, strand < 5%), all-beta length > 60, helix < 5%, strand > 45%), alpha/beta (length 60%, helix > 30%, strand > 20%), other (thresholds for classification from Refs. 78,99,250).
[k] Accuracy range: PSIPRED results were published for different conversions of the eight DSSP states to three states.

reported to be about 74% (2). This value may be overestimated. Nevertheless, HMMSTR is clearly one of the better prediction methods.

Plethora of New Concepts for Secondary Structure Prediction Explored Recently. The following five methods are a small subset of new ideas explored to improve secondary structure prediction.

1. Ouali and King (173) combine neural networks and rule-based statistics in a cascade of classifiers. Based on a similar data set they estimate a level of prediction accuracy comparable to that of JPred2 (see Table 1).

2. Chandonia and Karplus (174) combined simplified output schemes (two output states) with networks trained on different tasks and a particular variant of early stopping; inputs are non-divergent alignments picked from the safe zone (Fig. 1). Based on a protocol similar to the one applied by the Danish group (175), the authors estimate a level of over 76% accuracy, i.e., a level that, if it holds up, is similar to that of SSpro (Table 1).

3. Supposedly the simplest new method that claims to almost approach the performance of PHD combines the information for secondary structure formation contained in amino acid singlets, doublets, and triplets.

4. Schmidler et al. (176) use a simple statistical model; the novel aspect is to replace compiling statistics over fixed stretches of N residues by segments signifying regular secondary structure (helix, strand). The underlying formalism resembles a hidden semi-Markov model allowing one to explicitly incorporate explicitly particular propensies such as helix caps (177). Based on noncomparable data sets, the authors estimated prediction accuracy to be around 69%; if correct, this value is extremely impressive for a second-generation method.

5. Without claims to surprising levels of accuracy, Figureau et al. [178] combine cleverly chosen pentapeptides from the database to obtain the final prediction.

3.4 Caution: Overoptimism Has Become Even More Likely!*

Seemingly Improve Accuracy by Ignoring Short Segments. There are many ways to achieve higher levels of accuracy. Among the simplest for secondary structure prediction is to convert 3_{10} helices and beta-bulges as-

---

* This section covers "what not to do," since many of the recently published methods fall prey to one of the problems mentioned.

signed by DSSP (48) to nonregular structure. This yields higher levels of accuracy, since all methods—on average—are better at predicting the middle of helices and strands than their caps and hence are more accurate for longer regular secondary structure segments (49,174). When using predicted secondary structure to predict 3D structure, short helices are important. Thus, I suggest bearing with the more conservative conversion strategy.

Comparing Apples and Oranges, or Comparing Too Few Apples with One Another. To overstate the point: There is *no* value in comparing methods evaluated on different data sets. Most secondary structure prediction methods are available. Thus, developers may want to compare their results to public methods based on the same data set (not previously used for any of the two). Many methods predicting aspects of protein structure and function have to fight with limited data availability. This is not at all the case for secondary structure prediction. Hundreds of new protein structures are added every year (6). If, for whatever reason, small data sets have to be used, developers should painstakingly try to estimate what "significant difference" means for their data set. For example, about 20 new protein structures are clearly too few! This is the number of proteins that were available for the CASP4 meeting. Based on that set, all third-generation methods were equal!

Seemingly Achieve 100% Accuracy by Using Correlated Sets. Many publications on predicting secondary structural class from amino acid composition allowed correlations between "training" and testing sets. Consequently, levels of prediction accuracy published exceeded by far the theoretical possible margins [179]. A very simple operational definition for "independent sets" is the following: Two proteins, A and B, are correlated if the sequence similarity between A and B suffices to predict the structure of B knowing A's structure. Assume we have two uncorrelated sets of proteins, S1 and S2. Can we train the method on set S1 and develop it on set S2 without further ado? While developing PROF, I realized that the answer is negative. In fact, I trained neural networks on about 2000 structures that had no significant level of sequence similarity to our original set of 126 proteins (50). I used the 126 only after I had completed developing the method and found a prediction accuracy exceeding 80% (unpublished). When testing PROF on a set of about 200 new structures that had been added to PDB in the meantime (different to that given in Table 1), prediction accuracy dropped. Do the 126 differ from the set used for Table 1? I failed to answer this question.

EVA: Automatic Evaluation of Automatic Prediction Servers. In collaboration with Volker Eyrich (Columbia), Marc Marti-Renom, Andrej Sali (both at Rockefeller), Florencio Pazos, and Alfonso Valencia (both at CNB

Madrid), we have started to address the preceding problems through the automatic server EVA (180,181). Leszek Rychlewski (IIMCB Warsaw) and Dani Fischer (Ben-Gurion University) are implementing similar ideas in LiveBench (182). The simple concept is the following: take the N newest experimental structures added to PDB, send the sequences to all prediction servers, collect the results, and accumulate a continuous evaluation of prediction accuracy every week. EVA has been evaluating secondary structure prediction methods for more than six months now. I found it instructive to see how the "ranking" of methods initially changed from week to week due to too-small sets. Currently, EVA also provides results for evaluating comparative modeling (Sali group) and residue–residue contacts (Valencia group). We hope that EVA will eventually simplify life for developers, referees, editors, and users.

3.5   State-of-the-Art Secondary Structure Prediction

3.5.1   What Does 77% Accuracy Mean in Practice?

Prediction Accuracy Peaks at 77% Accuracy. The current best methods reach a level around 77% three-state per-residue accuracy (Table 1). This constitutes a sustained level about five percentage points above last century's best method not using diverged profiles (PHD in Table 1). Fortunately, the improvement is valid for helix, strand, and nonregular regions (information and correlation indices in Table 1). Furthermore, significantly fewer residues are confused between the helix and strand states (BAD score, Table 1). Finally, some new methods also improve in a more global sense by improving the accuracy of assigning the secondary structural class (all-alpha, all-beta, alpha/beta, other) based on the predicted content of regular secondary structure (Class score, Table 1).

Difference Between 60% and 70% Accuracy May Matter a Lot! Some of the third-generation methods for secondary structure prediction are clearly superior to previous methods: β-strands are predicted more accurately; predicted segments look like those observed; and the overall accuracy is about 10 percentage points higher. The advantage in practice is illustrated in Figure 7. Not only does the third-generation method (here PHD) get most segments right, but it also enables one to focus on more reliably predicted residues. The reliability index (*Rel* in Fig. 7) is compiled as the difference between the output unit with the highest value (winner unit) and the output unit with the next highest value [normalized to a scale from 0 (low) to 9 (high)]. All strongly predicted residues (* in Fig. 7) are predicted correctly.

Values for Expected Prediction Accuracy are Distributions. Statements such as "secondary structure is about 90% conserved within sequence

```
    SEQ   KELVLALYDYQERSPREVTMKKGDILFLLNSTMKDWNKVEVEDRQGFVPAAYVKXLD
    OBS   EEEE         E--E    EEEEEE      EEEEE   EEEEEEEHHHHHEEEE
1st C+F   HHHHHHH      HHHHHH  EEEEE       HHHHHH  EEEEEEHHHHHHHH
2nd GOR   HHHHHHHH     HHHH    EEEEEE      EEEEEH  HHH  HHHHHHH
3rd PHD   EEEEEE       EEE     EEEEEEEE    HHHHHH  EEEE HHEEEE
    Rel   948999972587775211443884899847697314344045955111321221558
          *  ******  ******          --  ....  ....          ....  ....
```

```
    SEQ   EGTELNKIDEEPIAFGLVALNVMVVVGDAEGGTEAAEESLSGIEGVSNIEVTDVRSLN
    OBS        EE    REE    EEEEEEEEE     GGGGHHHHHH     EEEEEEEEEEEE

  JPred2       HHH          EEEEEEEEEE    HHHHHHHH       EEEEHHHH
    PHD        EEEE   E HEHEHHHEEEEEEE    HHHHHHHHH      EEEEEEEEEHH
 PHDpsi        EEEE   EEEEEHEHHHEEEEEEE   HHHHHHHHH      EEEEEEHHHHH
   PROF        EEEE   EEEHHHHEEEEEEE      HHHHHHH        REEEEEEEEEE
 PSIPRED              HHEEEEEEEEEEEEEEE   HHHHHHHHHH     EEEEEEEEEE
   SSpro       EEE    HE HHHEEEHHEEE      HHHHHHHHHH     EEEEEEEEEH

  EVA-4        EEE    HE HHHEEEEEEEEE     HHHHHHHHHH     EEEEEEEEHH
```

Figure 7 Example of secondary structure prediction of first to third generation: *Top Panel*: SH3 structure (Ref. 184). The dashes indicate the continuation of the second strand that was missed by DSSP. The methods are first generation: $C + F$ (Ref. 73); second generation: *GOR* (Ref. 243) (= GORIII), and third generation: *PHD* (Ref. 7). The levels of three-state accuracy were: $C + F = 59\%$; GOR = 65%; and PHD = 72%. Whereas the first- and second-generation methods performed above their average accuracy (Fig. 1) for this protein, the PHD prediction was average (Figs. 1 and 7). The strength of the PHD prediction was reflected in the one-digit reliability index (*Rel*, 0 = low, 9 = high) correlated with prediction accuracy. All residues predicted at values of Rel > 4 (marked by *) were predicted correctly. *Lower Panel*: Translation elongation factor beta-1 (Ref. 247): shown are examples for methods exploring extended profile searches (see Table 1 for abbreviations). An N-terminal strand and helix (not shown) were correctly predicted by all methods. Although the combination of various methods (EVA-4) is better on average (Table 1), it is debatable as to which prediction is most useful here.

families" (51) refer to averages over distributions. The same holds for the expected prediction accuracy (Fig. 8). Such distributions explain why some developers have overestimated the performance of their tools using data sets of only tens of proteins (or even fewer). In general, single sequences yield accuracy values about 10 percentage points lower than multiple alignments (50,54,78). Note that for most proteins, some helix and strand residues are confused (BAD predictions in Fig. 8).

Reliability of Prediction Correlates with Accuracy. For the user interested in a particular protein U, the fact that prediction accuracy varies with the protein (Fig. 8) implies a rather unfortunate message: The accuracy for U could be lower than 40%, or it could be higher than 90% (Fig. 8). Is there any way to provide an estimate of the end of the distribution at which the

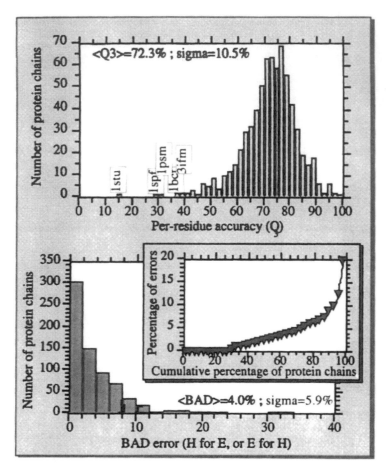

Figure 8 Expected variation of prediction accuracy with protein chain for PHD. *Top Panel*: Three-state per-residue accuracy [Eq. (1)]; PDB identifier given for the proteins predicted worst; percentage of BAD predictions, i.e., residues either predicted in helix and observed in strand or predicted in strand and observed in helix (introduced by Ref. 56). *Inset*: Cumulative percentage of proteins with BADly predicted residues (e.g., for 80% of the proteins the percentage of confusing helix and strand residues is under 7%; however, for only 30% of all proteins such a confusion never happened). Given: distributions (over 721 unique protein chains), averages, and one standard deviation. Distributions of all other third-generation methods given in Table 1 are qualitatively similar.

accuracy for U is likely to be? Indeed, the reliability index correlates with accuracy. In other words, residues with a higher reliability index are predicted with higher accuracy (7,50,78). Thus, the reliability index offers an excellent tool to focus on some key regions predicted at high levels of expected accuracy. Furthermore, the reliability index averaged over an entire protein correlates with the overall prediction accuracy for this protein (Fig. 9). (Note, however, that the reliability indices tend to be unusually high for alignments of sequence families without very divergent sequences.) Plotting the reliability of the prediction against accuracy (Fig. 9) also reveals that minor differences in overall accuracy may matter. For example, JPred2 and PROF differ by only two percentage points (Table 1); however, JPred2 reaches 88% accuracy for "only" 45% of all residues, whereas PROF reaches that level for more than 60% of all residues (Fig. 9).

Understandable Why Certain Proteins Predicted Poorly? For some of the worst predicted proteins, the low level of accuracy could be anticipated

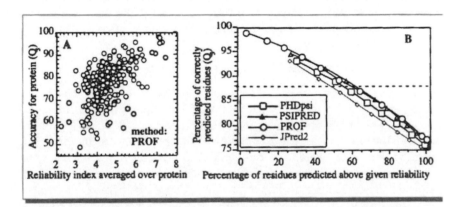

Figure 9 Correlation between reliability and accuracy. Residues predicted at higher reliability are predicted more accurately (7,50,78). In fact, proteins with higher average reliability index are predicted above average (A, method: PROF). For example, no protein predicted at an average reliability of 6 or more has less than 76% accuracy, and only 3 out of 201 are below 70% accuracy for an average index of 5 or more. PROF predictions were 5 or more on average for one-fourth of all proteins; for these the prediction accuracy was 83%. Reliability indices are now being used by most methods (B). They also enable users to spot particular regions predicted more accurately than others. For example, PROF and PSIPRED reach a level of accuracy similar to comparative modeling (around 88%, dotted line) for about 60% of all residues, and more than 93% of the quarter of the residues predicted at highest indices are correctly predicted. Note: The values in B are cumulative; e.g., 100% of all residues for PROF are predicted at 77.4% accuracy (Table 1).

from their unusual features, e.g., for crambin or the antifreeze glycoprotein type III. However, this procedure turned out to be rather arbitrary. First, some proteins with the same "unusual features" are predicted at high levels of accuracy. Second, similar proteins are occasionally predicted at very different levels of accuracy; e.g., both the phosphotidylinonitol 3-kinase (183) and the Src-homology domain of cytoskeletal spectrin have homologous structure (184) but prediction accuracy varies between less than 40% (pik) and more than 70% (spectrin). None of the conclusions from studying poor predictions has yet to yield a way to better predictions. Nevertheless, two observations may be added. First, bad alignments (i.e., noninformative and/or falsely aligned residues) result in bad predictions. Second, the BAD predictions (Fig. 8, Table 1), i.e., the confusion of helix and strand, are frequently observed in regions that are stabilized by long-range interactions. For example, the peptide around the fourth strand of SH3 (Fig. 7) forms a helix in solution (Luis Serrano, personal communication). Furthermore, helices and strands that are confused despite a high reliability index often have functional properties or are correlated with disease states (Rost, unpublished data). Regions predicted with equal propensity in two different states often correlate with "structural switches" (see ASP later).

3.5.2   What Is at the Base of the Recent Improvement?

Sources of Improvement: Four Parts Database Growth, Three Extended Search, Two Other. Jones suggested two causes for the improved accuracy: (1) training and (2) testing the method on PSI-BLAST profiles. Cuff and Barton examined in detail how different alignment methods improve (5). However, which fraction of the improvement results from the mere growth of the database, which from using more diverged profiles, and which from training on larger profiles? Using PHD from 1994 to separate the effects (8), we first compared a noniterative standard BLAST (150) search against SWISS-PROT (14) with one against SWISS-PROT + TrEMBL (14) + PDB (6). The larger database improves performance by about two percentage points (8). Second, we compared the standard BLAST against the big database with an iterative PSI-BLAST search. This yielded less than two percentage points of additional improvement (8). Thus, overall, the more divergent profile search against today's databases supposedly improves any method using alignment information by almost four percentage points (PHDpsi in Table 1). The improvement through using PSI-BLAST profiles to develop the method are relatively small: PHDpsi was trained on a small database of not very divergent profiles in 1994; e.g., in 2000, PROF was trained on PSI-BLAST profiles of a database 20 times larger. The two differ by only one percentage point (Table 1), and part of this difference resulted from implementing new concepts into PROF (Rost, unpublished; (9)).

Combination Improves on Nonsystematic Errors. Any prediction method has two types of errors: (1) systematic errors, e.g., through nonlocal effects, and (2) white noise errors caused by, e.g., the succession of the examples during training neural networks. Theoretically, combining any number of methods improves accuracy as long as the errors of the individual methods are mutually independent and are not just systematic (185). PHD—and more recently others (5,174,175)—utilized this fact by combining different neural networks. The idea of combining different prediction methods has been around in secondary structure prediction for a long time (186); Cuff and Barton (3,4) implemented it in JPred for different third-generation methods. In particular, JPred uses a simple expert rule for compiling the final average. King et al. (187) tested a variety of different combination strategies. Selbig et al. (188) compiled the jury through an elaborated decision-tree-based system. Guermeur et al. (189) used a more refined variant of the JPred idea of weighting methods. Overall, combinations of independent prediction methods seem to yield levels of accuracy higher than that of the single best method. In particular, combining the four current best methods (PROF, PSIPRED, SSpro, and PHDpsi) improved prediction accuracy to 77.8% (Table 1, EVA-4). However, for every protein, one method tends to be clearly superior to the combined prediction. Is it really wise to include significantly inferior methods in a combined prediction? No: Averaging over all methods used for EVA decreased accuracy over the best individual methods, although averaging over the better ones was better than averaging the best ones (data not shown). Is there any criterion for when to include a method and when not? Concepts weighting the individual methods based on their accuracy and "entropy" (175) appear successful only for large numbers of methods ((175), Rost, unpublished). Nevertheless, methods that are significantly overtrained can improve when combined (Krogh, unpublished). More rigorous studies for the optimal combination may provide a better picture. The technical problem of utilizing many methods in a public server is that the field is advancing too fast: Today's methods are more accurate than averages over yesterday's methods (hence the JPred server now returns JPred2 results by default).

3.5.3 Availability of Methods

Internet Prediction Services for Secondary Structure in General. Programs for the prediction of secondary structure available as Internet services have mushroomed since the first prediction service, PredictProtein, went online in 1992 (119,149) (a list of links is in Ref. 190). Our META-

PredictProtein server (191) enables users to access a number of the best prediction methods through one single interface. Unfortunately, not all available methods have been sufficiently tested, and some are not very accurate. We try to address this problem by maintaining EVA for the automatic evaluation of prediction servers (180,181). In general, prediction accuracy is significantly superior if predictions are based on multiple alignments (25,154,192).

Completely vs. Almost Automatic. The PHD/PROF prediction methods are automatically available via the Internet service PredictProtein (119) (use the Web interface at http://cubic.bioc.columbia.edu/predictprotein or e-mail the word *help* to PredictProtein@columbia.edu). Users have the choice between the fully automatic procedure taking the query sequence through the entire cycle and expert intervention into the generation of the alignment. Indeed, without spending much time, users typically can improve prediction accuracy easily by choosing "good" alignments.

3.6   Are Secondary Structure Predictions Useful in Practice?

Regions Likely to Undergo Structural Change Predicted Successfully. Young et al. (1) had uncovered an impressive correlation between local secondary structure predictions and global conditions. The authors monitor regions for which secondary structure prediction methods give equally strong preferences for two different states. Such regions are processed combining simple statistics and expert rules. The final method is tested on 16 proteins known to undergo structural rearrangements and on a number of other proteins. The authors report no false positives and identify most known structural switches. Subsequently, the group applied the method to the myosin family, identifying putative switching regions that were not known before but appeared reasonable candidates (193). I find this method quite remarkable in two ways: (1) It is the most general method using predictions of protein structure to predict some aspects of function, and (2) it illustrates that predictions may be useful even when structures are known (as in the case of the myosin family).

Classifying Proteins Based on Secondary Structure Predictions in the Context of Genome Analysis. Proteins can be classified into families based on predicted and observed secondary structure (28,194). However, such procedures have been limited to a very coarse-grained grouping only occasionally useful for inferring function. Nevertheless, in particular predictions of membrane helices and coiled-coil regions are crucial for genome analysis in particular. Recently, we came across an observation that may have important implications for structural genomics: More than one-fifth of all eukaryotic proteins appeared to have regions longer than 60 residues apparently lacking any regular secondary structure (195). Most of these regions were not of low complexity, i.e., not composition biased. Surprisingly, these regions appeared evolutionarily as conserved as all other regions in the respective proteins. This application of secondary structure prediction may aid in classifying proteins and in separating domains, possibly even in identifying particular functional motifs.

Aspects of Protein Function Predicted Based on Expert Analysis of Secondary Structure. The typical scenario in which secondary structure predictions help one to learn about function is when are experts combining combine predictions and their intuition, most often to find similarities to between proteins of known function but insignificant sequence similarity (40,196–207). Usually, such applications are based on very specific details about predicted secondary structure. Thus, these successful correlations of secondary structure and function appear difficult to incorporate into automatic methods.

Exploring Secondary Structure Predictions to Improve Database Searches. Initially, three groups independently applied secondary structure predictions for fold recognition, i.e., the detection of structural similarities between proteins of unrelated sequences (208–210). A few years later, almost every other fold recognition/threading method has adopted this concept (211–220). Two recent methods extended the concept not only by refining the database search, but by actually refining the quality of the alignment through an iterative procedure (171,221). A related strategy was implored explored by Ng et al. to improve predictions and alignments for membrane proteins (222).

From 1D Predictions to 2D and 3D Structure. Are secondary structure predictions accurate enough to help predicting higher-order aspects of protein structure automatically? Two-dimensional (interresidue contacts) predictions: Baldi, and coworkers (223) recently improved the level of accuracy in predicting beta-strand pairings over earlier work (152) through using another elaborate neural network system. Three-dimensional predictions: The following list of five groups exemplifies how secondary structure predictions have are now a popular first step toward predicting 3D structure. (1) Ortiz et al. (224) successfully use secondary structure predictions as one component of their 3D structure prediction method. (2) Eyrich et al. (225,226) minimize the energy of arranging predicted rigid secondary structure segments. (3) Lomize et al. (227) also start from secondary structure segments. (4) Chen et al. (228) suggest using secondary structure predictions to reduce the complexity of molecular dynamics simulations. (5) Levitt et al. (229,230) combine secondary structure-based simplified presentations with a particular lattice simulation, attempting to enumerate all possible folds.

3.7   And What is the Limit of Prediction Accuracy?

Eighty-Eight Percent is a Limit, But Shall We Ever Reach Close to That? Protein secondary structure formation is influenced by long-range interactions (46,47,231) and by the environment (1,232). Consequently, stretches of up to 11 adjacent residues (dubbed chameleon after Ref. 23) can be found in different secondary structure states (233–235). Implicitly, such nonlocal effects are contained in the exchange patterns of protein families. This is reflected in the fact that strand is predicted almost as accurately as helix (Table 1), although sheets are stabilized by more nonlocal interactions than helices. Local profiles can even suffice to identify structural switches (1,193). Surprisingly, we can find some traces of folding events in secondary structure predictions (236). Even more amazing is a study suggesting that alignment-based methods achieve similar levels of accuracy for chameleon regions as for all other regions (235). Secondary structure assignments may vary for two versions of the same structure. One reason is that protein structures are not rocks but dynamic objects, with some regions more mobile than others. Another reason is that any assignment method has to choose particular thresholds (e.g., DSSP chooses a cutoff in the Coulomb energy of a hydrogen bond). Consequently, assignments differ by about 5–15 percentage points between different X-ray versions or different NMR models for the same protein (Andersen and Rost, unpublished) and by about 12 percentage points between structural homologs (51). The latter number provides the upper limit for secondary structure prediction of error-free comparative modeling. I doubt that ab initio predictions of secondary structure will ever become more accurate than that. Hence, I believe a value around 88% constitutes an operational upper limit for prediction accuracy. After the recent advances, we reached above 76%. Thus, we need to increase by another 12 percentage points (or even less). What is the major obstacle to reaching another six percentage points higher? Is it the size of the experimental database, as suggested by Ref. 234? I doubt this, since PHDpsi trained on only 200 proteins using PSI-BLAST input is almost as accurate as PSIPRED trained on 2000 proteins (Table 1). Will the current explosion of sequences boost accuracy? In fact, current databases have fewer than 10 homologs for more than one-third of the 150 tested proteins (Table 1) and more than 100 for only 20% of the proteins. Although based on a set too small for conclusions, for these 20% highly populated families the accuracy of PROF was four percentage points above average (data not shown). Thus, larger databases may get us six percentage points higher, and they may not. The answer remains nebulous.

4 NOTES

The following notes resulted from nine years of experience running the PredictProtein server (119) and from various structure prediction workshops (237). Some comments apply in particular to the PHD/PROF methods (7,238). However, most hold also for using other secondary structure prediction methods (a detailed list of "Hints for users" is given on our Web site (119).

4.1 What Can You Expect from Secondary Structure Prediction?

How Accurate are the Predictions? The expected levels of accuracy (PROF $Q_3 = 77 \pm 10\%$) are valid for typical globular, water-soluble proteins when the multiple alignment contains many and diverse sequences. High values for the reliability indices indicate more accurate predictions (Fig. 9). However, for alignments with little variation in the sequences, the reliability indices adopt misleadingly high values. PHD/PROF predictions tend to be relatively accurate for porins (7); however, for helical membrane proteins other programs ought to be used (7,39,238).

Confusion Between Strand and Helix? PHD (as well as other methods) focuses on predicting hydrogen bonds. Consequently, strongly predicted (high-reliability-index) helices are occasionally observed as strands, and vice versa (Fig. 8, Table 1). In fact, some of these BAD predictions correspond to structural switching regions.

Strong Signal from Secondary Structure Caps? The ends of helices and strands contain a strong signal. However, PHD on average predicts the core of helices and strands more accurately than the caps (49). This is also true for the other methods listed in Table 1 (data not shown).

Internal Helices Predicted Poorly? Benner has indicated that internal helices are difficult to predict (53,137). On average, this is not the case for PHD predictions (239).

What About Protein Design and Synthesized Peptides? The PHD networks are trained on naturally evolved proteins. However, the predictions have been useful in some cases to investigate the influence of single mutations (e.g., for Chameleon (231,240) and for Janus (241), Rost, unpublished). For short polypeptides, users should bear in mind that the network input consists of 17 adjacent residues. Thus, shorter sequences may be dominated by the ends (which are treated as solvent by the current version of PHD).

4.2   How Can You Avoid Pitfalls?

Seventy Percent Correct Implies 30% Incorrect.   The most accurate methods for predicting secondary structure reach sustained levels of about 70% accuracy. When interpreting predictions for a particular protein it is often instructive to mark the 30% of the residues you suspect to be falsely predicted.

Special Classes of Proteins.   Prediction methods are usually derived from knowledge contained in proteins from subsets of current databases. Consequently, they should not be applied to classes of proteins not included in these subsets, e.g., methods for predicting helices in globular proteins are likely to fail when applied to predicting transmembrane helices. In general, results should be taken with caution for proteins with unusual features, such as proline-rich regions, or unusually many cysteine bonds or for domain interfaces.

Better Alignments Yield Better Predictions.   Multiple alignment-based predictions are substantially more accurate than single sequence-based predictions. How many sequences do you need in your alignment for an improvement? And how sensitive are prediction methods to errors in the alignment? The more divergent sequences contained in the alignment, the better (two distantly related sequences often improve secondary structure predictions by several percentage points). Regions with few aligned sequences yield less reliable predictions. The sensitivity to alignment errors depends on the methods; e.g., secondary structure prediction is less sensitive to alignment errors than accessibility prediction.

One-dimensional Structure May or May Not Be Sufficient to Infer 3D Structure.   Say you obtain as prediction for regular secondary structure: helix-strand-strand-helix-strand-strand (H-E-E-H-E-E). Assume, you find a protein of known structure with the same motif (H-E-E-H-E-E). Can you conclude that the two proteins have the same fold? Yes and no; your guess may be correct, but there are various ways to realize the given motif by completely different structures. For example, at least, 16 structurally unrelated proteins contain the secondary structure motif "H-E-E-H-E-E."

ACKNOWLEDGEMENTS

Particular thanks to Volker Eyrich for his crucial help with setting up the META-PP and EVA servers, without which most of the results presented here would not exist. Last but not least, thanks to all those who deposit their experimental data in public databases and to those who maintain these databases.

REFERENCES

1. Young, M., K. Kirshenbaum, K.A. Dill, and S. Highsmith. Predicting conformational switches in proteins. Prot. Sci. 8:1752–1764, 1999.
2. Bystroff, C., V. Thorsson, and D. Baker. HMMSTR: a hidden Markov model for local sequence–structure correlations in proteins. J. Mol. Biol. 301:173–190, 2000.
3. Cuff, J.A., M.E. Clamp, A.S. Siddiqui, M. Finlay, and G.J. Barton. JPred: a consensus secondary structure prediction server. Bioinformatics 14:892–893, 1998.
4. Cuff, J.A. and G.J. Barton. Evaluation and improvement of multiple sequence methods for protein secondary structure prediction. Proteins 34:508–519, 1999.
5. Cuff, J.A. and G.J. Barton. Application of multiple sequence alignment profiles to improve protein secondary structure prediction. Proteins 40:502–511, 2000.
6. Berman, H.M., J. Westbrook, Z. Feng, G. Gillliland, T.N. Bhat, H. Weissig, I.N. Shindyalov, and P.E. Bourne. The Protein Data Bank. Nucl. Acids Res. 28:235–242, 2000.
7. Rost, B. PHD: predicting one-dimensional protein structure by profile-based neural networks. Meth. Enzymol. 266:525–539, 1996.
8. Przybylski, D. and B. Rost. PSI-BLAST for Structure Prediction: Plug-In and Win. New York: Columbia University Press, 2001.
9. Rost, B. Better secondary structure prediction through more data. http:// cubic.bioc.columbia.edu/predictprotein, Columbia University, 2000.
10. Altschul, S., T. Madden, A. Shaffer, J. Zhang, Z. Zhang, W. Miller, and D. Lipman. Gapped Blast and PSI-Blast: a new generation of protein database search programs. Nucl. Acids Res. 25:3389–3402, 1997.
11. Jones, D.T. Protein secondary structure prediction based on position-specific scoring matrices. J. Mol. Biol. 292:195–202, 1999.
12. Karplus, K., C. Barrett, and R. Hughey. Hidden Markov models for detecting remote protein homologies. Bioinformatics 14:846–856, 1998.
13. Baldi, P., S. Brunak, P. Frasconi, G. Soda, and G. Pollastri. Exploiting the past and the future in protein secondary structure prediction. Bioinformatics 15:937–946, 1999.
14. Bairoch, A. and R. Apweiler. The SWISS-PROT protein sequence database and its supplement TrEMBL in 2000. Nucl. Acids Res. 28:45–48, 2000.
15. Gaasterland, T. and C.W. Sensen. MAGPIE: automated genome interpretation. TIGS 12:76–78, 1996.
16. Gaasterland, T. and C. Sensen. Fully automated genome analysis that reflects user needs and preferences - a detailed introduction to the MAGPIE system architecture. Biochimie 78:302–310, 1996.
17. Liu , J. and B. Rost. Analyzing all proteins in entire genomes: distribution of protein length. http://cubic.bioc.columbia.edu/genomes/RES/length/, CUBIC, Columbia University, Dept. of Biochemistry and Molecular Biophysics, 2000.

18. Bernstein, F.C., T.F. Koetzle, G.J.B. Williams, E.F. Meyer, M.D. Brice, J.R. Rodgers, O. Kennard, T. Shimanouchi, and M. Tasumi. The Protein Data Bank: a computer-based archival file for macromolecular structures. J. Mol. Biol. 112:535–542, 1977.

19. Liu, J. and B. Rost. Similar percentages of helical membrane proteins in all organisms. Prot. Sci. In submission, 2001.

20. Sanchez, R., U. Pieper, N. Mirkovic, P.I. de Bakker, E. Wittenstein, and A. Sali. MODBASE, a database of annotated comparative protein structure models. Nucl. Acids Res. 28:250–253, 2000.

21. CASP1. Special issue: First Meeting on Critical Assessment of Protein Structure prediction (CASP). Proteins 23:1995.

22. CASP2. Special issue: Second Meeting on Critical Assessment of Protein Structure prediction (CASP). Proteins Suppl. 2:1997.

23. CASP3. Special issue: Third Meeting on Critical Assessment of Protein Structure prediction (CASP). Proteins Suppl. 2:1999.

24. CASP4. Fourth meeting on the critical assessment of techniques for protein structure prediction. http://PredictionCenter.llnl.gov/casp4/Casp4.html, Prediction Center, Lawrence Livermore National Lab, 2000.

25. Rost, B. and C. Sander. Bridging the protein sequence–structure gap by structure predictions. Annu. Rev. Biophys. Biomol. Struct. 25:113–136, 1996.

26. Rost, B. and C. Sander. Structure prediction of proteins—where are we now? Curr. Opin. Biotech. 5:372–380, 1994.

27. Rost, B. Protein structure prediction in 1D, 2D, and 3D. In: PvR Schleyer, NL Allinger, T Clark, J Gasteiger, PA Kollman, HF Schaefer III, and PR Schreiner, eds. The Encyclopaedia of Computational Chemistry. Chichester, UK: Wiley, 1998, pp 2242–2255.

28. Gerstein, M. and M. Levitt. A structural census of the current population of protein sequences. Proc. Natl. Acad. Sci. U.S.A. 94:11911–11916, 1997.

29. Teichmann, S.A., C. Chothia, and M. Gerstein. Advances in structural genomics. Curr. Opin. Str. Biol. 9:390–399, 1999.

30. Frishman, D. PEDANT: protein extraction, description, and analysis tool. Max Planck Institute, Munich, 2000.

31. Liu, J. and B. Rost. Analyzing all proteins in entire genomes. http://cubic.-bioc.columbia.edu/genomes/, CUBIC, Columbia University, Dept. of Biochemistry & Molecular Biophysics, 2000.

32. Monne, M., M. Hermansson, and G. von Heijne. A turn propensity scale for transmembrane helices. J. Mol. Biol. 288:141–145, 1999.

33. Lio, P. and M. Vannucci. Wavelet change-point prediction of transmembrane proteins. Bioinformatics 16:376–382, 2000.

34. Pappu, R.V., G.R. Marshall, and J.W. Ponder. A potential smoothing algorithm accurately predicts transmembrane helix packing [published erratum appears in Nat. Struct. Biol. 6(2):1999]. Nat. Struct. Biol. 6:50–55, 1999.

35. Pilpel, Y., N. Ben-Tal, and D. Lancet. kPROT: a knowledge-based scale for the propensity of residue orientation in transmembrane segments. Application to membrane protein structure prediction. J. Mol. Biol. 294:921–935, 1999.

36. Pasquier, C., V.J. Promponas, G.A. Palaios, J.S. Hamodrakas, and S.J. Hamodrakas. A novel method for predicting transmembrane segments in proteins based on a statistical analysis of the SwissProt database: the PRED-TMR algorithm. Prot. Engin. 12:381–385, 1999.

37. Chou, K.C. and D.W. Elrod. Prediction of membrane protein types and subcellular locations. Proteins 34:137–153, 1999.

38. Kühlbrandt, W. and E. Gouaux. Membrane proteins. Curr. Opin. Str. Biol. 9:445–447, 1999.

39. Rost, B. and S.I. O'Donoghue. Sisyphus and prediction of protein structure. CABIOS 13:345–356, 1997.

40. de Fays, K., A. Tibor, C. Lambert, C. Vinals, P. Denoel, X. De Bolle, J. Wouters, J.J. Letesson, and E. Depiereux. Structure and function prediction of the *Brucella abortus* P39 protein by comparative modeling with marginal sequence similarities. Prot. Engin. 12:217–223, 1999.

41. Lupas, A. Predicting coiled-coil regions in proteins. Curr. Opin. Str. Biol. 7:388–393, 1997.

42. Wolf, E., P.S. Kim, and B. Berger. MultiCoil: a program for predicting two- and three-stranded coiled coils. Prot. Sci. 6:1179–1189, 1997.

43. O'Donoghue, S.I. and M. Nilges. Tertiary structure prediction using mean-force potentials and internal energy functions: successful prediction for coiled-coil geometries. Folding Design 2:S47–S52, 1997.

44. Kolinski, A., J. Skolnick, A. Godzik, and W.P. Hu. A method for the prediction of surface "U"-turns and transglobular connections in small proteins. Proteins 27:290–308, 1997.

45. Shepherd, A.J., D. Gorse, and J.M. Thornton. Prediction of the location and type of beta-turns in proteins using neural networks. Prot. Sci. 8:1045–1055, 1999.

46. Muñoz, V., P. Cronet, E. López-Hernández, and L. Serrano. Analysis of the effect of local interactions on protein stability. Folding Design 1:167–178, 1996.

47. Villegas, V., J. Zurdo, V.V. Filimonov, F.X. Aviles, C.M. Dobson, and L. Serrano. Protein engineering as a strategy to avoid formation of amyloid fibrils. Prot. Sci. 9:1700–1708, 2000.

48. Kabsch, W. and C. Sander. Dictionary of protein secondary structure: pattern recognition of hydrogen-bonded and geometrical features. Biopolymers 22:2577–2637, 1983.

49. Rost, B. and C. Sander. 1D secondary structure prediction through evolutionary profiles. In: H Bohr and S Brunak, eds. Protein Structure by Distance Analysis. Washington, DC: IOS Press, 1994, pp 257–276.

50. Rost, B. and C. Sander. Prediction of protein secondary structure at better than 70% accuracy. J. Mol. Biol. 232:584–599, 1993.

51. Rost, B., C. Sander, and R. Schneider. Redefining the goals of protein secondary structure prediction. J. Mol. Biol. 235:13–26, 1994.

52. Thornton, J.M., T.P. Flores, D.T. Jones, and M.B. Swindells. Prediction of progress at last. Nature 354:105–106, 1992.

53. Benner, S.A. and D.L. Gerloff. Predicting the conformation of proteins: man versus machine. FEBS Lett. 325:29–33, 1993.

54. Rost, B., C. Sander, and R. Schneider. Progress in protein structure prediction? TIBS 18:120–123, 1993.

55. Russell, R.B. and G.J. Barton. The limits of protein secondary structure prediction accuracy from multiple sequence alignment. J. Mol. Biol. 234:951–957, 1993.

56. Defay, T. and F.E. Cohen. Evaluation of current techniques for ab initio protein structure prediction. Proteins 23:431–445, 1995.

57. Rost, B. and C. Sander. Improved prediction of protein secondary structure by use of sequence profiles and neural networks. Proc. Natl. Acad. Sci. U.S.A. 90:7558–7562, 1993.

58. Zemla, A., C. Venclovas, K. Fidelis, and B. Rost. A modified definition of SOV, a segment-based measure for protein secondary structure prediction assessment. Proteins 34:220–223, 1999.

59. Rost, B. Twilight zone of protein sequence alignments. Prot. Engin. 12:85–94, 1999.

60. Kendrew, J.C., R.E. Dickerson, B.E. Strandberg, R.J. Hart, D.R. Davies, and D.C. Phillips. Structure of myoglobin: a three-dimensional Fourier synthesis at 2-Å resolution. Nature 185:422–427, 1960.

61. Perutz, M.F., M.G. Rossmann, A.F. Cullis, G. Muirhead, G. Will, and A.T. North. Structure of haemoglobin: a three-dimensional Fourier synthesis at 5.5-Å resolution, obtained by X-ray analysis. Nature 185:416–422, 1960.

62. Pauling, L. and R.B. Corey. Configurations of polypeptide chains with favored orientations around single bonds: two new pleated sheets. Proc. Natl. Acad. Sci. U.S.A. 37:729–740, 1951.

63. Pauling, L., R.B. Corey, and H.R. Branson. The structure of proteins: two hydrogen-bonded helical configurations of the polypeptide chain. Proc. Natl. Acad. Sci. U.S.A. 37:205–234, 1951.

64. Szent-Györgyi, A.G. and C. Cohen. Role of proline in polypeptide chain configuration of proteins. Science 126:697, 1957.

65. Blout, E.R., C. de Lozé, S.M. Bloom, and G.D. Fasman. Dependence of the conformation of synthetic polypeptides on amino acid composition. J. Am. Chem. Soc. 82:3787–3789, 1960.

66. Blout, E.R. The dependence of the conformation of polypetides and proteins upon amino acid composition. In: M Stahman, ed. Polyamino Acids, Polypeptides, and Proteins. Madison: Univ. of Wisconsin Press, 1962, pp 275–279.

67. Scheraga, H.A. Structural studies of ribonuclease III. A model for the secondary and tertiary structure. J. Am. Chem. Soc. 82:3847–3852, 1960.

68. Davies, D.R. A correlation between amino acid composition and protein structure. J. Mol. Biol. 9:605–609, 1964.

69. Schiffer, M. and A.B. Edmundson. Use of helical wheels to represent the structures of proteins and to identify segments with helical potential. Biophys. J. 7:121, 1967.

70. Pain, R.H. and B. Robson. Analysis of the code relating sequence to secondary structure in proteins. Nature 227:62–63, 1970.
71. Finkelstein, A.V. and O.B. Ptitsyn. Statistical analysis of the correlation among amino acid residues in helical, β-structural and nonregular regions of globular proteins. J. Mol. Biol. 62:613–624, 1971.
72. Robson, B. and R.H. Pain. Analysis of the code relating sequence to conformation in proteins: possible implications for the mechanism of formation of helical regions. J. Mol. Biol. 58:237–259, 1971.
73. Chou, P.Y. and U.D. Fasman. Prediction of protein conformation. Biochem. 13:211–215, 1974.
74. Lim, V.I. Structural principles of the globular organization of protein chains. A stereochemical theory of globular protein secondary structure. J. Mol. Biol. 88:857–872, 1974.
75. Rose, G.D. Prediction of chain turns in globular proteins on a hydrophobic basis. Nature 272:586–590, 1978.
76. Kabsch, W. and C. Sander. How good are predictions of protein secondary structure? FEBS Lett. 155:179–182, 1983.
77. Rost, B. and C. Sander. Secondary structure prediction of all-helical proteins in two states. Prot. Engin. 6:831–836, 1993.
78. Rost, B. and C. Sander. Combining evolutionary information and neural networks to predict protein secondary structure. Proteins 19:55–72, 1994.
79. Kabat, E.A. and T.T. Wu. The influence of nearest-neighbor amino acids on the conformation of the middle amino acid in proteins: comparison of predicted and experimental determination of β-sheets in concanavalin A. Proc. Natl. Acad. Sci. U.S.A. 70:1473–1477, 1973.
80. Maxfield, F.R. and H.A. Scheraga. Status of empirical methods for the prediction of protein backbone topography. Biochem. 15:5138–5153, 1976.
81. Robson, B. Conformational properties of amino acid residues in globular proteins. J. Mol. Biol. 107:327–356, 1976.
82. Nagano, K. Triplet information in helix prediction applied to the analysis of super-secondary structures. J. Mol. Biol. 109:251–274, 1977.
83. Garnier, J., D.J. Osguthorpe, and B. Robson. Analysis of the accuracy and implications of simple methods for predicting the secondary structure of globular proteins. J. Mol. Biol. 120:97-120, 1978.
84. Gibrat, J.-F., J. Garnier, and B. Robson. Further developments of protein secondary structure prediction using information theory. New parameters and consideration of residue pairs. J. Mol. Biol. 198:425–443, 1987.
85. Biou, V., J.F. Gibrat, J.M. Levin, B. Robson, and J. Garnier. Secondary structure prediction: combination of three different methods. Prot. Engin. 2:185–191, 1988.
86. Gascuel, O. and J.L. Golmard. A simple method for predicting the secondary structure of globular proteins: implications and accuracy. CABIOS 4:357–365, 1988.
87. Lupas, A., M. Van Dyke, and J. Stock. Predicting coiled coils from protein sequences. Science 252:1162–1164, 1991.

88. Viswanadhan, V.N., B. Denckla, and J.N. Weinstein. New joint prediction algorithm (Q7-JASEP) improves the prediction of protein secondary structure. Biochem. 30:11164–11172, 1991.

89. Juretic, D., B. Lee, N. Trinajstic, and R.W. Williams. Conformational preference functions for predicting helices in membrane proteins. Biopolymers 33:255–273, 1993.

90. Mamitsuka, H. and K. Yamanishi. Protein α-helix region prediction based on stochastic-rule learning. 26th Annual Hawaii International Conference on System Sciences, Maui, HI, 1993, pp 659–668.

91. Donnelly, D., J.P. Overington, and T.L. Blundell. The prediction and orientation of α-helices from sequence alignments: the combined use of environment-dependent substitution tables, Fourier transform methods and helix capping rules. Prot. Engin. 7:645–653, 1994.

92. Ptitsyn, O.B. and A.V. Finkelstein. Theory of protein secondary structure and algorithm of its prediction. Biopolymers 22:15–25, 1983.

93. Taylor, W.R. and J.M. Thornton. Prediction of super-secondary structure in proteins. Nature 301:540–542, 1983.

94. Cohen, F.E. and I.D. Kuntz. Tertiary structure prediction. In: GD Fasman, ed. Prediction of Protein Structure and the Principles of Protein Conformation. New York: Plenum Press, 1989, pp 647–706.

95. Rooman, M.J., J.P. Kocher, and S.J. Wodak. Prediction of protein backbone conformation based on seven structure assignments: influence of local interactions. J. Mol. Biol. 221:961–979, 1991.

96. Qian, N. and T.J. Sejnowski. Predicting the secondary structure of globular proteins using neural network models. J. Mol. Biol. 202:865–884, 1988.

97. Bohr, H., J. Bohr, S. Brunak, R.M.J. Cotterill, B. Lautrup, L. Nørskov, O.H. Olsen, and S.B. Petersen. Protein secondary structure and homology by neural networks. FEBS Lett. 241:223–228, 1988.

98. Holley, H.L. and M. Karplus. Protein secondary structure prediction with a neural network. Proc. Natl. Acad. Sci. U.S.A. 86:152–156, 1989.

99. Kneller, D.G., F.E. Cohen, and R. Langridge. Improvements in protein secondary structure prediction by an enhanced neural network. J. Mol. Biol. 214:171–182, 1990.

100. Stolorz, P., A. Lapedes, and Y. Xia. Predicting protein secondary structure using neural net and statistical methods. J. Mol. Biol. 225:363–377, 1992.

101. Zhang, X., J.P. Mesirov, and D.L. Waltz. Hybrid system for protein secondary structure prediction. J. Mol. Biol. 225:1049–1063, 1992.

102. Maclin, R. and J.W. Shavlik. Using knowledge-based neural networks to improve algorithms: refining the Chou–Fasman algorithm for protein folding. Machine Learning 11:195–215, 1993.

103. Chandonia, J.-M. and M. Karplus. Neural networks for secondary structure and structural class predictions. Prot. Sci. 4:275–285, 1995.

104. Mitchell, E.M., P.J. Artymiuk, D.W. Rice, and P. Willett. Use of techniques derived from graph theory to compare secondary structure motifs in proteins. J. Mol. Biol. 212:151–166, 1992.

105. Geourjon, C. and G. Deléage. SOPMA: significant improvements in protein secondary structure prediction by consensus prediction from multiple alignments. CABIOS 11:681–684, 1995.
106. Kanehisa, M. A multivariate analysis method for discriminating protein secondary structural segments. Prot. Engin. 2:87–92, 1988.
107. Munson, P.J. and R.K. Singh. Multibody interactions within the graph of protein structure. Fifth International Conference on Intelligent Systems for Molecular Biology, Halkidiki, Greece, 1997, pp 198–201.
108. King, R.D., S. Muggleton, R.A. Lewis, and M.J.E. Sternberg. Drug design by machine learning: the use of inductive logic programming to model the structure–activity relationships of trimethoprim analogues binding to dihydrofolate reductase. Proc. Natl. Acad. Sci. U.S.A. 89:11322–11326, 1992.
109. Muggleton, S., R.D. King, and M.J.E. Sternberg. Protein secondary structure prediction using logic-based machine learning. Prot. Engin. 5:647–657, 1992.
110. Frishman, D. and P. Argos. Knowledge-based protein secondary structure assignment. Proteins 23:566–579, 1995.
111. Zhu, Z.-Y. and T.L. Blundell. The use of amino acid patterns of classified helices and strands in secondary structure prediction. J. Mol. Biol. 260:261–276, 1996.
112. Asogawa, M. Beta-sheet prediction using interstrand residue pairs and refinement with Hopfield neural network. Ismb 5:48–51, 1997.
113. Yi, T.-M. and E.S. Lander. Protein secondary structure prediction using nearest-neigbor methods. J. Mol. Biol. 232:1117–1129, 1993.
114. Solovyev, V.V. and A.A. Salamov. Predicting α-helix and β-strand segments of globular proteins. CABIOS 10:661–669, 1994.
115. Salamov, A.A. and V.V. Solovyev. Prediction of protein secondary structure by combining nearest-neighbor algorithms and multiple sequence alignment. J. Mol. Biol. 247:11–15, 1995.
116. Kabsch, W. and C. Sander. Segment83. Unpublished, 1983.
117. Schneider, R. Sekundärstrukturvorhersage von Proteinen unter Berücksichtigung von Tertiärstrukturaspekten. PhD dissertation, University of Heidelberg, Germany, 1989.
118. Devereux, J., P. Haeberli, and O. Smithies. GCG package. Nucl. Acids Res. 12:387–395, 1984.
119. Rost, B. PredictProtein—internet prediction service. http://cubic.bioc.columbia.edu/predictprotein, Columbia University, New York, 2000.
120. Dao-pin, S., U. Sauer, H. Nicholson, and B.W. Matthews. Contributions of surface salt bridges to the stability of bacteriophage T4 lysozyme determined by directed mutagenesis. Biochem. 30:7142–7153, 1991.
121. Doolittle, R.F. Of URFs and ORFs: a primer on how to analyze derived amino acid sequences. Mill Valley, CA: University Science Books, 1986.
122. Chothia, C. and A.M. Lesk. The relation between the divergence of sequence and structure in proteins. EMBO J. 5:823–826, 1986.
123. Lesk, A.M. Protein Architecture—A Practical Approach. 1. New York: Oxford University Press, 1991, p. 287.

124. Sander, C. and R. Schneider. Database of homology-derived structures and the structural meaning of sequence alignment. Proteins 9:56–68, 1991.

125. Rost, B. Protein structures sustain evolutionary drift. Folding Design 2:S19–S24, 1997.

126. Yang, A.S. and B. Honig. An integrated approach to the analysis and modeling of protein sequences and structures. II. On the relationship between sequence and structural similarity for proteins that are not obviously related in sequence. J. Mol. Biol. 301:679–689, 2000.

127. Lichtarge, O., H.R. Bourne, and F.E. Cohen. An evolutionary trace method defines binding surfaces common to protein families. J. Mol. Biol. 257:342–358, 1996.

128. Pazos, F., L. Sanchez-Pulido, J.A. Garcia-Ranea, M.A. Andrade, S. Atrian, and A. Valencia. Comparative analysis of different methods for the detection of specificity regions in protein families. BCEC97: Bio-Computing and Emergent Computation, Skövde, Sweden, 1997, pp 132–145.

129. Dickerson, R.E., R. Timkovich, and R.J. Almassy. The cytochrome fold and the evolution of bacterial energy metabolism. J. Mol. Biol. 100:473–491, 1976.

130. Dickerson, R.E. The structure of cytochrome C and the rates of molecular evolution. J. Mol. Evol. 1:26–45, 1971.

131. Frampton, J., A. Leutz, T.J. Gibson, and T. Graf. DNA-binding domain ancestry. Nature 342:134, 1989.

132. Benner, S.A. Patterns of divergence in homologous proteins as indicators of tertiary and quaternary structure. Adv. Enzyme Regul. 28:219–236, 1989.

133. Bazan, J.F. Structural design and molecular evolution of a cytokine receptor superfamily. Proc. Natl. Acad. Sci. U.S.A. 87:6934–6938, 1990.

134. Benner, S.A. and D. Gerloff. Patterns of divergence in homologous proteins as indicators of secondary and tertiary structure of the catalytic domain of protein kinases. Adv. Enz. Reg. 31:121–181, 1990.

135. Niermann, T. and K. Kirschner. Improving the prediction of secondary structure of "TIM-barrel" enzymes. Protein Eng. 4:137–147, 1990.

136. Barton, G.J., R.H. Newman, P.S. Freemont, and M.J. Crumpton. Amino acid sequence analysis of the annexin supergene family of proteins. Eur. J. Biochem. 198:749–760, 1991.

137. Benner, S.A. Predicting de novo the folded structure of proteins. Curr. Opin. Str. Biol. 2:402–412, 1992.

138. Gibson, T.J. Assignment of α-helices in multiply aligned protein sequences—applications to DNA binding motifs. In: WR Taylor, ed. Patterns in Protein Sequence and Structure. Berlin: Springer-Verlag, 1992, pp 99–110.

139. Musacchio, A., T. Gibson, V.-P. Lehto, and M. Saraste. SH3—an abundant protein domain in search of a function. FEBS Lett. 307:55-61, 1992.

140. Barton, G.J. and R.B. Russell. Protein structure prediction. Nature 361:505–506, 1993.

141. Boscott, P.E., G.J. Barton, and W.G. Richards. Secondary structure prediction for homology modeling. Prot. Engin. 6:261–266, 1993.

142. Gerloff, D.L., T.F. Jenny, L.J. Knecht, G.H. Gonnet, and S.A. Benner. The nitrogenase MoFe protein. FEBS Lett. 318:118–124, 1993.

143. Gibson, T.J., J.D. Thompson, and R.A. Abagyan. Proposed structure for the DNA-binding domain of the helix-loop-helix family of eukaryotic gene regulatory proteins. Prot. Engin. 6:41–50, 1993.

144. Livingstone, C.D. and G.J. Barton. Secondary structure prediction from multiple sequence data: blood clotting factor XIII and versinia protein-tyrosine phosphatase. Int. J. Peptide Protein Res. 44:239–244, 1994.

145. Hansen, J.E., O. Lund, J.O. Nielsen, S. Brunak, and J.-E.S. Hansen. Prediction of the secondary structure of HIV-1 gp120. Proteins 25:1–11, 1996.

146. Valencia, A., T.J. Hubbard, A. Muga, S. Bañuelos, O. Llorca, J. Carrascosa, and J.M. Valpuesta. Prediction of the structure of GroES and its interaction with GroEL. Proteins 22:199–209, 1995.

147. Maxfield, F.R. and H.A. Scheraga. Improvements in the prediction of protein topography by reduction of statistical errors. Biochem. 18:697–704, 1979.

148. Zvelebil, M.J., G.J. Barton, W.R. Taylor, and M.J.E. Sternberg. Prediction of protein secondary structure and active sites using alignment of homologous sequences. J. Mol. Biol. 195:957–961, 1987.

149. Rost, B., C. Sander, and R. Schneider. PHD—an automatic server for protein secondary structure prediction. CABIOS 10:53–60, 1994.

150. Altschul, S.F. and W. Gish. Local alignment statistics. Meth. Enzymol. 266:460–480, 1996.

151. Schneider, R. Sequenz und Sequenz-Struktur Vergleiche und deren Anwendung für die Struktur- und Funktionsvorhersage von Proteinen. PhD dissertation, University of Heidelberg, 1994.

152. Hubbard, T.J.P. and J. Park. Fold recognition and ab initio structure predictions using hidden Markov models and β-strand pair potentials. Proteins 23:398–402, 1995.

153. Mehta, P.K., J. Heringa, and P. Argos. A simple and fast approach to prediction of protein secondary structure from multiply aligned sequences with accuracy above 70%. Prot. Sci. 4:2517–2525, 1995.

154. Di Francesco, V., J. Garnier, and P.J. Munson. Improving protein secondary structure prediction with aligned homologous sequences. Prot. Sci. 5:106–113, 1996.

155. Riis, S.K. and A. Krogh. Improving prediction of protein secondary structure using structured neural networks and multiple sequence alignments. J. Comp. Biol. 3:163–183, 1996.

156. Gerloff, D.L. and F.E. Cohen. Secondary structure prediction and unrefined tertiary structure prediction for cyclin A, B, and D. Proteins 24:18–34, 1996.

157. Frishman, D. and P. Argos. 75% accuracy in protein secondary structure prediction. Proteins 27:329–335, 1997.

158. Salamov, A.A. and V.V. Solovyev. Protein secondary structure prediction using local alignments. J. Mol. Biol. 268:31–36, 1997.

159. Levin, J.M., S. Pascarella, P. Argos, and J. Garnier. Quantification of secondary structure prediction improvement using multiple alignment. Prot. Engin. 6:849–854, 1993.
160. King, R.D. and M.J. Sternberg. Identification and application of the concepts important for accurate and reliable protein secondary structure prediction. Prot. Sci. 5:2298–2310, 1996.
161. Barton, G.J. Protein sequence alignment and database scanning. In: MJE Sternberg, ed. Protein Structure Prediction. Oxford, UK: Oxford University Press, 1996, pp 31–64.
162. Gribskov, M. and S. Veretnik. Identification of sequence patterns with profile analysis. Meth. Enzymol. 266:198–227, 1996.
163. Hughey, R. and A. Krogh. Hidden Markov models for sequence analysis: extension and analysis of the basic method. CABIOS 12:95–107, 1996.
164. Orengo, C.A. and W.R. Taylor. SSAP: sequential structure alignment program for protein structure comparison. Meth. Enzymol. 266:617–635, 1996.
165. Taylor, W.R. Multiple protein sequence alignment: algorithms and gap insertion. Meth. Enzymol. 266:343–367, 1996.
166. Higgins, D.G., J.D. Thompson, and T.J. Gibson. Using CLUSTAL for multiple sequence alignments. Meth. Enzymol. 266:383–402, 1996.
167. Eddy, S.R. Profile hidden Markov models. Bioinformatics 14:755–763, 1998.
168. Orengo, C.A., J.E. Bray, T. Hubbard, L. LoConte, and I. Sillitoe. Analysis and assessment of ab initio three-dimensional prediction, secondary structure, and contacts prediction. Proteins 37:149–170, 1999.
169. Karplus, K., C. Barrett, M. Cline, M. Diekhans, L. Grate, and R. Hughey. Predicting protein structure using only sequence information. Proteins S3:121–125, 1999.
170. Cuff, J.A., E. Birney, M.E. Clamp, and G.J. Barton. ProtEST: protein multiple sequence alignments from expressed sequence tags. Bioinformatics 16:111–116, 2000.
171. Jennings, A.J., C.M. Edge, and M.J.E. Sternberg. An approach to improve multiple alignments of protein sequences using predicted secondary structure. Prot. Engin. In press, 2000.
172. Reczko, M. Protein secondary structure prediction with partially recurrent neural networks. First International Workshop on Neural Networks Applied to Chemistry and Environmental Sciences, Lyon, France, 1993, pp 153–159.
173. Ouali, M. and R.D. King. Cascaded multiple classifiers for secondary structure prediction. Prot. Sci. 9:1162–1176, 2000.
174. Chandonia, J.M. and M. Karplus. New methods for accurate prediction of protein secondary structure. Proteins 35:293–306, 1999.
175. Petersen, T.N., C. Lundegaard, M. Nielsen, H. Bohr, J. Bohr, S. Brunak, G.P. Gippert, and O. Lund. Prediction of protein secondary structure at 80% accuracy. Proteins 41:17–20, 2000.
176. Schmidler, S.C., J.S. Liu, and D.L. Brutlag. Bayesian segmentation of protein secondary structure. J. Comp. Biol. 7:233–248, 2000.

177. Aurora, R. and G.D. Rose. Helix capping. Prot. Sci. 7:21–38, 1998.
178. Figureau, A., M. Angelica Soto, and J. Toha. Secondary structure of proteins and three-dimensional pattern recognition. J. Theor. Biol. 201:103–111, 1999.
179. Wang, Z.-X. and Z. Yuan. How good is prediction of protein structural class by the component-coupled method? Proteins 38:165–175, 2000.
180. Eyrich, V., M.A. Martí-Renom, D. Przybylski, A. Fiser, F. Pazos, A. Valencia, A. Sali, and B. Rost. EVA: continuous automatic evaluation of protein structure prediction servers. Bioinformatics, in submission, 2001.
181. Eyrich, V., M.A. Martí-Renom, D. Przybylski, A. Fiser, F. Pazos, A. Valencia, A. Sali, and B. Rost. EVA: continuous automatic evaluation of protein structure prediction servers. Columbia University, 2001, http://cubic.-bioc.columbia.edu/eva.
182. Rychlewski, L. and D. Fischer. LiveBench: continous benchmarking of prediction servers. http://BioInfo.PL/LiveBench/, IIMCB Warsaw, 2000.
183. Koyama, S., H. Yu, D.C. Dalgarno, T.B. Shin, L.D. Zydowsky, and S.L. Schreiber. Structure of the PI3K SH3 domain and analysis of the SH3 family. Cell 72:945–952, 1993.
184. Musacchio, A., M. Noble, R. Pauptit, R. Wierenga, and M. Saraste. Crystal structure of a Src-homology 3 (SH3) domain. Nature 359:851–855, 1992.
185. Hansen, L.K. and P. Salamon. Neural network ensembles. IEEE Trans. Pattern Anal. Machine Intel. 12:993–1001, 1990.
186. Rost, B. and C. Sander. Third-generation prediction of secondary structure. In: D Webster, ed. Protein Structure Prediction: Methods and Protocols. Totowa, NJ: Humana Press, 2000, pp 71–95.
187. King, R.D., M. Ouali, A.T. Strong, A. Aly, A. Elmaghraby, M. Kantardzic, and D. Page. Is it better to combine predictions? Prot. Engin. 13:15–19, 2000.
188. Selbig, J., T. Mevissen, and T. Lengauer. Decision tree–based formation of consensus protein secondary structure prediction. Bioinformatics 15:1039–1046, 1999.
189. Guermeur, Y., C. Geourjon, P. Gallinari, and G. Deleage. Improved performance in protein secondary structure prediction by inhomogeneous score combination. Bioinformatics 15:413–421, 1999.
190. Rost, B. WWW Services for Sequence Analysis. http://cubic.bioc.columbia.edu/doc/links_index.html, EMBL, 2001.
191. Eyrich, V. and B. Rost. The META-PredictProtein server. http://dodo.bioc.-columbia.edu/predictprotein/submit_meta.html, CUBIC, Columbia University, Dept. of Biochemistry & Molecular Biophysics, 2000.
192. Barton, G.J. Protein secondary structure prediction. Curr. Opin. Str. Biol. 5:372–376, 1995.
193. Kirshenbaum, K., M. Young, and S. Highsmith. Predicting allosteric switches in myosins. Prot. Sci. 8:1806–1815, 1999.
194. Przytycka, T., R. Aurora, and G.D. Rose. A protein taxonomy based on secondary structure. Nat. Struct. Biol. 6:672–682, 1999.
195. Liu T, J., H. Tan, and B. Rost. Genomes Full of Proteins with Long Nonstructured Regions? Columbia University Press, 2000.

196. Paquet, J.Y., C. Vinals, J. Wouters, J.J. Letesson, and E. Depiereux. Topology prediction of Brucella abortus Omp2b and Omp2a porins after critical assessment of transmembrane beta-strands prediction by several secondary structure prediction methods. J. Biomol. Struct. Dyn. 17:747–757, 2000.

197. Di Stasio, E., F. Sciandra, B. Maras, F. Di Tommaso, T.C. Petrucci, B. Giardina, and A. Brancaccio. Structural and functional analysis of the N-terminal extracellular region of beta-dystroglycan. Biochem. Biophys. Res. Commun. 266:274–278, 1999.

198. Juan, H.F., C.C. Hung, K.T. Wang, and S.H. Chiou. Comparison of three classes of snake neurotoxins by homology modeling and computer simulation graphics. Biochem. Biophys. Res. Commun. 257:500–510, 1999.

199. Laval, V., M. Chabannes, M. Carriere, H. Canut, A. Barre, P. Rouge, R. Pont-Lezica, and J. Galaud. A family of Arabidopsis plasma membrane receptors presenting animal beta-integrin domains. Biochim. Biophys. Ac. 1435:61–70, 1999.

200. Seto, M.H., H.L. Liu, D.A. Zajchowski, and M. Whitlow. Protein fold analysis of the B30.2-like domain. Proteins 35:235–249, 1999.

201. Xu, H., R. Aurora, G.D. Rose, and R.H. White. Identifying two ancient enzymes in Archaea using predicted secondary structure alignment. Nat. Struct. Biol. 6:750–754, 1999.

202. Jackson, R.M. and R.B. Russell. The serine protease inhibitor canonical loop conformation: examples found in extracellular hydrolases, toxins, cytokines and viral proteins. J. Mol. Biol. 296:325–334, 2000.

203. Stawiski, E.W., A.E. Baucom, S.C. Lohr, and L.M. Gregoret. Predicting protein function from structure: unique structural features of proteases. Proc. Natl. Acad. Sci. U.S.A. 97:3954–3958, 2000.

204. Shah, P.S., F. Bizik, R.K. Dukor, and P.K. Qasba. Active site studies of bovine alpha1 → 3-galactosyltransferase and its secondary structure prediction. Biochim. Biophys. Ac. 1480:222–234, 2000.

205. Brautigam, C., G.C. Steenbergen-Spanjers, G.F. Hoffmann, C. Dionisi-Vici, L.P. van den Heuvel, J.A. Smeitink, and R.A. Wevers. Biochemical and molecular genetic characteristics of the severe form of tyrosine hydroxylase deficiency. Clin. Chem. 45:2073–2078, 1999.

206. Davies, G.P., I. Martin, S.S. Sturrock, A. Cronshaw, N.E. Murray, and D.T. Dryden. On the structure and operation of type I DNA restriction enzymes. J. Mol. Biol. 290:565–579, 1999.

207. Gerloff, D.L., G.M. Cannarozzi, M. Joachimiak, F.E. Cohen, D. Schreiber, and S.A. Benner. Evolutionary, mechanistic, and predictive analyses of the hydroxymethyldihydropterin pyrophosphokinase family of proteins. Biochem. Biophys. Res. Commun. 254:70–76, 1999.

208. Fischer, D. and D. Eisenberg. Fold recognition using sequence-derived properties. Prot. Sci. 5:947–955, 1996.

209. Russell, R.B., R.R. Copley, and G.J. Barton. Protein fold recognition by mapping predicted secondary structures. J. Mol. Biol. 259:349–365, 1996.

210. Rost, B. TOPITS: Threading one-dimensional predictions into three-dimensional structures. Third International Conference on Intelligent Systems for Molecular Biology, Cambridge, England, 1995, pp 314–321.

211. de la Cruz, X. and J.M. Thornton. Factors limiting the performance of prediction-based fold recognition methods. Prot. Sci. 8:750–759, 1999.

212. Di Francesco, V., P.J. Munson, and J. Garnier. FORESST: fold recognition from secondary structure predictions of proteins. Bioinformatics 15:131–140, 1999.

213. Kelley, L.A., R.M. MacCallum, and M.J. Sternberg. Enhanced genome annotation using structural profiles in the program 3D-PSSM. J. Mol. Biol. 299:499–520, 2000.

214. Ayers, D.J., P.R. Gooley, A. Widmer-Cooper, and A.E. Torda. Enhanced protein fold recognition using secondary structure information from NMR. Prot. Sci. 8:1127–1133, 1999.

215. Hargbo, J. and A. Elofsson. Hidden Markov models that use predicted secondary structures for fold recognition. Proteins 36:68–76, 1999.

216. Jones, D.T. GenTHREADER: an efficient and reliable protein fold recognition method for genomic sequences. J. Mol. Biol. 287:797–815, 1999.

217. Panchenko, A., A. Marchler-Bauer, and S.H. Bryant. Threading with explicit models for evolutionary conservation of structure and sequence. Proteins Suppl 3:133–140, 1999.

218. Ota, M., T. Kawabata, A.R. Kinjo, and K. Nishikawa. Cooperative approach for the protein fold recognition. Proteins 37:126–132, 1999.

219. Koretke, K.K., R.B. Russell, R.R. Copley, and A.N. Lupas. Fold recognition using sequence and secondary structure information. Proteins 37:141–148, 1999.

220. Jones, D.T., M. Tress, K. Bryson, and C. Hadley. Successful recognition of protein folds using threading methods biased by sequence similarity and predicted secondary structure. Proteins 37:104–111, 1999.

221. Heringa, J. Two strategies for sequence comparison: profile-preprocessed and secondary structure-induced multiple alignment. Comput. Chem. 23:341–364, 1999.

222. Ng, P., J. Henikoff, and S. Henikoff. PHAT: a transmembrane-specific substitution matrix. Bioinformatics 16, In press, 2000.

223. Baldi, P., G. Pollastri, C.A. Andersen, and S. Brunak. Matching protein beta-sheet partners by feedforward and recurrent neural networks. Ismb 8:25–36, 2000.

224. Ortiz, A.R., A. Kolinski, P. Rotkiewicz, B. Ilkowski, and J. Skolnick. Ab initio folding of proteins using restraints derived from evolutionary information. Proteins Suppl. 3:177–185, 1999.

225. Eyrich, V.A., D.M. Standley, A.K. Felts, and R.A. Friesner. Protein tertiary structure prediction using a branch and bound algorithm. Proteins 35:41–57, 1999.

226. Eyrich, V.A., D.M. Standley, and R.A. Friesner. Prediction of protein tertiary structure to low resolution: performance for a large and structurally diverse test set. J. Mol. Biol. 288:725–742, 1999.

227. Lomize, A.L., I.D. Pogozheva, and H.I. Mosberg. Prediction of protein structure: the problem of fold multiplicity. Protein Suppl.:199–203, 1999.

228. Chen, C.C., J.P. Singh, and R.B. Altman. Using imperfect secondary structure predictions to improve molecular structure computations. Bioinformatics 15:53–65, 1999.

229. Samudrala, R., Y. Xia, E. Huang, and M. Levitt. Ab initio protein structure prediction using a combined hierarchical approach. Proteins Suppl.:194–198, 1999.

230. Samudrala, R., E.S. Huang, P. Koehl, and M. Levitt. Constructing side chains on near-native main chains for ab initio protein structure prediction. Prot. Engin. 13:453–457, 2000.

231. Minor, D.L.J. and P.S. Kim. Context-dependent secondary structure formation of a designed protein sequence. Nature 380:730–734, 1996.

232. Krittanai, C. and W.C.J. Johnson. The relative order of helical propensity of amino acids changes with solvent environment. Proteins 39:132–141, 2000.

233. Zhou, X., F. Alber, G. Folkers, G.H. Gonnet, and G. Chelvanayagam. An analysis of the helix-to-strand transition between peptides with identical sequence. Proteins 41:248–256, 2000.

234. Pan, X.M., W.D. Niu, and Z.X. Wang. What is the minimum number of residues to determine the secondary structural state? J. Prot. Chem. 18:579–584, 1999.

235. Jacoboni, I., P.L. Martelli, P. Fariselli, M. Compiani, and R. Casadio. Predictions of protein segments with the same aminoacid sequence and different secondary structure: a benchmark for predictive methods. Proteins 41:535–544, 2000.

236. Compiani, M., P. Fariselli, P.L. Martelli, and R. Casadio. Neural networks to study invariant features of protein folding. Theoretical Chemistry Accounts 101:21–26, 1999.

237. Rost, B. and A. Valencia. Pitfalls of protein sequence analysis. Curr. Opin. Biotech. 7:457–461, 1996.

238. Rost, B., R. Casadio, and P. Fariselli. Topology prediction for helical transmembrane proteins at 86% accuracy. Prot. Sci. 5:1704–1718, 1996.

239. Rost, B. Accuracy of predicting buried helices by PHDsec. http://www.embl-heidelberg.de/~rost/Res/96B-PredBuriedHelices.html, EMBL Heidelberg, 1996.

240. Rost, B. 1D structure prediction for Chameleon (IgG binding domain of protein G). http://www.embl-heidelberg.de/~rost/Res/96C-PredChameleon.html, EMBL Heidelberg, 1996.

241. Dalal, S., S. Balasubramanian, and L. Regan. Protein alchemy: changing β-sheet into α-helix. Nat. Struct. Biol. 4:548–552, 1997.

242. Chou, P.Y. and G.D. Fasman. Prediction of the secondary structure of proteins from their amino acid sequence. Adv. Enzymol. 47:45–148, 1978.

243. Garnier, J., J.-F. Gibrat, and B. Robson. GOR method for predicting protein secondary structure from amino acid sequence. Meth. Enzymol. 266:540–553, 1996.

244. Rost, B. Predicting protein structure: better data, better results! J. Mol. Biol. In submission, 2001.

245. Abagyan, R.A. and S. Batalov. Do aligned sequences share the same fold? J. Mol. Biol. 273:355–368, 1997.

246. Park, J., S.A. Teichmann, T. Hubbard, and C. Chothia. Intermediate sequences increase the detection of distant sequence homologies. J. Mol. Biol. 273:349–354, 1997.

247. Kozlov, G., I. Ekiel, N. Beglova, A. Yee, A. Dharamsi, A. Engel, N. Siddiqui, A. Nong, and K. Gehring. Rapid fold and structure determination of the archaeal translation elongation factor 1beta from Methanobacterium thermoautotrophicum. J Biomol NMR 17:187–194, 2000.

248. Rost, B., V.A. Eyrich, D. Przybylski, F. Pazos, A. Valencia, A. Fiser, M. Marti-Renom, R. Sanchez, and A. Sali. EVA—evaluation of automatic protein structure prediction services. http://cubic.bioc.columbia.edu/eva, Columbia University/Rockefeller University/CNB Madrid, 2000.

249. Matthews, B.W. Comparison of the predicted and observed secondary structure of T4 phage lysozyme. Biochim. Biophys. Ac. 405:442–451, 1975.

250. Zhang, C.-T. and K.-C. Chou. An optimization approach to predicting protein structural class from amino acid composition. Prot. Sci. 1:401–408, 1992.

9

Novel Fold and Ab Initio Methods for Protein Structure Generation

David J. Osguthorpe
University of Bath in Swindon, Swindon, United Kingdom

1 INTRODUCTION

Protein folding is still a major problem that is incompletely understood at the present time. We have known since the pioneering experiments of Anfinsen (1) in the early 1960s that the folding of most globular proteins is a purely physical phenomenon dependent only on the specific amino acid sequence of the protein and the solvent environment. Hence, it should be possible to define a force field based on the physics of the interactions among atoms, including the solvent, and to use a statistical mechanical energy surface searching method, such as molecular dynamics or Monte Carlo, to determine the most stable structure of the protein at a given temperature and solvent condition.

Since that time much effort has been devoted to creating a system for predicting protein structure from sequence alone, although this is still not a reliable process, even for globular proteins. Computational solutions to the problem have to address the major difficulty of protein folding, the large size of proteins and the long time scale of folding. Typical proteins fold in vivo in the range of 1 millisecond to 1 second. This is a long time for a molecule, where torsion angle rotations occur on the picosecond-to-nanosecond time scale. All-atom molecular dynamics simulations of proteins, the closest physical model of proteins (except for a quantum mechanical model), typically have a step size of 1 femtosecond (10^{-15}). So to fold a protein on the computer would require simulations of 10^{12}–10^{15} steps, which at 1 millisecond a step would take 31–31,000 years. Hence, to use the current most accurate physical model is essentially computationally not feasible at the moment. (This also rules out any form of quantum mechanical model, although most of the interactions in protein folding do not require a quantum mechanical model.)

As experimental structures of proteins became available it became clear that many proteins have a similar tertiary structure or pattern of the polypeptide chain in space; this is what is called the *fold*. It also became apparent that proteins with similar structure had similar sequences. If the unknown protein has an amino acid sequence that is similar enough to a known protein tertiary structure, then homology modeling techniques can be used (see Chapter 7). At weaker levels of sequence similarity, fold recognition or threading methods are viable (1a). However, the main goal is to predict the structure of proteins with arbitrary sequences, in particular those that have no identifiable sequence similarity to known structures. The "novel fold and ab initio" in the title of this chapter refers to methods that attempt to solve this problem, i.e., to generate protein tertiary structures that have not been seen in the structural database before. There are two basic approaches to the problem, statistical and physical. In the statistical approaches the fitness functions (equivalent to the potential in a physical model) are essentially determined by a statistical analysis of the known protein structure database. The physical approaches use potentials derived from the underlying forces involved. In this chapter, as in the recent CASP4 meeting (see later for more details about the CASP meetings), *novel fold* will be used to describe any method that attempts to generate tertiary structure from seqeuence, whereas *ab initio* will be reserved for those methods that are based on physical principles. For novel fold methods, there is a wide spectrum, depending on how much information is used from the known structure database. This can be in a direct form, for example, using fragments of known structures to actually generate the structure, and indirectly, via potentials derived from a statistical analysis of the database.

2 WHAT IS A FOLD?

A critical aspect of protein structure that is rarely discussed is the definition of a protein fold. The protein fold, i.e., the pattern of the polypeptide chain in space, is essentially a visual definition requiring a human being to analyze different structures visually. Although a number of attempts have been made to create computational definitions of folds (2,3) most classification schemes based on fold, e.g., SCOP (4) and CATH (5) are based on human analysis. Hence, current definitions of protein folds are extremely empirical and thus are subject to the many problems of human perception and subjectivity. As human beings we may attribute to visual features an importance they do not deserve, because they look visually appealing in some way. The main computational method used to measure structural similarity is the root mean square deviation or rms. Unfortunately, this is a very poor measure of fold similarity, since two structures with different folds can easily have the same rms. For example, one of the first folding simulations of pancreatic trypsin inhibitor (6) had a final C-α(CA) rms of 3.0 Å but was an incorrect fold. (C-α rms refers to the rms calculated for the C-α atoms of the protein only). My own work at the time demonstrated that only below 3 Å could the CA rms measure guarantee fold similarity; i.e., the path of the chain in space is visually similar to the native structure (7). My recent folding work has shown that proteins can fluctuate between 3 and 6 Å CA rms and are visually still in the same fold. In some of the results of CASP4 discussed later, the folds are still similar at the level of 8–9 Å CA rms.

To show some of the problems in comparing folds, Figure 1a shows an apparently successful prediction of the fold of target T0110 using my ab initio methods from the recent CASP4 meeting (Table 2 gives details of the proteins associated with the various targets mentioned in this chapter). At first sight this appears to be correct, with the secondary structure elements of the prediction following the path of the chain in the experimental structure (the CA rms is 9.16 Å). However, in Figure 1b the equivalent strands of the β-hairpin are highlighted and show in the prediction this β-hairpin is inverted.

Recently, Goddard et. al. (8) suggested a different method for classifying protein structures based on the concept of a *topomer*. When this concept is applied to the many decoy data sets (9–11), though they may have a large number of different structures by rms, the number of different folds is much smaller (D.J. Osguthorpe, unpublished results). Hence, passing such a decoy set is not as good a test of the ability of a potential to discriminate between folds as might appear at first.

Another aspect that fold comparison methods do not take into account is fold fluctuation. Unfortunately, the main structural method for proteins, X-ray crystallography, presents a single structure as representing the "structure" of a protein. This leads to the perception that this is the "true" structure. However, it has long been known that proteins are not fixed structures and are unfolding and refolding continuously, as shown by deuterium exchange studies (12). In these studies normal proteins are put in deuterated water and the rates of exchange of amide protons to deuterons measured, and even protons completely buried according to the X-ray structure can be seen to exchange with the solvent. Li and Woodward (12) give a

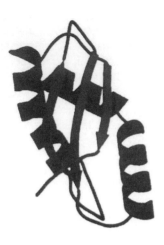 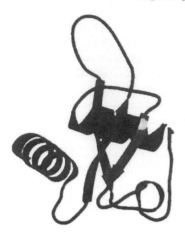

Experiment   Model

Figure 1a Comparison of the experimental and predicted structure of CASP4
target T0110, overall rms of 9.16 Å, showing the apparent similarity of the fold.

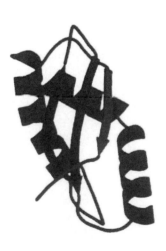 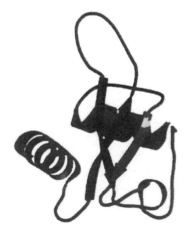

Experiment   Model

Figure 1b Same as Figure 1a, but highlighting the incorrect overlap of two strands
of the sheet.

very good description of the native state: "The native state ensemble fluctuates about an average approximated by the crystal structure, and on many time scales samples numerous additional conformers, many near the average in structure and energy, and some rare and far from the average in structure and/or energy." Unlike many protein folding methods that tend to deliver a single structural result, molecular dynamics allows such an ensemble to be generated, and my results using this technique do show large fluctuations in structure, as noted earlier. Rather than selecting the structure by the lowest value of the fitness or potential function, as is most commonly done, it may be important to compare the average value of the potential function of an ensemble of conformations to determine the native fold ensemble. Using the lowest value of a potential function is equivalent to comparing structures at 0 K. For example, if you have two potentials wells that have the same well depth, but with one wide and one narrow, the wide well is preferred on entropy grounds. Comparing the minimum energies of these two wells does not distinguish between them, whereas looking at the free energy, which can only be done using an ensemble of structures, would.

3 OUTLINE OF FOLDING METHODS

All protein folding methods have to solve three problems (13):

1. How to represent protein structure
2. How to represent the interactions involved
3. How to search this interaction space

In all three cases the primary concern is how much computer time is a particular choice going to require, for the ability to generate large numbers of different conformations and check their fitness function within a reasonable amount of computer time is crucial to the success of an algorithm.

3.1 Structure Representations

Two features dominate what structure representations can be used practically. The first is the number of particles representing the protein structure. These range from the all-atom model, the united-atom model, virtual-atom models with one, two, or at least two atoms per residue (14–16), and finally to models that use one atom to represent more than one residue (17). The second is the nature of the phase space, which can be either continuous (known as off-lattice models) or discrete (the lattice models) (18,19). Some models combine both continuous and discrete components, for example, rigid geometry models, in which some virtual internal degrees of freedom, such as virtual bond lengths, are fixed while others are continuous.

Each of these choices has implications for how long it will take to calculate the fitness (or potential) function having generated a structure and how easy it is to search this geometry space.

3.2   Force Fields and Fitness Functions

The second requirement for protein folding is a fitness function (or potential function in the ab initio case) and parameters. It is the potential function that, in the end, determines whether or not a method is capable of predicting the native structure of a protein. Currently fitness functions are dominated by those derived from statistical analyses of the known protein structures (20).

Statistical potentials can be split into two groups—those that use a purely statistical analysis, of which the potentials of Simons et al. (21) are a good example, and those that use an underlying physical model and the experimental data are used to parameterize that model, of which the UNRES force field of Liwo et al. is an example (22–24). The statistical potentials of Simons et al. (21) use a Bayesian statistical analysis and conditional probabilities to partition the information in the database, as originated by Robson (25) and used in the successful GOR secondary structure prediction algorithm (26). A slightly different approach was taken by Miyazawa and Jernigan (27,28), whose potentials are based on a chemical concept for the statistical analysis, though it is still a statistical analysis. Another physicochemical approach is based on a parameterization of the electrostatics of secondary structure formation (29–31). Of course, although there are many different algorithms for extracting statistical potentials, they all rely on essentially the same database and so contain the same information.

The vast majority of sequence-to-structure algorithms so far are based on the use of statistical potentials, even though there are two major problems with them. First, they are bounded by the database used to extract statistics. That is, as with all statistical methods, they will be reliable only as long as the protein whose structure is required is within the sequence–structure space of the database. Second, it is difficult to infer from the parameters the physical reasons why a particular structure exists, because many physical effects get combined and averaged in a single statistical parameter.

The second is the more fundamental problem with statistical potentials. Each term can reflect the combination of a number of different physical effects. For example, most of the side-chain contact potentials in present use are referred to as "hydrophobic potentials." Side-chain contact potentials also include interactions between charged and polar residues, where hydrogen bonding and electrostatic forces would also be included in the "hydrophobic" contact potentials. The hydrophobic effect is really composed of two different forces: the van der Waals interactions between atoms that are buried and totally excluded from water, and what can be called the "true" hydrophobic effect, which occurs only when water is present between the two atoms.

3.3 Potential Optimization

Many potentials, both statistical and physical, are then "optimized" using the known structure database to improve the gap between the native state and the nearby wrong structures, i.e., non-native structures whose fitness function is similar to the native, often known as Z-score optimization (32,33). A danger with these optimization approaches is that only sequences that fold are considered; it is equally important that a folding potential does not allow nonfolding sequences to fold. Maximizing the difference between the native and non-native structures for folding sequences may overstabilize the native structure. Most proteins in nature are only marginally stable; that is, they are as stable as required for the cellular function being performed in the natural environment, and no more.

3.4 Search Techniques

The third and final requirement for protein folding is a conformational search technique, although, of course, no amount of tinkering with search techniques can make up for a poor potential.

There are three major search techniques in use in protein folding: genetic algorithms, Monte Carlo, and molecular dynamics. The vast majority use some form of Monte Carlo method (34), and this is often a part of genetic algorithm methods. Monte Carlo methods are invariably used for lattice models of proteins and for statistical potentials, because it is not easy to define derivatives for these potentials; for example, they often rely on counting contacts around a particular residue.

4 PROTEIN FOLDING: THERMODYNAMIC OR KINETIC?

One of the major questions about protein folding can be posed succinctly: Is it thermodynamic, in which case the folding pathway is not important, or is it kinetic, in which case a structure generation program would also have to exactly follow the pathway of folding in vivo? Although for many proteins the thermodynamic hypothesis has been shown to be valid experimentally, they can be completely refolded in vitro from the denatured state, this is not true of all. Most searching techniques are essentially looking for a minimum value of the fitness function, which implies they are assuming the thermodynamic hypothesis.

Another thermodynamic issue for ab initio protein folding is the role of metals, hetero-groups, ion-binding sites, and disulphide bridges. One of the problems with ab initio folding based on physical principles is that, if only the sequence is included, then the folded structure generated is that of the apo-protein, that is, the protein without the ion, metal or hetero-group and so on. It would be invalid for a physical-principle protein folding method to correctly predict, for example, an ion-binding site if the ion itself is not included. An example of this is the structure of the second EPS15 homology domain (PDB code 1eh2 (35), CASP3 target T0074), which does contain a calcium-binding site and whose experimental structure was obtained with calcium present. In the experimental binding site there are charged aspartic acid and glutamic acid side-chain carboxyl groups located only 2.5 Å away from each other. This is possible only in the presence of the calcium; without the calcium these side chains must be further apart as a result of repulsive electrostatic interactions. Figure 2 presents the experimental structure and a predicted fold using my ab initio folding technique, with the side chains of the carboxylic acids shown, which clearly illustrates

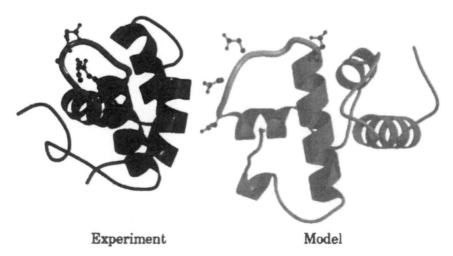

Experiment   Model

Figure 2 Comparison of the experimental and predicted structures of CASP3 target T0074, with the side chain shown explicitly for the four residues (3 Asp, 1 Glu) interacting with the bound calcium in the native structure, where the distance between carboxyls is around 2–3 Å. In the predicted structure of the apo-protein, these side chains are far apart.

this. The question arises as to at what stage of the folding process the calcium actually starts to interact with the side chains of the binding site residues; this is likely to be only after the initial collapse of the protein and some structure formation.

Disulphide bridge proteins have the problem that the formation of the disulphide bridge adds a large amount of free energy to the system that could therefore be the major determinant of the folded structure and predominate over the usual forces, such as hydrophobicity.

One area that is also overlooked is the experimental conditions of the structural study, which can have a dramatic effect on the structure of proteins. Crystallization media are not simple solutions, often containing a number of different chemicals at high concentrations. This is something that is important to define for ab initio folding studies, where it may lead to a change in the potentials used. Again, statistical potentials will simply average such effects or would require splitting the database into sections and generating statistics for each environment section. One example I have found is the protein pulmonary surfactant–associated polypeptide (PDB structure 1spf (36)). This originated from looking at proteins in the database that the PHD (37) secondary structure prediction algorithm did not predict well (B.H. Rost, personal communication). For 1spf, PHD predicts it as strand, but experimentally (NMR) it is helical; see Table 1.

The large percentage of valines would suggest a strand prediction, even by eye. However, the experimental conditions for the structure was a deuterated chloroform, methanol, and hydrochloric acid mixture in the proportions 32:64:5. Such a solution will have a very low dielectric constant compared to water, which is consistent with the fact this peptide is associated with membrane/surfactant systems. So, as one might expect for the low-dielectric environment of the membrane or this solution, the increase in strength of hydrogen bonds in such an environment can overcome the globular protein preference of valine for strand. It also points out the extreme importance of not using secondary structure prediction methods based on globular protein data for segments of protein sequences that may be in the membrane.

Although it is important to reproduce the overall fold, it is also important to reproduce the structure at functional sites (38) and methods may achieve the overall fold but not determine a more specific functional feature. For statistical potentials, whether such features are reproduced depends on whether the information required to generate the features is specifically maintained in the statistical analysis, in which case the feature would be expected to be reproduced, or whether the information is averaged, in which case it is unlikely the feature would be reproduced.

Table 1 PHD Predictions for 1SPF

```
        ........1.........2.........3....
AA   |  LRIPCCPVNLKRLLVVVVVLVVVVIVGALLMGL
Expt.|          HHHHHHHHHHHHHHHHHHHHHHH
PHD  |            EEEEEEEEEEEEEEEEEE
Rel  |  99712564223899999887753213499
```

5 THE CASP EXPERIMENTS

The Critical Assessment of Methods of Protein Structure Prediction (CASP) (39–42) meetings have become the premier forum for the comparison of protein structure prediction methods. To ensure unbiased evaluation of predictions, a double-blind test system is used, the structures of the sequences used for prediction are unknown to predictors, and the assessment is carried out without knowledge of the submitting group's identity. At CASP4, in December 2000, as usual there were three assessed sections—homology modeling, fold recognition, and novel fold—plus a section analyzing the results of automatic servers, CAFASP2. A personal review of the results in the novel fold section follows. The assessment of results in the novel fold section is difficult because if there is existing information about structure, there is no way of detecting whether predictors have used such information or not. Therefore, to assess the novel fold methods, only novel folds or folds that had no identifiable sequence similarity to known structures are used, to ensure that predictors could not have used pre-existing information in their submissions. However, when the experimental structures are known of some of these proteins that had no apparent sequence similarity, they are found to have structural similarity to parts of existing proteins. Hence, for the assessment, the targets are classified according to the difficulty using their known structure.

5.1 Overview of Novel Fold Results

In relative terms there was again significant improvement compared to CASP3. However, in absolute terms it is still not good. Of the 17 target proteins or domains selected for assessing the novel fold section, only four structures were truly successfully predicted. Three of the successful predictions had an overall CA rms of under 8 Å (CASP target numbers 91, 104 and the second domain of target 89). Table 2 gives the identification of proteins with their CASP target numbers, also found at http://PredictionCenter.llnl.gov/casp4/Casp4.html. These are getting larger; for example, target 91, with a smallest CA rms of 4.97 Å, has 105 amino acids, or target 104, with a smallest CA rms of 6.21 Å and 158 residues. (The smallest CA rms refers to the smallest rms achieved by any predictor in the novel fold section). Target 124, a protein consisting of long helices, which in one sense is not a standard globular protein, was also successfully predicted, even though the CA rms was 8.46 Å; due to the long helices, even a small misalignment would lead to a large rms deviation. This had 242 residues. A further three proteins were predicted with a CA rms between 8 and 9 Å, targets 97, 98, and 106. From comparing with the native structure,

Table 2 CASP4 Target Numbers Referred to in the Text and the Proteins
to Which They Refer

T0089	FTSA	FtsA, *T. maritima* (43)
		Second domain, residues 239–290
T0091	YBAB	Hypothetical protein H10442, *H. influenzae*
T0097	ER29	C-terminal domain of ERp29, rat
		PDB code 1G7D
T0098	SP0A	C-terminal domain of Spo0A, *B. stearothermophilus*
		PDB code 1FC3(44)
T0102	AS48	Bacteriocin AS-48, *E. faecalis*
		PDB code 1E68(45)
TO104	YJEE	Hypothetical protein H10065, *H. influenzae*
T0106	SFRP3	Secreted frizzled protein 3, mouse
T0110	RBFA	Ribosome-binding factor A, *H. influenzae*
T0124	PLCB	Phospholipase C beta C-terminus, turkey

the overall folds of these three targets were successfully predicted. Figure 3 shows the experimental structure and my prediction of target 98, overall CA rms of 9.89 Å, which is representative of the level of structural similarity that I have called a successful prediction of the fold for these three proteins. For the rest of the 10 structures, the CA rms was over 10 Å, with the average of the best rms for each of the 10 targets being 14.71. In these cases only some fractional substructure of the target was predicted well, although this amount has increased compared to CASP3.

The results do show that to some extent helical proteins are easier to predict than mixed helical-sheet proteins and that mainly sheet proteins are difficult to predict (the number of mainly sheet proteins was significantly higher in CASP4 than previously). It does appear for these proteins that getting the turns in the right place is critical to the structure of these proteins. Of the seven protein folds correctly generated, five were either all or mainly helical proteins.

Another major issue for novel fold methods is that there is still little consistency between the methods; i.e., the various methods do not predict the same targets well and others poorly, but seem to randomly get some targets well and others poorly.

On the positive side, novel fold methods have correctly predicted the structure of four difficult targets from sequence alone, with no prior knowledge of the structure, a significant achievement. Further, an additional two not-so-difficult targets were correctly predicted using novel fold methods. More significantly, the true ab initio methods managed to do as well as most of the methods using statistical potentials and/or known structure fragments.

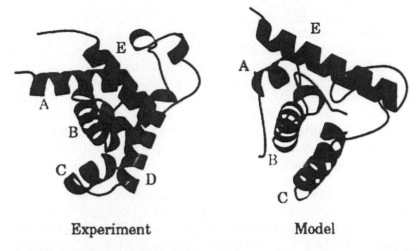

Experiment   Model

Figure 3 Comparison of the experimental and predicted structures of CASP4 target T0098, showing the level of fold similarity typical for an overall rms of 9.89 Å. The corresponding helices are labelled A, B etc. The predicted structure is topologically threaded correctly. The gap in the chain in the model structure is an artifact at a proline residue.

5.2   Comparison of Methods

The novel fold methods in use can be classified into three groups: those that use statistical potentials and structure fragments from known structures, those that use statistical potentials but generate all structure, and those that use physical potentials and generate all structure (only the last method is ab initio according to the definition given previously). Most methods seem to be similar to those the predictors used in CASP3, and although there were some new predictors, truly novel algorithms were not apparent.

The methods that seemed to generate more accurate subfragments, at CASP4 and CASP3, are those that use direct statistical potentials and generate structures by coupling together fragments of structures in the known structure database, so called minithreading methods. The method of Baker continues to impress (43,21), the main difference to CASP3 apparently simply generating more conformations for selection and the use of clustering to select the native structure based on the ideas of Shortle et al. (44). Shortle uses a method that seems very similar in principle, the selection of fragments from known structures, putting fragments together and selection via a potential, but he uses a different selection of fragments and potential compared to Baker. Skolnick's method (44a) is an example of the second type:

All structure is generated, the method does not use fragments directly, but the potentials are statistical. Additionally, a threading technique is used to generate potentials that add secondary and tertiary restraints; i.e., a distance bias is added between selected residues. Scheraga's method is a combination, starting with a low-resolution model and statistical parameters to generate clusters of conformations, followed by conversion to a united-atom model and using the ECEPP physical potential, with solvent interactions included via the SRFOPT potential rather than explicit waters (45). The method of Rose, which is a true ab initio method, uses a physical model (46,47) that is determined mainly by steric clashes, hydrogen bonding, and hydrophobic contacts to predict structure. Levitt's ab initio method started from predicted secondary structure and then used energy minimization from many random starting conformations with hydrophobic, hydrogen bond, and charge potentials to find the predicted native structure. The concepts behind the ab initio folding model I used are described in detail in the next section, but briefly it attempts to provide as accurate a model of the physics of the forces involved at the level of the simplified geometry used. Apart from the results of Baker, who predicted the most correct folds and correct fragments of folds, distinguishing between the results of other predictors who did well in the novel fold section was more of an issue of whose fragments of reasonably predicted structure were better than others. Most good novel fold predictors got the folds mainly correct of three or four proteins; the rest of the predictions were just fragments done well.

6 PHILOSOPHY OF A MODEL FOR AB INITIO PROTEIN FOLDING

My original idea in constructing models for protein folding was to start with as simple a model as possible. This model should at least be able to produce a number of plausible folded conformations for a protein, even if it was proved impossible for this model to select the native structure because of the approximations; i.e., the feature selecting for the native structure was not realizable in this model. Thus, a protein folding scenario would be to use the simple model to produce hundreds, or even thousands, of folded conformations, which would then be converted to a more detailed model for the final selection. All that would be required of the model is that the native structure be one of these 100 or 1000 conformations. There is also a more fundamental argument for a simplified model based on homology. Many different sequences have a similar fold or similar ordering in space of the secondary structure elements. One could argue that each different sequence has a highly specific set of interactions that just happen to lead to this similar structure. What appears more likely is that it is the contribution of residues to a global property that creates this similar structure, for example, the hydrophobicity of residues. In this case the specific details of each residue are unimportant, just the contribution to this global property, hence a simplified model would be able to generate the correct fold of a sequence, although the exact geometric details would be distorted.

6.1 Simplified Geometry Model

The model involves representing the backbone of each residue by one sphere, or "atom," and the side chains by up to three "atoms." The side chains of Ala, Val, Ile, Ser, Thr, and Pro are represented by one sphere, Leu, His, Asp, Glu, Asn, Gln, Cys, and Met by two spheres, and Phe, Tyr, Trp, Lys, and Arg by three spheres. The different number of spheres reflects the anisotropic nature of the average shape of the corresponding side chains. It also enables the assigning of different characteristics to parts of the side chain of a residue; for example, the side chain of Arg includes a hydrophobic chain and a polar/charged end. Although in this representation many residues have the same number of atoms, they do not lose their unique identity, since they have different potential parameters.

6.2 Simplified Potentials

The potentials required can be split into three major groups: the virtual internal potentials that stabilize the geometry of the protein (virtual bonds, angles, and torsion), secondary structure stabilization potentials, and the global potentials (nonbond interactions and solvation energy), which deal with the effects of the environment but do not require the environment to be modeled explicitly.

The potential energy function for the model is defined as:

$$E_{\text{Total}} = E_{\text{Internal}} + E_{\text{Secondary Structure}} + E_{\text{Global}}$$

6.2.1 Internal Potentials

The internal energy is defined in terms of virtual bond, angles, and torsions (or out of plane). A number of functional forms are used, the standard full-atom model harmonic terms, quadratic functions, and Gaussian functions, plus combinations of these terms. Additionally, an out-of-plane virtual-valence-angle cross-term is defined:

$$E_{\text{Internal}} = E_{\text{V.bond}} + E_{\text{V.angle}} + E_{\text{V.torsion}} + E_{\text{V.oop}} + E_{\text{V.oopXV.angle}}$$

Additionally, virtual angle–virtual angle–virtual torsion angle cross-terms are defined for dealing with correlations between the two internal valence angles of a torsion angle in the backbone. These are particularly important for turn conformations.

The values of the parameters were derived by emulating the energy surface calculated using a full-atom model and from observed distributions of the corresponding internals in experimental structures. An important consideration of using the database was to remove the artifacts in the distributions created by the occurrence of secondary structure. The two major secondary structures, α-helix and β-sheet, are associated with highly constrained values of the virtual valence and torsion angles, so using all virtual torsions and angles leads to distributions with large peaks at these values. In potential parameterization it is important to include physical effects only once, and the secondary structure energy, i.e., backbone hydrogen bonding, was to be included by separate potentials and so should not be included in these virtual internals. Hence, distributions for the virtual internals were constructed from only those residues that were not in helix, turn, or sheet according to DSSP (48) rules. These plots showed very different features compared to distributions that included all secondary structures. Another important point is that the virtual internals involving the backbone CA atom and the side-chain CB atom are the same for all amino acids except Gly and Pro, so no sequence-dependent effects can be introduced by them (in generating the observed distributions for these internals, all amino acid types were used). Backbone virtual internal potential forms and parameters were created for three amino acid types, Gly, Pro, and the rest in both cis and trans forms of the backbone amide bond.

6.2.2 Secondary Structure Energy/Backbone Hydrogen Bonding Potentials

With the simplified geometry model, only CA atoms exist for the backbone, and yet backbone hydrogen bonding is very important in the stabilization of the standard secondary structures. However, the standard secondary structures have a fixed and specific set of distances between the CA atoms. Hence the basic approach was to determine the equilibrium distances between CA atoms in 3–10 helices, α-helices, and parallel and antiparallel β-sheets and to use Gaussian functions to stabilize these distances.

$$E_{\text{Secondary Structure}} = E_{\text{Helix}} + E_{\text{Sheet}}$$

For the β-sheets it was also necessary to include some vector terms as well to ensure that only when the two strands were aligned was the potential strong. Further improvements to the sheet potentials were necessary to remove conformations that are never seen in real proteins but were created in trial folding runs.

It should be noted that in all cases the secondary structure potentials merely stabilize distances that are found; this is not a preimposition of secondary structure. The β-sheet potentials do a full search of all residue pairs to find any that are close enough to form sheets in each energy calculation.

6.2.3 Local Secondary Structure Energy

It has long been known that amino acids have a preference for either the helical or strand conformation, and these preferences are the basis of secondary structure prediction algorithms. One observation that all analyses of secondary structure preferences show is that residues that prefer the helical conformation have either no or only a single carbon attached to the Cα atom (apart from the Cβ atom), which is also not part of a bulky, planar ring system, i.e., Ala, Lys, Arg, Glu, Gln, Leu, and Met. Conversely, residues that prefer the strand (extended) conformation have two carbons on the Cα or a bulky group, Val, Ile, Thr, His, Phe, Tyr, Trp, and Cys. Even after many years of research on the subject there is still no clear physical explanation for this, with two main competing ideas. Srinivasan and Rose (47) use steric and entropy arguments as the basis for local secondary structure in their ab initio folding algorithm. Another explanation of this effect is electrostatic screening (29–31).

In both cases, this is a local effect, i.e., accounted for by short-range interactions in sequence along the protein chain and excluding short-distance but long-sequence-range interactions. Again, one of the problems with the statistical preferences from the database is that they include global effects and do not measure the local effects alone, whereas what is required in the potential is the local effect alone. The essence of the Srinivasan and Rose model is that the preference for helix is created by bad steric interactions of the bulky side chains with other side chains and the main chain when in the helix conformation, which reduces the number of side chain conformations available to these residues in the helical conformation. That is, it's not that the helix-preferring residues positively prefer (i.e., have a lower energy than) the helix; rather, the strand-preferring residues have a negative preference for helix (i.e., a higher energy). Note that in explanations of secondary structure on the basis of local interactions, the helix is preferred generally because it has local hydrogen bonds. The hydrogen bonds in sheets are considered to be global interactions, so the (extended) strand conformation has no local hydrogen bond component and is less favored, even though it is the most preferred conformation of residues according to the Ramachandran map (49). However, it is still possible to find side-chain torsion angles that do allow strand-preferring residues to be in the helical conformation. In a scan I performed of the structural database (PDB select 1997 (50) 25% homology, unpublished data) for the Trp, Phe or Tyr, Phe or Tyr, three-residue sequential combination, the vast majority of them occur in the strand (sheet) conformation, but there was one case (the photosynthetic reaction center, 1pcr (51)) where they were in the middle of a helix. A calculation of the energy of this tripeptide showed that there were no steric problems but only when the observed three side-chain χ-1 torsion angles were constrained to their observed values. Any attempt to change any one of the χ-1 torsion angles to another of the three minima led to clashes. So of the 27 possible χ-1 torsion angle combinations, only one is available in the helical conformation.

To explain this kind of local effect and other local properties, a separate energy term must be added explicitly, since local secondary structure is due to local interactions between the side-chain atoms and backbone atoms, some of which are missing in the model. An overall preference for any residue has been added by stabilizing virtual torsions and angles using $i - i + 2$, $i + 1 - i + 3$, and $i - i + 3$ distances and Gaussian functions for both the helical and strand conformations. Because individual residue conformations affect only the virtual valence angle, the overall preference is specifically increased only for contiguous pairs of residues that both prefer the helical conformation or that both prefer the strand conformation. That is, the two central CA's of a backbone virtual torsion must both prefer the helical or strand conformation to increase the local secondary structure potential of the virtual torsion:

$$E_{\text{Local Secondary Structure}} = E_{\text{Local Turn}} + E_{\text{Local Strand}}$$

One of the interesting aspects of CASP4 is that a number of targets had long helices (e.g., target 124, which is a bundle of three long helices) either with no typical globular protein structure or the helices stick out of the globular structure. All these helices show very strong local secondary structure preferences with long runs of helix-preferring residues. In comparison, typical helices in globular proteins do not show such strong helical preferences. This suggests that one of the requirements for globular proteins is that the secondary structure elements not have very strong secondary structure preferences and that overstabilizing secondary structure elements can destroy globular protein structure.

6.2.4   Global/Solvation Potentials

The remaining potentials are used to represent the nonbonded interactions of the residues with each other and the interactions with solvent. The fundamental idea behind the solvation potentials was to use fast approximations to the physical forces involved in real protein structures. Also, because molecular dynamics was seen as one of the primary tools to be used in the parameterization procedure and for first attempts at protein folding, the potentials had to have analytical derivatives for speed:

$$E_{Global} = E_{vander\,Walls} + E_{Hydrophobic} + E_{Electrostatic}$$

6.2.5 Physical Model Solvation Potentials—Solvation

The main idea for this potential model was that most protein atoms should not have an attractive interaction with other protein atoms, reflecting the fact that the real interactions with protein atoms would be replaced by solvent interactions if the atom became exposed, hence its overall energy would not change depending on whether it was buried or exposed. However, the atoms should still have excluded volume so a repulsion potential is required at short distances. Just removing the dispersion term from the Lennard–Jones is not good enough, for the repulsion component is well above zero at the minimum of the original Lennard–Jones potential. An offset Lennard–Jones potential is used, where the well depth is offset to zero at the Lennard–Jones radius and the energy is set to zero for distances between atoms greater than the Lennard–Jones radius. This potential is used for most atoms, in particular the CA backbone atoms and any atom that does not have a specific Lennard–Jones potential.

6.2.6 Physical Model Solvation Potentials—Hydrophobicity

The next effect to consider is the "hydrophobic" effect. I consider this to be associated with two parts, the van der Waals potential between atoms (which is attractive) and effects due to the interactions with water. When side chains are buried in the hydrophobic core of a protein, the only interactions available are the standard van der Waals interactions, because there is no water present. Calculations by Levitt have shown that the stability of proteins where mutations have been made only to residues in the core have a very good correlation with the van der Waals energy of the core (52). Hence side-chain atoms of hydrophobic groups were given a standard Lennard–Jones potential with an initial energy assignment for interactions between the atoms in the same side chain such that the total side chain–side chain interaction energy is close to the enthalpy of vaporization of the most similar hydrocarbon. This would reproduce the energy of the hydrophobic core when hydrophobic side chains are buried.

This determined the potential between the same side-chain atom types. For dissimilar side-chain atom types, an analysis of the distribution of side-chain atoms around an atom in known protein structures showed to a first approximation little difference in preference between the atoms. This distribution is not that created by normal combination rules for the Lennard–Jones potential, such as the geometric mean rules. A function was created that would give such a distribution, and this was used to generate the mixed terms for the Lennard–Jones parameters of hydrophobic side-chain atoms.

Having accounted for the potential of hydrophobic side chains when buried and away from water, a potential for hydrophobic atoms when exposed to water is required. It is only this term that is considered to be truly the "hydrophobic" part, in the sense that it reflects the effect of hydrophobic groups on water structure. This was done by introducing a hydrophobic sigmoid potential. (The initial folding work of Levitt (14) had used a sigmoid potential for hydrophobic residues.) In this type of potential, the distances from one atom to all other atoms of the same type are computed and converted through some form of sigmoid function before being summed to give the potential value for the atom. For CASP4 this sigmoid potential is used only between the aliphatic side-chain atoms, reflecting the different "hydrophobicity" of aliphatic and aromatic amino acids as seen in calorimetry studies (53).

A final adjustment to the "hydrophobicity" potential was to give certain groups in residues not normally considered hydrophobic a nonzero Lennard–Jones function so that an interaction existed between them and hydrophobic groups. These groups were not included in the sigmoid potential. Such groups were the Ala $C\beta$, the Thr $C\beta$ (because of the methyl group), the $C\beta$ of the charged amino acids Asp, Glu, Lys, and Arg, and Asn and Gln. It also included the $C\gamma$ atom of Lys and Arg. Observations of experimental structures and surface accessibility calculations show that these groups are as buried as any of the atoms in the classic hydrophobic side chains.

6.2.7 Physical Model Solvation Potentials—Electrostatics

This aspect of the potentials is mainly neglected by all current protein folding models:

$$E_{\text{Electrostatic}} = E_{\text{Self-energy}} + E_{\text{Coulombic}}$$

The correct way to compute electrostatics, without including all waters explicitly, is to use the Poisson–Boltzmann equations, and numerical methods to do this have been widely used (54,55). Honig's paper on model electrostatics (56) used the Kirkwood–Tanford model to describe some of the effects that need to be included to get a good approximation to the electrostatics. The Kirkwood–Tanford model (57) assumes a spherical "protein" that has a low dielectric constant in an environment with a high dielectric constant plus ionic effects, in which point charges are embedded. Their paper gives full formulas for the calculation of the electrostatic energy, including self-energy. My potential uses an inverse model, in which the electrostatic interactions between the charged groups are varied according to their local dielectric environment, evaluated by applying a sigmoid function as before to the count of surrounding nonpolar groups. To take into account ionic strength effects, which are assumed to play a role at large distances between charges but not at short range, a distance-dependent dielectric of the square of the distance was used (because the Debye–Huckel theory on which this aspect is based assumes an averaged ionic atmosphere around each charge, which is certainly not true for charges on the surface of a folded protein). Hence, electrostatic interactions were computed using a distance-cubed term.

6.2.8 Charge Self-Energy

The other feature of electrostatics that needs to be covered is the difficulty of burying charges, the self-energy. Significant energy is required to move a charged point from the high-dielectric region to the low-dielectric region; this is called the *self-energy* of the charge (56). This is the physical basis underlying the observation that charged residues are rarely buried in proteins. It is actually a much stronger rule of proteins that the charged group of charged residues is exposed than that the side chains of hydrophobic residues are buried. Charged groups are buried only if in a salt bridge or extensively hydrogen bonded. The simple electrostatic explanation for this is the self-energy of a charge, which says it requires a lot of energy to move a charge from a high-dielectric region into a low-dielectric region.

Because there is a big difference in surface accessibility among the charged residues, independent self-potentials are assigned for Lys, Asp, or Glu and Arg. The lysine charged end point is the most solvent-exposed group of proteins, with an average relative surface-accessible area greater than 50%. Glu is next, followed by Asp, both in the 45% region; Arg is the least exposed, at around 35%. This is what you would expect based on charge density considerations, the self-energy being much greater for a charge field that is small and highly charged. With only one heavy atom, the amine group of lysine is the smallest charged group, when compared with the carboxyl group of Glu or Asp, which spreads the charge further. The charged guanidinium group charge of Arg spreads the charge over a very large area (four heavy atoms). The same sigmoid function counting the number of nonpolar groups surrounding a charge is used as before, scaled by a potential constant that gives a positive energy for burying a charge.

6.2.9   Physical Model Solvation Potentials—Scaling

Dipole Dielectric Screening   The interaction between dipoles as they move from a high-dielectric region to a low-dielectric region is increased. This implies that the backbone hydrogen bonds of secondary structures get stronger as they are increasingly buried. This is supported by statistical analyses of protein structures. These show that hydrophobic residues are good predictors of the presence of secondary structure, which are essentially hydrogen bond networks (D.J. Osguthorpe, unpublished results). In the unfolded protein, the stability of backbone–backbone hydrogen bonds is likely to be similar to that of backbone–water hydrogen bonds, hence there should be no energy-stabilizing backbone hydrogen bonds. This effect has been included by scaling the backbone hydrogen bond energy term (E_{Helix} and E_{Sheet}) via a sigmoid function counting the number of surrounding nonpolar groups. Interestingly, protein folding has long been classified as a cooperative process, and this scaling creates a direct mechanism for such cooperativity.

Charge Dielectric Screening   A similar effect applies to the Coulombic interactions between charges. Interactions between charged pairs not surrounded by nonpolar groups (high dielectric) will be weak and strong when surrounded by nonpolars (low dielectric). It is this effect that allows the creation of buried salt bridges, for the Coulombic attraction between the buried opposing charges can overwhelm the self-energy of the charges. In this case the electrostatic interactions are scaled by the sigmoid function of surrounding nonpolar groups.

7   THE FUTURE OF NOVEL FOLD AND AB INITIO PROTEIN FOLDING

The next few years are going to be intensely exciting in this field, because the progress made so far suggests the definitive solution to the protein folding problem is very close. What is even more heartening is that physics-based ab initio methods are managing to keep up with most of the statistical methods. So not only will we be able to generate structure from sequence, but we will also understand why a sequence has adopted its particular fold.

REFERENCES

1. C. Anfinsen. Principles that govern the folding of polypeptide chains. Science 181:223–230, 1973.

1a. M.J. Sippl, P. Lackner, F.S. Domingues, A. Prilc, R. Malik, A. Andreeva, and M. Wiederstein. Assessment of the CASP4 fold recognition category. Proteins Struct. Funct. Genet. Suppl. 55–67, 2001.

2. L. Holm and C. Sander. Mapping the protein universe. Science 273:595–602, 1996.

3. J.F. Gibrat, T. Madel, and S.H. Bryant. Surprising similarities in structure comparison. Curr. Opin. Struct. Biol. 6:377–385, 1996.

4. A.G. Murzin, S.E. Brenner, T. Hubbard, and C. Chothia. SCOP: a structural classification of proteins database for the investigation of sequences and structure. J. Mol. Biol. 247:536–540, 1995.

5. C.A. Orengo, A.D. Michie, S. Jones, D.T. Jones, M.B. Swindells, and J.M. Thornton. CATH—a heirarchic classification of protein domain structures. Structure 5:1093–1108, 1997.

6. M. Levitt and A. Warshel. Computer simulation of protein folding. Nature 253:694–698, 1975.

7. D.J. Osguthorpe Ph.D. dissertation, University of Manchester, Manchester, U.K., 1979.

8. D.A. Debe, M.J. Carlson, and W.A. Goddard III. The topomer-sampling model of protein folding. Proc. Natl. Acad. Sci. USA 96:2596–2601, 1999.

9. B. Park and M. Levitt. Energy functions that discriminate X-ray and near-native folds from well-constructed decoys. J. Mol. Biol. 258:367–392, 1996.

10. K.T. Simons, C. Kooperberg, E. Huang, and D. Baker. Assembly of protein tertiary structures from fragments with similar local sequences using simulated annealing and Bayesian scoring functions. J. Mol. Biol. 268:209–225, 1997.

11. http://dd.stanford.edu

12. C. Woodward and R.H. Li. The hydrogen exchange core and protein folding. Protein Science 8:1571–1590, 1999.

13. D.J. Osguthorpe. Ab Initio Protein Folding. Curr. Opin. Struct. Biol. 146–152, 2000.

14. M. Levitt. A simplified representation of protein conformations for rapid simulation of protein folding. J. Mol. Biol. 104:59–107, 1976.

15. D.J. Osguthorpe. Analysis of the predicted structures of domain 1 of protein G3 (T0030) and NK-lysin (T0042). Proteins Suppl. 1:172–178, 1997.

16. D.J. Osguthorpe. Improved ab initio predictions with a simplified, flexible geometry model. Proteins Suppl. 3:186–193, 1999.

17. R. Samudrala, Yu Xia, E. Huang, and M. Levitt. Ab initio protein structure prediction using a combined hierarchical approach. Proteins Suppl:194–198, 1999.

18. B.A. Reva, D.S. Rykunov, A.V. Finkelstein, and J. Skolnick. Optimization of protein structure on lattices using a self-consistent approach. J. Comput. Biology 5:531–538, 1998.

19. D. Thirumalai and D.K. Klimov. Deciphering the timescales and mechanisms of protein folding using minimal off-lattice models. Curr. Opin. Struct. Biol. 9:197–207, 1999.

20. Ming-Hong Hao and H.A. Scheraga. Designing potential energy functions for protein folding. Curr. Opin. Struct. Biol. 9:184–188, 1999.

21. K.T. Simons, I. Ruczinski, C. Kooperberg, B.A. Fox, C. Bystroff, and D. Baker, Improved recognition of native-like protein structures using a combination of sequence-dependent and sequence-independent features of proteins. Proteins 34:82–95, 1999.

22. A. Liwo, S. Oldziej, M.R. Pincus, R.J. Wawak, S. Rackovsky, and H.A. Scheraga. A united-residue force field for off-lattice protein-structure simulations. I. Functional forms and parameters of long-range side-chain interaction potentials from protein crystal data. J. Comput. Chem. 18:849–873, 1997.

23. A. Liwo, S. Oldziej, M.R. Pincus, R.J. Wawak, S. Rackovsky, and H.A. Scheraga. A united-residue force field for off-lattice protein-structure simulations. II. Parameterization of short-range interactions and determination of weights of energy terms by Z-score optimization. J. Comput. Chem. 18:874–887, 1997.

24. A. Liwo, R. Kazmierkiewicz, C. Czaplewski, M. Groth, S. Oldziej, R.J. Wawak, S. Rackovsky, M.R. Pincus, and H.A. Scheraga. United-residue force field for off-lattice protein-structure simulations: III. Origin of backbone hydrogen-bonding cooperativity in united-residue potentials. J. Comput. Chem. 19:259–276, 1998.

25. B. Robson. Analysis of the code relating sequence to conformation in globular proteins. Biochem. J. 141:853–867, 1974.

26. J. Garnier, D.J. Osguthorpe, and B. Robson. Analysis of accuracy and implications of simple methods for predicting secondary structure of globular proteins. J. Mol.Biol. 120:97–120, 1978.

27. Sanzo Miyazawa and R.L. Jernigan. Estimation of effective interresidue contact energies from protein crystal structures: quasi-chemical approximation. Macromolecules 18:534–552, 1985.

28. Sanzo Miyazawa and R.L. Jernigan. Evaluation of short-range interactions as secondary structure energies for protein fold and sequence recognition. Proteins 36:347–356, 1999.

29. F. Avbelj and J. Moult. Role of electrostatic screening in determining protein main chain conformational preferences. Biochemistry 34:755–764, 1995.

30. F. Avbelj and L. Fele. Role of main-chain electrostatics, hydrophobic effect and side-chain conformational entropy in determining the secondary structure of proteins. J. Mol. Biol. 279:665–684, 1998.

31. F. Avbelj and L. Fele. Prediction of the three-dimensional structure of proteins using the electrostatic screening model and hierarchic condensation. Proteins 31:74–96, 1998.

32. A. Godzik, A. Kolinski, and J. Skolnick. De-novo and inverse folding predictions of protein structure and dynamics. J. Comput. Aid. Mol. Des. 7:397–438, 1993.

33. R.A. Goldstein, Z.A. Luthey-Schulten, and P.G. Wolynes. Protein tertiary structure recognition using optimized Hamiltonians with local interactions. Proc. Natl. Acad. Sci. USA 89:9029–9033, 1992.

34. U.H.E Hansmann and Y. Okamoto. New Monte Carlo algorithms for protein folding. Curr. Opin. Struct. Biol. 9:177–183, 1999.

35. T. De Beer, R.E. Carter, K.E. Lobel-Rice, A. Sorkin, and M. Overdun, Solution structure and Asn-Pro-Phe binding pocket of the Eps15 homology domain. Science 281:1357–1360, 1998.

36. J. Johansson, T. Szyperski, T. Curstedt, and K. Wuthrich. The NMR structure of the pulmonary surfactant-associated polypeptide SP-C in an apolar solvent contains a Valyl-rich alpha-helix. Biochemistry 33:6015–6023, 1994.

37. B. Rost and C. Sander. Combining evolutionary information and neural networks to predict protein secondary structure. Proteins 19:55–72, 1994.

38. L.P. Wei, E.S. Huang, and R.B. Altman. Are predicted structures good enough to preserve functional sites?. Structure Folding Design 7:643–650, 1999.

39. J. Moult, J.T. Pedersen, R. Judson, and K. Fidelis. A large scale experiment to assess protein-structure prediction methods. Proteins 23:R2–R4, 1995.

40. J. Moult, T. Hubbard, S.H. Bryant, K. Fidelis, and J.T. Pedersen. Critical Assessment of Methods of Protein Structure Prediction (CASP): Round II. Proteins Suppl. 1:2–6, 1997.

41. J. Moult, T. Hubbard, K. Fidelis, and J.T. Pedersen. Critical Assessment of Methods of Protein Structure Prediction (CASP): Round III. Proteins Suppl:2–6, 1999.

41a. J. Moult, K. Fidelis, A. Zemla, and T. Hubbard. Critical assessment of methods of protein structure prediction (CASP): round IV. Proteins Suppl. 2–7, 2001.

42. http://PredictionCenter.llnl.gov/

43. K.T. Simons, R. Bonneau, I. Ruczinski, and D. Baker. Ab initio protein structure predictions of CASP III targets using ROSETTA. Proteins Suppl:171–176, 1999.

44. D. Shortle, K.T. Simons, and D. Baker. Clustering of low-energy conformations near the native structure of small proteins. Proc. Natl. Acad. Sci. USA 95:11158–11162, 1998.

44a. J. Skolnick, A. Kolinski, D. Kihara, M. Betancourt, P. Rotkiewicz, and M. Boniecki. Ab initio protein structure prediction via a combination of threading, lattice folding, clustering, and structure refinement. Proteins Struct. Funct. Genet. Suppl. 149–156, 2001.

45. Jooyoung Lee, A. Liwo, D.R. Ripoll, J. Pillardy, and H.A. Scheraga. Calculation of protein conformation by global optimization of a potential energy function. Proteins Suppl:204–208, 1999.

46. R. Srinivasan and G.D. Rose. LINUS: A hierarchic procedure to predict the fold of a protein. Proteins 22:81–99, 1995.

47. R. Srinivasan and G.D. Rose. A physical basis for protein secondary structure. Proc. Natl. Acad. Sci. USA 96:14258–14263, 1999.

48. W. Kabsch and C. Sander. Dictionary of protein secondary structure: pattern recognition of hydrogen-bonded and geometrical features. Biopolymers 22:2577–2637, 1983.

49. G. N. Ramachandran and V. Sasisekharan. Adv. Protein Chem. 23:283, 1968.
50. U. Hobohm and C. Sander. Enlarged representative set of protein structures. Protein Science 3:522, 1994.
51. J. Deisenhofer, O. Epp, K. Mikki, R. Huber, and H. Michel. Structure of the protein subunits in the photosynthetic reaction centre of *Rhodopseudomonas viridis* at 3-Å resolution. Nature 318:618–624, 1985.
52. C. Lee and M. Levitt. Accurate prediction of the stability and activity effects of site-directed mutagenesis on a protein core. Nature 352:448–451, 1991.
53. P.L. Privalov. Thermodynamics of protein folding. J. Chem. Thermodynamics 29:447–474, 1997.
54. J. Warwicker. Continuum dielectric modelling of the protein-solvent systems, and calculation of the long-range electrostatic field of the enzyme phosphoglycerate mutase. J. Theor. Biol. 121:199–210, 1986.
55. A. Nicholls and B. Honig. A rapid finite-difference algorithm, utilizing successive over-relaxation to solve the Poisson–Boltzmann equation. J. Comput. Chem. 12:435–445, 1991.
56. M.K. Gilson, A. Rashin, R. Fine, and B. Honig. On the calculation of electrostatic interactions in proteins. J. Mol. Biol. 183:503–516, 1985.
57. C. Tanford and J.G. Kirkwood. Theory of protein titration curves. I. General equations for impenetrable spheres. J. Am. Chem. Soc. 79:5333–5339, 1957.

10

Identifying Errors in Three-Dimensional Protein Models

Brian D. Marsden and Ruben A. Abagyan
The Scripps Research Institute, La Jolla, California, U.S.A.

1 INTRODUCTION

Building a structural model for every protein from the proteome is an important aspect of understanding protein function and its differences between homologs, variants, mutants, etc. The task of generating hundreds of thousands of models does not seem impossible, due to progress in both experimental structure determination (1) and theoretical structure prediction by homology techniques (2). However, all models necessarily contain an elaborate network of errors of varying character and magnitude, depending on the derivation method. Understanding these errors is key to the utility of a model.

All structure generation technologies, experimental and theoretical, are becoming more automated. There have been a number of recent developments in many of the methods involved in X-ray crystallographic structure determination (3–5). It is now possible to perform partial automatic assignment of NMR spectra coupled with automatic structure calculation (6,7). Modeling techniques that employ a simple inheritance of the aligned backbone and a nominal placement of different side chains and loops can be performed in seconds (e.g., ICM (8,9), Swissmodel (10), Modeller (11)) and, therefore, models of tens of thousands of proteins of the proteome can easily be generated.

Automated techniques are now being employed to isolate and determine all possible protein folds by experimental methods (e.g., Joint Center for Structural Genomics (JCSG), http://www.jcsg.org). On these scales of data throughput, it is not possible to carefully hand-inspect each stage of the structure determination of each protein. Instead, automatic methods of structure error detection are becoming more and more necessary (12). Even though some basic quality control methods (which detect simple stereochemistry errors and large clashes) are often applied, the lack of more sophisticated quality control and model reliability annotation is the price that currently has to be paid for the demand for more structures more quickly. However, individual visual inspection is also not a panacea, since humans err. A very good analysis of errors in of structures in the Protein Structure Database (PDB) (13) can be found in the review by Hooft and coworkers (14).

In summary, automation of structure determination and prediction necessarily calls for the automation of error detection, which in turn requires better classification of errors.

"'What is truth?' asked jesting Pilat" (Francis Bacon). What is a true model? Proteins are complicated structural entities in continuous motion. Simply by virtue of representing them as one or several configurations we lose information. However, the loss of information does not constitute an introduction of error. What does constitute an error is a conformation, local or global, that is almost never adopted by the protein. A practical model is therefore one or several representative conformations of a statistical ensemble complemented by local average dynamic information (e.g., in the form of B-factors). Overall, for the sake of this chapter, we would like to assume that a local protein region can either have a *single* predominant conformation (the majority of the protein) or be unstructured to a different degree (the minority). Our definition of error will break down for proteins not satisfying these criteria.

The accuracy of a model may be predicted in terms of its global characteristics ("How wrong is this model?") or in terms of its local characteristics ("Which parts of this model are likely to be the most reliable?"). Models are not generated just for the sake of creating a set of coordinates. They are generated to derive or predict interesting biological information. However, any information taken from an erroneous local region of a model is likely to be erroneous itself. Clearly it is very important to be able to predict the local accuracy or confidence of the local accuracy of the model concerned in order to evaluate the significance of any model-derived information.

There are many scenarios where models of protein structures are determined in order to gain an understanding of their local characteristics. We need to be concerned about model errors in the following applications.

Small ligand docking to a model: For virtual ligand screening studies, where large numbers of small chemical molecules are evaluated for their ability to bind to a protein, it is often only important that the binding region of the protein target be determined as accurately as possible. An inaccurate structure in this region may result in a final library of possible ligands that are not significantly biologically active.

Protein/peptide docking to a model: Local areas of the surface of a protein structure may be important in docking with other proteins or smaller peptide ligands.

Structure–Function prediction: When a newly derived protein structure is determined, its function (if it is unknown) can sometimes be elucidated by the close examination of local regions of the structure, looking in particular for previously known structural motifs. A measure of the local accuracy of such motifs is critical in order to be confident that the predicted function is likely to be correct.

Catalytic mechanism: The composition and configuration of residue side chains in active sites in enzymes is key to the understanding of any chemical reaction the enzyme may catalyze. An inaccurately predicted side-chain orientation in a protein model may lead to an incorrect derivation of the chemical pathway that is involved in any chemical reaction.

Parameter derivation: The role of local accuracy of protein structural models is also important in more theoretical studies. In the development of new model-generation methods, it is critical that the data set of protein structures used to parameterize and refine the method include as little error as possible, otherwise the method will be flawed at best and useless at worst. Therefore, it is important that the local accuracy of the structures be measurable in some way.

Molecular replacement: The efficacy of the use of protein structural models as molecular-replacement templates in X-ray crystallography studies (15) is critically dependent upon the accuracy of the whole model. However, local structural accuracy predictions allow regions that are predicted to have poor accuracy to have their artificial B-factors down-weighted.

A key problem in the assessment of the accuracy of protein structural models is that a simple vacuum energy function is currently unable to reliably predict the accuracy of protein structural models, let alone local regions within a model (16). This forces us to derive more sophisticated energy functions (17) or use other empirical computational methods that focus on many separate aspects of the protein model to determine what, problems may exist, where, and perhaps why (18–22).

This chapter focuses upon the types of local errors that can occur in protein structural models. Local errors in protein structural models can be classified in two ways: by their geometrical manifestation and by their origin. By origin we mean a method, or procedure, computational or experimental, leading to a model. We first discuss local errors that can occur in all methods of protein structural model prediction as well as local errors that are method specific. Methods to detect and, where possible, quantify such errors will be described. The extent to which recovery from such errors can be made will be covered. Ways in which new prediction methods might be evaluated will also be discussed.

2   GEOMETRICAL CLASSIFICATION OF ERRORS

2.1   Errors in Covalent Geometry

Local chemical structure is characterized by bond lengths, bond angles, planarity, and chirality. Even small deviations of these values beyond their equilibrium values, especially for bond lengths, may lead to significant artificial energy strain. Typically, no experimental method for proteins is accurate enough to provide sufficient information about small deviations of covalent geometries from their idealized values, and the model values depend on the parameterization of the force field used to refine the model. These errors are trivial to detect.

2.2   Through-Space Atomic Clashes

A common local geometrical error relates to the nature of the packing of atoms within the model. Interatomic repulsion is a very steep function of a distance between neighboring atoms not connected by a covalent bond. The distances cannot be smaller than a sum of van der Waals radii, unless the two atoms are involved in a hydrogen bond. Strictly speaking the minimal distance between two atoms is not a simple sum of two van der Waals radii, as the combination rules in various force fields show (this in turn indicates that ultimately the energy-based error detection methods will be more accurate). The resulting clash is energetically very unfavorable. Clashes can occur between atoms due to experimental or theoretical restraints (11,23) that are incorrect or too severe. Incorrect restraints forcing atoms into non-native positions can result in other atoms being squeezed together, forming a clash (Fig. 1a). Clashes can manifest themselves either as scattered individual bumps or as multiple clashes between atom groups.

2.3 Errors in Torsion Angles

A torsion angle, defined as a dihedral between planes formed by two consecutive atom triplets in a chain, can deviate from its correct value (Fig. 1b). This can cause a side chain to point in the wrong direction or to orient incorrectly. Inaccurate side-chain torsion angles may occur due to incorrect experimental data (e.g., a number of poorly assigned NMR distance restraints involving atom(s) within the side chain) or to a poorly parameterized or poorly weighted force field (used to enforce "realistic" geometry during model optimization).

2.4 Peptide Flip Errors

Peptide bonds can adopt either the cis or trans form. Normally, only the sterically favorable trans form is found in protein structures, apart from proline residues, which can adopt the cis form. Clearly a cis form residue will lead to the backbone of the model to proceed in a different spatial direction (Fig. 1c). Such an error is known as a peptide flip (24). Again, as for side-chain rotamer errors, cis form residues may occur due to poor experimental data or poor model optimization (25).

2.5 Backbone Deviations

Finally, the local position of the backbone of the model may be inaccurate (Fig. 1d). This may be especially true in noncore regions of the model, where there is the greatest steric possibility of structural variation. The source of such an error may be a lack of data (e.g., a lack of NMR distance restraints or structural templates in homology modeling) or imprecise data (e.g., a poorly defined area of electron density in an X-ray crystallography study). It must be remembered, however, that the dynamic nature of backbones that form noncore coil structures implies that there may be not one preferred configuration in vivo. In this circumstance, it is impossible for a definitive configuration to be modeled (although since NMR protein structure solution methods result in a family of structures, a feel for the possible range of local backbone configurations may be obtained). Backbone deviation errors are difficult to predict and are also the most damaging in terms of the accuracy of a local region of a model.

3 ERRORS DEPENDANT ON THE MODEL DERIVATION PROCEDURE

Method-dependent errors result solely from assumptions, limitations, or errors that are inherent in the nature of the source data and the method

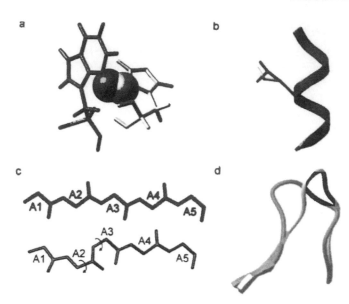

Figure 1 Examples of errors in covalent geometry. (a) Through-space atomic clash. Here, the Hε3 atom of a tryptophan residue and the Hδ1 atom of a histidine residue are too close together, resulting in an energetically unfavorable contact. (b) Torsion angle errors. The side chain of a leucine residue can adopt a number of preferred orientations (Ref. 46). Two of the most favored conformations occupy very similar regions of space, leading to possible error. (c) Peptide-flip. *Top*: A poly-alanine chain (side chains are shown with thinner lines). *Bottom*: The same chain but with a peptide flip between residues A2 and A3 due to inversions of the phi angle of A2 and the psi angle of A3 (shown by arrows). (d) Backbone deviation between two homologous protein structures.

used to produce the model from those data. Since the quantity and quality of data that is used to predict the structure of a protein are often the most critical determinants of the accuracy of a model, a discussion of these sources of errors is warranted.

3.1   Errors in X-ray Crystallography

This is the predominant experimental method in protein structure prediction, being able to solve structures of proteins made up of a few residues to many hundreds of residues. Over 80% of all structures in the PDB (13) have been solved using this method.

One of the most significant sources of error is the raw data itself. The error critically depends on the observation/parameter ratio, which typically is very low in macromolecular crystallography. At 2.8Å resolution, the ratio is only about 1 if the Cartesian coordinates and an isotropic temperature factor are determined. This ratio grows approximately as an inverse cubic dependency upon resolution and reaches a reasonable number of about 10 at 1.3 Å. At ratios under 3 it is very easy to "overfit" the data with a partially wrong model.

3.1.1 Tracing the Backbone

In the extreme case, when the resolution is poor but visible, registration errors (i.e., errors in assignment of residues to particular areas of density) can occur whereby one or more residues are shifted away from their correct location within the structures, including a complete mistracing (26). Another type of drastic problem occurs due to a lack of any clear electron density. In this situation some crystallographers will not provide a prediction of the local structure, whereas others will provide an arbitrary conformation of the unresolved fragment. Finally, even if the backbone is traced correctly over-all, the lack of local electron density quality may lead to ambiguities and errors in the exact values of phi, psi, and omega backbone dihedral angles. A frequent error is the peptide flip (Fig. 1c), which preserves the positions of the flanking side chains with incorrect orientation of the peptide group. In addition, in the case of small residues, the orientation of the $C\alpha$–$C\beta$ bonds, and therefore the local backbone conformation, may also be incorrect.

3.1.2 Fitting the Side Chains

Usually, it is difficult to accurately map the side chain of the noncore residues within the protein to local areas of electron density, leading to a locally inaccurate structure prediction or even to multiple conformations. At typical resolutions, a further common problem characteristic of macromolecular crystallography arises from its inability to see hydrogen atoms and to discriminate between similar-sized heavy atoms (e.g., carbon, nitrogen, and oxygen). Even at very high resolutions, it is often difficult to determine which way residues should be placed around the side chains of asparagine, glutamine, and histidine, since the difficulty of determining where the terminal carbon and nitrogen atoms are in the electron density map makes the side chains appear to be symmetrical.

3.1.3 Refinement

The final step in X-ray crystallographic structure prediction is the auto-mated refinement, in which the structure is optimized against the data, usually with additional empirical function terms representing conformational energy. This procedure involves some sampling of the conformational space, using either local or global optimization methods (e.g., molecular dynamics and simulated annealing), and can result in errors due to underlying assumptions in the objective function and/or insufficient sampling.

3.2   Errors in NMR Models

3.2.1   Atom-Atom Distance Determination

The NMR solution structure determination methods rely mainly on the nuclear Overhauser effect (NOE), which gives an estimate of the distance between two atoms in a molecule (23). However, the NOE effect is proportional to the inverse sixth power of the distance between the two atoms. As a consequence, this effect is measurable only for distances up to around 5 Å. Hence any structure determined using this method does not include any long-range information at all. This is not a significant problem for globular proteins, where there is usually a high density of distance restraints associated with the atoms in the core of the molecule.

Since an NOE gives only an estimate of the distance between two atoms, it is common practice to assign each NOE to two or more "bins," for example, between 1.8 and 2.7 Å, between 1.8 and 3.5 Å, and between 1.8 and 5.0 Å. Assignment of an NOE to the wrong bin will have a direct effect upon the final model, especially if the number of NOEs assigned to the atoms concerned is relatively small, since the restraint will be either too long or, worse still, too short. Misassignment of NOEs to the wrong atom is also a problem and will significantly affect the accuracy of the final model. These problems may be caused by poor peak dispersion in the NMR spectra or to human error when the spectra are being assigned.

3.2.2   Structure Calculation

A key problem with NMR solution structure determination methods is that regions of the molecule that undergo significant dynamics on time scales that are relatively slow (i.e., slower than a few nanoseconds) often do not provide enough information for the structure calculation method to assign a unique or preferred conformation to that region (even if one exists). Because of this and because of the error introduced into the calculation by the binning procedure of the interatomic restraints, it is common practice to supply a family of structural models rather than one model, (as in an X-ray crystallographic study), in order to reflect the range of possible conformations the protein may be adopting in solution.

Ratnaparkhi et al. (27) have shown that the degree of packing of NMR solution structures is often unreliable using current methods. By comparing the degree of packing of 70 structures solved both by NMR and X-ray crystallographic techniques, the normalized packing values for the NMR structures were often found to be substantially under- and (in some cases) overestimated relative to the corresponding X-ray-derived structures. This can be accounted for by the fact that, in general, the energy function used to calculate the structure contains no attractive components apart from the pseudo-energy term describing the effect of the NOE distance restraints. It is therefore energetically more favorable for the structure to expand rather than to contract (28–30). Further, they showed that NMR solution structures of the same protein, solved by different laboratories, showed significant differences in the degree of packing. This suggests that artifacts may be introduced into current NMR solution structure determination techniques at one or more of the data collection, analysis, or structure calculation steps.

The consequences of this experimental technique's inability to accurately produce structures that reflect the native packing density are not always clear. However, it is likely to have significant implications for local structure accuracy and may have a direct effect upon the modeling of important motifs, for example, the geometry of binding pockets. This is especially true in regions of the model structure where the NOE restraint density is low, since the local contribution of the NOE pseudo-energy term to the total energy function in these areas will be proportionally smaller.

3.3 Errors in Homology Models

There are a number of critical points within a typical homology modeling procedure (Fig. 2). Here we discuss the effects of each error at each point in the procedure.

3.3.1 Poor Template Choice

The theoretical approach to protein structure prediction relies on the availability of one or more structures (templates) of homologous proteins that have been previously solved, usually by an experimental method such as NMR or X-ray crystallography. The choice of the most appropriate and accurate templates to base a protein structural model upon is becoming easier as more experimentally derived protein structural models are placed in the PDB (13). However, if the function of the molecule is not known a priori or if there is little sequence homology with any previously solved structure, it is difficult to be sure that the most appropriate template is

Template Choice

Wrong 3D topology
Effects of local errors in templates

Sequence - Structure Alignment

Secondary structure misalignment

Modeling

Backbone errors in vicinity of Insertions/Deletions
Side-chain mispredictions
Plastic large-scale deformations

Figure 2 Flow diagram of critical points in the homology modeling procedure where any resulting error will become unresolvable.

being used (if it exists at all). Clearly an incorrect template will lead to an irretrievably inaccurate model, both locally and globally.

3.3.2 Alignment Errors

A key source of error in models predicted by homology modeling is the (multiple) sequence alignment that is used to map the features of the template residues to the target structures. Whole local regions of the target structure can be incorrectly predicted if the sequence alignment between the template and target sequences is structurally inaccurate. For example, a one-residue shift of a template structure from the correct alignment will lead to the backbone of the target structure also being shifted by one residue, producing side-chain placement errors (especially in secondary structural elements) and inaccurate backbone conformations.

3.3.3 Inheritance of Errors from the Template

The selection of appropriate templates is no guarantee of success. Since the resulting model is built using the characteristics of the template structures, any errors in these structures (such as those just discussed) are likely to be propagated into the final model.

3.3.4   Backbone Conformational Errors

If the degree of sequence similarity is particularly low (e.g., below the "twilight zone" of around 25% (31,32)), it is likely that local areas of the target structure may be predicted to form incorrect secondary structure or even an incorrect fold.

3.3.5   Backbone Errors Around Deletions in Alignment

The template structure sequences are never identical to the target sequence. Deletions within the final model relative to the template structure(s) are also a major source of error. The inherent discontinuity along the backbone in the template structure must be resolved in the final modeled structure. Deletions relative to the template structures most often occur outside the core of the structure to be modeled, and it is here that most backbone deviations occur, resulting in prediction errors.

3.3.6   Backbone Errors in and Around Insertions in Alignment

Assuming that reasonable template structures are chosen, and that an accurate sequence alignment is created, the next major source of error arises within parts of the final model where there are no homologous template structures available to base the modeled structure upon (i.e., insertions). Again, these features usually occur upon the surface of the protein rather than the core.

3.3.7   Side-Chain Mispredictions

For residues in the target structure that have poor sequence homology with the equivalent residues in the templates structures, there is often little, or even incorrect, information that can be used about the geometry of the residue's side chains in the target structure. This can lead to problems of poor packing in the core of the structure. Specifically, side-chain packing can change considerably, leading side chains in the final model to adopt very erroneous conformations and to the possibility that biologically important side chains will be incorrectly exposed or buried in the surface of the structure.

3.3.8   Plastic Large-Scale Topological Deformations

Even without any insertions and deletions, the model backbone may differ from the template conformation due to cumulative nonlocal deviations that may be necessary to resolve otherwise irreconcilable structural problems in the homology model. It is fair to say that currently these changes are impossible to predict reliably.

4   THE DETECTION AND PREDICTION OF ERRORS

The detection of local error in model structure has two goals. (1) to alleviate the errors as far as possible; (2) to annotate the final model to give an estimate of its local reliability. Knowing what sort of errors can occur in a model of a protein, how does one detect their existence in the model and perhaps identify their source in the context of the model as a whole or a local region of the model? It is not entirely trivial to perform such an analysis. Although it is relatively easy to detect regions of a model that might be erroneous, it is not always as easy to say what the source of the error is. Further, the use of knowledge-based error detection methods (discussed later) can lead to cases where apparent errors are just unusual, yet accurate, substructures.

Local error detection methods generally take one of two approaches: an attempt to compare the protein model to the data used to create the model, or only taking the model itself and using some form of statistical or energetic approach to measure local accuracy.

In this section we will focus upon error detection methods that are available to the modeler. Once again we will divide the methods into method-specific and method-independent approaches. We will attempt to point out what we consider to be the benefits and disadvantages of each method. Procedures that might be employed to avoid or alleviate errors will also be discussed.

4.1   Geometrical Error Detection

All protein structural models can suffer from errors in covalent geometry, as discussed earlier. The detection of such errors can often indicate the existence of a greater underlying error, or errors, in the local structure of the model. There are a number of programs available that are able to detect the most common forms of covalent geometry errors and report their existence in an easy-to-digest format. Recently, there has been a concerted effort to validate a number of error detection packages (33), which has resulted in a number of improvements in their implementation.

It important to stress that the model covalent geometry in most cases results from the model-building procedure and/or the bond-stretching, bond angle, and dihedral-bending force field parameters used in refinement. For example, NMR models built by DYANA (34) will always have ideal covalent geometry since the building procedure does not allow the initial "ideal" values to change. If the angle and bond length values are to change, the detection of the covalent geometry problems should be performed with respect to the ideal parameters used in the refinement (e.g., the Engh and Huber parameters (35)). Unfortunately, no geometrical procedure is currently using this approach. However, an energy detection approach (see later) resolves this problem. Only covalent geometry that is not restrained during the modeling procedure is unbiased and is a legitimate target of covalent error-detection (36).

PROCHECK (37) is a widely used suite of programs that compares a wide range of a model's geometric characteristics with a database of geometric characteristics from a set of high-resolution protein structures. The coordinates of the model structure are supplied to the program in a PDB-format file. By default, a number of postscript files are then created, along with a text summary file, indicating the results of the analysis. Errors such as abnormal bond lengths, angles, dihedral angles, and puckered rings are pinpointed. Side-chain torsion angles are calculated and presented in χ^1/χ^2 per-residue plots. Indicators of the number of bad contacts, omega angle standard deviation, $C\alpha$ tetrahedral angle distortion, and side-chain dihedral angles in the context of the expected resolution of the final model structure (supplied by the user) are also provided, giving a feel for the quality of the model as a whole. The backbone geometry of a model is also represented by a Ramachandran plot, with outliers from the most populated regions labeled with residue numbers (Fig. 3). A useful feature is the production of a summary of the most important geometric features per residue, which allows one to gauge the regions of the model that are likely to contain the most significant errors. NMR solution structure families of models are also accommodated by PROCHECK, using the PROCHECK_NMR program (37). This takes a PDB-format file of all models and is able to produce similar plots for each model, along with plots indicating the number of models with errors in each residue.

WHATCHECK (14) also takes a PDB-format file of a model but, in addition to checking the nomenclature used in the file, performs a wider range of geometric tests. Many of these tests, such as packing quality and Ramachandran plot quality, result in a value that characterizes the whole model rather than local regions of the model. The results are output to a text file along with a number of postscript plots. Local tests performed by

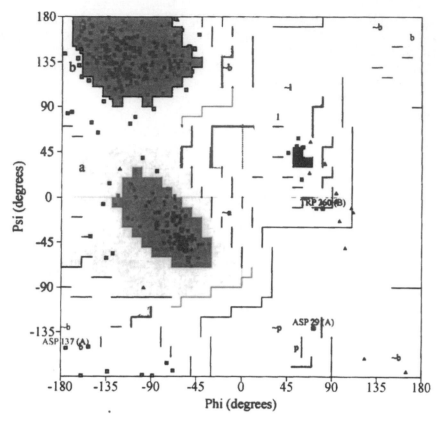

Figure 3   Example of a Ramachandran plot as produced by PROCHECK. Residues (apart from glycine) with unusual backbone geometry are annotated within the plot, giving a quick view of the location of possible local errors.

WHATCHECK include checks for unusual bond lengths, bond and torsion angles, deviation of the backbone omega angles from 180°, ring planarity, and proline puckering, as well as checks for atoms that may be too close to each other ("bumps"). The chirality of atom groups is checked by calculating the "improper" dihedral angles, which should not deviate greatly from ±35° for nonplanar groups and 0° for planar groups.

It should be noted that both PROCHECK and WHATCHECK use a database of high-resolution structures from which typical stereochemical characteristics are derived. These are then used for comparison with the characteristics of the model. Hence it should be kept in mind that any characteristic that is said to be an outlier by either of these programs is not necessarily in error; rather, it is merely uncommon. Although this interpretation may sometimes be correct, it is clearly important to check such characteristics carefully to make sure this is the case. These correct deviations often occur in functionally important regions of a structure.

A number of error detection methods analyze the local interactions around residues or atoms. Since these are not restrained (apart from those interactions restrained by NMR NOE-derived distance restraints, for example), this is often a sensitive approach to error detection. These approaches do not identify the exact nature of any local error, but merely detect the effect of the error upon the local structure. As such, these methods are most useful when local errors that have been detected by methods described earlier have been identified and explored.

The local distribution of atoms in protein structures has been investigated, and it has been found that atom–atom interactions occur with nonrandom frequencies (38). This result is the basis of the ERRAT program (38), which is able to detect local errors in a model using a nine residue sliding window. Deviations from the expected C–C, C–N, C–O, N–N, N–O, and O–O interactions are calculated within this window and displayed as a graph, giving an indication of where there are likely to be local modeling errors. The method was able to successfully detect errors in obsolete PDB models, and the authors conclude that ERRAT is able to detect backbones errors down to 1.5 Å. However, they also conclude that unrefined models are likely to score badly, suggesting that this method should be used only once local errors detected by other methods have been dealt with.

The PROVE program (36) calculates atomic volumes of completely buried atoms using the Voronoi method and compares the results to a database of expected values derived from a set of 64 X-ray structures whose resolution is 2 Å or less. A Z-score (the difference between the actual and expected values, divided by the standard deviation of the expected distribution) is then calculated, giving a normalized measure of the deviation of the group of atoms concerned (e.g., within a residue) from the expected value. The results from this method can be confusing, since high Z-scores may result from errors that propagated from residues that are neighbors in space but not sequence. However, this can be seen as a benefit of the method, since PROCHECK (for example) is unlikely to detect such errors. The recent evaluation of PROVE by the EU 3D Validation Network [33] found that this method reliably detects local errors when the Z-score is greater than 2.5, although care needs to be taken when multiple conformations in X-ray models exist.

4.2   Error Detection Using Mean-Force/Statistical Approaches

The Eisenberg group has created a profile method that is implemented in their program, VERIFY3D (39,40). The local environment of each residue in the model structure is determined, including details such as the buried area, local secondary structure, and what fraction of the side chain is covered by polar atoms. This is used to calculate the "compatibility" of the local structure with its sequence by using a 21-residue sliding window. The results are displayed in a profile window plot, giving an indication of where there may be local errors in the model.

Empirically derived potentials of mean force (41) have been derived by Sippl (22) to assess the local accuracy of model structures by comparing the environment within the structure. The PROSAII program, which employs this empirical potential, is commonly used to detect misfolded models but may also be helpful in identifying potentially erroneous regions of a model.

A similar but more recent method using an atomic mean-force potential is employed by the ANOLEA program (42). The potential in this method has been derived from a set of 180 protein chains that have less than 25% sequence identity and better than 3 Å resolution. The effects of any local stereochemistry and the effects of local secondary structure that might bias the calculation are removed by considering only interactions between atoms that are more than 11 residues apart in the sequence but less than 7 Å apart in space. An energy plot along the length of the sequence is created, giving an indication of where there may be errors in the model. The application of this potential was found to be sensitive to errors such as might be caused by misaligned target/template sequences as used by homology modeling.

A question has been raised about the theoretical validity of mean force potential approaches (43), and yet their application has had some success (e.g., Ref. 44).

4.3   Energy-Based Error Detection

The use of physical energy potentials has also been explored for the detection of local errors in models. Maiorov and Abagyan's method (45), which uses the molecular mechanic facilities provided by the ICM program (46,47), begins by regularizing the model structure. This involves adding missing atoms (for example, protons in X-ray model structures) and the imposition of idealized geometry, followed by a number of rounds of energy relaxation. For each residue in the model structure, the average energy for the residue, empirically derived from a set of 277 high-resolution structures, is subtracted from the observed energy of the residue and then divided by the standard deviation of the residue energy found in the database of structures. This normalized residue energy (NRE) for each residue in the model structure can then be used to create an annotated backbone representation of the model, indicating local regions of the model that are energetically strained (Fig. 4).

4.4 Method-Specific Error Detection

4.4.1 Detection of Crystallographic Model Errors

These errors are well studied (e.g., see an excellent review by Klewegt in Ref. 25). If the electron density is clear, there is not much chance for error. However, the density may be missing or ambiguous in areas ranging from small groups to significant areas of protein structure (Fig. 5). In those cases, a crystallographer is confronted with a need to make a decision.

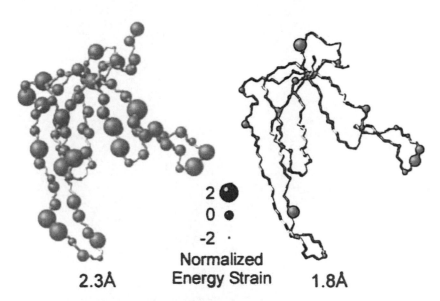

Figure 4 Calculation of backbone energy strain can be useful in detecting local errors. On the left is a backbone representation of the 2.3Å structure of gene V binding protein (PDB code 2gn5); on the right is a backbone representation of a higher-resolution structure (1.8 Å, PDB code 1bgh). At each residue position is a sphere whose size is related to the calculated normalized residue energy. It can be seen that the higher-resolution structure possesses a significantly less energy-strained backbone than the lower-resolution structure.

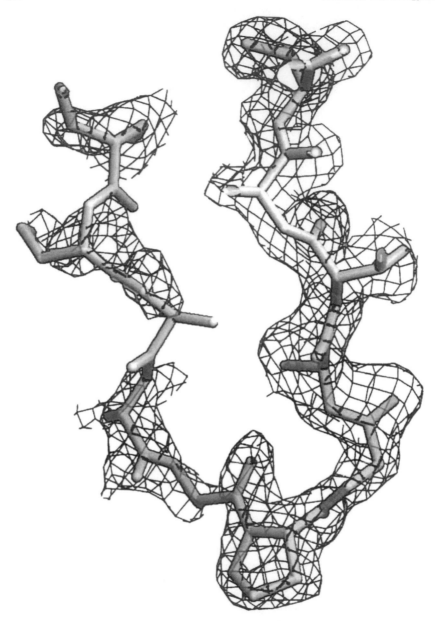

Figure 5 Example of regions of poor electron density (left) that might lead to errors in atom placement.

If a crystallographer has little or no clear density in a part of the model, he or she faces two arbitrary choices:

- Either to build some chain into this area or to break the chain and not build any atoms into the uncertain area.
- If the decision in the previous step is to build, the next choice is to assign either a low occupancy or high B-factor. In most cases the refinement programs optimize only the three-dimensional coordinates and the B-factor, but not the occupancy parameters.

In either case, errors will result due to either nonexistent atoms, unrealistic conformational representations, or inaccurate occupancy parameters. Therefore any atom with a high B-factor should be regarded as being a possible source of error (Fig. 6).

The fit of the model's residues to the electron density can be estimated by using "real-space" parameters such as the $R_{residue}$ factor (48) or a linear correlation coefficient, CC. The $R_{residue}$ parameter is more often employed because it is not so dependent upon the strength of the electron density (49).

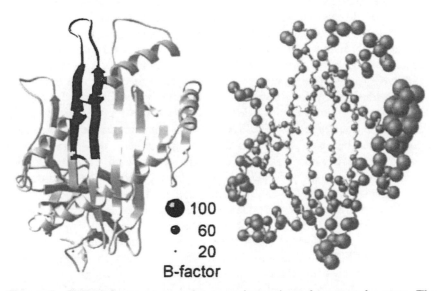

Figure 6 High B-factors may point to regions where there may be error. The structure of the H-2DD MHC Class I protein (PDB code 1bii) is shown on the left. On the right, the backbone of the structure is shown, with each residue studded with a sphere whose size is related to the magnitude of the residue's B-factor. It can be seen that the short, solvent-exposed alpha-helix has particularly high B-factors compared with the rest of the structure.

However, these methods are not sensitive to subtle errors in the model (i.e., errors of less than 2Å rmsd) (50). Zhou and Mowbray (51) have derived a "real-space" correlation coefficient function, R_{ED}, that gives a sensitive measure of the match between local areas of the model and the electron density. This method is able to detect some errors at the atomic level, which makes this approach, in conjunction with other measures of accuracy such as the indirect B-factor, very powerful. But the authors note that even if such a combined approach is used, 30–40% of errors are likely to be missed. However, with the use of other error detection methods in conjunction with this approach, such as the stereochemical indicators discussed later, this value is likely to be significantly smaller.

Another set of methods that measure the local fit of the model to the electron density are provided by the software package SFCHECK (52). SFCHECK takes the predicted atomic coordinates of the protein structure model and the structure–factor amplitudes. In addition to calculating a number of global accuracy measures, such as the R-factor, it also calculates five parameters that evaluate the local agreement between the electron density map and the model.

A normalized average displacement value is calculated that gives a measure of the tendency of the atom or atoms concerned to move away from their predicted positions in the model, given the local electron density. This therefore measures the likelihood that the atom or atoms will be inaccurately placed in the model. SFCHECK also calculates a number of values that give an indication of where errors may exist in the protein model. An electron density map for a given group of atoms is calculated and compared with the experimental electron density, giving a relative measure of where the electron density is low. The average B-factor per residue is also calculated. From this it is possible to deduce regions of a well-refined model where there are high B-factors associated with high electron density, which might imply the possibility of error in the model. The continuity of electron density along the chain in the electron density map is also evaluated. Discontinuities along the chain suggest regions of low electron density or where registration errors may have occurred.

Given a PDB-format file of the protein structure model, the program WHATCHECK (14) is able to detect a number of X-ray-specific errors. Peptide bond flips are detected by comparing the backbone geometry in the model with a database of backbone geometries from a set of high-resolution structures. If most of the database geometries are different from the model's geometry, it may indicate that the peptide plane needs to be flipped.

WHATCHECK also checks the orientation of asparagine, histadine, and glutamine residues using a hydrogen bond force field (53) and predicts the protonation states of histadine residues.

Crystal contacts can distort protein conformations and lead to some conformational differences due to different crystal environments. These differences were evaluated by looking at the differences between CAD values (28) (see Sec. 5.7) and backbone rmsd (see Sec. 5.2) for 27 pairs of structures related by noncrystallographic symmetry. It was found that the average CAD error is approximately 5% (28).

In terms of avoiding the creation of many of the errors already mentioned, we recommend that one places a large emphasis upon both the visual inspection of data and the refinement stage of the modeling procedure. The more refinement that takes place, the fewer local errors there are likely to be in the final model. We also advocate the use of the latest methods available—a method from 10 years ago is less likely to perform as well as one that has been available for only one or two years.

4.4.2 Detection of NMR Model Errors

The errors in NMR structure determination come from false-positive NOEs, false-negative NOEs, ambiguous assignments, and the transformation from an NOE intensity to an interatomic distance. Also, large-scale topological deformation artifacts may result from the local and relative nature of experimental information, in contrast to the absolute atom locations in crystallography.

As discussed earlier, the binning of distance restraints based upon NOE data can lead to a significant source of error. The cumulative effect of under- and overestimated distance restraints can mean atoms are pulled into inaccurate conformations in the predicted structure. Programs such as XPLOR (54) and CNS (55) have facilities to perform the back-calculation of the NOE pattern from the protein model. Differences in this pattern compared with the experimental NOE spectrum can then allow one to pinpoint regions of the molecule that are not accurately satisfying the experimental data. The reassignment of the affected NOEs or rebinning of the restraints concerned can then be performed, the protein structure recalculated, and the NOE back-calculation reperformed to deduce what effect the changes have made upon the accuracy of the protein structure model.

An equivalent measure to the X-ray R-factor value has been defined in a number of ways for NMR models that allows for a comparison of simulated and experimental NOE patterns. One of the most sensitive measures has been developed by Gronwald et al. (56). Their RFAC program calculates an R-factor based upon such patterns but also includes within the analysis NOE experimental peaks that are not assigned to any atom in the protein. A further key feature of this program is its ability to peak pick and integrate the experimental spectrum automatically.

A common measure of model accuracy used in the publication of NMR protein structure models is to quote the number of violated distance restraints and dihedral angle restraints (derived from J-coupling data). Standard structure calculation scripts used in XPLOR (54) and CNS (55) output such violations for each model in an ensemble or family of models. AQUA (37) goes a step further by analyzing the whole ensemble of models for violations. The results can then be interfaced with PROCHECK-NMR (37) (see later for more about this program) to provide a graphical representation of where there are consistent violations—a good indication of regions that are being inaccurately predicted.

A lack of NOEs, and therefore distance restraints, for a particular region of a protein structure, particularly on the surface of the protein, inevitably leads to conformational heterogeneity within the family of models that this prediction method produces. It is common practice to analyze the number of restraints assigned to each residue in the molecule, allowing one to predict regions of the molecule that are relatively underrestrained, and therefore possibly inaccurate, due either to conformational dynamics or to experimental error. These regions can then be further analyzed using NMR relaxation data in the form of the "model-free" method (57,58). This method provides an estimate of the dynamic character of each residue in terms of its motional restriction (the generalized order parameter, S^2) and an estimate of the internal correlation time of the motion. Such an analysis is not trivial, and it is uncommon for the model-free parameters to be accurately predicted for each residue. However, this approach allows one to deduce if a region of a model is likely to be inaccurate due to conformational dynamics or is an artifact of the experimental procedure.

The lack of long-range restraints inevitably leads to a lack of long-range order, which can lead local regions of a model to be inaccurate relative to regions further away. Recently new techniques have been developed to introduce long-range information based upon how the molecule tumbles in the liquid crystal phase (59,60). The protein sample is placed in two different low-concentration solutions of bicelles (typically 5–7.5%), sometimes doped with a charged group (for example, Ref. 61). Using high-field NMR spectrometers it is possible to measure residual dipolar couplings as a consequence of the protein molecules' being trapped between the bicelles and their rotation becoming slightly anisotropic. These data can then be exploited through an additional pseudo-potential in the structure calculation, which restrains internuclear vectors with respect to an external alignment tensor axis frame. The use of this external frame of reference makes all restrained vectors interdependent, leading to the introduction of long-range information. A similar technique can be used to incorporate the information from the T_1 and T_2 relaxation times of ^{15}N nuclei in axially symmetrical molecules (62). The addition of both of these additional restraints into a structure calculation is not trivial, since a number of parameters, which are very sensitive to one another, have to be optimized in the calculation procedure. Indeed, almost all reports of the use of these restraints have used only one of the two types of restraints rather than both. However, it has been shown that although the rmsd of the NOE restraints increases, suggesting an increased deviation of the structure from the NOE restraints, the rmsd of the ensemble of models decreases (for example, Ref. 63). This implies that the precision of the models improves, reducing the magnitude of local errors in the models.

The problem of atom packing in NMR protein structural models has been addressed by Kuszewski et al. (29), who have proposed the use of an additional pseudo-energy potential in the structure calculation procedure that attempts to restrain the radius of gyration (R_{gyr}) of a specified subset of atoms in a molecule to a supplied value. There are a number of issues that one must be aware of when using this potential. First, unless one has an optimal R_{gyr} derived from small-angle X-ray scattering data, one must rely on an empirical relationship that relates the optimal R_{gyr} to the number of atoms considered (64). Second, as Kuszewski et al. indicate, it is very important that the atom selection restrained by this potential be overall globular in nature. Unstructured regions on the surface of the protein may not be locally globular in nature, so restraining these along with more globular core atoms will result in the collapse of these unstructured regions, which may be inaccurate. Third, if the protein to be modeled is made up of more than one domain or exhibits subdomains that may not be entirely dynamically coupled, care should be taken that these are restrained separately. This is possible in the implementation of this potential in the program CNS (55). The authors of this work show that for a number of different globular proteins, imposition of such a restraint improves the fit of the resulting models with models of the same proteins derived from X-ray crystallographic data.

Similar to our comments about avoidance of errors in NMR models, we recommend that as much refinement of the model be performed as possible, since this will eliminate a significant number of local problems in the structure. Again, we also advocate that those methods that have been made available most recently be used. Also, it is important that older force-field parameterizations are avoided, since newer versions have many improvements and errors removed (for example, Ref. 65).

4.4.3 Prediction of Homology Model Errors

In a previous section we described the main sources of model errors inherent in homology models. Here we will talk about ways to detect and possibly avoid those errors.

Template Recognition. Typically models are built only from sequences that have significant similarity to known structures. Therefore, the recognition process is not normally a source of error. However, in the case where there is more than one template available, how does one choose between structures of varying sequence similarity to the target sequence, number of sequence insertions/deletions, differing resolution, or determination method, to minimize the degree of error in the resulting model? Useful criteria, in order of preference are:

1. Smallest number of local insertions/deletions (ideally none)
2. Local sequence identity
3. X-ray crystallographic model preferable to an NMR or theoretical model
4. Greatest overall resolution
5. Smallest number of local errors

Instead of trying to reconcile this list for a single template, one may instead create a chaemeric template incorporating fragments of several identified templates that, together, satisfy the criteria better (8).

If no suitable template is easily found, one should resort to sensitive remote-similarity methods, such as ICM ZEGA (see Fig. 7 for an example script) and the hidden Markov model (HMM) methods (e.g., Ref. 66). However, the quality of the alignment is bound to be low, so the only hope for reducing model error is to build local fragments that have higher local similarity.

Minimizing Alignment Errors. Simplistically, a model is as good as the alignment. It is important to be aware that the sequence alignments that might be produced in the template recognition search are unlikely to accurately reflect the actual structural alignment of the target and template sequences, especially if the sequence identity is less than 40% (31,67). As such, the (multiple) sequence alignment used to map the template features onto the target structure should be recreated from scratch, placing particular emphasis on achieving an accurate structural alignment. Useful characteristics to enhance the sequence alignment include secondary structure, surface accessibility, and functional residues.

The choice of scoring matrix and gap function plays an important role in the creation of the template/target sequence alignment. It is important to realize that parameters that are optimal for the template search are not necessarily optimal for a structurally accurate sequence alignment. To achieve the best alignments it is useful to experiment with different gap penalty values and multiple sequence alignments.

```
# Specify ZEGA method
alignMethod="ZEGA"
# Load in target sequence (in FASTA format)
read sequence "target.seq" name="target"
# Find possible templates in PDB
find database "pdb" target
# Read in the hits
read sequence "pdb.seq"
# Group all sequences...
group sequence str_align
# ... in order to perform a tentative multiple sequence
# alignment
align str_align
# Show the alignment
str_align
# Write the alignment to the file "str_align.all" so that we
# can alter it by hand
write alignment str_align
quit
```

Figure 7 ICM script for finding remote structural homologs in the PDB using the ZEGA method.

Figure 8 shows an example of a poor alignment between target and template sequences. Particular care needs to be taken around parts of the alignment where there are insertions or deletions relative to the target sequence. In addition, a good structural alignment should properly pair residues involved in secondary structural elements. Sequences that form beta-strands that are misaligned by a one-residue shift will result in side chains that point in the opposite direction, resulting in a significant change in packing in the target structure. Misalignments of alpha-helices will also result in the same type of error. Gaps in the sequences within secondary structural elements also should be avoided.

It is important that the resulting sequence alignment be checked and even altered by hand to attain an optimal structural alignment. The local ZEGA pP profile (31,67) may be used to determine if an alteration within the alignment may be considered to give an improvement in terms of the structural accuracy of the alignment. However, the ultimate criterion of how the accuracy of the alignment has changed is the close examination of the model structure itself, since an analysis of the model will be more accurate than analysis of the alignment. Here, errors, such as the secondary structure element misalignments just mentioned, will be obvious in comparison with the template structures. It is often useful to repeatedly model the structure,

Sequence Alignment

```
3bto        ...RLDTMVTALSCCQEAYGVSVIVGVPPDSQNLSMNPMLLLSGRTW_____KG...
1ykf        ...NADIMATAVKIVKPG_____GTIANVNYFGEGEVLPVPRLEWGCGMAHK...
2ary 3bto   _HHHHHHHHHHB_____EEEE_____GHHHH___EE_____EE
2ary 1ykf   _GGHHHHHHHB_____EEEE_____GGG____
```

Structural Alignment

```
3bto        ...RLDTMVTALSCCQEAYGVSVIVGVPRDSQNLSMNPMLL___LSGRTWK...
1ykf        ...NADIMATAVKIVK_PGGTIANVNYFGEGEVLPVPRLEWGCGMAHKTIK...
2ary 3bto   _HHHHHHHHHHB_____EEEE_____GHHH___H___EEE
2ary 1ykf   _GGHHHHHHHB_____EEEE_____GGG____EEE
```

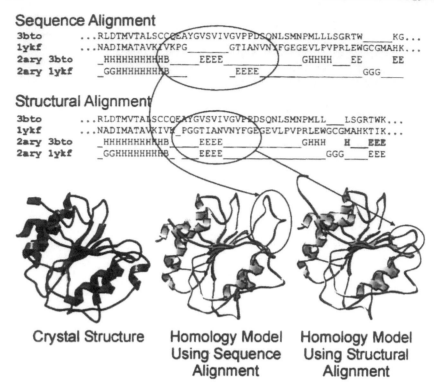

Crystal Structure   Homology Model   Homology Model
                       Using Sequence   Using Structural
                       Alignment   Alignment

Figure 8 Example of the effects of misalignment of target/template sequences. Here it can be seen that the misalignment of part of the 1ykf sequence to the template sequence of 3bto leads to the incorrect modeling of a loop.

analyze the model, and then make changes to the alignment based upon the analysis. It should be noted that it is often possible to have more than one structural alignment that can be considered correct (68,69).

Once an acceptable alignment has been created, the prediction of the target structure can take place. There are a number of approaches to predicting a protein structure by homology modeling, such as the use of spatial restraints derived from the alignment in conjunction with geometric restraints (e.g., the program MODELLER (11)); the assembly of rigid-body segments; the reconstruction of small lengths of peptide based upon a database of structural preferences. The most error-prone part of homology modeling is the modeling of insertions where there is no, or little, structural information from template structures. Currently, there are no methods available that are able to accurately predict a preferred conformation of such a segment if the number of residues is greater than 5 (70,71).

Though the methods described so far in this section attempt to detect where errors occur, the method of Cardozo et al. (72) takes a different approach. They took a benchmark set of sequence–structure alignments and derived scoring functions that predict whether the local backbone of the target model might be expected to deviate from the template structure. These functions are made up of a linear combination of a number of measures of local characteristics of the template structure and target sequences. These include: the distance to the closest insertion; the sequence distance to the closest linear gap (not including N- and C-terminal gaps); the local deviation of the packing density from the packing density of the whole template structure; the B-factors of the local region of the template structure; the angle between the first and last three residues in a local region; the difference between the region's accessible surface area and the mean accessible surface area of the ungapped parts of the template structure; the local multiple sequence alignment score; and the "contact sequence alignment" score (CSA), which is the ZEGA score of a pseudo-alignment of residues whose atoms are within 2.5 Å of any atom in the region of the template with the equivalent residues in the target sequence. Therefore, given a target sequence, template structure(s), target model structure, and multiple sequence alignment, this method provides the basis for the annotation of the backbone of the model structure.

Since this method does not detect the existence of errors in the model but predicts local regions where backbone deformations might be expected, it can be used to pinpoint regions where particular attention needs to be taken during the error detection and resolution procedures.

In order to avoid the forms of local errors we have discussed, we believe that it is essential that more research be made into techniques better than those currently available. Loop-modeling methods are especially important in this regard. Also, longer simulations during the final modeling procedure can only help in the removal of local errors.

5 MEASURES TO COMPARE A MODEL WITH A "TRUE" STRUCTURE

First, given a protein structure prediction method and a structure of a protein that is to be taken as a "standard of truth," how does one assess the success of the prediction method at predicting the structure of the protein? This is a problem not just for those who work on finding new and improved methods of protein structure prediction, but also for those who need to assess available methods. Second, there are normal structure variations and alterations, e.g., alternative loop conformations, or domain rearrangements, which need to be measured. In those situations, measures to compare two conformations and identify the differences are necessary. The Critical Assessment of Structure Prediction (CASP) experiments (73–75) provide a good benchmark for the evaluation of the current state of theoretical structure prediction and have utilized a variety of geometrical error measures (2,71,76,77).

Here we describe nine different measures of structural differences between two models of the same molecule. If one model is taken as a standard of truth and the other is a generated model, these measures will quantify the geometrical errors. Historically, rmsd was the most commonly used measure, even though it is really applicable only in a limited number of situations. Each measure has its optimal application domain.

5.1   All-Heavy-Atom Coordinate rmsd

This number is calculated upon optimal superposition of the equivalent set of heavy atoms. Analytical algorithms for the identification of the rotation and translation, which optimizes the root mean square deviation of a fixed set of equivalent atom Cartesian coordinates, were derived by McLachlan (78) and Kabsch (79). Each contributing pair of atoms can be weighted. The resulting rmsd is calculated as follows:

$$\text{rmsd} = \sqrt{\frac{\sum_{i=1}^{n} d_i^2}{n}}$$

where d_i is the distance between two equivalent heavy atoms, i, and there are n equivalent atoms.

A nontrivial but critical part of the rmsd calculation is to take residue symmetries into account. For example, a phenylalanine side chain has a twofold symmetry, which leads chemically identical atoms with different names to occupy the same space. This concerns the following residues (equivalent atoms are given in parentheses): tyrosine (Cδ, Cϵ); phenylalanine (Cδ, Cϵ; valine (Cγ1, Cγ2); leucine (Cδ1, Cδ2); arginine (NH1, NH2); aspartate (Oδ1, Oδ2); glutamate (Oϵ1, Oϵ2). To find the correct rmsd, one must swap the indices of specified atoms 1 and 2 and choose a resulting configuration with lower rmsd.

The rmsd works reasonably well if there is no plastic deformation of the overall structure and all the individual atomic deviations are of the same order of magnitude. Otherwise, the rmsd value will be dominated by the largest deviation in a frequently unimportant region (e.g., a surface lysine side chain) and will not be interpretable.

To address the problem of plastic deformations or domain rearrangements, some methods attempt to identify a subset of aligned pairs that produce the best rmsd after superposition. For example, Lackner et al.

(80) recently have devised a method (ProSup) able to accurately superimpose structures that are remotely related in terms of structure while allowing the quality of a number of structural fits to be ranked purely on the basis of the number of aligned residue pairs. A filter is also used on aligned residue pairs whose side chains are incompatible (e.g., in beta-strands that are misaligned by one residue). ProSup supplies a range of possible structural alignments, which may be useful in the derivation of new, empirically based error detection methods. ProSup was applied to the results of CASP3 (81).

5.2 Backbone and Cα Coordinate rmsd

This measure also relies on a global static superposition of all the equivalent atoms at the same time. The backbone conformation is a more structurally conservative feature than the side chains. Therefore, measuring the rmsd of the backbone is a better indicator of significant structural deformations. However, the foregoing limitations concerning the relative domain shifts and plastic deformations still apply. In addition, movements of large flexible loops will create a problem with the backbone rmsd, which is equivalent, in essence, to the long side-chain deviations that plague heavy-atom rmsd, i.e., the loop deviation will dominate the overall backbone rmsd.

Both backbone and all-heavy-atom measures are global in nature and do not discriminate between evenly and unevenly distributed deformations. Secondly, in the case of an uneven distribution of the deformation, it does not tell us where the deformation occurs. Analysis of the individual contributions to the total rmsd resolves the problem.

5.3 Local (Fragment) Coordinate rmsd

The main limitation of the previous two measures is their reliance on a global superposition of all equivalent atoms. However, frequently this superposition does not make sense, e.g., in a multidomain protein where the constituent domains shift with respect to each other without changing their internal structure. Superimposing only a protein fragment, e.g., 10–25 residues, before calculating the local rmsd partially resolves this problem. The choice of the window size will depend upon the scale of the structural changes of interest. The net result of this calculation is an array of deviation values that can be mapped onto the protein backbone.

5.4 Fraction-Correct Measure Based on Local rmsd Profile

Predictions of larger proteins frequently lead to a mosaic pattern of correct and completely wrong topologies. The best way to characterize the overall quality of such a model is to define what fraction of the topology is correct. To do that, we need to postulate a threshold for the local rmsd value. If a cutoff value is applied to the error profile calculated by the fragment rmsd calculation just described, one can then easily calculate the ratio of the residues below the threshold.

5.5   Angular rmsd

The previous calculations were based on optimal superposition of equivalent pairs of atoms followed by the measurement of the deviations of absolute Cartesian positions of atoms. However, the use of the internal coordinates, such as torsion angles of the backbone and side chains, avoids the need for structural superposition and is free from the effects of plastic deformations. For example, the backbone angular rmsd is calculated as:

$$\text{rmsd} = \sqrt{\frac{\sum_{i=1}^{n}(\Delta\phi_i^2 + \Delta\psi_i^2)}{n}}$$

where n is the number of equivalent residues, $\Delta\phi_i$ is the difference between the phi angles of the equivalent pair of residues, i, and $\Delta\psi_i$ is the difference between the psi angles of the same equivalent pair of residues.

A similar approach can be applied to the internal coordinates describing secondary structure topology (82).

5.6   Distance rmsd

Interatomic distances are the third way—and probably the most physical in nature—to characterize protein conformation. Therefore, analyzing changes of those distances leads us to the distance rmsd measure. A straightforward measure relying on interatomic distances is the all-atom distance rmsd. However, the large distances are not as significant in terms of local error and can be filtered out. Contact maps and contact map differences can be derived to evaluate the conformational changes and errors. A matrix with all Cα–Cα distances is calculated for each of the two structures. Then the two matrices can be compared and the difference contact map derived. A single number can also be derived to characterize the deviation.

5.7   Contact-Area Difference

Contact-area difference (CAD) (28) is a normalized sum of absolute differences of residue–residue contact surface areas calculated between the model and the "true" structure. Since this approach reflects not only backbone topology but also side-chain packing, and is smooth, continuous, threshold free, and not affected by plastic deformation, it can be successfully used to detect differences between two structures that backbone rmsd is sometimes unable to discover. And CAD can also be used with a fixed window length to create a profile showing local regions of a model that are significantly different compared to the "true" structure.

5.8 Static rmsd

In both global and local rmsd, the *same* set of atoms is used for super-position and calculation of the deviations. However, some applications, e.g., measuring loop errors or peptide placement errors or position of a small domain with respect to a larger domain, call for a different calculation. In this case the superposition is first performed over the atoms that are different from those in the area where an error or deviation is expected. Then the rmsd is calculated only over the atoms of interest. This measure is called static rmsd, for lack of a better name.

5.9 Relative Displacement Error

The relative displacement error is a measure that can be used to evaluate the accuracy of a loops that can be partially correct. In this case, the local profile is calculated with a static rmsd procedure, threshold (similar to the fraction-correct method earlier) is defined, and the number of correctly predicted loop residues is calculated.

6 OUTLOOK

The move toward more automated and higher-throughput methods of pro-tein structure prediction and experimental determination provides new chal-lenges to the protein modeler. On these large scales of data throughput, it is not possible to carefully hand-inspect each stage of the structure determina-tion of each protein. This lack of "quality-control" will inevitably lead to less accurate models than those models that are hand-determined by a per-son with an experienced eye.

The current lack of consistent error annotation for all generated or predicted models is akin to the lack of expiration dates on food product-s—you might end up drinking milk that is far past its best, with nasty consequences! Similarly, a model should be labeled similar to: "Protein structure health warning: the use of fragments 10–24 and 152–200 is hazar-dous for your predictions and may lead to a sudden lack of employment!"

Therefore it is becoming increasingly important that new methods for error detection and prediction be created that can automatically annotate model structures, giving an indication of the local reliability of the model.

Better statistics on erroneous structures, new, and more accurate, force fields, better global optimization algorithms, and combination approaches will lead to a better, more useful models.

ACKNOWLEDGEMENTS

We would like to thank Maxim Totrov, Sergei Batalov, and Wen Hwa Lee for interesting discussions and help in the preparation of this chapter. We would like to thank Molsoft LLC for providing the ICM package with which most figures in this chapter were generated. Finally we would like to thank the NIH, DOE, and the Wellcome Trust for their financial support.

REFERENCES

1. Ferentz, A.E. and G. Wagner. NMR spectroscopy: a multifaceted approach to macromolecular structure. Q Rev Biophys 33(1):29–65, 2000.
2. Jones, T.A. and G.J. Kleywegt. CASP3 comparative modeling evaluation. Proteins 37(S3):30–46, 1999.
3. Brünger, A.T., P.D. Adams, and L.M. Rice. Recent developments for the efficient crystallographic refinement of macromolecular structures. Curr Opin Struct Biol 8(5):606–11, 1998.
4. Adams, P.D. and R.W. Grosse-Kunstleve. Recent developments in software for the automation of crystallographic macromolecular structure determination. Curr Opin Struct Biol 10(5):564–568, 2000.
5. Stevens, R.C. High-throughput protein crystallization. Curr Opin Struct Biol 10(5):558–563, 2000.
6. Xu, Y., J. Wu, D. Gorenstein, and W. Braun. Automated 2D NOESY assignment and structure calculation of Crambin(S22/I25) with the self-correcting distance geometry-based NOAH/DIAMOD programs. J Magn Reson 136(1):76–85, 1999.
7. Mumenthaler, C., P. Guntert, W. Braun, and K. Wuthrich. Automated combined assignment of NOESY spectra and three-dimensional protein structure determination. J Biomol NMR 10(4):351–362, 1997.
8. Abagyan, R., S. Batalov, T. Cardozo, M. Totrov, J. Webber, and Y. Zhou. Homology modeling with internal coordinate mechanics: deformation zone mapping and improvements of models via conformational search. Proteins Suppl(1):29–37, 1997.
9. Cardozo, T., M. Totrov, and R. Abagyan. Homology modeling by the ICM method. Proteins 23(3):403–414, 1995.
10. Guex, N. and M.C. Peitsch. SWISS-MODEL and the Swiss-PdbViewer: an environment for comparative protein modeling. Electrophoresis 18(15):2714–2723, 1997.
11. Sali, A. and T.L. Blundell. Comparative protein modeling by satisfaction of spatial restraints. J Mol Biol 234(3):779–815, 1993.

12. Sanchez, R. and A. Sali. Large-scale protein structure modeling of the *Saccharomyces cerevisiae* genome. Proc Natl Acad Sci USA, 95(23):13597–13602, 1998.
13. Berman, H.M., T.N. Bhat, P.E. Bourne, Z. Feng, G. Gilliland, H. Weissig, and J. Westbrook. The Protein Data Bank and the challenge of structural genomics. Nat Struct Biol 7 Suppl:957–959, 2000.
14. Hooft, R.W., G. Vriend, C. Sander, and E.E. Abola. Errors in protein structures. Nature 381(6580):272, 1996.
15. Howell, P.L., S.C. Almo, M.R. Parsons, J. Hajdu, and G.A. Petsko. Structure determination of turkey egg-white lysozyme using Laue diffraction data. Acta Crystallogr B 48(Pt 2):200–207, 1992.
16. Novotny, J., R. Bruccoleri, and M. Karplus. An analysis of incorrectly folded protein models. Implications for structure predictions. J Mol Biol 177(4):787–818, 1984.
17. Novotny, J., A.A. Rashin, and R.E. Bruccoleri. Criteria that discriminate between native proteins and incorrectly folded models. Proteins 4(1):19–30, 1988.
18. Kocher, J.P., M.J. Rooman, and S.J. Wodak. Factors influencing the ability of knowledge-based potentials to identify native sequence-structure matches. J Mol Biol 235(5):1598–1613, 1994.
19. Jones, D.T. and J.M. Thornton. Potential energy functions for threading. Curr Opin Struct Biol 6(2):210–216, 1996.
20. Bryant, S.H. and S.F. Altschul. Statistics of sequence–structure threading. Curr Opin Struct Biol 5(2):236–244, 1995.
21. Wodak, S.J. and M.J. Rooman. Factors influencing the ability of knowledge-based potentials to identify native sequence-structure matches. Curr. Opin. Struct. Biol. 3:247–259, 1993.
22. Sippl, M.J. Recognition of errors in three-dimensional structures of proteins. Proteins, 17(4):355–362, 1993.
23. Wuthrich, K. NMR of Proteins and Nucleic Acids. New York: Wiley, 1986.
24. Jones, T.A., J.Y. Zou, S.W. Cowan, and Kjeldgaard. Improved methods for binding protein models in electron density maps and the location of errors in these models. Acta Crystallogr A 47(Pt 2):110–119, 1991.
25. Kleywegt, G.J. Validation of protein crystal structures. Acta Crystallogr D Biol Crystallogr 56(Pt 3):249–265, 2000.
26. Kleywegt, G.J. Validation of protein models from C-alpha coordinates alone. J Mol Biol, 273(2):371–386, 1997.
27. Ratnaparkhi, G.S., S. Ramachandran, J.B. Udgaonkar, and R. Varadarajan. Discrepancies between the NMR and X-ray structures of uncomplexed barstar: analysis suggests that packing densities of protein structures determined by NMR are unreliable. Biochemistry 37(19):6958–6966, 1998.
28. Abagyan, R.A. and M.M. Totrov. Contact area difference (CAD): a robust measure to evaluate accuracy of protein models. J Mol Biol 268(3):678–685, 1997.

29. Kuszewski, J., A.M. Gronenborn, and G.M. Clore. Improving the packing and accuracy of NMR structures with a pseudopotential for the radius of gyration. J Am Chem Soc 121(10):2337–2338, 1999.

30. Gronenborn, A.M. and G.M. Clore. Structures of protein complexes by multidimensional heteronuclear magnetic resonance spectroscopy. Crit Rev Biochem Molec Biol 30(5):351–385, 1997.

31. Rost, B. Twilight zone of protein sequence alignments. Protein Eng 12(2):85–94, 1999.

32. Chothia, C. and A.M. Lesk. The relation between the divergence of sequence and structure in proteins. Embo J 5(4):823–826, 1986.

33. Network, E.-D.V. Who checks the checkers? Four validation tools applied to eight atomic resolution structures. EU 3-D Validation Network. J Mol Biol 276(2):417–436, 1998.

34. Guntert, P., C. Mumenthaler, and K. Wuthrich. Torsion angle dynamics for NMR structure calculation with the new program DYANA. J Mol Biol 273(1):283–298., 1997.

35. Engh, R.A. and R. Huber. Accurate bond and angle parameters for X-ray protein structure refinement. Acta Cryst A47:400–404, 1991.

36. Pontius, J., J. Richelle, and S.J. Wodak. Deviations from standard atomic volumes as a quality measure for protein crystal structures. J Mol Biol 264(1):121–136, 1996.

37. Laskowski, R.A., J.A. Rullmannn, M.W. MacArthur, R. Kaptein, and J.M. Thornton. AQUA and PROCHECK-NMR: programs for checking the quality of protein structures solved by NMR. J Biomol NMR, 8(4):477–486, 1996.

38. Colovos, C. and T.O. Yeates. Verification of protein structures: patterns of nonbonded atomic interactions. Protein Sci 2(9):1511–1519, 1993.

39. Luthy, R., J.U. Bowie, and D. Eisenberg. Assessment of protein models with three-dimensional profiles. Nature 356(6364):83–85, 1992.

40. Eisenberg, D., R. Luthy, and J.U. Bowie. VERIFY3D: assessment of protein models with three-dimensional profiles. Methods Enzymol 277:396–404, 1997.

41. Sippl, M.J. Calculation of conformational ensembles from potentials of mean force. An approach to the knowledge-based prediction of local structures in globular proteins. J Mol Biol 213(4):859–883, 1990.

42. Melo, F. and E. Feytmans. Assessing protein structures with a nonlocal atomic interaction energy. J Mol Biol 277(5):1141-1152, 1998.

43. Ben-Naim, A. Statistical potentials extracted from protein structures: are these meaningful potentials? J. Chem. Phys. 107(9):3698–3706, 1997.

44. Miwa, J.M., I. Ibanez-Tallon, G.W. Crabtree, R. Sanchez, A. Sali, L.W. Role, and N. Heintz. lynx1, an endogenous toxin-like modulator of nicotinic acetylcholine receptors in the mammalian CNS. Neuron 23(1):105–114, 1999.

45. Maiorov, V. and R. Abagyan. Energy strain in three-dimensional protein structures. Fold Des 3(4):259–269, 1998.

46. Abagyan, R. and M. Totrov. Biased probability Monte Carlo conformational searches and electrostatic calculations for peptides and proteins. J Mol Biol 235(3):983–1002, 1994.

47. Abagyan, R.A., M. Totrov, and D. Kuznetsov. ICM—A new method for protein modeling and design: applications to docking and structure predicition from the distorted native conformation. J. Comp. Chem. 15(5):488–506, 1993.

48. Branden, C.I. and T.A. Jones. Between objectivity and subjectivity. Nature 343(6260):687–689, 1990.

49. Read, R.J. Improved Fourier coefficients for maps using phases from partial structures with errors. Acta Cryst. A42:140–149, 1986.

50. Jones, T.A., J.-Y. Zou, C.S. W., and K. M. Improved methods for building protein models in electron density maps and the location of errors in these models. Acta Cryst. A47:110–119, 1991.

51. Zhou, J. and S.L. Mowbray. An evaluation of the use of databases in protein structure refinement. Acta Cryst. D50:237–249, 1993.

52. Vaguine, A.A., J. Richelle, and S.J. Wodak. *SFCHECK*: a unified set of procedures for evaluating the quality of macromolecular structure–factor data and their agreement with the atomic model. Acta Cryst D55:191–205, 1999.

53. Hooft, R.W., C. Sander, and G. Vriend. Positioning hydrogen atoms by optimizing hydrogen-bond networks in protein structures. Proteins 26(4):363–376, 1996.

54. Brünger, A.T. XPLOR Version 3.1. A system for X-ray Crystallography and NMR. New Haven, CT: Yale University Press, 1992.

55. Brünger, A.T., P.D. Adams, G.M. Clore, W.L. DeLano, P. Gros, R.W. Grosse-Kunstleve, J.-S. Jiang, J. Kuszewski, M. Nilges, N.S. Pannu, R.J. Read, L.M. Rice, S. T., and W.G. L. Crystallography NMR system: a new software suite for macromolecular structure determination. Acta Cryst. D54:922–937, 1998.

56. Gronwald, W., R. Kirchhofer, A. Gorler, W. Kremer, B. Ganslmeier, K.P. Neidig, and H.R. Kalbitzer. RFAC, a program for automated NMR R-factor estimation. J Biomol NMR 17(2):137–151, 2000.

57. Lipari, G. and A. Szabo. Model-Free approach to the interpretation of nuclear magnetic resonance relaxation in macromoloecule. 2. Analysis of experimental results. J Am Chem Soc 104(17):45590-4570, 1982.

58. Lipari, G. and A. Szabo. Model-free approach to the interpretation of nuclear magnetic resonance relaxation in macromoloecule. 1. Theory and range of validity. J Am Chem Soc, 104(17):4546–4559, 1982.

59. Tjandra, N. and A. Bax. Direct measurement of distances and angles in bio-molecules by NMR in a dilute liquid crystalline medium. Science 278(5340):1111–1114, 1997.

60. Tjandra, N., J.G. Omichinski, A.M. Gronenborn, G.M. Clore, and A. Bax. Use of dipolar 1H-15N and 1H-13C couplings in the structure determination of magnetically oriented macromolecules in solution. Nat Struct Biol 4(9):732–738, 1997.

61. Zweckstetter, M. and A. Bax. Predicition of sterically induced alignment in a dilute liquid crystalline phase: aid to protein structure determination by NMR. J Am Chem Soc 122:3791–3792, 2000.

62. Tjandra, N., D.S. Garrett, A.M. Gronenborn, A. Bax, and G.M. Clore. Defining long range order in NMR structure determination from the dependence of heteronuclear relaxation times on rotational diffusion anisotropy. Nat Struct Biol 4(6):443–449, 1997.

63. Schwalbe, H., S.B. Grimshaw, A. Spencer, M. Buck, J. Boyd, C.M. Dobson, C. Redfield, and L.J. Smith. A refined solution structure of hen lysozyme determined using residual dipolar coupling data. Protein Sci 10(4):677–688, 2001.

64. Skolnick, J., A. Kolinski, and A.R. Ortiz. MONSSTER: a method for folding globular proteins with a small number of distance restraints. J Mol Biol 265(2):217–241, 1997.

65. Linge, J.P. and M. Nilges. Influence of nonbonded parameters on the quality of NMR structures: a new force field for NMR structure calculation. J Biomolec NMR 13(1):51–59, 1999.

66. Bateman, A., E. Birney, R. Durbin, S.R. Eddy, R.D. Finn, and E.L. Sonnhammer. Pfam 3.1: 1313 multiple alignments and profile HMMs match the majority of proteins. Nucleic Acids Res 27(1):260–262, 1999.

67. Abagyan, R.A. and S. Batalov. Do aligned sequences share the same fold? J Mol Biol 273(1):355–368, 1997.

68. Feng, Z.K. and M.J. Sippl. Optimum superimposition of protein structures: ambiguities and implications. Fold Des 1(2):123–132, 1996.

69. Godzik, A. The structural alignment between two proteins: is there a unique answer? Protein Sci, 5(7):1325–1338, 1996.

70. Fiser, A., R.K. Do, and A. Sali. Modeling of loops in protein structures. Protein Sci 9(9):1753–1773., 2000.

71. Martin, A.C., M.W. MacArthur, and J.M. Thornton. Assessment of comparative modeling in CASP2. Proteins Suppl(1):14–28, 1997.

72. Cardozo, T., S. Batalov, and R.A. Abagyan. Estimating local backbone structural deviation in homology models. Computers Chemistry 24:13–31, 2000.

73. Moult, J., J.T. Pedersen, R. Judson, and K. Fidelis. A large-scale experiment to assess protein structure prediction methods. Proteins 23(3):ii–v., 1995.

74. Moult, J., T. Hubbard, S.H. Bryant, K. Fidelis, and J.T. Pedersen. Critical assessment of methods of protein structure prediction (CASP): round II. Proteins Suppl(1):2–6, 1997.

75. Moult, J., T. Hubbard, K. Fidelis, and J.T. Pedersen. Critical assessment of methods of protein structure prediction (CASP): round III. Proteins Suppl(3):2–6, 1999.

76. Mosimann, S., R. Meleshko, and M.N. James. A critical assessment of comparative molecular modeling of tertiary structures of proteins. Proteins 23(3):301–317, 1995.

77. Venclovas, C., A. Zemla, K. Fidelis, and J. Moult. Criteria for evaluating protein structures derived from comparative modeling. Proteins Suppl(1):7–13., 1997.

78. McLachlan, A.D. Gene duplications in the structural evolution of chymotrypsin. J.Mol. Biol. 128:49–79, 1979.

79. Kabsch, W. A solution for the best rotation to relate two sets of vectors. Acta Cryst. A32:922, 1976.

80. Lackner, P., W.A. Koppensteiner, M.J. Sippl, and F.S. Domingues. ProSup: a refined tool for protein structure alignment. Protein Eng 13(11):745–752, 2000.

81. Lackner, P., W.A. Koppensteiner, F.S. Domingues, and M.J. Sippl. Automated large-scale evaluation of protein structure predictions. Proteins 37(S3):7–14, 1999.

82. Abagyan, R.A. and V.N. Maiorov. An automatic search for similar spatial arrangements of alpha-helices and beta-strands in globular proteins. J Biomolec Strut Design 6(6):1045–1060, 1989.

11

Comparative Analysis and Evolutionary Classification of Protein Structures

Liisa Holm
University of Helsinki, Helsinki, Finland

1 INTRODUCTION

Nothing in biology makes sense except in the light of evolution.
— T. Dobzhansky (1)

This chapter describes concepts and algorithms of the Dali (distance matrix alignment) method. Specific problems addressed are structural alignment and domain decomposition, culminating in the automated detection of remote homology. In each case, the computational problem conceptually boils down to determining the optimal size and number of clusters by optimizing a cost function, a general approach with applications in many partition problems and related to ideas of information theory. Our key thesis is that the *economy of description*—the objective of the clustering—reflects an underlying *economy of conception* in molecular evolution and thereby yields biologically relevant results.

In the era of high-throughput and genome-scale studies, categorizing and correlating the huge amounts of new information with what is already known is an important task. Structural genomics studies, for example, generate new protein structures so quickly that the biochemical and functional characterization can lag behind. You can hypothesize about the function of these proteins on the basis of their structures by examining their similarities

315

and potential evolutionary relationships with other, well-characterized proteins. Classifying a new protein in a superfamily is important for focusing experiments on its most likely functions. Such classification, often performed by hand, has now been fully automated based on the methods described here. Correct functional and evolutionary classification of a new structure is difficult for distantly related proteins and error-prone using simple statistical scores based on sequence or structure similarity. The sophisticated new approach takes into account not only alignment scores but also a number of other computable attributes, such as functional sites deduced from sequence conservation patterns. This automated approach should be useful in providing functional hypotheses that can be tested experimentally.

2   STRUCTURE ALIGNMENT

Structure alignment is an optimization problem that requires the transformation of intuitive notions of structural similarity into objective quantities, with suitable choices of parameters. Meaningful distance measures, in our view, are difficult to construct in this context, because extensive structural decorations are supported outside the common core. An extreme example of structural decorations is the superfamily that includes glycogen phosphorylase and T4 beta-glucosyltransferase. The latter is a protein of ~ 340 residues, and its structure is completely embedded in that of glycogen phosphorylase, which has evolved to a size of over 800 residues by the insertion of long loops and subdomains (Fig. 1). Many measures of structural similarity are in use, often based on intermolecular distances upon rigid-body superimposition (2–7). In a 3D comparison, one explicitly rotates and translates one molecule relative to the other and measures intermolecular distances between equivalent points in the two chains. The objective is to find the rigid-body superimposition (translation and rotation of one molecule relative to another) such that it accommodates the largest possible number of equivalent points within small deviations, typically less than 2–3 Å.

The Dali method is based on a sensitive measure of geometrical similarities defined as a weighted sum of similarities of intramolecular distances (8). Three-dimensional shape is described with a matrix of all intramolecular distances between the C-alpha atoms. Such a distance matrix is independent of coordinate frame but contains more than enough information to reconstruct the 3D coordinates, except for overall chirality, by distance geometry methods. Imagine sliding one (transparent) distance matrix on top of another. Depending on the register of the two matrices, similar substructures will stand out as submatrices with similar patterns (Fig. 2).

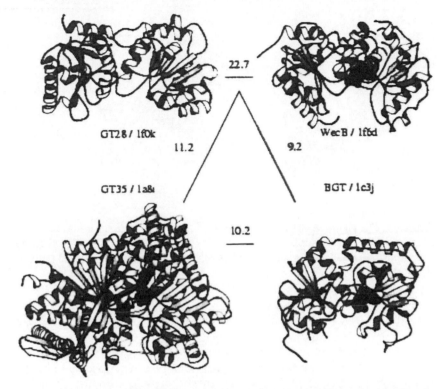

Figure 1 Structural divergence within a glucosyltransferase superfamily that includes glycogen phosphorylase (lower left) and T4 beta-glucosyltransferase (lower right). Edge weights are Dali Z-scores. The structures have been superimposed and translated apart.

Structurally equivalent regions can be filtered out with a fixed cutoff on acceptable differences of intramolecular distances or, as we prefer, with a continuous function defined in terms of relative distance deviations. The common structure is revealed when two distance matrices are brought into register by keeping only rows or columns corresponding to the structurally equivalent residues.

The geometrical score S is defined as a sum over all pairs of residues i, j in the common structural core of proteins A, B:

$$S(A, B) = \sum \sum (\theta - \Delta(d_{ij}^A, d_{ij}^B))\omega(d_{ij}^A, d_{ij}^B) \tag{1}$$

where Δ is the deviation of intramolecular C-alpha to C-alpha distances between (i^A, j^A) and (i^B, j^B) relative to their arithmetic mean d, θ is the threshold of similarity, set empirically to 0.2 (20%), the envelope function

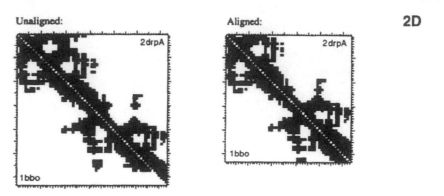

Figure 2 The common structural core of two zinc finger structures that both contain two domains is revealed by removing rows and columns from the full C-alpha–C-alpha distance matrices on the left side so that only structurally aligned pairs are left on the right side.

$\omega = \exp(-d^2/r^2)$, where $r = 20$ Å, downweights contributions from distant pairs.

Dali's weighted sum of intramolecular distance difference matrices captures the strong conservation of functionally constrained motifs, e.g., in the surroundings of an active site, but at the same time it allows for structural deviations between more distant parts of the molecules. For example, Dali aligns different TIM barrel structures over 200 residues corresponding to the $(\beta/\alpha)_8$ core. This is despite variable ellipticity of the barrel cross sections that leads to high root mean square distance deviations in rigid-body 3D superimposition. The one-dimensional alignment of amino acid strings of remote homologs deriving from the structural alignment reveals conserved functional residues (Fig. 3).

The statistical significance of the comparison score for two proteins can be assessed with empirical criteria (calibrated on a large number of known examples). The mean and standard deviations of Dali similarity scores were calibrated against pairwise all-on-all comparisons in a database 220 proteins as a function of protein size. Shape similarity quantified with the distance matrix comparison scores can then be expressed in terms of normalized Z-scores, that is, standard deviations above the mean (9). The relationship between mean score m and size $L = (L^A L^B)^{1/2}$ is closely approximated by the polynomial

$$m(L) = 7.95 + 0.71L - 2.59e^{-4}L^2 - 1.92e^{-6}L^3, \qquad L \leq 400 \qquad (2)$$

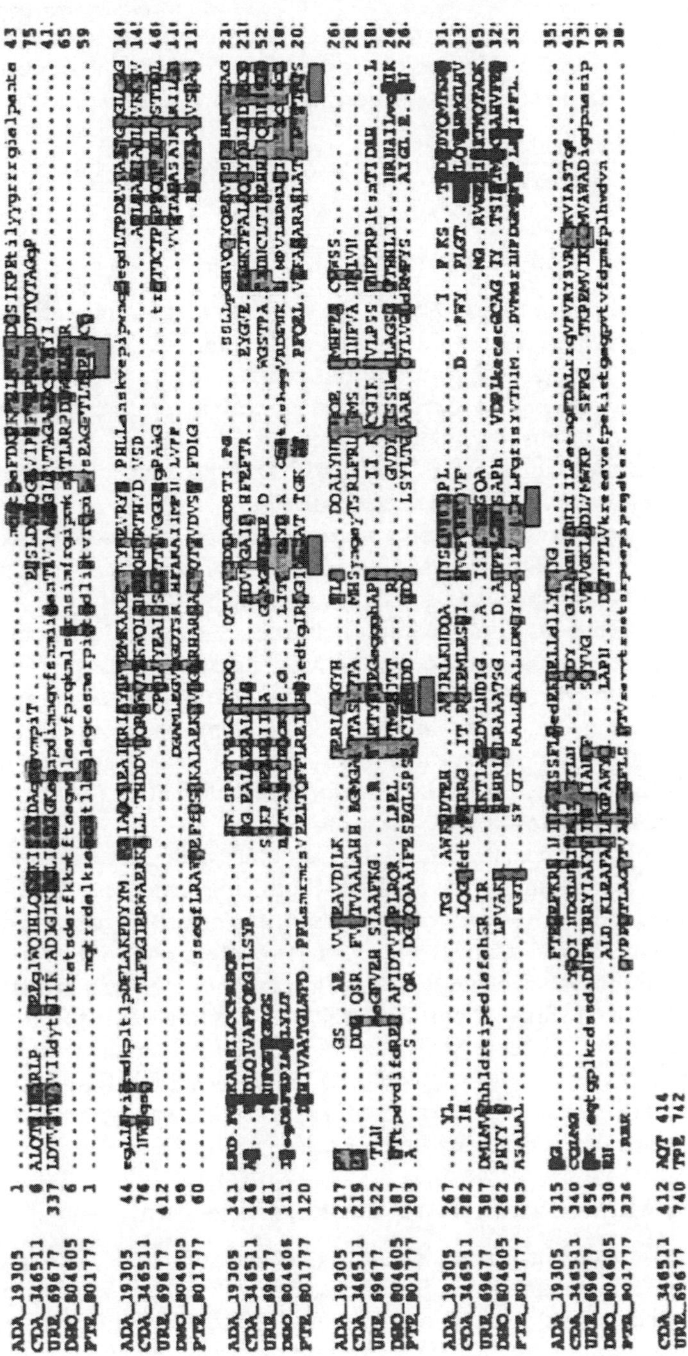

Figure 3 Structural alignment of a diverse hydrolase superfamily that includes adenosine deaminase (ADA), cytosine deaminase (CDA), urease (URE), dihydroorotase (DHO), and phosphotriesterase (PTE). Active site residues are underlined. The lysine conserved in URE, DHO, and PTE is carbamoylated and involved in binuclear sites, but the lysine is not conserved in ADA and CDA, which are mononuclear. (Based on Ref. 42.)

Above $L = 400$, $m(L)$ is extrapolated using a linear increment over $m(400)$ because there were too few data points for calibration. Using a smoothed estimate of the average standard deviation, the Z-score is defined as

$$Z(A, B) = \frac{S(A, B) - m(L)}{0.50m(L)} \tag{3}$$

2.1 Searching Three-Dimensional Databases

Many algorithms have been adapted to the problem of geometrical shape comparison of proteins, including branch-and-bound algorithms, brute force systematic searches, subgraph isomorphism algorithms, stochastic optimization by Monte Carlo or simulated annealing protocols, genetic algorithms, look-up or hashing methods, dynamic programming, and clustering. For most practical purposes, the algorithmic problem of 3D shape comparison of proteins can be considered solved.

Whatever the measure and search variables, the search landscape contains very many local optima due to the recurrence of secondary structure elements (helices and strands) and small tertiary structural motifs, i.e., associations of two, three, or four helices or strands. However, in practical applications it is not necessary to locate the absolute optimum of the objective function in each pair comparison. This is because one is usually interested in only those matches that involve a large common folding pattern that makes up an entire structural domain. In particular, for a protein structure used as a query, researchers want to see all matches that score above some similarity threshold.

Our strategy for efficient searches in the database of 3D structures is first to scan for obvious similarities using fast (but, in general, less accurate) procedures and then to rescan for more subtle similarities using more sophisticated (but slower) algorithms. Next, two algorithms based on a concise representation of protein structure in terms of secondary structure elements are described. These algorithms deliver a starting point for a final optimization of the Dali score [Eq. (1)] by Monte Carlo refinement (8), which removes any restrictions on gaps and extends the alignment to loops. Sequential ordering of the aligned segments is required as a constraint. This constraint is motivated esthetically.

2.2 Greedy Three-Dimensional Lookup Algorithm

The 3D lookup is a fast heuristic algorithm that catches easy-to-find structural similarities and is part of the Dali 3D search server (10). In principle, the search for the optimal translation-rotation operators is a problem with six degrees of freedom. Our fast 3D lookup circumvents this complication by making an educated guess for the optimal superimposition. The guess is based on the observation that an optimal superimposition in terms of residue centers (C-alpha atoms) typically produces a close spatial coincidence of secondary structural element (SSE) vectors in the two proteins. Due to the way in which amino acid mutations are accommodated in protein structure, the positions and directions of the SSEs can indeed be better conserved than the position of the residue centers that define them. Turning this around, superimposing a subset of such well-matching SSEs is sufficient to *approximately* regenerate the desired rigid-body transformation of the entire structures. In other words, the idea is to recover the whole from a comparison of the essential parts.

The key procedural step is to compare the spatial arrangements of SSEs in two proteins by superimposing appropriate internal coordinate frames, one for each protein. We define such internal coordinate frames in terms of the axis of one leading SSE and the direction to a second SSE (centering one SSE at the origin, aligning it with the y-axis, and rotating the molecule around this axis so that the center of a second SSE is in the positive xy-plane). It is not known beforehand which frame to select in either protein. Fortunately, the number of possible coordinate frames is small enough to allow exhaustive testing of all frames for one structure against all frames for the other structure. For larger proteins, we limit this number by excluding coordinate frames generated by pairs of SSEs that have a mutual center-to-center distance larger than 12 Å.

The lookup step consists of counting, for each coordinate frame of the query protein, how many SSEs match (within specific tolerance) in each database protein and in which coordinate frame. The preorientation defined by the maximal SSE match is then used as the starting point for an iterative extension of a residue-wise alignment (Fig. 4). This iterative procedure is similar to dynamic programming used in pairwise sequence alignment except that the scores for residue pairings are derived from their intermolecular distance in the current superimposition. After each iteration, the superimposition of the structures is recomputed to minimize the least squares distance of equivalent residues from the previous alignment.

The algorithm described here is meant to be fast, if not complete. Although the present method will not find all neighbors of a query structure in the database, it saves time in the identification of easy-to-find hits. The search of one structure against the structure database of several thousand structures typically takes only about 5 min on a computer workstation Other simplified methods achieve similar speed. In this way, a large portion (about 90%) of all significant protein–protein shape similarities can be found. If a strong hit is found, then the database search using more sensitive

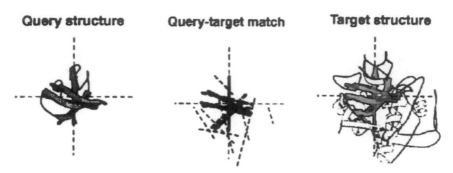

Query structure   **Query-target match**   **Target structure**

Figure 4   3D lookup algorithm identifies an SH3-like domain in papain (target structure). Bars denote vector representation of secondary structure elements. The common elements are shaded in the ribbon representation.

but slower search methods can be restricted to this structural neighborhood (known from previous exhaustive comparison of all proteins in the database). This strategy of using multiple algorithmic approaches to the structure comparison problem makes sure that nothing is missed while the overall procedure becomes much more efficient.

2.3   Divide-and-Conquer Algorithm

The general problem of finding the global best alignment of two protein traces with respect to a sum-of-pairs objective function has the complexity of an NP-hard problem. Algorithmic solutions must either settle for an approximate solution or risk sifting through an exponentially large search space (approximately N^M possible alignments of a sequence of N residues onto a structure consisting of M segments of protein trace). To solve this problem to a reasonable approximation, we have adapted the elegant branch-and-bound algorithm by Lathrop and Smith (11) that was originally developed for sequence–structure alignment (to optimally fit the sequence of protein A into the structure of protein B). The complexity of the structure alignment problem is much reduced by considering only nongapped segment pairs. A natural segmentation uses the secondary structure elements of the query structure (12). Our adaptation of the branch-and-bound procedure replaces the sequence of protein A by the trace of residue centers of protein A and thus tests all ways of placing ungapped segments of protein A at strategically chosen positions in the structure of protein B (at the beginning of all secondary structure segments, for example).

Figure 5 illustrates the algorithmic principle. Rather than sifting through each possible combination of segment pairings explicitly, the branch-and-bound algorithm estimates an upper bound on the score in a

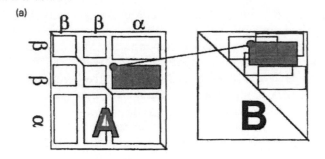

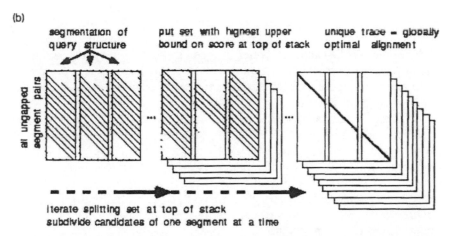

Figure 5 Branch-and-bound search. (a) The algorithm tests all possible placements of ungapped segments from protein B onto strategic positions in structure A (such as the beginning of secondary structure elements). (b) Diagonal lines represent non-gapped segment pairings between segments of the query structure (horizontal) and the protein being aligned to it (vertical). The divide-and-conquer strategy is guaranteed to find the globally optimal solution.

pool of possible candidate pairings and iteratively splits alignment search space into ever smaller subsets of candidate pairings. The objective function (Dali score) evaluates not only interactions within segments but also interactions between segments. For example, if the query structure consists of segments 1–3, the score is the sum of involving distance submatrices $(1,1)$, $(1,2)$, $(1,3)$, $(2,1)$, $(2,2)$, $(2,3)$, $(1,2)$, $(2,3)$, and $(3,3)$ in the distance matrix of the query structure and their counterparts in the distance matrix of the aligned structure (Fig. 5a). The upper bound on the sum of pairs is the sum of the maximal value of each term in the sum within the subset of candidate pairings under consideration. Eventually, the subset with the highest bound contains only a unique solution, the optimal alignments (Fig. 5b). As a result, most placements of residues in protein A onto segments in protein B are pruned before they are examined explicitly. For example, comparing the structures of transducin-alpha [Protein Data Bank code 1tag, 16 segments] with that of Ras p21 [5p21, 166 residues] leads to a nominal search of 10^{35} spatial arrangements, although the best solution is found after only 11 s on a fast computer workstation.

A few approximations have been introduced to reduce the combinatorial complexity of the search and to increase speed. If the search landscape is so flat that 10,000 splittings of the search space have not resulted in a unique solution, the 90% of lowest scoring subsets are discarded. Segments of protein A may be truncated from either end or both ends or deleted entirely as they are placed onto secondary structures in protein B. Continuing the branch-and-bound procedure past the global optimum yields suboptimal solutions in monotonically decreasing order. In our implementation, suboptimal alignments cannot reuse residue pairs used in any higher-scoring alignment.

A significant match between two proteins is very likely to contain significant matches between well-chosen substructures. We steer the search toward matches of compact substructures (described in Sec. 3.1) using a hierarchical build-up procedure. The pairwise comparison of two structures first applies the branch-and-bound algorithm to the nodes of a tree of compact folding units of the query structure. All segment pairings from alignments that scored above a threshold are pooled when moving up the hierarchical tree of folding units.

2.4   Generating Multiple Structure Alignments

The T-Coffee program (13) is used to generate multiple alignments such that the placement of residues in columns is maximally supported by the underlying library of pairwise alignments. The pairwise alignment library is the result of Dali structure comparisons. A reliability score is computed to indicate well-defined regions (the structural core) and regions where structural equivalences are ambiguous (e.g., loops of different length and different conformations). Technically, T-Coffee improves alignment quality in a few known cases of functional families where active site residues were inconsistently aligned in some pairwise Dali comparisons. Scientifically, the definition of functional families and reliable multiple structure alignments opens the door to sensitive sequence database searches using position-specific profiles and benchmarking the accuracy of threading predictions.

2.5 Availability

The database search methodology containing the foregoing algorithms, plus other tools, is made available over the Internet to users with a coordinate data set describing a 3D protein structure in hand. The Dali server (http://www.embl-ebi.ac.uk/dali) is routinely used to compare newly solved structures against those in the Protein Data Bank, to compare ab initio predicted structures to the real structure (e.g., CASP), and to maintain the Dali Domain Dictionary classification of protein folds (14). A stand-alone program package, DaliLite, is available for academic researchers to compare large numbers of structures for specialized projects efficiently and locally (15).

3 DELINEATING DOMAINS IN THREE-DIMENSIONAL STRUCTURES

Structural similarities within the set of proteins with unique sequences are typically restricted to only parts of the protein structure. Similar substructures, with relatively sharp boundaries, may recur between several proteins; conversely, many proteins can be economically described as combinations of recurrent substructures (domains). The notion of such economical description is related to that of minimal encoding in information theory and, in this context, refers to the intuitive goal of defining a small set of large substructures in terms of which most protein structures can be described. In one attempt to achieve this goal, we have combined the notions of compactness and recurrence of domains. A *compact* domain has minimal surface and maximal interior residue–residue contacts. A *recurrent* domain is one that appears several times as a recognizably similar substructure in different proteins (Fig. 6). This leads to an operational definition of substructures that makes use (1) of a physical decomposition of protein structure into a tree of putative folding units at all size levels and (2) of the property that normalized distance matrix similarity scores are strongest for complete overlap of large units. Given a database of protein shapes, pairwise structural similarities, and alternative decompositions into substructures, the notion of maximal recurrence is implemented by selection of a set of substructures for which the sum of similarities is maximized across the database.

3.1 Compactness

Many ingenious techniques have been invented for locating structural domains in 3D structures, including but not limited to: inspection of distance maps, clustering, neighborhood correlation, plane cutting, minimization of interface area, maximization of buried surface area, minimization of

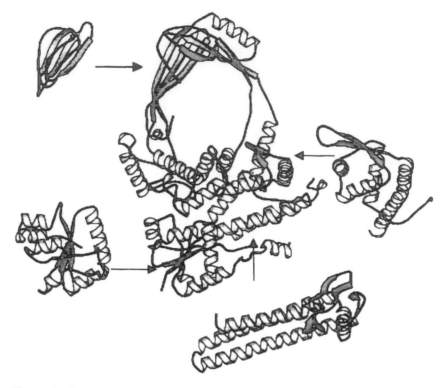

Figure 6 Recurrent domains in topoisomerase (1ecl). The structural neighbors are shown alongside the matching domains. The middle DNA-binding domain with a winged-HTH fold is duplicated in topoisomerase.

specific volume, maximization of compactness, and searching for mechanical hinge points (9,16–22).

Common to most approaches are the assumptions that folding units are compact and that the interactions between them are weak. These notions can be made quantitative, for example, by counting interactomic contacts and by locating domain borders by a (binary) partition into groups such that the number of contacts between groups is minimized. In a harmonic approximation model (23), protein unfolding begins with the separation of two compact domains D_1 and D_2. Domains D_1 and D_2 interact via non-bonded atomic interactions at their interface I_{12}, and their relative motion is governed by the strength of the interface and the distribution of masses. The most likely domain separation involves units for which the time constant of relative motion (τ) is largest. τ squared is proportional to $[N_1 N_2/(N_1 + N_2)]/I_{12}$, where $N_{1,2}$ are the numbers of nonhydrogen atoms 343 in domains $D_{1,2}$ and I_{12} is the number of atomic contacts across the interface. A putative order of folding (or unfolding) events can be inferred starting from the complete structure and recursively cutting it (in silico) into smaller and smaller substructures (16). Alternatively, one may start from the residues or secondary structure element level and successively associate the most strongly interacting groups. These procedures involve two optimization problems.

The first optimization problem is algorithmic and concerns finding the optimal subdivisions. This problem is complicated by the possibility that the polypeptide chain may pass several times from one domain to another. In other words, the domain is composed of discontinuous segments along the polypeptide chain. Without the constraint of sequential continuity, there is a combinatorial number of possibilities for dividing a set of residues into subsets. This hurdle has been overcome by fast heuristics (16,20,22).

The second optimization problem is concerned with the definition of termination criteria for recursive algorithms. Can we pinpoint physical criteria that distinguish between autonomous and nonautonomous folding units? It has proven difficult to formulate such criteria, because most physical measures related to compactness do not have a clear biomodal distribution. For this reason, most domain assignment algorithms (16–19,21,24) use empirical cutoff parameters that have been fine-tuned against an external reference set of domain definitions.

3.2 Recurrence

It seems natural to assume that domain boundaries should be conserved in evolution between closely and even more distantly related members of a protein family or superfamily. However, compactness algorithms that are used to analyze a protein coordinate set in isolation may produce different results for homologs or even for different conformers of the same protein. Concerns for consistency in the context of large-scale structural classifications have led to a reformulation of the domain assignment problem. Consequently, the goals have moved away from (imprecise) physical models of stable folding units and toward recognizing such units phenomenologically in the database of known structures through recurrence. The concept of recurrence has long been the cornerstone of domain assignments by experts who recognize domains by visual inspection (25). In computational terms, the key ingredients of the optimization problem are a gain associated with reusing a previously declared substructure and a cost associated with using many different substructures as building blocks to describe a protein. An analogy can be found in the writing of a scholarly text. It is cheap to copy blocks of text from earlier scholarly works, but it takes some thought and effort to glue many fragments together in a fluent narrative.

With a suitably defined cost function, recurrence can be used to select an optimal set of substructures from the folding or unfolding trees generated by compactness criteria. Thus, the unsatisfactorily solved problem of defining termination criteria for compactness algorithms can be turned into an optimization problem that does not rely on any external reference and leads to an internally consistent set of domain definitions. The key difficulty in this approach is in quantifying the notion of *economy* so that it leads to a selection of substructures of "appropriate" size, that is, globular folds and not, for example, supersecondary structural motifs. One cost function, which is physical nonsense but has the desired qualitative behaviour, is defined as the sum of the Dali Z-scores over all pairwise domain–domain comparisons, where domains are the selected units from the unfolding tree of proteins in a representative set of protein structures (9). This cost function quantifies recurrence in terms of the statistical significance of structural similarity for all pairs of candidate domains in a representative database. The statistical significance is highest for structural similarities that (1) involve large units and (2) completely cover a substructure unit that has been chosen as a candidate domain. Exploiting these effects, the sum-of-pairs objective function favors recurrences of large substructures with distinct topological arrangement and packing of secondary structure elements (high Z-scores) and disfavors small substructures consisting of one or two secondary structure elements (very low Z-scores) despite their higher frequency of recurrence.

Though other formulations of the optimization problem are possible, this empirically chosen objective function combined with a simple greedy algorithm for optimization delivers a useful set of domain definitions without human intervention (9).

4   A MAP OF FOLD SPACE

As more and more protein structures are determined experimentally, automation of the comparison and classification process becomes indispensable. Which basis set represents fold space? Conceptually, each protein structure may be imagined as a point in an abstract, high-dimensional fold space where the coordinates of a query protein are determined by its structural similarity with a representative set of structures. Multivariate scaling methods can now be used to illustrate the overall distribution of domains. At long range, the overall distribution of folds is dominated by five densely populated regions, which we call *attractors* (Fig. 7). At intermediate range, clusters are related by shape similarity that does not necessarily reflect similarity of biological function (for example, globins and colicin A). At close

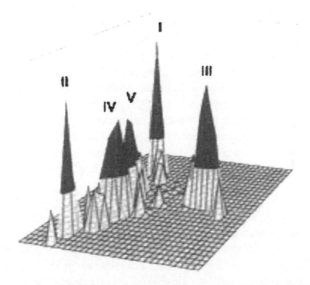

Figure 7 Density distribution of domains in fold space according to Dali. Quantification of the pairwise structural similarities in an all-on-all comparison of protein structures allows one to position each structure relative to the others in an abstract, high-dimensional fold space (shape space). The height of the peaks reflects population density (of folds in fold space). The horizontal axes are the two dominant eigenvalues, and the vertical axis represents the number of protein shapes per unit area (logarithmic scale, arbitrary units). The long-range distribution of different architectures is revealed in a projection down onto the plane based on multivariate scaling, so proximity in the plot corresponds to correlated structural neighborhoods. See text for explanation of roman numerals.

range in this fold space, clusters represent protein families related through strong functional constraints (for example, hemoglobin and myoglobin).

The five dominant peaks in the distribution of domains in the 2D projection of shape space contain domains with similar secondary structure composition and characteristic topological motifs (secondary structure elements plus loop connections). The five attractor regions correspond to remarkably simple pathways of collapsing α-helix and β-strand elements into globular proteins. In the folded structures, the shared motifs are not exposed to solvent, so they are likely to form early on in the folding process and may represent nucleation sites. All folds with sheets of mainly parallel β-strands map to attractor I. The parallel β folds contain a β-x-β unit, where the intervening segment (x) is required to reverse chain direction so that the strands are parallel. The β-α-β unit has a preferred handedness determined by polymer physics and the natural twist of β-strands. Attractor II contains a variety of helical folds. The connectivity of elements in the folds of attractors III and IV contains meander motifs suggestive of the collapse of a long hairpin, either of β-strands only or of β-strands alternating with a helical pair $(\beta\text{-}\alpha\text{-}\beta)_2$. The β-zigzag motif of attractor V is simply a series of antiparallel hairpin connections between sequentially adjacent strands. Elementary polymer physics indicates that interactions in space between regions of the chain that are close in sequence are much more probable than those between sequence-distant regions. The β-zigzag motif occurs in both flat sheets and barrels, and there is considerable variation in the length of strands (about four residues in propeller blades, about 13 in porin barrels).

A partition at the next level of granularity leads to an operational definition of fold type. Fold types are defined as clusters of structural neighbors in fold space with average pairwise Dali Z-scores above 2. The threshold has been chosen empirically and groups together structures that have topological similarity. Higher Z-scores correspond to structures that agree more closely in architectural detail (Fig. 8). The population of fold types is highly skewed (Fig. 9). Forty percent of all known domains (protein substructures) are covered by 16 fold classes. Although each fold class has individual features, most fold classes map to five attractor regions (peaks I through V).

5   DELINEATING THE BOUNDARIES OF SUPERFAMILIES

Domains are classified in the same superfamily if there is compelling evidence of a common ancestor. This evidence is often based on features like the conservation of unusual structural features, clusters of conserved residues (giving especially sharp signatures in enzyme active sites), sequence similarity through bridging intermediates (leading to elongated clusters in protein space (26)), or functional similarities (conserved molecular protocols). The deciding factors can be quite subtle, and this is why evolutionary classification has traditionally been subjective. Indeed, some consider this field impossible or inappropriate to address using numerical methods. Undaunted, a number of research groups have developed numerical criteria to make evolutionary and functional classification objective.

The goal is to derive, or invent, scoring functions that discriminate homologous from unhomologous pairs with minimal overlap. A key difficulty is that the boundary between apparent homologs and analogs (unhomologous or convergent folds) corresponds to a very broad range of values in sequence similarity, structural similarity, and functional similarity in different protein families. It seems difficult to find feature sets for classifiers that would have a low error rate together with high coverage (27–31). For

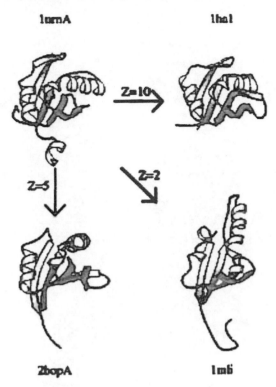

Figure 8 Structural neighbors of 1urnA (top left). 1 mli (bottom right) has the same topology even though there are shifts in the relative orientation of secondary structure elements.

example, whereas fold types could be defined using a uniform cutoff in structural similarity (Dali Z-scores), a vertical cut through the structural similarity dendrogram is a poor classifier when it comes to discriminating homologous proteins from unhomologous ones (Fig. 10). How to interpret this disappointing result? The structural similarity tree is derived using a measure for the statistical significance of observing the same 3D arrangement of structural elements (across many length scales). The larger the protein, the larger is the space of possible configurations and hence the smaller the probability of the same configuration of a large number of elements. Thus, there is a built-in size factor in the structural similarity score so that large domains get much higher Z-scores than small and less compact ones. On the other hand, different superfamilies may have genuinely different rates of structural divergence.

Does this make the Dali measure of structural similarity useless in evolutionary classification? Far from it. We just have to examine the situa-

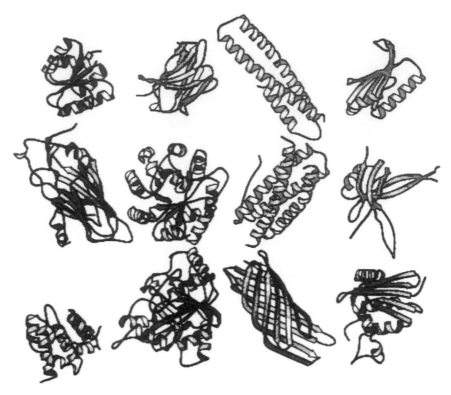

Figure 9 Top 12 fold types with the largest number of superfamilies in the Dali classification ("superfolds").

tion from the perspective of an underlying evolutionary model (Fig. 11). The key observation is that the topology (branching pattern) of the structural similarity tree gives a good representation of evolutionary relationships. The members of a superfamily (as defined in Ref. 32) tend to occupy monophyletic branches of the structural similarity tree. This means that we can limit possible partitions of protein space into superfamilies to branches of the structural similarity tree. But in order to be able to partition the tree, we need to complement structure similarity with additional measures of functional similarity (similar to the way in which 2D gel electrophoresis is better at separating the contents of a cell by using two different criteria, i.e., the isoelectric point and molecular weight). We describe functional similarity by so-called feature vectors, which measure properties such as sequence identity of the structural alignment, conserved residues in contact with ligands, and annotation keyword similarity. A neural network integrates scores based on these disparate data. The neural network was trained to recognize homo-

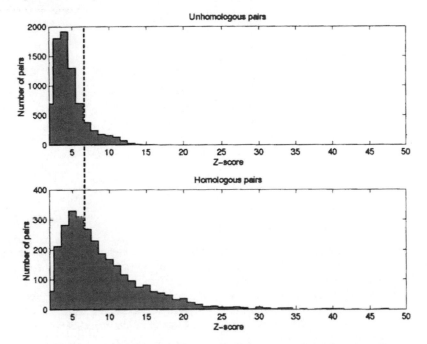

Figure 10 The standard assessment method in remote homolog detection uses a manual classification (SCOP) as a reference of "truth." A good scoring function discriminates between homologous and unhomologous pairs. The dotted line represents a threshold value in the scoring function. Here, the Z-score of Dali is used. False positives are unhomologous test examples to the right of the threshold line, at the top. False negatives are homologous test examples to the left of the threshold line, on the bottom. Coverage is defined as the fraction of homologous test examples that are on the right side of the threshold line, on the bottom.

logous proteins and to discriminate them from analogs and presents a single numerical value per protein pair. The partition procedure locates the optimal boundary between folds and superfamilies based on the intra- and intercluster functional similarities. This has the advantage that missing data for particular pairs can be compensated for by strong similarities between enclosing neighbors in the tree.

The result is a new method (33) that identified 77% of homologous pairs with 92% reliability in jackknife validation against the SCOP database (Fig. 12). This is an almost twofold increase over other automated classifiers. Coverage is limited mostly by disagreement with SCOP's fold definitions and to a smaller extent by unknown functional attributes. Interestingly, functional annotations in databases were found to be often redundant with strong sequence motifs. This means that the method should

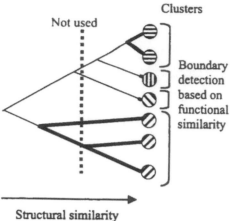

Figure 11 The topology of a structural similarity tree is highly informative about evolutionary relationships. A universal threshold in the structural similarity score (indicated by the dotted vertical line) is not meaningful, because the radius (structural divergence) of families varies over a wide range, depending on their functional constraints. The tree can be partitioned into clusters of homologs using other kinds of information, such as functional attributes. In this example, there seem to be four clusters with distinct patterns.

be useful in the classification of structures of hypothetical proteins and in providing first-pass functional hypotheses that can be tested experimentally. Inspection indicates the lack of evidence (undefined functional features) as a limiting factor. New information may support further mergers of superfamilies in the future. It will also be technically straightforward to add more functional attributes to the feature vectors. In particular, data from functional genomics provide new ways of quantifying functional similarity, e.g., in terms of the similarity of transcriptional profiles of two genes in a large number of experimental conditions.

5.1 Neural Network Classifier for Homology

The boundaries of superfamilies in the fold dendrogram are identified based on functional similarity. A neural network was trained against the fold to superfamily transition in SCOP, using the different functional attributes listed in Table 1 as input. The output of the neural network ranges from zero (analogous pairs) to 1 (homologous pairs) and is defined as our measure of functional similarity, ϕ. Though many homologous pairs are more functionally similar than most analogous pairs, the distributions of functional similarity (ϕ) values of homologs and analogs are broad and overlap.

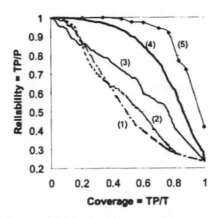

Figure 12 Jackknife evaluation of the accuracy of remote homolog detection. The prediction accuracy is summarized by coverage and reliability. The tested examples are rank-ordered according to the neural network output, with the strongest predictions at the top. The training set consisted of 11,907 unrelated pairs (same SCOP fold but different superfamily) and 3,635 related pairs (same SCOP superfamily) from a representative set of single-domain PDB structures. $N = 15,542$ training runs were made, each using $(N - 1)$ examples for training and testing the example left out. Let us consider the P (positive) highest-scoring examples. In this set, reliability is defined as TP/P, where TP (true positive) is the number of positive examples that are correctly identified as related, and coverage is defined as TP/T, where T (true) is the number of related pairs in the whole test set. P varies from 1 to N along each curve. A perfect classifier would rank all true pairs above the first false pair, driving the curve to the top-right corner of the graph. Ranking by (1) sequence identity alone; (2) structure similarity alone; (3) keyword similarity alone; (4) neural network output; (5) correspondence to optimal partitions obtained at different values of θ in upcoming Eq. (4), i.e., using the context in the fold dendrogram as a noise filter on neural network predictions.

The feature vector inputs are derived from structural conservation, sequence conservation, and sequence annotation, exploiting sequence alignments and structure superimposition to transfer position-specific information from sequence homologs to the query structures. "Keyword similarity" is the dot product of vectors representing the frequency of occurrence of Swissprot keywords in sequence homologs of either query structure. Noninformative keywords such as "3D-structure" are excluded. "Functional preference" is defined per amino acid type and is summed over all residues in a 3D cluster of conserved residues (Table 2). Feature computation is described at depth in Ref. 33.

The Dali Z-score, functional preference, and keyword similarity are open scales of similarity and were linearly rescaled to zero mean and a

Table 1 Feature Vector for the (2pth, 1cfzA) Pair

Feature	Evidence	Value
Z-score	Dali structural alignment	10.2
Sequence identity	Dali structural alignment	14%
Sequence family overlap	No common Blast sequence neighbors	"no"
Identical conserved residues in contact with ligand	No ligand information for 2pth	"unknown"
Functional preference	2pth N10 and 1cfzA N10 are structurally equivalent, conserved and in spatial proximity	0.38
Keyword similarity	2pth: 1/13 "sporulation", 12/13 "hydrolase"; 1cfzA: 12/12 "protease", 12/12 "hydrolase"	0.93
Common E.C. numbers	2pth: E.C.3.1.1.29, 1cfzA: E.C.3.4.–.–	1
Overlap of annotated sites	2pth G100D is a temperature-sensitive mutation and structurally equivalent to 1cfzA G72; both residues are conserved	"yes"

Table 2 Functional Preference of
Amino Acid Types

Amino acid	Functional preference
H	0.367
C	0.204
S	0.129
K	0.095
T	0.093
N	0.076
R	0.052
E	0.050
Q	0.047
D	0.039
A	0.018
M	0.015
I	−0.010
Y	−0.042
V	−0.068
G	−0.075
F	−0.115
W	−0.147
L	−0.189
P	−0.199

standard deviation of 1. The problem of missing values in specific components of the input vectors is severe in our case. For example, the similarity of enzyme classification codes is a strong feature, but it is defined for only 20% of the pair examples in the training set. There are various heuristics in the literature for dealing with missing data in classification problems. We filled the missing values for the enzyme classification codes with the mean value for all known pairs. Similarly, ligand information is unavailable or incomplete for many structures in the PDB. The feature "identical conserved residues in contact with a ligand" was therefore encoded as "yes," "no," or "unknown."

Layered feed-forward neural networks were optimized by a backpropagation algorithm (34–37). Networks of widely different architectures were tested using one layer of hidden units, where the number of hidden units was initially set to

$$2 \times (\text{number of input units}) + 1$$

and reduced until an optimum was reached. The final architecture had 9 input units, 10 units in the hidden layer, and 1 output unit, leading to a total of

$$9 \times 10 + 10 \times 1 = 100$$

adjustable weights. All weights in the neural network were randomly initialized to a value from the interval $[-1, 1]$ prior to network training. The early-stopping technique was used to prevent overfitting of the free parameters of the network (34). During training, the error function (difference between desired and obtained outputs) of the training set falls continuously until it converges on some value. An independent validation set consists of examples not in the training set. The error function of the validation set is usually higher than that of the training set; it falls initially but then rises again as overfitting sets in. Training of the neural network is stopped at the minimum.

5.2 Optimal Partitioning of Protein Space

Our goal is to partition the fold dendrogram so that the observed functional similarities (strong neural network predictions) are concentrated as much as possible within the selected clusters. The clusters are branches of the tree and are interpreted as superfamilies. The objective function imposes thresholds on the neural network outputs so that there is a gain from including "similar" pairs and a penalty for including "dissimilar" pairs in a cluster. This definition is reminiscent of that of the Dali score [Eq. (1)]. More formally, the optimal partitioning of the fold dendrogram results in a set of superfamily-ancestor nodes $\{C\}$, over which the sum of node scores $S(C)$ is maximal:

$$S(C) = \sum_{i=1}^{N_c} \sum_{j=1}^{N_c} [\phi(i,j) - \theta] \tag{4}$$

The node score $S(C)$ is summed over all pairs of descendants (i,j) of a superfamily ancestor node C. The set of descendants of node C is called a cluster and forms a superfamily. $\phi(i,j)$ is the output from the neural network for a protein pair (i,j), N_c is the number of members in the cluster, and θ is the threshold parameter. The merging of two branches of the fold dendrogram is favored if their average connection strength is above θ. Algebraically, if a cluster C consists of two subsets (branches) A and B, then

$$s(C) = s(A) + s(B) + 2s(AB)$$

where $s(AB)$ denotes the sum over pairs where one structure belongs to subset A and the other belongs to subset B. The condition for merging A

and B is $s(C) > s(A) + s(B)$, which clearly holds only if $s(AB) > 0$. A straightforward tree traversal algorithm yields the optimal partition. Algorithmically, the goal is to select a set of nodes covering all leaves such that the sum of node scores is maximal. Initially, select all leaf nodes and set

$$S_{max}(\text{leaf}) = S(\text{leaf}) = 1.00 - \theta$$

with the self-comparison $\phi(i, j)$ set to 1.00. Then the algorithm traverses the fold tree from leaves to root. For each node C with children A and B, compute two scores: $S(C)$ from Eq. (4) and $S_{max}(C)$, defined as

$$S_{max}(C) = \max[S(C), S_{max}(A) + S_{max}(B)] \tag{5}$$

If $S(C)$ is equal to $S_{max}(C)$, then node C overrides any descendant nodes in the optimal partition, where no subdivision or merger increases the sum of node scores s over the selected set of nodes.

Figure 13 illustrates partitions in interesting regions of the structure similarity tree. Partitions at $\theta = 0.33$ gave a best retroprediction of SCOP superfamily assignments.

In conclusion, we have proposed a numerical taxonomy that applies uniform criteria leading to a robust automatic evolutionary classification of protein structures. The topology of protein space is probed using structural similarity. Searching for clusters of structural neighbors where the members consistently share many functional attributes leads to an optimal partitioning of protein space that corresponds well to the analog/homolog boundaries drawn by biologists. A continuously updated domain dictionary should be a valuable Web resource (http://www.embl-ebi.ac.uk/dali/domain). The next section demonstrates applications of the automatic evolutionary classification to the generation of functional hypotheses in non-hypothesis-driven structural genomics efforts.

6 FROM STRUCTURE TO FUNCTION

The automated classification uses a limited set of generic functional attributes to determine superfamily membership. Once superfamily membership is established, detailed functional predictions can be based on *judicious* carryover of the functional properties of experimentally characterized members within a superfamily. For example, RecA, helicases, F1F0-ATPase, and TrwB are members of a ubiquitous superfamily involved in diverse cellular functions. Members of the superfamily function as DNA pumps in recombination, replication, repair, transcription, and bacterial conjugation and as the proton pump that generates ATP. Although the sequences of these proteins have diverged greatly, aspects of their organization into hexameric

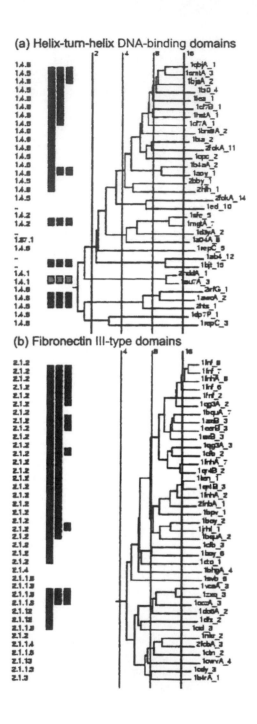

Figure 13

(c) Glycosylhydrolase TIM barrels

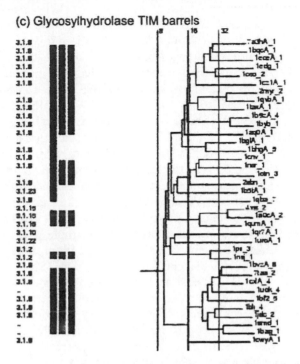

Figure 13 Evolutionarily related families are automatically unified. SCOP labels are shown on the left. Dali domains without a similarly defined domain in SCOP are shown as '..'. The results of unification at different values of the θ parameter (from left to right: 0.33, 0.60, 0.90) are shown by vertical bars. The horizontal axis is the Dali Z-score. (a) For example, $\theta = 0.33$ unifies the domains from 1qbjA_1 to 2fhf_1, inclusive. At higher values of θ, it splits into a larger number of unified families. The other unified families (e.g., 1sfe_5 and 1rngA_7) have strong signals and are identified already at very strict θ values. (b) All fibronectin III-type domains (SCOP 2.1.2), with one exception, occupy a monophyletic branch of the Dali fold dendrogram. The main branch is successfully unified by the automatic classifier (at $\theta = 0.33$). (c) The fold dendrogram suggests that the glycosylhydrolase TIM barrel superfamily (SCOP 3.1.8) consists of structurally distinct subgroups (top and bottom, with different SCOP classes in the middle).

rings have been preserved. For example, the conserved pumping action of the foregoing superfamily has led to reassessment of the proposed cellular function of some proteins first assigned as helicases (38). This example illustrates how complex molecular protocols are frequently reused in evolution. Correct evolutionary classification is bioinformaticians' free lunch with regard to predicting nontrivial aspects of protein function.

Structure-based evolutionary classification can be useful in generating hypotheses about hypothetical proteins. Table 3 is a digest of 15 recently solved structural genomics targets from representatives in the FSSP database (April 2001). Criteria for selection were that the structures were not used for training the neural network and that they contain the term "STRUCTURAL GENOMICS" or "UNKNOWN FUNCTION" in the PDB header record. Four of these were without structural neighbors. Three structures had structural neighbors but insufficient functional similarity for grouping them into a superfamily. Interestingly, biochemical experiments to test for functional similarity to the closest structural neighbors of Mth538 and Mth175 were inconclusive (39), indicating that classification into a new family is probably a correct decision. Eight structures joined existing and emerging superfamilies, leading on to hypotheses about biochemical function that could be tested experimentally. For example, the unification of MTH152 and *A. fulgidus* ferric reductase AF0830 prompted further investigation into the putative molecular function of MTH152. Several lines of evidence point to MTH152 being an FMN:NADP oxidoreductase by analogy with ferric reductase but of unknown substrate specificity (Fig. 14).

The neural network detects the evolutionary relationship at high confidence ($\phi = 0.99$). The active features are a high Z-score of 18.5, pairwise sequence identity of 15%, sequence family overlap (a strong feature), and a modest function preference of 0.05 identical conserved residues in the structural core (shown as sticks). Surprisingly, the feature "identical conserved residues in contact with a ligand" is silent, because the contacts with FMN are mostly from the backbone of nonconserved residues. MTH152 and AF0830 do in fact belong to a large structurally defined superfamily of FMN-binding domains, including (1axj, 1ci0A) and the ferredoxin reductase-like FAD-linked domains. The latter group has a cyclic permutation of the beta-barrel. Independent sequence analysis has MTH152 and AF0830 in COG1853. However, it is not enough merely to carry over the annotation of the nearest neighbor (by structure or sequence search); one must assess the position of the query protein in the phylogenetic tree of the superfamily and ideally check for the presence of sequence signatures for substrate specificity. The active site of MTH152 is defined by the superimposed FMN cofactors and NADP+ in ferric reductase. A sulphate ion binds to MTH152 in a position structurally equivalent to that of the NADP diphosphate. His144 of MTH152 is equivalent to His126, which makes contacts with the NADP in ferric reductase. This histidine is only semiconserved in COG1853 but segregates in phylogenetic trees based on a multiple alignment of the members. Twenty-one of 22 sequences of one subgroup have got the histidine and the remaining 11 outlier sequences have not (cf. http://www.ncbi.nlm.-nih.gov/COG/). His126 is a likely marker of the NADP-dependent enzy-

Table 3 Classification of Recently Solved Structural Genomics Targets

Protein	PDB	Author's functional classification	Evolutionary classification[a] (this work)
Mth1615	1eijA	DNA-binding, putative transcription factor	New fold
Mth1184	1gh9A	Putative metal-binding protein	New fold
Hi1434	1dbuA	Putative nucleotides or oligonucleotide-binding domain	New fold
E. coli YrdC	1hruA	Putative dsRNA-binding protein	New fold
Mth538	1eiwA	Unknown	New family
Mth1175	1eoIA	Unknown	New family
Clostridium CipC	1ehxA	Scaffolding protein and the first prokaryotic member of the I set of the immunoglobulin superfamily	New family
B. subtilis maf	1ex2A	Nucleotide binding, putative NTPase	Same superfamily as with Mj0226 pyrophosphatase (1b87A)
Mth152	1ejeA	FMN- and nickel-binding protein	Same superfamily as ferric reductase (1i0rA)
Mj0541	1f9aA	NMN adenyltransferase	Same superfamily as two nucleotidylyl transferases (1b6tA, 1cozA)
Mouse doppel	1i17A	Paralog of the cellular prion protein but with a distinct physiological role and distinct pathology	Same superfamily as prion proteins (1b10A, 1qlzA)
Yeast Ure2	1g6wa	Prion protein, lacks GST activity	Same superfamily as 6 glutathione S-transferases (GSTs)
Mj0882	1dusA	Unpublished	Same superfamily as 16 methyltransferases
E. coli CyaY	1ew4A	Belongs to the frataxin family, which is linked to the neurodegenerative disease Friedreich ataxia	Same superfamily as frataxin (1dlxA)
Mth649	1i81A	Belongs to the SnRNP Sm protein family; 37% sequence identity to 1d3bA	Same superfamily as small nuclear ribonucleo-proteins (SnRNPs)

[a]Superfamilies defined at $\theta = 0.33$. Folds defined by cutting the fold dendrogram at $Z = 2$.

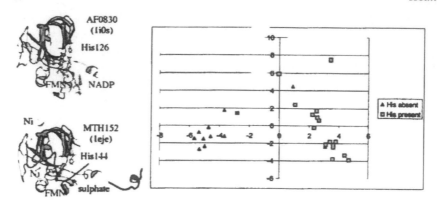

Figure 14 Phylogenetic analysis supports the prediction of a more precise function to the FMN-binding protein Mth152 function (namely, that it is an NADP-dependent oxidoreductase) based on its unification with *A. fulgidus* ferric reductase. *Left*: structural superimposition. *Right*: SequenceSpace analysis (Ref. 43) of COG1853. MTH152 is the square dot on the left side. AF0830 is located on the right side.

matic mechanism proposed for ferric reductase. The sequences are too diverse to resolve the base of the phylogenetic tree, and MTH152 may have a different substrate from ferric compounds. Indeed, there is another *A. fulgidus* gene, AF1706, which at 28% sequence identity is more similar to MTH152 than to AF0830. COG1853 also contains a second member from *M. thermoautotrophicum*. MTH1574 lacks the histidine marker and is predicted to be NADP-independent.

7 COMPLETING THE PROTEIN MAP

The growth of sequence and function data from genome projects and 3D structures from experimental structural biology should yield a complete catalog of all proteins soon. Orphan sequences, with no known relatives detectable by sequence alignment, are already diminishing in number, and observations of the recurrence of similar substructures in remotely related proteins are more frequent. As more experimentally determined proteins structures become available and computational tools improve, model building by homology will yield a rapidly increasing fraction of all possible 3D models of natural proteins.

Structural genomics is the idea of solving a covering set of protein structures so that any protein sequence (the target) comes within model-building distance of a known structure (the template). The principal limitations of model-building by homology are (1) detecting homology, (2) structural divergence between template and modeled protein, and (3) the quality of alignment. Structure comparison is more powerful than sequence comparison in detecting homology. This is because similarity of shape remains detectable even though the sequence may have changed beyond recognition in the course of evolution. Comparing protein shapes rather than protein sequences is like using a bigger telescope that looks farther into the protein universe, and thus farther back in time, opening the door to detecting the most remote and most fascinating evolutionary relations. However, protein sequence comparison is simpler than shape comparison and is routinely used in studies of protein evolution; shape comparison can be used only if 3D structures are available—currently still in a few percent of all cases. The structural divergence between template and target structures is an impediment to accurate modeling of many surface regions, but superfamilies with many known structures show remarkable conservation in and around active sites. Indeed, the relationship between rmsd as a function of the number of residues structurally aligned has been suggested as one way to identify the active site of proteins of unknown function (40). Reproducing the structural alignments of superfamilies using only sequence information is an important challenge to sequence alignment technology. It is a commonly held belief that 30% sequence identity is required for reasonable modeling accuracy (41). The ability to generate accurate alignments of proteins across large evolutionary distances is important for the study of sequence–function correlations. It will also have an economic impact on structural genomics as a result of fewer solved structures yielding useful 3D models for a larger number of sequences.

In time, computational biologists will move beyond the mere description of evolutionary relations to a quantitative and predictive model of the evolution of proteins. The increasingly complete knowledge of protein structure will be used as a basis for detailed modeling of protein function, protein–protein interactions, and metabolic or signaling pathways. Mapping the protein universe by surveying and classifying protein shapes is a key contribution to these endeavors.

REFERENCES

1. T Dobzhansky. Nothing in biology makes sense except in the light of evolution. Am Biol Teacher 35:125–129, 1973.
2. K Diederichs. Structural superposition of proteins with unknown alignment and detection of topological similarity using a six-dimensional search algorithm. Proteins 23:187–195, 1995.
3. L Holm, C Sander. Mapping the protein universe. Science 273:595–603, 1996.
4. A Falicov, FE Cohen. A surface of minimum area metric for the structural comparison of proteins. J Mol Biol 258:871–892, 1996.

5. IN Shindyalov, PE Bourne. Protein structure alignment by incremental combinatorial extension (CE) of the optimal path. Protein Eng 11:739–747, 1998.
6. JV Lehtonen, K Denessiouk, AC May, MS Johnson. Finding local structural similarities among families of unrelated protein structures: a generic nonlinear alignment algorithm. Proteins 34:341–355, 1999.
7. WR Taylor. Protein structure comparison using iterated double dynamic programming. Protein Sci 8:654–665, 1999.
8. L Holm, C Sander. Protein structure comparison by alignment of distance matrices. J Mol Biol 233:123–138, 1993.
9. L Holm, C Sander. Dictionary of recurrent domains in protein structures. Proteins 33:88–96, 1998.
10. L Holm, C Sander. 3-D lookup: fast protein structure database searches at 90% reliability. Proc Int Conf Intell Syst Mol Biol 3:179–187, 1995.
11. RH Lathrop, TF Smith. Global optimum protein threading with gapped alignment and empirical pair score functions. J Mol Biol 255:641–665, 1996.
12. W Kabsch, C Sander. Dictionary of protein secondary structure: pattern recognition of hydrogen-bonded and geometrical features. Biopolymers 22:2577–2637, 1983.
13. C Notredame, DG Higgins, J Heringa. T-Coffee: A novel method for fast and accurate multiple sequence alignment. J Mol Biol 302:205–217, 2000.
14. S Dietmann, J Park, C Notredame, A Heger, M Lappe, L Holm. A fully automatic evolutionary classification of protein folds: Dali Domain Dictionary version 3. Nucleic Acids Res 29:55–57, 2001.
15. L Holm, J Park. DaliLite workbench for protein structure comparison. Bioinformatics 16:566–567, 2000.
16. L Holm, C Sander. Parser for protein folding units. Proteins 19:256–268, 1994.
17. SA Islam, J Luo, MJ Sternberg. Identification and analysis of domains in proteins. Protein Eng 8:513–525, 1995.
18. S Jones, M Stewart, A Michie, MB Swindells, C Orengo, JM Thornton. Domain assignment for protein structures using a consensus approach: characterization and analysis. Protein Sci 7:233–242, 1998.
19. AS Siddiqui, GJ Barton. Continuous and discontinuous domains: an algorithm for the automatic generation of reliable protein domain definitions. Protein Sci 4:872–884, 1995.
20. MH Zehfus. Identification of compact, hydrophobically stabilized domains and modules containing multiple peptide chains. Protein Sci 6:1210–1219, 1997.
21. R Sowdhamini, SD Rufino, TL Blundell. A database of globular protein structural domains: clustering of representative family members into similar folds. Fold Des 1:209–220, 1996.
22. L Wernisch, M Hunting, SJ Wodak. Identification of structural domains in proteins by a graph heuristic. Proteins 35:338–352, 1999.
23. C Sander. Physical criteria for folding units of globular proteins. In: M Balaban, ed. Structural aspects of recognition and assembly of biological

macromolecules, Vol. I. Proteins and protein complexes, fibrous proteins. Jerusalem: Alpha Press, 1981, pp 183–195.

24. Y Xu, D Xu, HN Gabow. Protein domain decomposition using a graph-theoretic approach. Bioinformatics 16:1091–1104, 2000.
25. JS Richardson. The anatomy and taxonomy of protein structure. Adv Protein Chem 34:167–339, 1981.
26. JM Smith. Natural selection and the concept of a protein space. Nature 225:563–564, 1970.
27. RB Russell, MA Saqi, RA Sayle, PA Bates, MJ Sternberg. Recognition of analogous and homologous protein folds: analysis of sequence and structure conservation. J Mol Biol 269:423–439, 1997.
28. T Kawabata, K Nishikawa. Protein structure comparison using the Markov transition model of evolution. Proteins 41:108–122, 2000.
29. Y Matsuo, SH Bryant. Identification of homologous core structures. Proteins 35:70–79, 1999.
30. TC Wood, WR Pearson. Evolution of protein sequences and structures. J Mol Biol 291:977–995, 1999.
31. L Holm, C Sander. Decision support system for the evolutionary classification of protein structures. Proc Int Conf Intell Syst Mol Biol 5:140–146, 1997.
32. L Lo Conte, B Ailey, TJ Hubbard, SE Brenner, AG Murzin, C Chothia. SCOP: a structural classification of proteins database. Nucleic Acids Res 28:257–259, 2000.
33. S Dietmann, L Holm. Identification of homology in protein structure classification. Nat Struct Biol 8:953–957, 2001.
34. CM Bishop. Neural networks for pattern recognition. New York: Oxford University Press, 1995, pp 482.
35. P Baldi, S Brunak. Bioinformatics: the machine learning approach. Cambridge: MIT Press, 1998, pp 351.
36. SE Fahlmann, C Lebiere. The cascade-correlation learning architecture. Advances in neural information processing systems. San Mateo, CA: Morgan Kaufmann, 1990, pp 524–532.
37. S Theodoridis, K Koutroumbas. Pattern Recognition. San Diego: Academic Press, 1999.
38. EH Egelman. Structural biology. Pumping DNA. Nature 409:573, 575, 2001.
39. D Christendat, et al. Structural proteomics of an archaeon. Nat Struct Biol 7:903–909, 2000.
40. JA Irving, JC Whisstock, AM Lesk. Protein structural alignments and functional genomics. Proteins 2:378–382, 2001.
41. D Vitkup, E Melamud, J Moult, C Sander. Completeness in structural genomics. Nat Struct Biol 8:559–566, 2001.
42. L Holm, C Sander. An evolutionary treasure: unification of a broad set of amidohydrolases related to urease. Proteins 28:72–82, 1997.
43. G Casari, C Sander, A Valencia. A method to predict functional residues in proteins. Nat Struct Biol 2:171–178, 1995.

12

Automated Genome Functional Annotation for Structural Genomics

Sophia Tsoka and Christos A. Ouzounis
EMBL–European Bioinformatics Institute, Hinxton, Cambridgeshire, United Kingdom

1 LARGE-SCALE PROTEIN SEQUENCE, STRUCTURE, AND FUNCTION ANALYSIS

The onset of genome sequencing has brought about significant changes in the way biological data are accumulated and has radically transformed the process of biological discovery. Before the availability of complete genome sequences from unicellular or multicellular organisms, biological observations were conducted predominantly by means of an experiment that generally focused on the study of a *single* gene or gene product. With the entire genetic inventory of organisms available, molecular biologists and biochemists are faced with the task of analyzing the actions and interactions of *hundreds or thousands* of molecular components. This enormous task is feasible due to an impressive collection of sophisticated data-mining and -analysis tools that biologists depend on as well as an ever-increasing acceptance of computational analyses of their system of study. The ultimate goal of such analyses is to produce precise molecular models to support and justify detailed maps of biochemical functions and interactions at the cellular level.

Given a newly sequenced genome, a series of computational analyses are typically performed to detect and functionally characterize the pieces of the cellular machinery (1). Once genes have been identified and translated, proteins are compared against databases of protein sequences or structures. Given the evolutionary links between organisms, if a suitably homologous protein of known function is identified, many features can be transferred to the new, previously uncharacterized sequence (2).

The primary sequence of a protein largely determines its secondary structure features as well as its three-dimensional conformation. Generally, sequence identity of pairwise sequence comparison higher than 30% is required for assigning structure to genome sequences through *homology* or *comparative modeling*. For lower sequence identity, structure prediction is based on determining whether a sequence adopts an already known protein fold (*fold recognition*) (3,4). Several databases exist for classifying the structural properties of the currently known structures (5,6).

The sequence and structural properties of a protein molecule establish the biological role of the molecule within the cell, its evolutionary relations to other protein molecules, and its potential as a drug target (7). Usually, it is preferred that functional assignments be done on the basis of structure rather than sequence, for two main reasons: (1) structural features are generally more conserved than primary sequence, and (2) structure allows a more rational basis of functional transfer.

However, the procedure of annotating a protein sequence by homology is currently performed largely on the basis of sequence rather than structural similarity, mainly due to the fact that sequences vastly outnumber the available structures. Currently the nonredundant database of protein sequences contains 791,165 entries (NRDB; October 2001). Swiss-Prot (8), a protein database with manually curated functional annotations, contains 101,602 sequences (release 40). The Protein Databank (PDB) (9), a database of three-dimensional coordinates for macromolecules, consists of 16,306 entries (2001). These numbers indicate two major bottlenecks in protein sequence and structure analysis, namely, the manual curation of genome sequences and the experimental determination of protein structure. Yet this large discrepancy between sequences and structures is likely to change as more structures are gathered and the molecular principles of biochemical function are discovered. In fact, it is anticipated that the sequence and structural libraries will gradually coalesce to form an integrated resource that records the interaction of structural models with functional features (7).

2 THE IMPACT OF STRUCTURAL GENOMICS ON FUNCTION ANNOTATION

To accelerate the determination of protein structure and to avoid redundancy, a number of initiatives have been developed to foster collaboration and sharing of resources, in analogy with similar initiatives in genome sequencing. These activities, known as *structural genomics*, are steered by academic and industry consortia and aim to solve as many structures as possible in the most efficient way.

It is expected that these initiatives will generate a representative set of the number of protein folds in nature, accompanied by an understanding of the molecular principles of biochemical function. Such knowledge has the potential to fuel further development of computational methods for mapping sequence to function (e.g., through homology modeling) rapidly and cost effectively (10). Structural genomics projects may have a variety of goals, according to the biological questions at hand. For instance, they may focus on the determination of protein structures for entire biochemical pathways, including the detection of active sites and mechanisms of catalytic action (11), the systematic analysis of certain fold types, such as $(\alpha/\beta)_8$ barrels (12), and the delineation of structural types within entire genome sequences (13–15).

Advances in purification and measurement science as well as computational methods for structure determination have significantly increased the rate of structure deposition in databases. However, a greater acceleration of structure determination would be desirable, because the exponential increase in genome sequences is threatening to widen the gap between the sequence and structure blueprints of genomes. Automated systems for functional annotation can help in this direction because they have been designed to aid rapid analysis of genome sequences. Next we explore the use of such a system in a structural genomics context giving examples of target identification and validation.

3 AUTOMATED GENOME SEQUENCE ANNOTATION: THE GENEQUIZ SYSTEM

Automated genome functional assignment systems such as GeneQuiz have stemmed from the need to handle the influx of large amounts of genome sequence data (16). The analysis of such data requires the use of multiple pieces of software and databases, which are flexibly embodied in the workflow configuration of the system (17). This approach to precalculated information at such scale is only possible due to the underlying decisions for full automation, thus freeing expert and nonexpert users to focus on the validation and interpretation of results, obtained in a uniform and objective manner. Moreover, because no intermediate steps require any manual intervention, analyses are reproducible and comparable across different datasets and time points.

GeneQuiz suggests high-quality annotations along with the ability to trace the reasoning process for each assignment. Finally, it should be mentioned that the system is not intended to replace human experts, but rather to encapsulate human expertise by using a set of state-of-the-art computational biology methods with optimized parameter settings. In short, the system is both a vast resource for genome annotation and an interesting experiment in encapsulating human expertise for computational genomics.

3.1 Structure of the GeneQuiz System

A GeneQuiz run requires as input an arbitrary set of protein sequences, typically representing the content of an entire genome. The output is functional annotation for each protein, lists of homologs in the database, various functional features, matches to motif collections, and assignment into a functional class—with full records of the evidence that has led to such assignments. The analysis is performed by four modules: GQupdate, GQsearch, GQreason, and GQbrowse. A broad overview of the system is provided next. For a more detailed description of GeneQuiz, the reader is referred to the relevant literature (17–18).

3.1.1 GQupdate: Maintainance and Update of Molecular Biology Databases

GQupdate maintains a list of up-to-date, nonredundant protein (19) and nucleotide sequence databases that are derived from a collection of public databases. Table 1 shows the biological databases queried by GeneQuiz.

3.1.2 GQsearch: Sequence Search Against Biological Databases

Each sequence from the query set in turn triggers the GQsearch module. This module first detects and masks low-complexity regions that usually distort the database search statistics. Two algorithms for the detection of

Table 1   List of Databases Used for Functional Annotation by GeneQuiz

Protein sequences	Swiss-Prot, Swiss_new, Ensembl, WormPep, Pironly
Nucleotide sequence translations	TreEMBL, TrEMBL_new
Nucleotide sequences	EMBL, EMBL_new, GenGank, dbEST
Protein motifs	Prosite, Blocks
Protein structures	PDB
Protein families	PFam

Reference sources for these databases are not given, but they can be found in the *Nucleic Acids Research* special Database Issue, published each year.

low-complexity regions are used: seg (20) and CAST (21). The masked sequence is subsequently used as the input to standard search algorithms in order to detect sequence similarities in the databases. A list of significantly similar sequences is built using both the BLAST (22) and FASTA algorithms (23).

Sequence analysis is complemented by other diagnostic methods performed for identification of patterns, the creation of alignments between the query sequence and its homologs (24), and the extraction of structural features. For secondary structure features in particular, the predictions include identification of transmembrane regions, connecting loop topology, and solvent accessibility (25). Table 2 lists all computational methods run by GeneQuiz for the characterization of each input sequence.

Given an alignment with high similarity between the query sequence and a sequence of known structure, construction of a three-dimensional model of the query sequence may be performed using the WHATIF program for homology modeling (26). The program uses a sequence alignment between the target sequence and the homologous sequence of known structure and generates a three-dimensional structure for the corresponding part of the input sequence, as identified by the sequence alignment.

3.1.3 GQreason: Functional Assignment and Inference

The processes of functional assignment and classification are performed by the GQreason module. This module involves the encoding of several rules to analyze the information accumulated for each sequence in a manner analogous to the evaluation performed by a human expert. The goal is twofold: (1) to designate a specific function to the query sequence on the basis of the detected similarities to database entries, and then (2) to classify this function into a particular category of cellular processes.

To assign a functional annotation, GeneQuiz first estimates the reliability of transferring the function of each of the homologs. This is done by

Table 2 Computational Methods Invoked by the GQsearch Module of GeneQuiz

Low-complexity detection	seg, CAST
Sequence comparison	BLASTP, FASTA
Support methods	Repeats, coils, blimps, proseach, MaxHom, MView
	PredictProtein (secondary structure, accessibility, transmembrane), WHATIF

References to these programs can be found in the original paper, Ref. 17, or the Web site.

sorting the list of homologs according to (1) sequence similarity to the query, (2) confidence in the quality of annotation in databases, and (3) scores from search algorithms. The following ranking is currently used for the annotation quality of databases: Swiss-Prot, PIR, TREMBL, GenPept, EMBL, and GenBank. The scores of search algorithms are combined, with BLAST preferred over FASTA, according to a complex, empirically derived, scheme that takes into account score values from the two algorithms and derives a reliability value for each assignment (Table 5 in Ref. 17).

The sorted list of annotations is then used to perform lexical analysis in order to discard meaningless terms (e.g., hypothetical protein, predicted conserved protein). Of the annotations that remain, the one with the highest reliability score is assigned to the query, and the reliability of annotation is designated by the terms *clear, tentative*, and *marginal*.

Subsequently, the query is assigned to one of 14 functional classes that specify distinct cellular processes, derived from Riley's functional classification (27). Table 3 lists the functional classes used by GeneQuiz. Functional classification is based on the mapping of a list of keywords (dictionary) corresponding to each functional class. Because each input sequence inherits the keywords and the annotation of the putative homologs, classifying this sequence to a functional class involves a look-up operation that associates the query sequence's keywords to a functional class (28).

Table 3 Functional Classes in GeneQuiz (in alphabetical order)

Amino acid biosynthesis
Biosynthesis of cofactors, prosthetic groups, and carriers
Cell envelope
Cellular processes
Central intermediary metabolism
Energy metabolism
Fatty acid and phospholipid metabolism
Purines, pyrimidines, nucleosides, and nucleotides
Regulatory functions
Replication
Transcription
Translation
Transport and binding proteins
Unknown

3.1.4 GQbrowse: Result Access and Browsing

GQbrowse assembles the results of any GeneQuiz analysis in Web-browsable reports. Reports take the form of analysis results for each individual input protein as well as precomputed queries for all the input proteins.

Individual protein report pages contain the evidence that led to a specific functional assignment. This includes the results of all diagnostic methods runs, the list of homologs identified (together with relevant alignments), details of structural features, as well as the three-dimensional model, if available. Links to relevant database entries are also included. Through this information (browsing-search results and statistics, motif searches, lists of homologs and alignments), the user can evaluate the assignment(s) made by the program.

The system also provides precomputed queries performed on the whole set of proteins, usually corresponding to a specific genome. Examples of the results for such queries are shown in Figure 1, which illustrates the front page of a GeneQuiz run for *Aeropyrum pernix* (29). An overview of the current functional content for a given genome is represented by an "information clock" (Fig. 1). The different sections indicate the number of sequences that have (1) homologs of known structure, (2) homologs of known function, (3) homologs of unknown function, and (4) no homologs. Also, precomputed queries allow users to access genome information by functional class, reliability of assignment, novel assignments not previously detected, as well as a number of ad hoc queries using text or sequence information (Fig. 1).

3.2 Assessment of System Annotation Performance

The quality of annotations obtained from automated systems such as GeneQuiz is largely dependent on the quality of annotation in the public databases. Issues such as misleading annotations, heterogeneous use of the various fields of entries (particularly important if multiple databases are used), and lack of standards and controlled vocabularies for function description are potential sources of error for any system that attempts to perform functional assignments with minimal manual intervention (2). Some of these issues are addressed in GeneQuiz by performing sensitive sequence comparisons together with lexical analysis on the annotations. The reduction of false positives is achieved through strict cutoffs in search algorithms (E-value threshold of 10^{-10} for BLASTP and score threshold of 130 for FASTA) and a conservative assignment of sequence into functional classes. The functional content of annotation is assessed on the basis of a dictionary of words with no specific functional significance and a well-defined algorithm for lexical analysis of annotations (28).

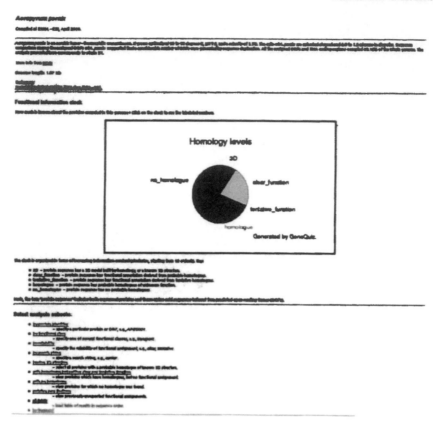

Figure 1 GeneQuiz report page for the *Aeropyrum pernix* genome. A typical page contains some information on the biology of the organism, an information clock indicating the different levels of annotation, and various ways of accessing the database, such as by protein name, functional class membership, and reliability of annotation (http://juva.ebi.ac.uk8765/ext-genequiz//genomes/ap0004/index.html).

Performance of the GeneQuiz system has been extensively validated. Such studies include whole genome analyses of *Mycoplasma genitalium* (30), *Methanococcus jannaschii* (31), and *Chlamydia trachomatis* (32). The error in functional classification is estimated to be approximately 5%, with a tendency to increase over time as the sequence databases grow. This increase may be attributed to erroneous assignments in databases spreading through transitive annotation procedures. Experimental characterization of the biochemical functions of proteins using high-throughput approaches has the potential to reverse this undesirable trend (2).

4 TARGET SELECTION FOR STRUCTURAL GENOMICS USING ANNOTATED GENOMES

The goal of target selection in structural genomics is to identify candidate (families of) molecules that have certain desirable properties. These targets are selected according to a number of criteria, the most popular of which include: (1) proteins with a large number of uncharacterized homologs; (2) proteins with few or no homologs that are perhaps species- or even strain-specific; (3) proteins that are not transmembrane and are predicted to be globular; (4) proteins likely to have new folds that have not been previously observed. Obviously, these properties are not mutually exclusive. However, to arrive at a final selection of targets, researchers need to perform multiple analyses that may be independent of each other. In that respect, the availability of an integrated resource containing various pieces of information is crucial. Ironically, the process of target selection relies on the maximum available knowledge, in order to successively eliminate (rather than select) targets likely to yield redundant structural information.

The massive annotation information for entire genome sequences that is available through the GeneQuiz Website* can be successfully used for target selection. The resource can be queried according to the criteria mentioned earlier either directly or in combination with other information, such as family detection or fold predictions. Apart from the usual criteria, other information can be very useful, for instance, presence of certain motifs, phylogenetic distribution in various species, keywords associated with the annotation, and general functional classes that correspond to specific cellular processes. In all, the more integrated and up to date the information available for each molecule is, the more reliable the final target selection is likely to be. Herein, we provide some examples of advanced usage of GeneQuiz, illustrating target selection for structural genomics using an extensive set of features for individual genes or whole genomes.

4.1 Comparable Analyses

One of the advantages of GeneQuiz is the ability to perform functional/ structural assignments on a genome-wide scale. Due to the automated nature of the analysis, GeneQuiz analyses are precisely specified, thus reproducible, and the results of different analyses are directly comparable. Such comparisons have the potential to reveal the level of knowledge for a set of species whose genome has been sequenced. For example, comparisons between different strains of the same species may identify the genetic basis of

---

*http://www.genomes.org/genequiz.html

strain-specific properties (33). Comparisons between pathogenic and non-pathogenic strains, in particular, may reveal the origin of virulence properties (34). Finally, whole-genome analysis and structural genomics should always result in a set of molecules suitable as drug targets (35).

Full, automatically updatable, annotation is critical in the process of target selection, because it can always point to the most recent information regarding a set of molecules. Comparisons of whole-genome analyses are particularly informative because they permit tracing progress over time, obtaining snapshots of the annotation level for a set of proteins, and allow comparisons of functional and structural assignments across species.

Recently, we have performed such a comparison using the genome sequence from 31 species and obtained the level of structural and functional annotation for each species (36) (Fig. 2). The range of species included in the analysis varies from some of the most well-characterized organisms (such as *Escherichia coli*, *Saccharomyces cerevisiae*, and *Bacillus subtilis*) to some less well-studied ones, including hyperthermophiles (e.g., *Archaeoglobus fulgidus*, *Aeropyrum pernix*) and medically important microorganisms (*Haemophilus influenzae*, *Neisseria meningitidis*).

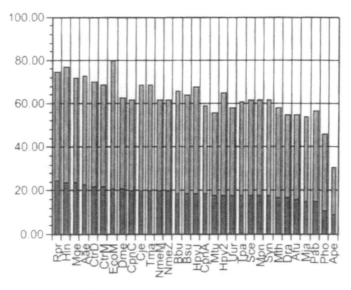

Figure 2 Analysis of 31 entire genome sequences using GeneQuiz. Species are sorted by the percentage of total structure assignment (dark gray). The level of functional annotation for each genome is also shown (light gray). It is evident that structurally the most well-characterized genomes are *Rickettsia prowazekii* and *H. influenzae* and that the least characterized genomes are predominantly archaeal species.

This analysis covers genomes from 31 species, containing 73,729 genes in total. A significant proportion of those corresponding to 45,681 proteins (62%) can be functionally annotated with clear homology to database entries, out of which 13,927 (19%) also have a homolog of known three-dimensional structure. These numbers imply that there are an additional 59,802 proteins encoded in those genomes, which await structural characterization. This example illustrates the challenge that structural genomics is facing: analyses should sift through tens of thousands of molecules in search of a good target. Overall, proteins with at least one segment related to one or more known structures ranged from 9% to 24.5% (expressed as percent of the total number of genome entries) in the 31 genomes studied.

Archaea seem to be the least well characterized group of organisms structurally; proteins with a homolog of known structure ranged from 9% for *A. pernix* to 17% for *Methanobacterium thermoautotrophicum*. The only two eukaryotic organisms in our collection, *S. cerevisiae* and *Drosophila melanogaster*, are found around the average, at 18% and 22% of the total number of proteins, respectively. Bacterial species represent the main corpus of our results. Of these, 15 species demonstrate above average percentage for proteins with homologs of known structure. These species include mostly small genomes, such as *M. genitalium* and *Rickettsia prowazekii*, species that are well characterized experimentally (*E. coli*, 21%, *B. subtilis*, 20%), or species that are significantly similar to well-characterized ones (*H. influenzae*, 24%, similar to *E. coli*). These differences, in the context of proteins that have not been characterized structurally, open up opportunities for target selection work; some of the less well-studied species represent a gold mine for structure targets, as has recently been shown in practice (13).

It seems that genome sequencing has benefited function prediction much more than structure characterization, as indicated by the higher percentage of average genome functional annotation (63% vs. 19%). Similar patterns apply here: Archaea are much less characterized, since function prediction ranges from 31% for *A. pernix* to 58% for *Pyrococcus abyssi*. Eukaryotes are again around average: 61% for *S. cerevisiae* and 63% for *D. melanogaster*. For the bacteria, there is a huge variation. The best-characterized species is *E. coli*, with function prediction reaching 80% of its proteins, closely followed by *H. influenzae* (78%), a species closely related to *E. coli*. With the recent appearance of more genomes, some improvement on these figures is expected (unpublished observations). However, it is highly likely that a significant breakthrough in function assignment will be achieved only with the availability of results from functional and structural genomics experiments and their incorporation into the relevant databases.

Thus, comparative analyses of this scale, and the opportunity to obtain genuine snapshots of the annotation level from the full database at any given point in time, represent valuable ways of focusing attention on particular species in a rational and comprehensive manner. Especially in the case of pathogenic organisms, this type of functional knowledge may be helpful for the acceleration of drug development (37).

4.2   Functional Class Assignment

Functional classification in GeneQuiz progresses from merely describing the level of homology between each query protein and targets in the database and the functional role of input sequences, to actually designating each functional assignment to one of 14 prespecified functional classes representing distinct cellular processes. Coupled with structural and other functional features, the purpose of such functional classification is to summarize the representation of individual biological processes (e.g., biosynthesis of amino acids, fatty acid metabolism, translation) and the refinement of hypotheses of genome biology with specific functional networks. Given both functional classifications and structural properties, questions may be answered such as the type of protein folds required for performing specific biochemical functions, the evolution of functional networks, e.g., by identifying cases of structure–function convergence and divergence (38–39).

Structural genomics initiatives have occasionally focused on the experimental structural characterization of proteins within a particular functional group in the hope of augmenting the phenotypic effect with molecular knowledge (40). An example of such structural genomics strategies is the determination of enzymes in individual biosynthetic pathways, such as sterol/isoprenoid biosynthesis (41). Such efforts may further fuel research into determining those functional attributes that are related to structural features, such as interaction sites, ligand–ligate affinity constants, turnover numbers (e.g., in the case of catalytic conversions), complex organization.

GeneQuiz was the first automated functional annotation project to adopt a fully automated mode of generating not only functional assignments for individual proteins but also partitions of entire genomes into several functional categories. Assignment employs the functional annotation string as well as database keywords associated with the query in order to allocate each protein to a particular functional group, as described earlier. Evidently, some cellular processes are better defined than others—e.g., proteins involved in energy metabolism are generally better understood than those involved in the cell envelope—and this will be reflected in the sensitivity and specificity of the assignment outcome. Generally, the system favors a conservative form of protein allocation into functional groups, to reduce false positives at the expense of possibly increasing the number of false negatives (i.e., unclassified proteins).

The GeneQuiz database management system offers the possibility of associating functional classification with structural information on the members of each functional class. The outcome permits one to answer the question of how well structural genomics projects have characterized each functional network at a particular time point. To showcase this capability with a particular example, we have formulated a query to select all *H. influenzae* proteins with a known (or inferred) structure for each of the 14 functional classes using the latest GeneQuiz run for *H. influenzae* (performed in October 2001, NRDB size 789,199 sequences). Of the total 1,707 ORFs, functional annotations were generated for 83% of the genome proteins and 33% of them also had a structural homolog defined. With regard to functional classification, 1,025 proteins (60% of total) were classified into the 14 functional classes. Most structurally resolved protein cases fall within a known functional class: Of the 565 structures currently available for the genome of *H. influenzae*, only 38 (6.7%) were found among the 682 unclassified sequences. Unclassified proteins are excluded from the following discussion.

We explored the level of structural determination of functional classes (Fig. 3). The most well-characterized functional classes were found to have around 60% of their members structurally determined: energy metabolism

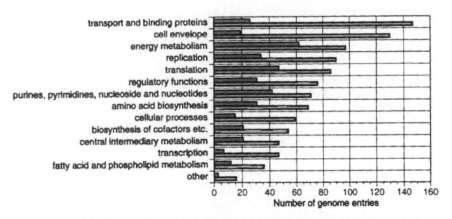

Figure 3 Assessment of structural determination for the functional classes represented in the genome of *H. infuenzae*. Proteins with a known structure or structural homolog (dark gray bars) are shown against the total number of sequences (light gray bars) classified in the corresponding functional class (classes are sorted according to this number). It is clear that classes such as amino acid biosynthesis are better characterized than classes such as cell envelope.

(63.9%), purines, pyrimidines, and nucleotides (59.1%), and translation (54.6%). Classes with around 40% of structure over the total were: amino acid biosynthesis (44.9%), central intermediary metabolism (44.7%), regulatory functions (40.8%), and biosynthesis of cofactor prosthetic groups and carriers (38.9%). Fatty acid and phospholipid metabolism and cellular processes are less well represented in terms of structure prediction, with 33.3% and 25.4% of structural homologs, respectively. Transport and binding proteins (17.7%) and cell envelope (14.6%) have the smallest number of structures identified, possibly due to the large number of transmembrane proteins involved in these processes. Finally, it is interesting that the functional class benefiting most from structural genomics studies appears to be transcription, with only 14.9% of the corresponding proteins having a structural homolog.

These discrepancies in structural determination among functional classes can be attributed to the following reasons. Specific functional processes have received significantly more research interest due to the ease of experimental system setup or direct association to medical/industrial applications; for example, compound biosynthesis is significantly better understood than transport and binding. Additionally, sequence conservation within each functional class has a profound effect on structure prediction by homology; homology modeling is more successful in defining functional groups where molecular structure is highly conserved. Finally, certain functional groups present particular difficulties in structure determination due to the presence of transmembrane segments (i.e., transport proteins) or problems in purification and crystallization.

4.3 Functional and Structural Assignment Progress Tracking and Update

The difficulties associated with the management of distributed efforts of structural and functional genomics can be alleviated by the availability of objective and reproducible analysis protocols. Systems such as GeneQuiz may be useful in progress monitoring and reporting on the amount of annotation quality and improvement over time. To this end, automatic updates of functional annotations for entire genomes can support disparate activities on function/structure assignment by tracking progress.

Comparisons of genome-wide analyses across different time periods is illustrated for the case of *H. influenzae*, the first entire genome sequenced (42). *Haemophilus influenzae* has attracted some attention as a structural genomics microbial target (15) due to its small genome, ease of manipulation of mutant strains, and the lack of unusual codons. GeneQuiz analyses have been repeated five times over six years, an overview of annotation performance is shown in Figure 4.

During this time period and especially during the last two years, there has been a clear trend of an increasing number of sequences with either a known structure or a homolog of known structure. This desirable effect can be attributed to (1) the well-planned strategies for selecting structural genomics targets, (2) the higher turnover in terms of structures being determined experimentally during the last few years, and, consequently, (3) the increasing success of homology modeling.

In contrast to structure prediction, Figure 4 suggests that function prediction has not been equally benefited by high-throughput genomics research, for it seems that function assignment through sequence homology has reached a saturation point. Clearly, significant benefits could be gained here by embracing the paradigm of worldwide, well-planned policies of experimental delineation of function, such as the ones followed by structural genomics projects and the incorporation of functional genomics results into the databases.

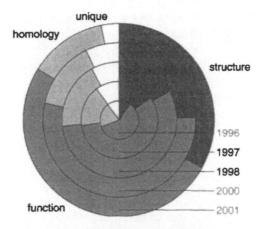

Figure 4 Progress of structure and function prediction over time illustrated in the case of *H. influenzae*. *Structure* denotes the number of sequences with structural homologs, *function* denotes the sequences with clear functional assignments, *homology* denotes the conserved sequences with no function assigned, and *unique* corresponds to species-specific sequences (no homologs in the database). The year of the analysis is indicated.

4.4 Determination of a Structure for 7,8-Dihydroneopterin Aldolase

As described earlier, given a suitably similar sequence of known structure, the WHATIF module of GeneQuiz uses the alignment of the query and target sequences to build a structural model of the query sequence automatically. Here, we provide an example of structural modeling by GeneQuiz. As an example, we use protein slr1626 of *Synechocystis* sp. (strain PCC6803), which was classified as a hypothetical protein in the original genome sequence. GeneQuiz identified a homolog in the Protein Structure Database (PDB) from *Staphylococcus aureus* with dihydroneopterin aldolase activity (PDB identifier: 1DHN) that has led to function as well as structure chracterization.

Dihydroneopterin aldolase (DHNA) catalyzes the conversion of 7,8-dihydroneopterin to 6-hydroxymethyl-7,8-dihydroneopterin during the synthesis of folic acid from guanosine triphosphate. DHNA activity is important to the manufacture of antiinfective drugs and has been detected in several other bacterial species, such as *Escherichia coli* and *Streptococcus pneumoniae*. The protein coding for dihydroneopterin aldolase in *Synechocystis* sp. (Swiss-Prot accession number P74342) has a 40% identity to the equivalent protein in *Staphylococcus aureus* (P56740) that has been biochemically and structurally analyzed (43). Based on this homology, the DHNA homolog for *Synechocystis* sp. has been modeled (Fig. 5).

The molecule is composed of eight monomer molecules; a "head-to-head" assembly is formed by two tetrameric rings (43). Analysis of conserved residues in amino acid sequences from different bacterial species reveals that the active site lies between the two adjacent subunits of the tetramer. The secondary structure features of the DHNA monomer include an antiparallel beta-sheet and two long alpha-helices; with the side chains of these secondary structure groups forming the hydrophobic core (Fig. 5).

5 CONCLUSIONS

We have illustrated how GeneQuiz can be used as a comprehensive database of functional annotations for large-scale genome analysis. It aids target identification by integrating cellular, functional, and structural information and providing the means for sophisticated queries on variable sources of information. We have demonstrated that the system can identify both which targets to select and which to avoid in structural genomics studies. Because currently one skilled person determines 5–10 structures per year (44), such resources provide the means to maximize output for structural genomics.

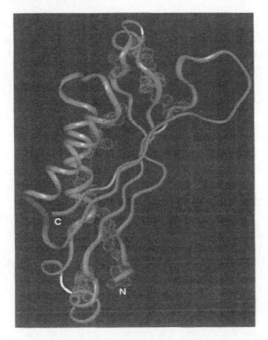

Figure 5 Structural model of protein slr1626 from *Synechocystis* sp. generated by GeneQuiz using homology modeling (PDB identifier of the reference protein: 1DHN). Only the structure of the monomer is shown. Details on molecule activity, structural features, and the original structure are given in the text. The C-alpha trace is represented by the ribbon, the shorter loop in slr1626 (gap of one residue in the alignment) is shown in dark gray, and the side chains of the invariant residues between the two proteins are shown as a light gray "cloud" around the C-alpha trace. The N- and C-terminus residues are also indicated.

Finally, the automatic extraction of functional features from protein structures is highly desirable for the future, but it is unlikely that structural information alone will be adequate for function prediction. Therefore, integrated functional and structural resources (as implemented in GeneQuiz) will always be a successful data model for computational biology databases (7).

REFERENCES

1. P Bork, T Dandekar, Y Diaz-Lazcoz, F Eisenhaber, M Huynen, Y Yuan. Predicting function: from genes to genomes and back. J Mol Biol 283:707–725, 1998.

2. S Tsoka, CA Ouzounis. Recent developments and future directions in computational genomics. FEBS Lett 480:42–48, 2000.
3. SA Teichmann, C Chothia, M Gerstein. Advances in structural genomics. Curr Opin Struct Biol 9:390–399, 1999.
4. D Baker, A Sali. Protein structure prediction and structural genomics. Science 294:93–96, 2001.
5. L Lo Conte, SE Brenner, TJ Hubbard, C Chothia, AG Murzin. SCOP database in 2002: refinements accommodate structural genomics. Nucleic Acids Res 30:264–267, 2002.
6. CA Orengo, JE Bray, DW Buchan, A Harrison, D Lee, FM Pearl, I Sillitoe, AE Todd, JM Thornton. The CATH protein family database: a resource for structural and functional annotation of genomes. Proteomics 2:11–21, 2002.
7. JM Thornton. From genome to function. Science 292:2095–2097, 2001.
8. A Bairoch, R Apweiler. The SWISS-PROT protein sequence database and its supplement TrEMBL in 2000. Nucleic Acids Res 28:45–48, 2000.
9. FC Bernstein, TF Koetzle, GJ Williams, EE Meyer Jr, MD Brice, JR Rodgers, O Kennard, T Shimanouchi, M Tasumi. The Protein Data Bank: a computer-based archival file for macromolecular structures. J Mol Biol 112:535–542, 1977.
10. D Vitkup, E Melamud, J Moult, C Sander. Completeness in structural genomics. Nat Struct Biol 8:559–566, 2001.
11. H Erlandsen, EE Abola, RC Stevens. Combining structural genomics and enzymology: completing the picture in metabolic pathways and enzyme active sites. Curr Opin Struct Biol 10:719–730, 2000.
12. N Wu, Y Mo, J Gao, EF Pai. Electrostatic stress in catalysis: structure and mechanism of the enzyme orotidine monophosphate decarboxylase. Proc Natl Acad Sci USA 97:2017–2022, 2000.
13. D Christendat, A Yee, A Dharamsi, Y Kluger, A Savchenko, JR Cort, V Booth, CD Mackereth, V Saridakis, I Ekiel, G Kozlov, KL Maxwell, N Wu, LP McIntosh, K Gehring, MA Kennedy, AR Davidson, EF Pai, M Gerstein, AM Edwards, CH Arrowsmith. Structural proteomics of an archaeon. Nat Struct Biol 7:903–909, 2000.
14. R Sanchez, A Sali. Large-scale protein structure modeling of the *Saccharomyces cerevisiae* genome. Proc Natl Acad Sci USA 95:13597–13602, 1998.
15 E Eisenstein, GL Gilliland, O Herzberg, J Moult, J Orban, RJ Poljak, L Banerjei, D Richardson, AJ Howard. Biological function made crystal clear—annotation of hypothetical proteins via structural genomics. Curr Opin Biotechnol 11:25–30, 2000.
16. M Scharf, R Schneider, G Casari, P Bork, A Valencia, C Ouzounis, C Sander. GeneQuiz: a workbench for sequence analysis. Proc Int Conf Intell Syst Mol Biol 2:348–353, 1994.
17. MA Andrade, NP Brown, C Leroy, S Hoersch, A de Daruvar, C Reich, A Franchini, J Tamames, A Valencia, C Ouzounis, C Sander. Automated genome sequence analysis and annotation. Bioinformatics 15:391–412, 1999.

18. S Hoersch, C Leroy, NP Brown, MA Andrade, C Sander. The GeneQuiz Web server: protein functional analysis through the Web. Trends Biochem Sci 25:33–35, 2000.

19. L Holm, C Sander. Removing near-neighbor redundancy from large protein sequence collections. Bioinformatics 14:423–429, 1998.

20. JC Wootton, S Federhen. Analysis of compositionally biased regions in sequence databases. Methods Enzymol. 266:554–571, 1996.

21. VJ Promponas, AJ Enright, S Tsoka, DP Kreil, C Leroy, S Hamodrakas, C Sander, CA Ouzounis. CAST: an iterative algorithm for the complexity analysis of sequence tracts. Complexity analysis of sequence tracts. Bioinformatics 16:915–922, 2000.

22. SF Altschul, W Gish, W Miller, EW Myers, DJ Lipman. Basic local alignment search tool. J Mol Biol 215:403–410, 1990.

23. WR Pearson, DJ Lipman. Improved tools for biological sequence comparison. Proc Natl Acad Sci USA 85:2444–2448, 1988.

24. NP Brown, C Leroy, C Sander. MView: a Web-compatible database search or multiple alignment viewer. Bioinformatics 14:380–381, 1998.

25. B Rost. PHD: predicting one-dimensional protein structure by profile-based neural networks. Methods Enzymol 266:525–539, 1996.

26. G Vriend. WHAT IF: a molecular modeling and drug design program. J Mol Graph 8:52–56, 1990.

27. M Riley. Functions of the gene products of *Escherichia coli*. Microbiol Rev 57:862–952, 1993.

28. J Tamames, C Ouzounis, G Casari, C Sander, A Valencia. EUCLID: automatic classification of proteins in functional classes by their database annotations. Bioinformatics 14:542–543, 1998.

29. Y Kawarabayasi, et al. Complete genome sequence of an aerobic hyper-thermophilic crenarchaeon, *Aeropyrum pernix* K1. DNA Res 6:83–101, 145–152, 1999.

30. C Ouzounis, G Casari, A Valencia, C Sander. Novelties from the complete genome of *Mycoplasma genitalium*. Mol Microbiol 20:898–900, 1996.

31. M Andrade, G Casari, A de Daruvar, C Sander, R Schneider, J Tamames, A Valencia, C Ouzounis. Sequence analysis of the *Methanococcus jannaschii* genome and the prediction of protein function. Comput Appl Biosci 13:481–483, 1997.

32. I Iliopoulos, S Tsoka, MA Andrade, AJ Enright, M Carroll, P Poullet, V Promponas, T Liakopoulos, G Palaios, C Pasquier, S Hamodrakas, J Tamames, AT Yagnik, A Tramontano, D Devos, C Blaschke, A Valencia, D Brett, D Martin, C Leroy, C Sander, CA Ouzounis. Evaluation of genome sequence annotation using the *Chlamydia trachomatis* genome. Submitted, 2002.

33. PJ Janssen, B Audit, CA Ouzounis. Strain-specific genes of *Helicobacter pylori*: distribution, function and dynamics. Nucleic Acids Res 29:4395–4404, 2001.

34. NT Perna, et al. Genome sequence of enterohaemorrhagic *Escherichia coli* O157:H7. Nature 409:529–533, 2001.
35. S Dry, S McCarthy, T Harris. Structural genomics in the biotechnology sector. Nat Struct Biol 7 Suppl:946–949, 2000.
36. I Iliopoulos, S Tsoka, MA Andrade, P Janssen, B Audit, A Tramontano, A Valencia, C Leroy, C Sander, CA Ouzounis. Genome sequences and great expectations. Genome Biol 2: INTERACTIONS0001, 2000.
37. L Shapiro, T Harris. Finding function through structural genomics. Curr Opin Biotechnol 11:31–35, 2000.
38. AE Todd, CA Orengo, JM Thornton. Evolution of function in protein superfamilies, from a structural perspective. J Mol Biol 307:1113–1143, 2001.
39. S Tsoka, CA Ouzounis. Functional versatility and molecular diversity of the metabolic map of *Escherichia coli*. Genome Res 11:1503–1510, 2001.
40. SE Brenner. Target selection for structural genomics. Nat Struct Biol 7 Suppl:967–969, 2000.
41. JB Bonanno, C Edo, N Eswar, U Pieper, MJ Romanowski, V Ilyin, SE Gerchman, H Kycia, FW Studier, A Sali, SK Burley. Structural genomics of enzymes involved in sterol/isoprenoid biosynthesis. Proc Natl Acad Sci USA 98:12896–12901, 2001.
42. RD Fleischmann, MD Adams, O White, RA Clayton, EF Kirkness, AR Kerlavage, CJ Bult, JF Tomb, BA Dougherty, JM Merrick, et al. Whole-genome random sequencing and assembly of *Haemophilus influenzae* Rd. Science 269:496–512, 1995.
43. M Hennig, A D'Arcy, IC Hampele, MG Page, C Oefner, GE Dale. Crystal structure and reaction mechanism of 7,8-dihydroneopterin aldolase from *Staphylococcus aureus*. Nat Struct Biol 5:357–362, 1998.
44. J Skolnick, JS Fetrow, A Kolinski. Structural genomics and its importance for gene function analysis. Nat Biotechnol 18:283–287, 2000.

13

The Importance of Structure-Based Function Annotation to Drug Discovery

Susan M. Baxter, Stacy Knutson, and Jacquelyn S. Fetrow
GeneFormatics, Inc., San Diego, California, U.S.A.

1 INFORMATION ABOUT PROTEIN FUNCTION IS KEY TO DRUG DISCOVERY

The genome-sequencing projects have been tremendously successful in providing a vast amount of protein sequence information for drug discovery efforts going forward. The fundamental challenge of the postgenomic era will be how to incorporate this deluge of protein sequence information into drug discovery strategies. Large-scale efforts to identify validated protein drug targets use cell-based methods, such as expression monitoring (1) as well as whole-organism genetic studies to identify essential genes or functions (2) for therapeutic intervention. These approaches will provide crucial biological validation, but it is not necessarily straightforward to match candidate lead compounds to target proteins based on this level of biological or functional annotation. Efficient lead discovery strategies will likely springboard from existing medicinal chemistry experience in designing small-molecule inhibitors or modulators of protein function. For rational and efficient lead optimization or even for virtual screening and computational docking strategies (3), knowledge of the physicochemical and structural features of the protein target are invaluable. That knowledge will be based on detailed information about target structure and the molecular function or functions encoded by that particular protein fold or structure.

The protein structure initiatives under way worldwide promise the availability of new protein structures (4,5), and those structures should provide a solid foundation for drug discovery in the postgenomic era. X-ray crystallographic, NMR spectroscopic, or even electron microscopic methods (6) will provide high-quality representative structures for both current and new pharmaceutical targets. The availability of sufficient public and private funding (7,8) ensures that many of the current technical hurdles and difficulties in protein structure determination will be tackled and eventually solved. Representative structures provide templates for comparative modeling and knowledge-based potentials for ab initio methods so that new structure models can be generated for protein sequences with high (> 30%) sequence similarity, thus filling out the structural space relative to the experimental templates. The accuracy of these computationally derived models should be detailed enough to provide valuable functional site information for lead discovery. With protein domain information in hand, workable leads can be developed in the context of the structure and chemistry of the binding sites identified in the protein structure. For instance, chemical compounds that bind a particular site on a representative protein structure can be used as starting scaffolds for generating leads that target proteins closely related in sequence and structure.

However, a significant problem with this approach is that tertiary structure information is not necessarily enough to determine the function of a protein or to identify potential small-molecule binding sites. Proteins have evolved specialized functional, or active, sites to carry out the biological complexity required by life. These functions and their integration far outnumber the estimated number (9–11) of domain structures available. As a result, the tempting practice of automatically transferring the functional annotation from one protein structure to another can lead to misannotation and misinterpretation (12). Unfortunately, as demonstrated by sequence genomics, automatic annotation transfer (13) works only some of the time. A series of surveys (14) of currently available structures illustrates that functional inference can correctly predict molecular function for roughly half of the proteins analyzed (15–17).

A complicating factor is the recognition that proteins, especially eukaryotic proteins, will likely carry out multiple functions on the molecular level. Multiple-domain proteins can carry out distinct functions (i.e., catalysis and protein–protein interaction) that reside in separate domains. Alternatively, multifunctionality can be incorporated in a single protein domain, for example, a cofactor-binding site proximal to a catalytic site. Each functional site provides a handle for inhibiting or modulating protein activity. Gerstein and coworkers (18) surveyed fold space and reported that common protein scaffolds, easily recognized based on sequence similarities, tended to be multifunctional. Furthermore, they discovered that function annotation for multidomain proteins can be accurately transferred with only 35% certainty for pairs of proteins sharing one domain but not necessarily sharing the entire protein architecture.

As structural genomics initiatives produce new protein structures in a large-scale effort to describe fold diversity, there will be structures solved for which molecular function is unknown. Early reports (19) from experimental structural genomics efforts indicate that it is not straightforward to identify biochemical function or functional sites for unannotated proteins, even with high-resolution structures in hand. From a biochemical perspective, Gerlt and Babbitt (20) describe the complexity in comparing enzymatic function, recognizing that even proteins categorized into functional families can be divergent in substrate specificity and mechanistic detail. Specifically, Wise and coworkers (21) compared the sequences and structures of two $(\beta/\alpha)_8$-barrel enzymes, orotidine 5'-monophosphate (OMPDC) and 3-keto-L-gulonate 6-phosphate decarboxylase (KGPDC). They discovered that the two proteins share significant active-site residues and structure, but the replacement of a conserved lysine in OMPDC to a glutamate in KGPDC contributes to a different function, with no mechanistic relationship to OMPDC. These seemingly fine details are of fundamental importance in designing specific and selective inhibitors or modulators of function as part of the process of developing small-molecule drug candidates. In addition to three-dimensional protein structures, then, methods are most urgently required for accurate identification of both functional residues and active site structures in proteins that can lead to testable hypotheses toward understanding the molecular and even biological role of a protein.

2 CONSERVED FUNCTIONAL MOTIFS IN PROTEIN STRUCTURE

Protein scientists recognized early that protein structures were more conserved than the identities of the amino acids of the underlying primary sequence (22,23). As more protein structures were solved, the bioinorganic chemists discovered conserved structure motifs for metal-binding sites. These motifs were three-dimensional arrangements of amino acids that were not necessarily close in primary sequence. The metal-binding motifs encoded important functionality by providing proper metal coordination for reactivity or structural stability (Fig. 1A, B). For instance, proteins that functioned as DNA-binding proteins used zinc-finger structure motifs to specifically target cognate DNA substrates (24). The EF hand proteins modulate signaling pathways, using a conserved structure motif that is exquisitely tuned by amino acid identities to bind calcium differentially

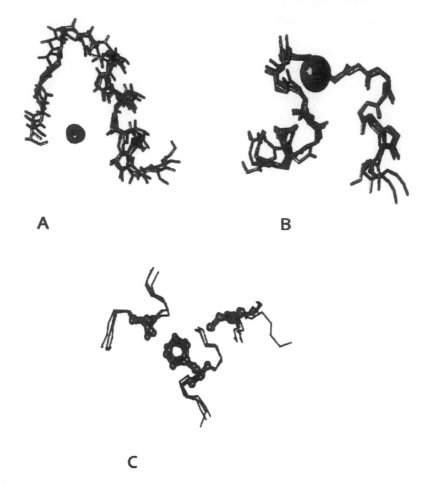

A

B

C

Figure 1 Three examples of function motifs that are structurally conserved across proteins. (A) Three examples of a zinc finger motif that is commonly found in proteins for which one function is DNA binding. The three proteins shown here are mouse zif268 zinc finger/DNA complex (1aay), yeast swi5 zinc-finger domain 1 (1ncs), and yeast transcription factor adr1 (1ard). The beta strand and alpha helix that contain the functionally important zinc ligands are structurally conserved in these three proteins. (B) Three examples of the EF hand calcium-binding motif that is found in many proteins involved in cell signaling. The three proteins shown here are human calmodulin (1cll), rabbit troponin C (1tcf), and pike parvalbumin (1pva). Two helices and the connecting loop, which contains the calcium-binding ligands, are structurally conserved in this functional motif. (C) Three examples of the catalytic triad that is key to the functioning of many serine hydrolases. The three proteins shown are human chymase, a carboxypeptidase (1pjp), human thrombin, a serine protease (1qur), and staphylokinase (1bui). The strict conservation of not only backbone structure, but also the conformations of the side chains of the catalytically important serine, histidine, and aspartic acid are apparent in this figure.

among family members (25). Structural motifs that bind metal ions are not necessarily independently folding domains, but they are identified in a wide variety of protein folds across phylogeny. These motifs have provided valuable lessons about protein folds and, as a result, have enabled elegant protein design and engineering studies (26–29).

The most highly conserved amino acids tend to be those involved directly in protein function (30,31). This observation is illustrated best by the conserved catalytic triad, serine-histidine-aspartate, that carries out the enzymatic activity of the serine proteases (32–34). The spatial arrangement of these residues allows precise positioning of substrate near the hyperreactive serine nucleophile (Fig. 1C). Again, this active site structure motif is not necessarily an independently folding domain (10), but it is supported in a wide variety of protein scaffolds. The surrounding structure and amino acid differences near the catalytic triad give rise to a great diversity of proteins that are defined by this enzymatic active-site motif, including trypsin proteases, lipases, and other α/β hydrolases (Fig. 2).

It is important to note that conserved functional site motifs, like the serine-histidine-aspartate triad, may not even incorporate information about spatially related elements of secondary structure. That is, a functional site can be composed of a conserved array of side chains that are arranged in three-dimensional space without relationship to primary sequence, secondary structure motifs, or supersecondary structure elements. For this reason, the serine proteases continue to serve as the quintessential model of a well-studied catalytic activity within a diverse set of sequences and structures. However, this property is not unique to the serine proteases. The low molecular weight phosphatases and classical protein tyrosine phosphatases share a common set of catalytic residues that are brought together in space by different arrangements of primary sequences and different overall protein architectures (Fig. 3). Nature has decided to conserve not only protein folds and domains, but also active site geometries. As a result, functional sites that carry out particular mechanisms—represented by all EC classes—are found repeated throughout protein fold space. The similarities in the active sites drive the catalysis and chemistry, while differences in the surrounding structure serve to modulate activity and affect specificity for each individual protein function as well as allowing the protein to fold and remain stable in the cellular milieu.

3 THE IMPORTANCE OF BIOCHEMICAL FUNCTION TO THE DRUG DISCOVERY PROCESS

Structural and mechanistic studies of the serine proteases, and other conserved pharmaceutically interesting protein families, have produced key

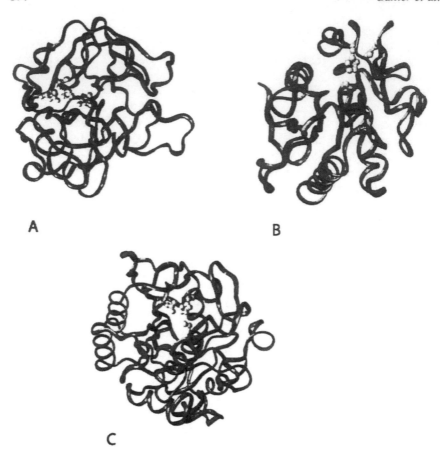

Figure 2 Three protein structures demonstrate that the serine-histidine-aspartate catalytic triad can be found in different protein architectures but carry out the same serine hydrolase function. This active site can be accurately identified by structural motifs, such as FFFs, that are designed to recognize the residues and their relative arrangement in three-dimensional space. (A) Activated protein C, a trypsin fold (1aut); (B) lipase (1cug); and (C) thermitase (1thm).

information for the design of compound libraries and specific inhibitors targeting medicinally interesting protein classes. Similarly, rich structural information about peripheral cofactor-binding geometries has provided alternate design strategies for inhibitors targeting kinases (35) and phosphatases (36). Therefore, biochemical function identification is important at (at least) two discernable stages of drug discovery.

Functional annotation of protein sequences becomes important first at the target discovery level. For instance, when sequencing or expression-

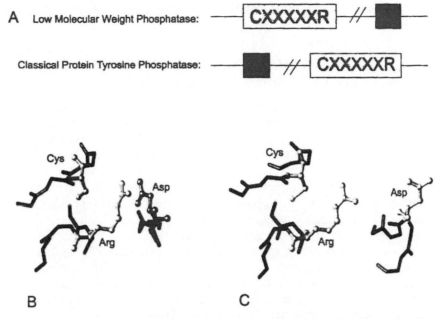

Figure 3 Comparing the protein tyrosine phosphatases to the low-molecular-weight phosphatases highlights similarities in active site geometry and key catalytic residues but differences in their order in the primary sequence. (A) The phosphatase sequence motif, CXXXXXR, is conserved in both families of phosphatases. However, the catalytically important aspartate, supplied by a loop, is arranged in a different sequential order along the primary sequence. The three-dimensional structural arrangement of key catalytic residues in the low-molecular-weight phosphatase (B, 1phr) and protein PTP1B tyrosine phosphatase (C, 2hng) active site. Comparison of these two functional sites clearly indicates the structural similarity of the functional site, even though the key amino acids are arranged differently along the primary sequence.

monitoring projects link sequences with biological pathway or tissue specificity data, biochemical or molecular function information can drive assay development for high-throughput screening or other strategic experiments that promote proteins further as therapeutic targets. Secondly, functional information is needed at the lead discovery stage, when specific information about a functional site (or even neighboring modulatory site) chemistry, and structure is needed for library design or inhibitor design and optimization. Functional site identification can also be useful for structural biology studies and proteomics projects analyzing structures with unknown function or unrecognized functional complexity. The remainder of the chapter will discuss structure-based methods for functional annotation of both protein structures and protein sequences aimed at addressing these drug discovery needs.

4 METHODS FOR IDENTIFYING FUNCTIONAL SITES IN PROTEIN STRUCTURE COORDINATES

Since the early 1990s, methods for comparing three-dimensional protein structures have been developed to ease the complex task of analyzing new structures against the ever-increasing database of protein folds, domains, and structures at the Protein Data Bank (37). For instance, Alexey Murzin and coworkers (37a) have built the Structural Classification of Proteins (SCOP) database based on expert comparisons of overall fold, not sequence similarity. Other, more automated methods (9,38) of structure comparison are more completely discussed elsewhere in this volume. However, the primary aim of structural or domain comparison methods is to classify protein structure, not necessarily to assign protein function. While evolutionary relationships and common ancestry (39,40) give some validity to using structural homology to transfer functional annotations, structure similarity does not necessarily imply functional similarity, especially at the mechanistic or molecular level, as discussed earlier in this chapter.

Recognizing the annotation value of identifying the conserved catalytic triad, serine-histidine-aspartate, that characterizes serine proteases, researchers have focused on this set of mechanistically important residues to design algorithms to probe protein structure coordinates, assign function, and identify active sites. Artymiuk and coworkers (41) used a search method based on graph theory to map out user-defined patterns of side chains in protein structures. They were able to automatically identify catalytic triads, zinc-binding sites, and nuclease active sites in the PDB, suggesting that the approach could be generalized. Wallace and coworkers (42) used a geometric hashing method to automatically derive a three-dimensional active site template describing the serine-histidine-aspartate catalytic triad and later (43) expanded the technique to identify nucleophile-histidine-electrostatic arrangements of side chains so that α/β hydrolases, cysteine proteases, and esterases could be identified from the PDB data set.

Fischer and coworkers (44,45) first used geometric hashing to represent entire protein structures as unconnected atoms in space, allowing the design of automatic searches for repeating structural motifs in the PDB that did not require user-defined searches for patterns of amino acids. This algorithm promised the ability to identify unrecognized and unexpected patterns of residues in protein structures. Due to the complexity of interpreting the output, however, the method was best suited to identifying supersecondary structures, such as helix-turn-helix or EF hand motifs, but improvements to the algorithm (45) allowed detection of protease active sites, specifically.

Russell (46) recognized that the search for functional sites was simplified by incorporating structure information already available in the PDB. He also recognized that the sensitivity of the search could be improved by ignoring sets of residues "unlikely to be involved" in function. He outlined an all-against-all search of the PDB for groups of residues shared by two protein structures and qualified the matches using distance geometry and statistical significance metrics. The method was used to probe the SCOP database for unrecognized yet conserved and functional residue patterns. One-third of the patterns detected were conserved residue geometries at metal-binding sites. Additionally, the method uncovered salt-bridge patterns and packing arrangements probably better correlated with protein fold maintenance, not functionality, suggesting that the automatic filter for selected residues served to overrepresent residues important for folding or structure stability. Nonetheless, this study proved that the structure databases, even though their coverage of fold space is not yet complete, provide a rich source of information for motif searches and comparison.

Narrowing structure searches to functionally important residues remains a difficult problem. In 1996 Karlin and coworkers (46a) presented a useful method to identify statistically significant clusters of residues in protein structure databases. Recognizing the utility of Karlin's methods, Jonassen and coworkers (47) were successful in identifying motifs and patterns of conserved amino acids involved in local packing interactions, some of which were protease catalytic triads. More recently, Friedberg and Margalit (48) decided to narrow the search for conserved motifs further by arraying a group of structures with conserved folds but very low sequence identity in an effort to identify "persistently conserved" positions and analyze their roles in preserving function. Key residues involved in active site structure and function were identified for a pair of sequence-dissimilar hydrolases, but the study still ran into the problem of overrepresented amino acids, even in the reduced test set.

The evolutionary trace (ET) method (49) was developed recently to identify key functional residues at binding surfaces. Invariant amino acids, or evolutionary traces, are identified from a multiple sequence alignment and a phylogenetic clustering analysis and then mapped onto the three-dimensional protein structure. Evolutionary traces for SH2, SH3, and nuclear hormone receptors successfully map to single, dominant patches or spatial arrays on the protein surface that coincided well with known binding sites and residues important for binding specificity. Similarly, de Rinaldis and coworkers (50) constructed three-dimensional profile templates, based on multiple sequence alignments of conserved, solvent-exposed residues at surface binding pockets, were used to screen the PDB and selectively identified the known SH2 and SH3 structures. Neither of these approaches was automatic and both relied on visual inspection of sequence alignments and dendograms to select sets of key residues. Nonetheless, the ET output, when mapped on three-dimensional structures, illuminates potential binding sites and functional sites on protein structures.

Kasuya and Thornton (51) used sequence patterns to search protein sequences in the PDB and recognized that sequence motifs might be used to functionally annotate protein structures. The combination of structural fold and sequence patterns, based on either experimental data from the literature or multiple sequence alignments, promised added sensitivity and selectivity to structure database searches. Subsequently, Jonassen and coworkers (52) also used functional information embedded in the PROSITE sequence fingerprints to simplify the search of the PDB for functional sites. Importantly, Jonassen and coworkers recognized that protein structures identified by their SapPat scans were matched in a new manner that does not correlate with global fold family classifications, reiterating the evolutionary disconnect between functional sites and overall protein fold.

Rather than using sequence patterns that incorporate residues important for structure, folding, and/or function, descriptors of active sites, termed "fuzzy functional forms," or FFFs, have been developed (53). These structural descriptors incorporate only functionally important residues and geometric information to describe their relative location in space. These FFFs are based on experimentally determined structures and incorporate the known physicochemical and structural features of functional sites (53); such information, identified right up-front, is key to the drug discovery process. The FFFs are not automatically generated but are based on mutational analyses, mechanistic studies, and other structural data available in the literature. However, FFFs can be used to automatically screen protein coordinates and identify functional sites, key functional residues, and their arrangement in three-dimensional space. The FFFs were used to screen the PDB for T1 ribonuclease, disulfide oxidoreductase (53), and α/β hydrolase (54) active sites. A search of the PDB using an oxidoreductase FFF (55) uncovered a putative, regulatory site in a subfamily of the serine/threonine protein phosphatases that appears to be selectively conserved in that particular family of phosphatases. This study highlights the usefulness and importance of identifying unrecognized, ancillary functional sites in protein structures.

5 METHODS FOR IDENTIFYING FUNCTIONAL MOTIFS IN PROTEIN SEQUENCES FROM GENOME ANALYSIS AND EXPRESSION MONITORING STUDIES

Methods for identifying structural motifs important for protein function were reviewed in the previous section. Most of these methods are trained and tested on known protein structures—those structures determined by NMR spectroscopy or X-ray crystallography that are available in the PDB. Very few methods have been applied on a genomic scale or even on a large scale to sequences and the structures that can be modeled from them. This limits the applicability of methods that map functional sites only on protein structure coordinates. Sequence motifs have been applied in this "genomic fashion" to proteins for many years now, often before the meaning of the sequence motif was known in the context of a protein structure or even the protein's function. Notable protein families, such as the homeodomains (56) and the WW proteins (57), were characterized first by nucleic acid or protein sequence similarities and homology. The genome-sequencing projects, along with other projects such as the compilation of curated data at Swiss-Prot (58) and protein structures at the PDB, have provided a critical mass of information so that conserved sequence patterns and motifs and even small groups of amino acids (like the serine-histidine-aspartate triad) can be correlated with structure or function. This section reviews an attempt to apply these structural motifs on a genomic scale.

Databases of conserved sequence patterns, such as Pfam (59), Prints (60), Blocks (61), COGs (62), and SMART (63), have been constructed to identify protein domains, families, and orthologs and are reviewed in the database issue of *Nucleic Acids Research* periodically. Embedded in these conserved sequence motifs, patterns, and signatures is information about key functional residues. In general, functionally important residues and the active sites they comprise are unevenly retained and identified in the construction of database sequence patterns. New approaches, such as CYRCA (64), are aimed at addressing the redundancy and incompleteness of the sequence pattern databases that lead to the conundrum of identifying key residues involved in structure and/or function. Aloy and coworkers (65) recognized that linked database content would enable more accurate functional annotation. They undertook the tedious task of establishing equivalencies between the SMART (63) and Pfam (59) databases by correlating the sequence signatures to structure families and classes identified by the SCOP (37a) database. For example, using the correlated data to analyze the sequence of a yeast protein of unknown function but whose structure was available (1ct5, 1b54), they predicted that the protein is involved in amino acid synthesis. The detection of family and motif relationships was based on statistical significance of structure-based sequence alignments; however, the synthesis of all the information was not automatic and required scientist interpretation, as do all the sequence pattern–based tools.

Evolutionary trace (ET) approaches, described earlier, have been used to predict important functional sites in proteins using sequence information as input, in the absence of structure information. Lichtarge and coworkers used the ET method to predict binding surfaces in G protein (49) and regulators of G-protein signaling (66) sequences that were later confirmed experimentally (67–69). Functional hot spots in SH2 and phosphotyrosine–binding sites have been identified (70) using a modified ET approach, called ConSurf, that incorporated physicochemical distance for more accurate tree reconstruction. Madabushi and coworkers (71) also amended the ET method to address functional annotation on a large scale by using statistical assessment of clustering and new gap treatment to extract ET signatures from a wide variety of protein folds and functions.

Despite the proven generality of the ET methods, they could not be applied to large-scale studies since they required human interaction at several points in the process. Another weakness of the ET-type methods is the reliance on phylogenetic analysis to identify clusters of residues. These methods select the highest-scoring cluster, disregarding the possibility that a query protein sequence might have several functional sites. In an effort to automate the ET approach, Aloy and coworkers (72) replaced the dendogram generation and visual inspection with a nearest neighbor clustering algorithm. To simplify further they mapped only invariant polar residues onto representative structures. They benchmarked the approach against structures in the PDB for which polar residues reside in the binding site. About half of the time, the automated ET method identified clusters of surface residues that overlapped 50% in volume with known binding sites. Landgraf and coworkers (73) decided to use three-dimensional cluster analysis to evaluate protein sequences from 35 different protein families with structural representatives available. Using a scoring function to describe sequence conservation of surrounding structure, on average 67% of known residues at protein–protein interface surfaces were identified. Thus, the ET methods promise great power in identifying active sites for otherwise uncharacterized protein sequences. This kind of information is obviously important for ligand prediction and thus, for lead discovery.

Recognition of functionally important clusters of residues in protein structures can be extended to predict function for protein sequences. Kleywegt (74) developed a pair of programs named SPASM and RIGOR, which incorporate spatial motifs based on PROSITE patterns to search the protein structure databases. The method was used to identify a motif belonging to the fatty acid–binding protein family in a protein of unknown function and structure. Although the approach can functionally annotate uncharacterized proteins, it cannot identify active sites, since PROSITE patterns do not necessarily describe spatially clustered functional sites.

The availability of a growing number of experimentally determined structures makes the task of correctly predicting protein folds for related (> 30% identity) sequences on a large scale increasingly feasible. However, many methods reviewed here, which depend on these closely related family members, ignore the probability of functionally similar sites in more distantly related sequences or even similar functional sites in analogous proteins (examples of both are shown in Figs. 2 and 3). In the absence of related protein structures, sequence-to-structure (or threading) alignments (53,75) provide structural information and a basis for function annotation of uncharacterized, or more distantly related, protein sequences. The *Escherichia coli* genome was searched using FFF descriptors (76) to identify proteins exhibiting glutaredoxin/thioredoxin disulfide oxidoreductase activity, demonstrating that automated structural predictions and functional assignments could be made on a large scale. Importantly, in addition to functional annotation of the protein sequence, the FFF-based method identified key amino acids involved in enzymatic catalysis, metal binding, and ligand binding on a large scale, on distantly related and possibly analogous proteins. This approach provides important molecular structure and functional site characterization for a potential protein target very early in the drug discovery process.

6 FUNCTION ANNOTATION AT THE BIOCHEMICAL, SYSTEMS, AND CLINICAL LEVELS—GOING FORWARD INTO THE POSTGENOMIC ERA

Efficient or rational compound library and drug design still requires biochemical and mechanistic information. This information is provided by understanding the structure and physicochemical properties of functional sites in proteins, but genomic-scale approaches of methods to identify these properties are still limited. New methods are needed to identify the key similarities and differences at functional sites in all related proteins in a genome (77–79). This kind of information offers the opportunity to design specificity into compounds from the beginning of the drug development cycle. Combined computational approaches to predict protein structure and the physicochemical details of an active site before an experimental structure is available offer exciting ways to speed lead development. Clearly, progress in these goals is tightly linked to the availability of representative protein structures. While great progress is being made in tackling soluble protein structures, we all await the inevitable, but necessary, experimental breakthroughs for routinely determining membrane-associated and membrane-bound protein and receptor structures and their drug complexes.

While function annotation of protein sequences and structures is currently of considerable interest, another fundamental challenge over the next several decade(s) will be to describe the biological role of a protein and to link that information to the biochemical and molecular functioning of a protein. Structural proteomics projects still tend to trap our focus on an individual protein target, but the availability of proteomic methods (80) to systematically break down and analyze protein pathways will provide impetus to correlate protein structure data with functional pathways and biological systems. Several groups have already mapped protein structures onto interaction networks (81,82) in an attempt to predict protein–protein partners and, perhaps, specific participation in a particular pathway. This will be of immense importance in adding biological validation to protein targets and, at the same time, yield important information for therapeutic strategies, but biochemical functional information is still key to rational or efficient compound library and drug design.

Finally, many pundits have promised the age of pharmacogenomics, where the genetic makeup of an individual drives therapeutic treatments prescribed for her. Making sense of the ever-accumulating clinical and genetic population data will be the key that allows this individualized approach to disease detection and intervention. Protein structure and biochemical function information, not just one-dimensional sequence information, is key to linking these data to drug discovery. Based on methods described in this chapter and already appearing in the literature (83,84), it seems completely plausible that we will be able to analyze the effects of polymorphisms, splicing, and translocations on protein structure and function and thus to infer something about the effectiveness of a particular treatment.

The seemingly fine details of biochemical function are of fundamental importance in designing inhibitors or modulators as part of the process of developing small-molecule drug leads. Development of methods to recognize the similarities and differences in the physicochemical properties of functional sites and application to all members in protein functional families is key to successfully utilizing the vast amounts of genomic sequence information that are available. Methods are urgently required for accurate identification of both functional residues and active site structures in proteins. These methods will lead to testable hypotheses aimed at understanding the molecular, and even biological, role of a protein. Successful identification of this information is essential to designing specificity into lead compounds early in the drug discovery process, thus allowing pharmaceutical researchers to truly recognize the promise of the human genome–sequencing projects.

REFERENCES

1. DJ Lockhart, EA Winzeler. Genomics, gene expression and DNA arrays. Nature 405:827–836, 2000.
2. EA Winzeler, DD Shoemaker, A Astromoff, H Liang, K Anderson, B Andre, R Bangham, R Benito, JD Boeke, H Bussey, AM Chu, C Connelly, K Davis, F Dietrich, SW Dow, M El Bakkoury, F Foury, SH Friend, E Gentalen, G Giaever, JH Hegemann, T Jones, M Laub, H Liao, RW Davis, et al. Functional characterization of the *S. cerevisiae* genome by gene deletion and parallel analysis. Science 285:901–906, 1999.
3. BA Grzybowski, AV Ishchenko, CY Kim, G Topalov, R Chapman, DW Christianson, GM Whitesides, EI Shakhnovich. Combinatorial computational method gives new picomolar ligands for a known enzyme. Proc Natl Acad Sci USA 99:1270–1273, 2002.
4. S Bhattacharyya, B Habibi-Nazhad, G Amegbey, CM Slupsky, A Yee, C Arrowsmith, DS Wishart. Identification of a novel archaebacterial thioredoxin: determination of function through structure. Biochemistry 41:4760–4770, 2002.
5. D Christendat, A Yee, A Dharamsi, Y Kluger, M Gerstein, CH Arrowsmith, AM Edwards. Structural proteomics: prospects for high-throughput sample preparation. Prog Biophys Mol Biol 73:339–345, 2000.
6. T Mielke, C Villa, PC Edwards, GF Schertler, MP Heyn. X-ray diffraction of heavy-atom-labelled two-dimensional crystals of rhodopsin identifies the position of cysteine 140 in helix 3 and cysteine 316 in helix 8. J Mol Biol 316:693–709, 2002.
7. M Norin, M Sundstrom. Structural proteomics: developments in structure-to-function predictions. Trends Biotechnol 20:79–84, 2002.
8. GT Montelione. Structural genomics: an approach to the protein folding problem. Proc Natl Acad Sci USA 98:13488–16489, 2001.
9. WR Taylor. A "periodic table" for protein structures. Nature 416:657–660, 2002.
10. RR Copley, T Doerks, I Letunic, P Bork. Protein domain analysis in the era of complete genomes. FEBS Lett 513:129–134, 2002.
11. J Liu, B Rost. Comparing function and structure between entire proteomes. Protein Sci 10:1970–1979, 2001.
12. SM Baxter, JS Fetrow. Sequence- and structure-based protein function prediction from genomic information. Curr Opin Drug Discov Devel 4:291–295, 2001.
13. CA Wilson, J Kreychman, M Gerstein. Assessing annotation transfer for genomics: quantifying the relations between protein sequence, structure and function through traditional and probabilistic scores. J Mol Biol 297:233–249, 2000.

14. AE Todd, CA Orengo, JM Thornton. Evolution of function in protein super-families, from a structural perspective. J Mol Biol 307:1113–1143, 2001.

15. A Kumar, PM Harrison, KH Cheung, N Lan, N Echols, P Bertone, P Miller, MB Gerstein, M Snyder. An integrated approach for finding overlooked genes in yeast. Nat Biotechnol 20:58–63, 2002.

16. H Hegyi, M Gerstein. Annotation transfer for genomics: measuring functional divergence in multi-domain proteins. Genome Res 11:1632–1640, 2001.

17. WA Koppensteiner, P Lackner, M Wiederstein, MJ Sippl. Characterization of novel proteins based on known protein structures. J Mol Biol 296:1139–1152, 2000.

18. H Hegyi, J Lin, D Greenbaum, M Gerstein. Structural genomics analysis: characteristics of atypical, common, and horizontally transferred folds. Proteins 47:126–141, 2002.

19. A Yee, X Chang, A Pineda-Lucena, B Wu, A Semesi, B Le, T Ramelot, GM Lee, S Bhattacharyya, P Gutierrez, A Denisov, CH Lee, JR Cort, G Kozlov, J Liao, G Finak, L Chen, D Wishart, W Lee, LP McIntosh, K Gehring, MA Kennedy, AM Edwards, CH Arrowsmith. An NMR approach to structural proteomics. Proc Natl Acad Sci USA 99:1825–1830, 2002.

20. JA Gerlt, PC Babbitt. Divergent evolution of enzymatic function: mechanistically diverse superfamilies and functionally distinct suprafamilies. Annu Rev Biochem 70:209–246, 2001.

21. E Wise, WS Yew, PC Babbitt, JA Gerlt, I Rayment. Homologous (beta/alpha)8-barrel enzymes that catalyze unrelated reactions: orotidine 5'-monophosphate decarboxylase and 3-keto-L-gulonate 6-phosphate decarboxylase. Biochemistry 41:3861–3869, 2002.

22. MG Rossmann, P Argos. Exploring structural homology of proteins. J Mol Biol 105:75–95, 1976.

23. JS Richardson, DC Richardson, KA Thomas, EW Silverton, DR Davies. Similarity of three-dimensional structure between the immunoglobulin domain and the copper, zinc superoxide dismutase subunit. J Mol Biol 102:221–235, 1976.

24. DL Merkle, JM Berg. Metal requirements for nucleic acid binding proteins. Methods Enzymol 208:46–54, 1991.

25. MR Nelson, E Thulin, PA Fagan, S Forsen, WJ Chazin. The EF-hand domain: a globally cooperative structural unit. Protein Sci 11:198–205, 2002.

26. A Lombardi, CM Summa, S Geremia, L Randaccio, V Pavone, WF DeGrado. Inaugural article: retrostructural analysis of metalloproteins: application to the design of a minimal model for diiron proteins. Proc Natl Acad Sci USA 97:6298–6305, 2000.

27. JS Marvin, HW Hellinga. Conversion of a maltose receptor into a zinc bio-sensor by computational design. Proc Natl Acad Sci USA 98:4955–4960, 2001.

28. HW Hellinga, JP Caradonna, FM Richards. Construction of new ligand-binding sites in proteins of known structure. II. Grafting of a buried transition metal binding site into *Escherichia coli* thioredoxin. J Mol Biol 222:787–803, 1991.

29. M Klemba, KH Gardner, S Marino, ND Clarke, L Regan. Novel metal-binding proteins by design. Nat Struct Biol 2:368–373, 1995.

30. P Argos, RM Garavito, W Eventoff, MG Rossmann, CI Branden. Similarities in active center geometries of zinc-containing enzymes, proteases and dehydrogenases. J Mol Biol 126:141–158, 1978.

31. RM Garavito, MG Rossmann, P Argos, W Eventoff. Convergence of active center geometries. Biochemistry 16:5065–5071, 1977.

32. DM Blow, JJ Birktoft, BS Hartley. Role of a buried acid group in the mechanism of action of chymotrypsin. Nature 221:337–340, 1969.

33. CS Wright, RA Alden, J Kraut. Structure of subtilisin BPN' at 2.5-angstrom resolution. Nature 221:235–242, 1969.

34. WR Kester, BW Matthews. Comparison of the structures of carboxypeptidase-A and thermolysin. J Biol Chem 252:7704–7710, 1977.

35. MJ Morin. From oncogene to drug: development of small-molecule tyrosine kinase inhibitors as anti-tumor and anti-angiogenic agents. Oncogene 19:6574–6783, 2000.

36. ZY Zhang. Protein tyrosine phosphatases: structure and function, substrate specificity, and inhibitor development. Annu Rev Pharmacol Toxicol 42:209–234, 2002.

37. HM Berman, J Westbrook, Z Feng, G Gilliland, TN Bhat, H Weissig, IN Shindyalov, PE Bourne. The Protein Data Bank. Nucleic Acids Res 28:235–242, 2000.

37a. L Lo Conte, SE Brenner, TJ Hubbard, C Chothia, AG Murzin. SCOP database in 2002: refinements accommodate structural genomics. Nucleic Acids Res 30:264–267, 2002.

38. S Dietmann, L Holm. Identification of homology in protein structure classification. Nat Struct Biol 8:953–957, 2001.

39. H Hegyi, M Gerstein. The relationship between protein structure and function: a comprehensive survey with application to the yeast genome. J Mol Biol 288:147–164, 1999.

40. EV Koonin, YI Wolf, L Aravind. Protein fold recognition using sequence profiles and its application in structural genomics. Adv Protein Chem 54:245–275, 2000.

41. PJ Artymiuk, AR Poirrette, HM Grindley, DW Rice, P Willett. A graph-theoretic approach to the identification of three-dimensional patterns of amino acid side chains in protein structures. J Mol Biol 243:327–344, 1994.

42. AC Wallace, RA Laskowski, JM Thornton. Derivation of 3D coordinate templates for searching structural databases: application to Ser-His-Asp catalytic triads in the serine proteinases and lipases. Protein Sci 5:1001–1013, 1996.

43. AC Wallace, N Borkakoti, JM Thornton. TESS: a geometric hashing algorithm for deriving 3D coordinate templates for searching structural databases. Application to enzyme active sites. Protein Sci 6:2308–2323, 1997.

44. D Fischer, O Bachar, R Nussinov, H Wolfson. An efficient automated computer vision–based technique for detection of three-dimensional structural motifs in proteins. J Biomol Struct Dyn 9:769–789, 1992.

45. D Fischer, H Wolfson, SL Lin, R Nussinov. Three-dimensional, sequence order–independent structural comparison of a serine protease against the crystallographic database reveals active site similarities: potential implications to evolution and to protein folding. Protein Sci 3:769–778, 1994.
46. RB Russell. Detection of protein three-dimensional side-chain patterns: new examples of convergent evolution. J Mol Biol 279:1211–1227, 1998.
46a. S Karlin, Z Zhu. Characterizations of diverse residue clussters in protein three-dimensional clusters. Proceed Natl Acad Sci USA 93:8344–8349, 1996.
47. I Jonassen, I Eidhammer, WR Taylor. Discovery of local packing motifs in protein structures. Proteins 34:206–219, 1999.
48. I Friedberg, H Margalit. Persistently conserved positions in structurally similar, sequence-dissimilar proteins: roles in preserving protein fold and function. Protein Sci 11:350–360, 2002.
49. O Lichtarge, HR Bourne, FE Cohen. An evolutionary trace method defines binding surfaces common to protein families. J Mol Biol 257:342–358, 1996.
50. M de Rinaldis, G Ausiello, G Cesareni, M Helmer-Citterich. Three-dimensional profiles: a new tool to identify protein surface similarities. J Mol Biol 284:1211–1221, 1998.
51. A Kasuya, JM Thornton. Three-dimensional structure analysis of PROSITE patterns. J Mol Biol 286:1673–1691, 1999.
52. I Jonassen, I Eidhammer, SH Grindhaug, WR Taylor. Searching the protein structure databank with weak sequence patterns and structural constraints. J Mol Biol 304:599–619, 2000.
53. JS Fetrow, J Skolnick. Method for prediction of protein function from sequence using the sequence-to-structure-to-function paradigm with application to glutaredoxins/thioredoxins and T1 ribonucleases. J Mol Biol 281:949–968, 1998.
54. B Zhang, L Rychlewski, K Pawlowski, JS Fetrow, J Skolnick, A Godzik. From fold predictions to function predictions: automation of functional site conservation analysis for functional genome predictions. Protein Sci 8:1104–1115, 1999.
55. JS Fetrow, N Siew, J Skolnick. Structure-based functional motif identifies a potential disulfide oxidoreductase active site in the serine/threonine protein phosphatase-1 subfamily. Faseb J 13:1866–1874, 1999.
56. WJ Gehring, M Affolter, T Burglin. Homeodomain proteins. Annu Rev Biochem 63:487–526, 1994.
57. M Sudol, K Sliwa, T Russo. Functions of WW domains in the nucleus. FEBS Lett 490:190–195, 2001.
58. A Bairoch, R Apweiler. The SWISS-PROT protein sequence database and its supplement TrEMBL in 2000. Nucleic Acids Res 28:45–48, 2000.
59. A Bateman, E Birney, L Cerruti, R Durbin, L Etwiller, SR Eddy, S Griffiths-Jones, KL Howe, M Marshall, EL Sonnhammer. The Pfam protein families database. Nucleic Acids Res 30:276–280, 2002.
60. TK Attwood, MJ Blythe, DR Flower, A Gaulton, JE Mabey, N Maudling, L McGregor, AL Mitchell, G Moulton, K Paine, P Scordis. PRINTS and

PRINTS-S shed light on protein ancestry. Nucleic Acids Res 30:239–241, 2002.

61. JG Henikoff, S Pietrokovski, CM McCallum, S Henikoff. Blocks-based methods for detecting protein homology. Electrophoresis 21:1700–1706, 2000.

62. DA Natale, MY Galperin, RL Tatusov, EV Koonin. Using the COG database to improve gene recognition in complete genomes. Genetica 108:9–17, 2000.

63. I Letunic, L Goodstadt, NJ Dickens, T Doerks, J Schultz, R Mott, F Ciccarelli, RR Copley, CP Ponting, P Bork. Recent improvements to the SMART domain-based sequence annotation resource. Nucleic Acids Res 30:242–244, 2002.

64. V Kunin, B Chan, E Sitbon, G Lithwick, S Pietrokovski. Consistency analysis of similarity between multiple alignments: prediction of protein function and fold structure from analysis of local sequence motifs. J Mol Biol 307:939–949, 2001.

65. P Aloy, B Oliva, E Querol, FX Aviles, RB Russell. Structural similarity to link sequence space: new potential superfamilies and implications for structural genomics. Protein Sci 11:1101–1116, 2002.

66. ME Sowa, W He, TG Wensel, O Lichtarge. A regulator of G protein signaling interaction surface linked to effector specificity. Proc Natl Acad Sci USA 97:1483–1488, 2000.

67. ME Sowa, W He, KC Slep, MA Kercher, O Lichtarge, TG Wensel. Prediction and confirmation of a site critical for effector regulation of RGS domain activity. Nat Struct Biol 8:234–237, 2001.

68. R Onrust, P Herzmark, P Chi, PD Garcia, O Lichtarge, C Kingsley, HR Bourne. Receptor and betagamma binding sites in the alpha subunit of the retinal G protein transducin. Science 275:381–384, 1997.

69. KC Slep, MA Kercher, W He, CW Cowan, TG Wensel, PB Sigler. Structural determinants for regulation of phosphodiesterase by a G protein at 2.0 Å. Nature 409:1071–1077, 2001.

70. A Armon, D Graur, N Ben-Tal. ConSurf: an algorithmic tool for the identification of functional regions in proteins by surface mapping of phylogenetic information. J Mol Biol 307:447–463, 2001.

71. S Madabushi, H Yao, M Marsh, DM Kristensen, A Philippi, ME Sowa, O Lichtarge. Structural clusters of evolutionary trace residues are statistically significant and common in proteins. J Mol Biol 316:139–154, 2002.

72. P Aloy, E Querol, FX Aviles, MJ Sternberg. Automated structure-based prediction of functional sites in proteins: applications to assessing the validity of inheriting protein function from homology in genome annotation and to protein docking. J Mol Biol 311:395–408, 2001.

73. R Landgraf, I Xenarios, D Eisenberg. Three-dimensional cluster analysis identifies interfaces and functional residue clusters in proteins. J Mol Biol 307:1487–1502, 2001.

74. GJ Kleywegt. Recognition of spatial motifs in protein structures. J Mol Biol 285:1887–1897, 1999.

75. J Skolnick, D Kihara. Defrosting the frozen approximation: PROSPECTOR—a new approach to threading. Proteins 42:319–331, 2001.

76. JS Fetrow, A Godzik, J Skolnick. Functional analysis of the *Escherichia coli* genome using the sequence-to-structure-to-function paradigm: identification of proteins exhibiting the glutaredoxin/thioredoxin disulfide oxidoreductase activity. J Mol Biol 282:703–711, 1998.

77. G Muller. Towards 3D structures of G protein-coupled receptors: a multidisciplinary approach. Curr Med Chem 7:861–888, 2000.

78. AJ Turner, RE Isaac, D Coates. The neprilysin (NEP) family of zinc metalloendopeptidases: genomics and function. Bioessays 23:261–269, 2001.

79. M Ridderstrom, I Zamora, O Fjellstrom, TB Andersson. Analysis of selective regions in the active sites of human cytochromes P450, 2C8, 2C9, 2C18, and 2C19 homology models using GRID/CPCA. J Med Chem 44:4072–4081, 2001.

80. AC Gavin, M Bosche, R Krause, P Grandi, M Marzioch, A Bauer, J Schultz, JM Rick, AM Michon, CM Cruciat, M Remor, C Hofert, M Schelder, M Brajenovic, H Ruffner, A Merino, K Klein, M Hudak, D Dickson, T Rudi, V Gnau, A Bauch, S Bastuck, B Huhse, C Leutwein, MA Heurtier, RR Copley, A Edelmann, E Querfurth, V Rybin, G Drewes, M Raida, T Bouwmeester, P Bork, B Seraphin, B Kuster, G Neubauer, G Superti-Furga. Functional organization of the yeast proteome by systematic analysis of protein complexes. Nature 415:141–147, 2002.

81. P Aloy, RB Russell. Interrogating protein interaction networks through structural biology. Proc Natl Acad Sci USA 23:23, 2002.

82. I Xenarios, D Eisenberg. Protein interaction databases. Curr Opin Biotechnol 12:334–339, 2001.

83. D Chasman, RM Adams. Predicting the functional consequences of nonsynonymous single nucleotide polymorphisms: structure-based assessment of amino acid variation. J Mol Biol 307:683–706, 2001.

84. PC Ng, S Henikoff. Predicting deleterious amino acid substitutions. Genome Res 11:863–74, 2001.

14

The Protein Data Bank

Helen M. Berman, John Westbrook, and Christine Zardecki
Rutgers, The State University of New Jersey, Piscataway, New Jersey, U.S.A.

Philip E. Bourne
University of California, San Diego, La Jolla, California, U.S.A.

1 INTRODUCTION

The Protein Data Bank (PDB) (1) is the single international repository for the three-dimensional structure data of biological macromolecules determined experimentally. Resources for depositing, extracting, and analyzing data from the PDB are available at no cost from PDB mirrors worldwide. This chapter describes the history and current state of the PDB, the systems that manage the data, and the future plans of the PDB.

2 HISTORY

In 1971, the Protein Data Bank began as a simple archive of seven crystal structures (2) that was made available on digital tape. Since then, the PDB has developed into a sophisticated resource with scalable systems that manage a high influx of data. At the time of this writing, the database contained over 14,500 entries. As the repository for the three-dimensional data of biological macromolecules, the PDB is responsible for the curation and dissemination of these data; it additionally provides tools for analyzing and understanding these structures.

The PDB began out of a grassroots movement among crystallographers. At crystallography meetings held in the early 1970s, informal discussion began about the creation of a repository that would disseminate information about protein structure. Through these conversations, the Protein Data Bank was born, with the mission to collect, archive, and disseminate data about the three-dimensional structures of biological macromolecules. Walter Hamilton of the Brookhaven National Laboratory and Olga Kennard of the Cambridge Structural Database (CSD) (3) collaborated to manage the resource (4), which was housed at Brookhaven.

By 1976, the PDB had emerged as a full-fledged international resource that had funding from the National Science Foundation and contained 23 entries in the archive. A relatively simple file format was created to hold the available information about a structure. Data in this format were distributed to 31 laboratories during that year.

In the 1980s, the number of structures in the PDB began to grow as the technology used for experiments and structure determination began to improve. The user community started to discuss mandatory depositions and guidelines that needed to be in place. By the mid-1990s, the PDB began to substantially increase in size (Fig. 1). This was due to the improved technology for all aspects of the crystallographic process, the addition of structures determined by nuclear magnetic resonance (NMR) methods, and changes in the community views about data sharing. By the early 1990s the majority of journals required a PDB accession code, and at least one funding agency (National Institute of General Medical Sciences) adopted the guidelines published by the International Union of Crystallography (IUCr) requiring data deposition for all structures. The information that needed to be recorded began to strain against the limits of the PDB format;

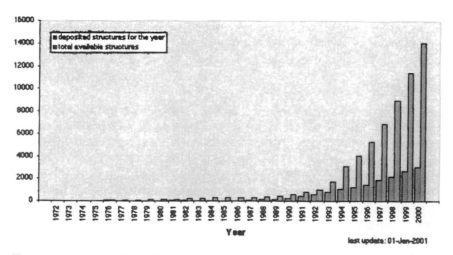

Figure 1   Growth of the PDB.

as a result, the Macromolecular Crystallographic Information File format was developed (mmCIF) (5). The mmCIF format is based upon the mmCIF dictionary, which is an ontology of 1700 terms that define macromolecular structure and the crystallographic experiment.

In October 1998, the management of the PDB became the responsibility of the Research Collaboratory for Structural Bioinformatics (RCSB). The vision of the RCSB is to create a resource based on the most modern technology that facilitates the use and analysis of structural data and thus creates an enabling resource for biological research. The PDB is operated by Rutgers, the State University of New Jersey, the National Institute of Standards and Technology, and the San Diego Supercomputer Center at the University of California, San Diego—three members of the RCSB.

3 CURRENT PDB HOLDINGS

The PDB contains structures determined by X-ray diffraction, NMR, theoretical modeling, and other techniques, such as cryoelectron microscopy. The structures include proteins, peptides, viruses, nucleic acid–containing structures, and carbohydrates. The distribution of these structures is shown in Table 1.

The data are collected from the depositors, who determine the structures. These data include the three-dimensional coordinates and general information specific to each entry (Table 2). Information specific to X-ray and NMR experiments is recorded, and unique data items to be collected from other types of experiments are being developed. The data collected are made available in each entry's released structure file and through various output options made possible by the PDB search engines.

Table 1 PDB Holdings as of March 6, 2001

	Proteins, peptides, and viruses	Nucleic acid complexes	Nucleic acids	Carbohydrates	Total
X-ray diffraction and other	10,926	521	552	14	12,013
NMR	1,810	70	354	4	2,238
Theoretical modeling	278	19	21	0	318
Total	13,014	610	927	18	14,569

Table 2 Content of Data in the PDB

Content of all depositions (X-ray and NMR)

Source: specifications such as genus, species, strain, or variant of gene (cloned or synthetic); expression vector and host, or description of method of chemical synthesis
Sequence: full sequence of all macromolecular components
Chemical name and formula of cofactors and prosthetic groups
Names of all components in structure
Qualitative description of characteristics of structure
Literature citations for the structure submitted
Three-dimensional coordinates

Additional items: X-ray depositions	Additional items: NMR depositions
Temperature factors and occupancies assigned to each atom	Designation of an energy-minimized average model or ensemble. If an ensemble is provided, the model number for each coordinate set that is deposited and an indication if one should be designated as a representative.
Crystallization conditions, including pH, temperature, solvents, salts, methods	Data collection information describing the types of methods used, instrumentation, magnetic field strength, console, probe head, sample tube
Crystal data, including the unit cell dimensions and space group	Sample conditions, including solvent, macromolecule concentration ranges, concentration ranges of buffers, salts, other components, isotopic composition
Presence of noncrystallographic symmetry	Experimental conditions, including temperature, pH, pressure, and oxidation state of structure determination and estimates of uncertainties in these values
Data collection information describing the methods used to collect the diffraction data, including instrument, wavelength, temperature, and processing programs	Noncovalent heterogeneity of sample, including self-aggregation, partial isotope exchange, conformational heterogeneity resulting in slow chemical exchange

Additional items: X-ray depositions	Additional items: NMR depositions
Data collection statistics, including data coverage, R_{sym}, data above 1, 2, 3 sigma levels, and resolution limits	Chemical heterogeneity of the sample (e.g., evidence for deamidation or minor covalent species)
Refinement information including R factor, resolution limits, number of reflections, method of refinement, sigma cutoff, geometrical targets, rmsd's, and sigmas	A list of NMR experiments used to determine the structure, including those used to determine resonance assignments, NOE/ROE data, dynamical data, scalar coupling constants, and those used to infer hydrogen bonds and bound ligands. The relationship of these experiments to the constraint files are given explicitly
Structure factors: h, k, l, Fobs, σ Fobs	Constraint files used to derive the structure

4 DATA DEPOSITION, VALIDATION, AND PROCESSING

The data contained in the PDB are deposited directly by the author. In many cases, data deposition is a requirement for publication and funding. The current deposition system is shown in Figure 2. The user deposits the atomic coordinates and the experimental data (with an optional validation step), generally using the AutoDep Input Tool (ADIT (6)). The entry is then annotated by the PDB staff using ADIT according to the steps listed next (Fig. 2).

When a depositor completes an ADIT deposition session, a PDB identifier is immediately returned to the author (Step 1). The information about the structure is loaded into the internal core database, and the PDB staff uses ADIT to help diagnose errors or inconsistencies in the files. The completely annotated entry as it will appear in the PDB resource, together with the validation information, is sent back to the depositor (Step 2). After reviewing the processed file, the author sends any revisions (Step 3). Depending on the nature of these revisions, Steps 2 and 3 may be repeated. All aspects of data processing, including the author communications, are recorded and stored in a correspondence archive. Once approval is received from the author (Step 4), the entry and the tables in the internal core

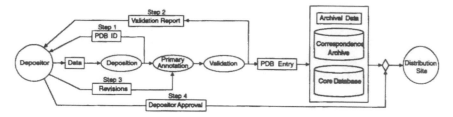

Figure 2   Data-processing steps, from depositor to release.

database are ready for distribution. The schema of this core database is a subset of the conceptual schema specified by the mmCIF dictionary.

The integrated ADIT system helps to ensure that the data submitted are consistent with the mmCIF dictionary, which defines data types, enumerates ranges of allowable values where possible, and describes allowable relationships between data values.

ADIT's validation step involves assessing the quality of deposited atomic models (geometric validation) and how well these models fit the experimental data (experimental validation). The PDB validates structures using accepted community standards as part of ADIT's integrated data-processing system (Table 3). The structure is also run through PROCHECK (7), NUCheck (8), and SFCHECK (9). The results of these checks are summarized in a report and sent to the author for review. As a result, changes can be incorporated in an entry before release. A summary atlas page and molecular graphics are also produced for review by the PDB annotator.

These checks and reports can also be run independently by the user before a structure is deposited to the PDB. The Validation Server is available over the Web at http://deposit.pdb.org/validate/. The software will also be made available online for downloading.

5   DATABASE ARCHITECTURE

The data are stored and organized into an integrated system of heterogeneous databases (Fig. 3). Queries to the PDB using the query interfaces are sent to the appropriate database in a way that is transparent to the user. This is achieved through a common gateway interface (CGI). The databases in this system include:

> *Keyword searching*: A Netscape LDAP server is used to provide keyword searching.

Table 3 Validation Checks

Covalent bond distances and angles	Proteins are compared against standard values from Engh and Huber (Ref. 23); nucleic acid bases are compared against standard values from Clowney et al. (Ref. 25); sugar and phosphates are compared against standard values from Gelbin et al. (Ref. 26).
Stereochemical validation	All chiral centers of proteins and nucleic acids are checked for correct stereochemistry.
Atom nomenclature	The nomenclature of all atoms is checked for compliance with IUPAC standards (Ref. 27) and is adjusted if necessary.
Close contacts	The distances between all atoms within the asymmetric unit of crystal structures and the unique molecule of NMR structures are calculated. For crystal structures, contacts between symmetry-related molecules are checked as well.
Ligand atom nomenclature	Residue and atom nomenclature is compared against the PDB dictionary (ftp://ftp.rcsb.org/pub/pdb/data/monomers/het_dictionary.txt) for all ligands as well as standard residues and bases. Unrecognized ligand groups are flagged, and any discrepancies in known ligands are listed as extra or missing atoms.
Sequence comparison	The sequence given in the PDB SEQRES records is compared against the sequence derived from the coordinate records. This information is displayed in a table where any differences or missing residues are marked. During structure processing, a BLAST (Ref. 28) search is used to find the best match of the given sequence and the sequence database references. Any conflict between the PDB SEQRES records and the sequence derived from the coordinate records is resolved by comparison with various sequence databases. Unresolved discrepancies are noted.
Distant waters	The distances between all water oxygen atoms and all polar atoms (oxygen and nitrogen) of the macromolecules, ligands, and solvent in the asymmetric unit are calculated. Distant solvent atoms are repositioned using crystallographic symmetry such that they fall within the solvation sphere of the macromolecule.

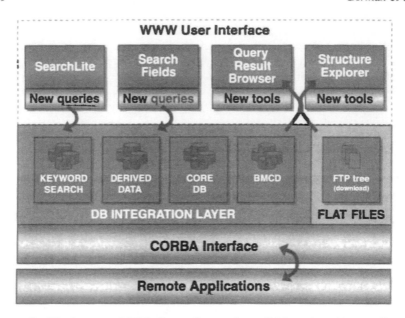

Figure 3 The integrated PDB Query System is available at http://www.pdb.org/ pdb/. A user query (from SearchLite or SearchFields) is transparently passed on to one or more of several underlying databases optimized to efficiently return different types of data (Query Result Browser and Structure Explorer pages). An interface for use by other databases and applications is currently under development, as well as new query capabilities and analysis tools.

Derived data: The POM (Property Object Model) (10) database contains indexed objects with native and derived properties. The indexing system saves considerable user access time.

A core database: The central database is a relational database managed by Sybase (11). It contains the primary experimental and coordinate data in tabular form.

BMCD: The Biological Macromolecule Crystallization Database (12) contains macromolecular, crystal, and summary data organized as a relational Sybase database.

FTP tree: The released files in final curated form (in mmCIF and PDB formats) are contained in the archive for downloading via FTP and access by the database system.

6 DATA QUERY AND REPORTING

The PDB provides a portal to general information about single structures, substructures, multiple structures, and their interrelationships. The site offers several different interfaces that can be used to query the database. The simplest search is performed by entering the PDB ID of the desired molecule. PDB IDs are generally published in the papers that describe the structure. If a user does not know the PDB ID of a particular structure or would like to search for a group of structures, two other search interfaces are available.

SearchLite provides a simple keyword search function. A single form is provided to search for all textual information contained within the PDB files. The user can enter a word or phrase, such as "protein kinase," and SearchLite will return a list of all of the files that contain it. The searches can be iterative and can also be constructed to limit the keyword searching to certain PDB file attributes, such as Author and Experimental Technique.

SearchFields is used for more detailed searches. The user can build the interface by selecting the fields, which are specific data items or areas, on which to search. The default interface includes the options for searching on citation author, chain type (i.e., protein, enzyme, nucleic acid), and compound information. Other fields available for searching include data items for general information (including deposition and release dates, EC number and classification), sequence and secondary structure (including chain length, FASTA search, sequence pattern, secondary structure content), and crystallographic experimental information (resolution, space group, unit cell dimensions, and refinement parameters).

The results of these searches can be explored by examining individual structures or by reporting on a set of multiple structures. Each structure in the PDB has a *Structure Explorer* entry, which provides several different ways of looking at a structure on different pages. The *Summary Information* page outlines general details of an entry: structural, citation, and experimental information. Interactive displays and prepared static images are available from the *View Structure* page. PDB structures can be interactively viewed using VRML, RasMol (13,14), Chime (MDL Information Systems, Inc.), Protein Explorer (http://proteinexplorer.org/), and a Java applet called QuickPDB (Shindyalov and Bourne, unpublished). Prepared images produced from MolScript (15) and Raster3D (16,17) are available in customizable sizes. The *Download/Display File* option provides quick access to the coordinate file in mmCIF or PDB format. The *Structural Neighbors* page provides access to the most common methods for finding and analyzing structures that have 3D structural similarity to the protein currently being explored, including CATH (18), CE (19), FSSP (20), SCOP (21), and VAST

(22). The *Geometry* section gives details of the geometry of the structure under study in either tabular or graphical form. Bond lengths, bond angles, and dihedral angles for proteins are compared to values determined from small-molecule data of amino acids, peptides, and small proteins (23). The *Other Sources* page cross-links to external resources for macromolecular structure data (Table 4). Each PDB entry is processed through the Molecular Information Agent (MIA; http://mia.sdsc.edu/) to generate a set of links or references pertaining to that particular structure. The results are then stored in a database that is accessed by the *Other Sources* page. These links are updated periodically. *Sequence Details* for each chain, including molecular weight, are provided and can be downloaded in FASTA format. For structures that are also in the NDB, the *NDB Atlas Entry* and *Quick Reports* for backbone torsion angles, base pair parameters, and groove dimensions are available. Links to the experimental data and/or any previous version of the entry are provided.

The *Query Result Browser* allows a user to examine multiple structures in a query result as a set. Customizable tabular reports and predefined tabular reports for cell dimensions, primary citation, structure identifier, sequence, experimental technique, and refinement information can be created. The entire set of data files can be downloaded as mmCIF or PDB structure files, as can the sequences in FASTA format. Further queries can also be done on the selected set of structures. Each structure in the *Query Result Browser* can also be examined using the *Structure Explorer* pages.

The *Structure Explorer* and *Query Result Browser* interfaces are accessible to other data resources through a simple CGI application programmer interface (API) described at http://www.rcsb.org/pdb/linking.html. The remote user or application program simply provides one or more PDB IDs as part of a URL Web address.

7   DISTRIBUTION

Data are released from the PDB FTP and Websites. These sites are updated weekly with the latest release of coordinate files, structure factor files, and NMR constraint data. The Website additionally provides resources and links to structural genomics sites. PDB mirrors, located around the world, are listed at http://www.rcsb.org/pdb/mirrors.html. The PDB is also distributed quarterly on CD-ROM. Details are available at http://www.rcsb.org/pdb/cdrom.html.

Table 4 Cross-Links to Other Data Resources Currently Provided by the PDB

Resource	Information content
3dee (Ref. 29)	Structural domain definitions
BMCD (Ref. 12)	Crystallization information about biomacromolecules
castP (Ref. 30)	Identification of protein pockets and cavities
CATH (Ref. 18)	Structural classifications
CE (Ref. 19)	Complete PDB and representative structure comparison and alignments
Columbia Picture Gallery (http://trantor.bioc.columbia.edu/GRASS/surfserv_info.cgi)	Static surface images generated by GRASP (Ref. 31)
CSU (Ref. 32)	Analysis of interatomic contacts in protein entries
DSSP (Ref. 33)	Secondary structure classification
EMBL (Ref. 34)	Nucleotide sequence database
Enzyme Structures Database (http://www.biochem.ucl.ac.uk/bsm/enzymes/)	Enzyme classifications and nomenclature
FSSP (Ref. 20)	Structurally similar families
GenBank (Ref. 35)	Nucleotide sequence database
GeneCensus (Ref. 36)	Genome occurrence of fold
GRASS (Ref. 37)	Graphical representation and analysis
HSSP (Ref. 38)	Homology-derived secondary structures
Image (Ref. 39)	Image library of biological macromolecules
LPC (Ref. 32)	Analysis of interatomic contacts in ligand–protein complexes

Table 4 *Continued*

Resource	Information content
MMDB (Ref. 40)	Database of three-dimensional structures
Medline (Ref. 41)	Direct access to Medline at NCBI
NCBI Taxonomy (Refs. 35 and 42)	Taxonomy
NDB (Ref. 43)	Database of three-dimensional nucleic acid structures
PDBObs (Ref. 44)	Obsolete-structures database
PDBREPORT (Ref. 45)	WHATCHECK reports
PDBSum (Ref. 46)	Summary information about protein structures
PIR (Ref. 47)	Sequence data
PQS (Ref. 48)	Quaternary structures of macromolecules
PROCHECK (Ref. 49)	Structure summary
ProClass (Ref. 50)	Family information
PRODOC (Ref. 51)	Prosite information
PRODOM (Ref. 52)	Graphic output of domain arrangements
PROMOTIF (Ref. 53)	Analyzing protein structural motifs
ProfileScan (http://www.isrec.isb-sib.ch/software/PFSCAN_form.html)	Profile search
PROSITE (Ref. 51)	Protein signature
Protomap (Ref. 54)	Family and cluster information
ScanProsite (Ref. 55)	Prosite pattern search
SCOP (Ref. 21)	Structure classifications

Resource	Information content
STING (Ref. 56)	Simultaneous display of structural and sequence information
SWISS-MODEL (Ref. 57)	Structure model
SWISS-PROT (Ref. 58)	Sequence data
Tops (Ref. 59)	Protein structure motif comparisons and topological diagrams
VAST (Ref. 22)	Vector alignment search tool (NCBI)

8 EDUCATION AND OUTREACH

The PDB is dedicated to providing a better understanding of biological macromolecules. A collaboration with David Goodsell of the Scripps Institute produces the PDB's *Molecule of the Month*, which explores and illustrates a key biological molecule for a general audience. The PDB continually develops its education section, which brings together basic information on proteins and nucleic acids for general audiences and resources for more advanced audiences.

The PDB Website is updated weekly with news of interest to PDB users. PDB newsletters are distributed quarterly in electronic and print form (see http://www.rcsb.org/pdb/forum.html for more information). Questions and comments about the PDB should be sent to info@rcsb.org.

9 FUTURE

These are exciting and challenging times to be responsible for the collection, curation, and distribution of macromolecular structure data. It is expected that improved technologies and experimental methods will accelerate the growth of the number of structures in the coming years. It is estimated that the PDB could grow to approximately 35,000 structures by 2005, which would nearly triple its size in less than five years. One major factor in this growth is the advent of structural genomics, whose goal is to determine the structures of as many of the proteins accessible from a given genome in the shortest time possible. This promises to greatly increase the amount of information that needs to be archived within the PDB, presenting a huge challenge to the timely distribution of high-quality data. The PDB's approach of using modern data-management practices should permit it to scale to accommodate a large data influx (24). The application of modern data-mining methods to the growing archive will provide new and perhaps unexpected information about biological structure and function.

ACKNOWLEDGEMENTS

The PDB is supported by funds from the National Science Foundation, the Office of Biology and Environmental Research at the Department of Energy, and two units of the National Institutes of Health: the National Institute of General Medical Sciences and the National Library of Medicine.

At the time of writing, current RCSB PDB staff include the authors indicated and Peter Arzberger, T.N. Bhat, Gary Gilliland, Bryan Bannister, Tammy Battistuz, Wolfgang Bluhm, Kyle Burkhardt, Li Chen, Haiyan Cheng, Victoria Colflesh, Nita Deshpande, Zukang Feng, Ward Fleri, Douglas Greer, Michahel Gribskov, Diane Hancock, Lisa Iype, Shri Jain, Jessica Marvin, Gnanesh Patel, Veerasamy Ravichandran, Bohdan Schneider, David Padilla, Lynn F. Ten Eyck, Michael Tung, Rosalina Valera, Lincong Wang, and Helge Weissig. PDB staff are listed at http://www.rcsb.org/pdb/rcsb-group.html.

REFERENCES

1. Berman, H. M., Westbrook, J., Feng, Z., Gilliland, G., Bhat, T. N., Weissig, H., Shindyalov, I. N., and Bourne, P. E. (2000) The Protein Data Bank. Nucleic Acids Res. 28:235–242.
2. Bernstein, F. C., Koetzle, T. F., Williams, G. J., Meyer, E. E., Brice, M. D., Rodgers, J. R., Kennard, O., Shimanouchi, T., and Tasumi, M. (1977) Protein Data Bank: a computer-based archival file for macromolecular structures. J. Mol. Biol. 112:535–542.
3. Allen, F. H., Bellard, S., Brice, M. D., Cartright, B. A., Doubleday, A., Higgs, H., Hummelink, T., Hummelink-Peters, B. G., Kennard, O., Motherwell, W. D. S., Rodgers, J. R., and Watson, D. G. (1979) The Cambridge Crystallographic Data Centre: computer-based search, retrieval, analysis and display of information. Acta Crystallogr. B35:2331–2339.
4. (1971) Protein Data Bank. Nature New Biol. 233:223.
5. Bourne, P., Berman, H. M., Watenpaugh, K., Westbrook, J. D., and Fitzgerald, P. M. D. (1997) The macromolecular Crystallographic Information File (mmCIF). Meth. Enzymol. 277:571–590.
6. Westbrook, J., Feng, Z., and Berman, H. M. (1998) ADIT—The AutoDep Input Tool. Department of Chemistry, Rutgers, University, New Brunswick, NJ.
7. Laskowski, R. A., McArthur, M. W., Moss, D. S., and Thornton, J. M. (1993) PROCHECK: a program to check the stereochemical quality of protein structures. J. Appl. Cryst. 26:283–291.

8. Feng, Z., Westbrook, J., and Berman, H. M. (1998) NUCheck. Rutgers University, New Brunswick, NJ.

9. Vaguine, A. A., Richelle, J., and Wodak, S. J. (1999) SFCHECK: a unified set of procedures for evaluating the quality of macromolecular structure–factor data and their agreement with the atomic model. Acta Crystallogr. D55:191–205.

10. Shindyalov, I. N., and Bourne, P. E. (1997) Protein data representation and query using optimized data decomposition. CABIOS 13:487–496.

11. Sybase, Inc. (1995) SYBASE SQL server release 11.0. Emeryville, CA.

12. Gilliland, G. L. (1988) A Biological Macromolecule Crystallization Database: a basis for a crystallization strategy. J. Cryst. Growth 90:51–59.

13. Sayle, R., and Milner-White, E. J. (1995) RasMol: biomolecular graphics for all. Trends Biochem. Sci. 20:374.

14. Bernstein, H. J. (2000) Recent changes to RasMol, recombining the variants. Trends Biochem. Sci. 25:453–455.

15. Kraulis, P. (1991) MOLSCRIPT: a program to produce both detailed and schematic plots of protein structures. J. Appl. Cryst. 24:946–950.

16. Bacon, D. J., and Anderson, W. F. (1988) A fast algorithm for rendering space-filling molecule pictures. J. Mol. Graphics 6:219–220.

17. Merrit, E. A., and Bacon, D. J. (1997) Raster3D: photorealistic molecular graphics. Meth. Enzymol. 277:505–524.

18. Orengo, C. A., Michie, A. D., Jones, S., Jones, D. T., Swindells, M. B., and Thornton, J. M. (1997) CATH—a hierarchic classification of protein domain structures. Structure 5:1093–1108.

19. Shindyalov, I. N., and Bourne, P. E. (1998) Protein structure alignment by incremental combinatory extension of the optimum path. Protein Eng. 11:739–747.

20. Holm, L., and Sander, C. (1998) Touring protein fold space with Dali/FSSP. Nucleic Acids Res. 26:316–319.

21. Murzin, A. G., Brenner, S. E., Hubbard, T., and Chothia, C. (1995) SCOP: a structural classification of proteins database for the investigation of sequences and structures. J. Mol. Biol. 247:536–540.

22. Gibrat, J.-F., Madej, T., and Bryant, S. H. (1996) Surprising similarities in structure comparison. Curr. Opin. Struct. Biol. 6:377–385.

23. Engh, R. A., and Huber, R. (1991) Accurate bond and angle parameters for X-ray protein structure refinement. Acta Crystallogr. A47:392–400.

24. Berman, H. M., Bhat, T. N., Bourne, P. E., Feng, Z., Gilliland, G., Weissig, H., and Westbrook, J. (2000) The Protein Data Bank and the challenge of structural genomics. Nat. Struct. Biol. 7:957–959.

25. Clowney, L., Jain, S. C., Srinivasan, A. R., Westbrook, J., Olson, W. K., and Berman, H. M. (1996) Geometric parameters in nucleic acids: nitrogenous bases. J. Am. Chem. Soc. 118:509–518.

26. Gelbin, A., Schneider, B., Clowney, L., Hsieh, S.-H., Olson, W. K., and Berman, H. M. (1996) Geometric parameters in nucleic acids: sugar and phosphate constituents. J. Am. Chem. Soc. 118(3):519–528.

27. IUPAC-IUB Joint Commission on Biochemical Nomenclature. (1983) Abbreviations and symbols for the description of conformations of polynucleotide chains. Eur. J. Biochem. 131:9–15.

28. Altschul, S. F., Gish, W., Miller, W., Myers, E. W., and Lipman, D. J. (1990) Basic local alignment search tool. J. Mol. Biol. 215:403–410.

29. Siddiqui, A., and Barton, G. (1996) 3Dee—a domain database. Perspectives on Protein Engineering 1996 2, (CD-ROM edition; Geisow, M.J. ed.) BIODIGM Ltd (UK).

30. Liang, J., Edelsbrunner, H., and Woodward, C. (1998) Anatomy of protein pockets and cavities: measurement of binding site geometry and implications for ligand design. Protein Sci. 7:1884–1897.

31. Nicholls, A., Bharadwaj, R., and Honig, B. (1993) GRASP: a graphical representation and analysis of surface properties. Biophys. J. 64:166–170.

32. Sobolev, V., Sorokine, A., Prilusky, J., Abola, E. E., and Edelman, M. (1999) Automated analysis of interatomic contacts in proteins. Bioinformatics 15:327–332.

33. Kabsch, W., and Sander, C. (1983) Dictionary of protein secondary structure: pattern recognition of hydrogen-bonded and geometrical features. Biopolymers 22:2577–2637.

34. Hamm, G. H., and Cameron, G. N. (1986) The EMBL data library. Nucleic Acids Res. 14:5–10.

35. Benson, D. A., Karsch-Mizrachi, I., Lipman, D. J., Ostell, J., Rapp, B. A., and Wheeler, D. L. (2000) GenBank. Nucleic Acids Res. 28:15–18.

36. Gerstein, M. (1998) How representative are the known structures of the proteins in a complete genome? A comprehensive structural census. Fold Des. 3:497–512.

37. Nayal, M., Hitz, B. C., and Honig, B. (1999) GRASS: A server for the graphical representation and analysis of structures. Protein Sci. 1999:676–679.

38. Dodge, C., Schneider, R., and Sander, C. (1998) The HSSP database of protein structure–sequence alignments and family profiles. Nucleic Acids Res. 26:313–315.

39. Sühnel, J. (1996) Image library of biological macromolecules. Comput. Appl. Biosci. 12:227–229.

40. Hogue, C., Ohkawa, H., and Bryant, S. (1996) A dynamic look at structures: WWW-Entrez and the Molecular Modeling Database. Trends Biochem. Sci. 21:226–229.

41. National Library of Medicine. (1989) MEDLINE [database online]. Bethesda, MD. Updated weekly. Available from: National Library of Medicine; OVID, Murray, UT; The Dialog Corporation, Palo Alto, CA.

42. Wheeler, D. L., Chappey, C., Lash, A. E., Leipe, D. D., Madden, T. L., Schuler, G. D., Tatusova, T. A., and Rapp, B. A. (2000) Database resources of the National Center for Biotechnology Information. Nucleic Acids Res. 28:10–14.

43. Berman, H. M., Olson, W. K., Beveridge, D. L., Westbrook, J., Gelbin, A., Demeny, T., Hsieh, S. H., Srinivasan, A. R., and Schneider, B. (1992) The

Nucleic Acid Database—a comprehensive relational database of three-dimensional structures of nucleic acids. Biophys. J. 63:751–759.

44. Weissig, H., Shindyalov, I. N., and Bourne, P. E. (1998) Macromolecular structure databases: past progress and future challenges. Acta Cryst. 54:1085–1094.

45. Hooft, R. W., Vriend, G., Sander, C., and Abola, E. E. (1996) Errors in protein structures. Nature 381:272.

46. Laskowski, R. A., Hutchinson, E. G., Michie, A. D., Wallace, A. C., Jones, M. L., and Thornton, J. M. (1997) PDBsum: a Web-based database of summaries and analyses of all PDB structures. Trends Biochem. Sci. 22:488–490.

47. Barker, W. C., Garavelli, J. S., Haft, D. H., Hunt, L. T., Marzec, C. R., Orcutt, B. C., Srinivasarao, G. Y., Yeh, L. S. L., Ledley, R. S., Mewes, H. W., Pfeiffer, F., and Tsugita, A. (1998) The PIR-International Protein Sequence Database. Nucleic Acids Res. 26:27–32.

48. Henrick, K., and Thornton, J. M. (1998) PQS: A protein quarternary file server. Trends Biochem. Sci. 23:358–361.

49. Laskowski, R. A., Rullmann, J. A., MacArthur, M. W., Kaptein, R., and Thornton, J. M. (1996) AQUA and PROCHECK-NMR: programs for checking the quality of protein structures solved by NMR. J. Biomol. NMR 8:477–486.

50. Wu, C., Shivakumar, S., and Huang, H. (1999) ProClass protein family database. Nucleic Acids Res. 27:272–274.

51. Hofmann, K., Bucher, P., Falquet, L., and Bairoch, A. (1999) The PROSITE database, its status in 1999. Nucleic Acids Res. 27:215–219.

52. Corpet, F., Gouzy, J., and Kahn, D. (1999) Recent improvements of the ProDom database of protein domain families. Nucleic Acids Res. 27:263–267.

53. Hutchinson, E. G., and Thornton, J. M. (1996) PROMOTIF—a program to identify and analyze structural motifs in proteins. Protein Sci. 5:212–220.

54. Yona, G., Linial, N., Linial, M., and Tishby, N. (1998) A map of protein space—an automatic hierarchical classification of all protein sequences. ISMB 6:212–221.

55. Appel, R. D., Bairoch, A., and Hoschstrasser, D. F. (1994) A new generation of information retrieval tools for biologists: the example of the ExPASy WWW server. Trends Biochem. Sci. 19:258–260.

56. Neshich, G., Togawa, R., Vilella, W., and Honig, B. (1998) STING (Sequence To and withIN Graphics) PDB_Viewer. Protein Data Bank Quarterly Newsletter 85:6–7.

57. Guex, N., and Peitsch, M. C. (1997) SWISS-MODEL and the Swiss-PdbViewer: an environment for comparative protein modeling. Electrophoresis 18:2714–2723.

58. Bairoch, A., and Boeckmann, B. (1994) The SWISS-PROT protein sequence databank: current status. Nucleic Acids Res. 22:3578–3580.

59. Westhead, D., Slidel, T., Flores, T., and Thorton, J. (1998) Protein structural topology: automated analysis and diagrammatic representation. Protein Sci. 8:897–904.

15

The European Bioinformatics Institute Macromolecular Structure Database (E-MSD)

Dimitris Dimitropoulos, Peter A. Keller, Kim Henrick,
John Ionides, Eugene Krissinel, Philip McNeil, and
Sameer S. Velankar
EMBL–European Bioinformatics Institute, Hinxton, Cambridgeshire,
United Kingdom

The European Bioinformatics Institute (http://www.ebi.ac.uk) was established in 1995 as a home for a large set of biological databases covering a broad range of topics, from nucleotide sequence to protein function. From its inception the EBI hosted the EMBL nucleotide sequence database (1) and TREMBL-SWISSPROT (2). The E-MSD (EBI-Macromolecular Structure Database, http://msd.ebi.ac.uk) was set up in 1996 to give Europe an autonomous facility to collect, organize, and make available data about macromolecular structures and to integrate better biological macromolecular coordinate data with the other databases already at the EBI. Since then, the E-MSD group has been working in three main areas:

> Accepting and processing depositions to the Protein Data Bank (PDB)
> Transforming the PDB flat file archive to a relational database system
> Developing services to search the PDB

1 ACCEPTING AND PROCESSING DEPOSITIONS TO THE PROTEIN DATA BANK (PDB)

In 1996 the PDB franchise was held by Brookhaven National Laboratories (BNL). One of the first projects at the E-MSD was to set up a local copy of

AutoDep, the PDB Web deposition interface developed at BNL, in order to improve the ease of deposition to the PDB for European groups. From early 1998 the E-MSD essentially provided a mirror that, at the end of the deposition process, forwarded the raw data files to BNL, where they were compiled into a PDB entry. During 1998 there were 2201 depositions to the PDB, 534 (24%) of which were routed through EBI in this fashion.

During 1999 the PDB franchise was transferred to the current holders, the RCSB (http://www.rcsb.org), who had developed the ADIT deposition interface (3). At the same time, AutoDep at the E-MSD was upgraded so that by June 1999 the raw files produced by AutoDep were processed to complete PDB entries locally and the finished PDB files were forwarded to the RCSB for inclusion in the weekly public release. Since then 1148 of the 7149 new depositions to the PDB have been processed by the E-MSD and integrated into the PDB archive in this manner, and currently 20% of depositions are processed at the EBI.

As soon as there is more than one deposition site feeding in to the PDB, it becomes critical that mechanisms are put in place to ensure that the archive maintains its unity. This was a particular concern for the PDB because the PDB file format is not rigorously defined and easily lends itself to a multiple interpretations. The model that the E-MSD and the RCSB have adopted is to define the set of mmCIF (4) data items that must be present to define a PDB format entry. This so-called *exchange dictionary* is maintained as an mmCIF dictionary extension and so defines the set of mmCIF items that would be required to reconstruct a PDB entry. PDB entries processed at the EBI are sent to the RCSB in mmCIF format, and the PDB format archive is best considered as a view on the mmCIF-format archive. Any deposition interface that can supply these items can therefore feed into the PDB, but there is no restriction against a given interface collecting more data or developing new annotation methods.

An upgraded version of AutoDep was released in April 2001. The new version, AutoDep 3.0, is considerably simplified; it no longer requests information that can be derived from the coordinates (e.g., secondary structure and disulphide bonds), and the vast majority of the data fields may be populated directly from uploaded CNS and CCP4 harvest files. These modifications have drastically reduced the time it takes to complete a deposition; a deposition will typically take 45 minutes, and for 95% of depositions a processed review copy and a report on the processing procedure is sent back to the depositor in less than one working day.

Some of the new techniques utilized by AutoDep 3.0 and the subsequent processing are detailed next. Many of these methods are also closely linked to the development of the relational database version of the PDB described in Section 2.

1.1 Data Harvesting

Data harvesting is the model by which the different software packages used in the structure solution process output a deposition file containing details of the method used and results obtained. When the user wishes to deposit the coordinates, there should be a collection of these "harvest" files holding details of how the model was obtained. The file collection can then be sent directly to the deposition center, bypassing much of the manual processing needed by a Web-based deposition interface.

Data harvesting eradicates typing and cutting/pasting errors as well as allowing more information to be archived without placing an additional burden on the depositor. E-MSD and CCP4 have cooperated on the initial ideas for data harvesting (5). AutoDep 3.0 reads CNS and CCP4 harvest files.

1.2 Extending Data Deposition of NMR and Cryoelectron Microscopy

The PDB has its roots in structures determined using X-ray crystallography and still represents X-ray structures better than those derived using other methods, such as nuclear magnetic resonance (NMR) and cryoelectron microscopy (cryo-EM). Part of the reason for this difference is that these other methods are relatively new and issues of data representation have not been widely addressed. E-MSD has been very active in the UK BBSRC-funded CCPN project to develop a data model for NMR data, and it coordinates an EU-funded project, IIMS, to integrate cryo-EM data into the PDB where possible and to set up an archive equivalent to the PDB for cryo-EM volume data.

1.3 Recognition of Chemical Species

Of the about 15,000 entries in the PDB, at least half contain metal ions or other nonpolypeptide groups. These chemical entities include substrates, products, inhibitors, and prosthetic groups. PDB conventions dictate that each chemical entity be identified by a three-letter code that is consistent across the entire archive. For example, every occurrence of β-glucose should be labeled GLC. The PDB requires the additional check that the atom names for all residues must be compliant with the PDB hetgroup dictionary and be presented in a set order defined in that same dictionary.

The correct recognition of the chemistry for each of these entities is a complicated procedure, not least because the methods used to determine macromolecular structure do not give accurate structures for the bound small molecules. The E-MSD has put in place a system for matching all the chemical constituents of the entry against the PDB hetgroup dictionary. Graph isomorphism approaches are used to match against a graph derived from the PDB hetgroup dictionary extended to include stereochemical detail such as chirality, ring atom definition, and cis/trans double-bond information.

For new ligands, procedures are in place to automatically generate the new dictionary entry. Generating a new dictionary entry automatically from the deposited coordinates is not easy, because, for example, bond orders and protons must be assigned. Many of the procedures are built around the CACTVS software suite (6). In addition, algorithms have been developed for matching fragments of molecules against fragments of the molecules in the PDB hetgroup dictionary (subgraph–subgraph isomorphism). These procedures are extremely useful for trying to ensure that families of compounds are handled in a consistent manner.

The completed chemical descriptions are exchanged with the RCSB on a daily basis to further ensure PDB consistency between entries processed at the two different sites.

1.4   Building of Cross-References from Primary Sequence

Deposition and annotation steps are taken to ensure that the data are not only consistent within a PDB entry and consistent across the PDB archive but also are consistent with other databases that contain related information. For a PDB entry the coordinates contain only the observed atom positions, and in many cases the atom sites do not necessarily represent the complete sequence of the protein studied. We work closely with SWISS-PROT for procedures that match atom records to the experiment sequences and to the sequence databases. SWISS-PROT information is to be used to generate appropriate HEADER, COMPND, DBREF, SEQADV, MODRES, and SOURCE records in the PDB entry. Determination of the correct sequence database reference is vital, for much of the subsequent data are dependent on the correct sequence. PDB information on chains, fragment sequences, and journal references are to be passed back to the SWISS-PROT database team at EBI to maintain consistency between the structure and protein sequence archives.

1.5   Recognition of Oligomeric State

Quaternary structure is defined as that level of form in which units of tertiary structure aggregate to form homo- or heteromultimers. Consideration of the presence of a quaternary state is important in the understanding of a protein's biological function. For a PDB entry determined using X-ray crystallography, the deposited coordinates usually consist of the contents of the asymmetric unit (ASU). The deposited coordinates may therefore contain one or more complete macromolecule(s), some parts of which may require crystallographic symmetry operations to be applied in order to generate the complete macromolecule(s). Algorithms (7,8) have been developed to determine the most likely oligomeric state, taking into account the symmetry-related chains. These algorithms form the basis of the Protein Quaternary Structure (PQS) server (http://pqs.ebi.ac.uk). An example taken from the PQS server is shown in Figure 1. Figure 1a shows the structure of ascorbate oxidase from zucchini as deposited to the PDB (9, PDB entry 1aoz). The two arms, at the top and the bottom left, are well ordered, and PQS finds an alternative dimer in which these two arms interlock at the dimer interface, as shown in Figure 1b. Interestingly, ascorbate oxidase is also found in higher oligomeric states, and so both the interfaces shown in Figure 1 are likely to be biologically significant. Such results make PQS a very useful tool for the annotation of PDB entries.

1.6 Recognition of Secondary Structure Elements

In the PDB, secondary structure is represented by the HELIX, SHEET, and TURN records. In AutoDep 2.0 the depositor was asked to provide secondary structure assignments. However, these assignments were frequently found to be inconsistent with the coordinates, due either to typing errors or to inappropriate cutting/pasting from other entries. Therefore AutoDep 3.0 does not ask for secondary structure, instead, a secondary structure is generated during processing, using a single program that integrates DSSP (10) and the Promotif suite (11) and is included in the copy of the PDB entry the

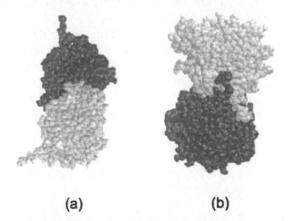

(a)   (b)

Figure 1 Structure of ascorbate oxidase (1aoz). (a) Dimer as deposited in asymmetric unit; (b) dimer determined using PQS. (From Ref. 9.)

depositor is sent for review. Any changes to the secondary structure that the depositor wishes to make are incorporated at this stage.

1.7 Validation

A key aspect of making the PDB useful to the interests of a diverse community of researchers is that the data should be accurate, consistent, and machine-readable and carry clear indicators of quality. Data are more useful if they are associated with meaningful confidence criteria and if they can be retrieved in a form that indicates the degree of confidence that can be placed on any observation.

Both AutoDep and the subsequent processing stages contain a validation component that is targeted primarily at determining deviations from what is normally observed. This is achieved by comparison with a knowledge base to identify unusual features. WHATCHECK (12) is run as part of AutoDep and a validation report prepared as part of the AutoDep procedures. Deviations from standard geometry and expected backbone torsion angles are generated, using in-house software, that are used to populate REMARK 500 in the PDB format files. As X-ray structures are increasingly deposited with structure factors, E-MSD will integrate validation against structure factor information in the deposition procedure.

It is anticipated that validation during deposition will become more important as high-throughput approaches for structure determination are developed and the solving of structures becomes separated from the analysis. The E-MSD works closely with the European software groups CCP4 (for X-ray structure determination) and CCPN (for NMR techniques) as well as the EU-funded NMRQUAL project for developing validation criteria for structure determined using NMR.

Ideally all the validation checks that are run during deposition would have been run before the deposition process starts. To encourage this, the E-MSD runs the CRITQUAL validation service (http://biotech.ebi. ac.uk:8400; Ref. 14). CRITQUAL, the European 3D Validation Network, has devised a series of geometrical and structure factor tests that may be used to assess how well a crystal structure fits the observed data and how well its geometry agrees with target values.

2 TRANSFORMING THE PDB FLAT FILE ARCHIVE TO A RELATIONAL DATABASE

For many uses the structural archive is limited by the fact that it is built around flat files in PDB format. Although a formal specification for the PDB format was produced in 1998 (http://www.rcsb.org/pdb/docs/format/

pdbguide2.2/guide2.2_frame.html), so many different dialects of PDB format had developed by that stage that trying to maintain an internally consistent archive in PDB format was, in practice, impossible. In an attempt to force the legacy archive into a more usable form and to ensure that these problems do not propagate into the future, E-MSD has been working on developing a relational database for structural data.

The database has been designed using the Oracle Designer CASE tool, which has been invaluable for tracking the development of such a highly complex set of tables (around 400 tables linked by 1000 relationships). The database performs two key functions. For legacy data it provides a filter that forces the legacy PDB data into a consistent framework (thus forming the basis for the development of search services, described later), for new data it provides a versatile way of handling the data provided during deposition through an interface such as AutoDep.

3 DEVELOPING SERVICES TO SEARCH THE PDB

Currently E-MSD runs a search interface to the PDB called OCA (http://oca.ebi.ac.uk) that was developed by Jaime Prilusky at the Weizmann Institute. OCA provides a Web interface to indexed flat files.

The E-MSD is developing search interfaces built around the database. Relational databases are very appealing for these services because they not only provide very efficient, scalable indexing but also subdivide the data so that it is relatively easy to manipulate the information returned from a query. Search interfaces built around indexed flat files are limited mostly to returning a subset of those files. Once the data are fully atomized in a relational database, however, it becomes a relatively simple matter to return a range of formats that are assembled on the fly, as well as tabular subsets of the data.

However, the normalized database described earlier is not ideal for searching, because the interesting data are spread out over many different tables that are slow to join together. In addition, the normalized database is tied to Oracle because it is tightly coupled to the development environment. Therefore, the normalized database is then transformed into a denormalized *data warehouse* structure for searching. This both speeds up the search and can be transformed to a more generic SQL form suitable for a variety of database engines. E-MSD was expecting to release a preliminary search interface built around the data warehouse, as well as distributing versions of the denormalized database, early in 2002.

4 FUTURE

The EMSD database is part of the EU-funded TEMBLOR project. TEMBLOR will be a new-generation bioinformatics project, centered on an integrated layer for the exploitation of genomic and proteomic data (Integr8) by drawing on databases maintained at major bioinformatics centers in Europe and by creating new, important resources for protein–protein interaction (IntAct), macrostructural (EMSD), and microarray (DESPRAD) data. Integr8 will enable text-, structure-, and sequence-based searches against a gene-centric view of all completed genomes. Zooming in on the sequence data linked to the gene will allow the user to see genomic, transcriptional, and protein sequences linked together. Each transcript will be linked "down" to the genomic sequence from which it is transcribed and "up" to the protein sequence into which it is translated. Each level will give direct access to the whole body of scientific knowledge about a given gene, transcript, or protein.

All this will be linked to the scientific literature and patent information, as well as to information on biological materials (in particular, gene libraries, individual clones, high-density clone filters, DNA and protein filters, clone and DNA pools, etc.). In addition to creating an integration layer to existing resources, it will be necessary to create some new components in the envisaged data backbone. Major projects within TEMBLOR are IntAct, to create a database for protein–protein interaction data; EMSD, to enhance the European Macrostructural Database; and DESPRAD, to establish a microarray data repository. Within TEMBLOR the EBI will develop new algorithms exploiting the integrative layer and adding value to the existing body of data

ACKNOWLEDGEMENTS

Many thanks to the many people who have provided input to this project, including Geoff Barton, Harry Boutsalikis, Richard Newman, Jorge Pineda, John Tate, Janet Thornton, and the RCSB. E-MSD is gratefully supported by the Wellcome Trust (GR062025MA), the EU (TEMBLOR, NMRQUAL and IIMS), and EMBL. EK is supported by CCP4.

REFERENCES

1. Hamm, G. H., and Cameron, G. N. (1986) The EMBL data library. Nucleic Acids Res.14:5–10. (http://www.ebi.ac.uk/embl/)
2. Bairoch, A., and Boeckmann, B. (1994) The SWISS-PROT protein sequence databank: current status. Nucleic Acids Res. 22:3578–3580. (http://www.ebi.ac.uk/swissprot/)

3. Berman, H. M., Westbrook, J., Feng, Z., Gilliland, G., Bhat, T. N., Weissig, H., Shindyalov, I. N. and Bourne, P. E. (2000) The Protein Data Bank. Nucleic Acids Res. 28:235–242.

4. Bourne, P., Berman, H. M., Watenpaugh, K., Westbrook, J. D., and Fitzgerald, P. M. D. (1997) The macromolecular Crystallographic Information File (mmCIF). Meth. Enzymol. 277:571–590. (http://pdb.rutgers.edu/mmcif/)

5. Reports on CCP4/E-MSD progress with harvesting: http://www.dl.ac.uk/CCP/CCP4/newsletter36/03_harvest.html; http://www.dl.ac.uk/CCP/CCP4/newsletter37/13_harvest.html.

6. Ihlenfeldt, W. D., Takahashi, Y., Abe, H., and Sasaki, S. (1994) Computation and management of chemical properties in CACTVS: an extensible networked approach toward modularity and flexibility J. Chem. Inf. Comp. Sci. 34:109–116. (http://www2.chemie.uni-erlangen.de/software/cactvs/index.html)

7. Henrick, K., and Thornton, J. M. (1998) PQS: A Protein Quarternary File Server. Trends Biochem. Sci. 23:358–361. (http://pqs.ebi.ac.uk)

8. Ponstingl, H., Henrick, K. and Thornton, J. M. (2000) Discriminating between homodimeric and monomeric proteins in the crystalline state. Proteins 41:47–57.

9. Messerschmidt, A., Ladenstein, R., Huber, R., Bolognesi, M., Avigliano, L., Petruzzelli, R., Ross, A, and Finazzi-Agro, A. (1992) Refined crystal structure of ascorbate oxidase at 1.9-Å resolution. J Mol Biol. 224(1):179–205.

10. Kabsch, W., and Sander, C. (1983) Dictionary of protein secondary structure:- pattern recognition of hydrogen-bonded and geometrical features. Biopolymers 22:2577–2637. (http://www.cmbi.kun.nl/gv/dssp/)

11. Hutchinson, E. G., and Thornton, J. M. (1996) PROMOTIF—a program to identify and analyze structural motifs in proteins. Protein Sci. 5:212–220. (http://www.biochem.ucl.ac.uk/~gail/promotif/promotif.html)

12. Hooft, R. W. W., Vriend, G., Sander, C., and Abola, E. E. (1996) Errors in protein structures. Nature 381:272–272.

13. Dodson, E. (1998) The role of validation in macromolecular crystallography Acta Cryst. D54:1109–1118.

16

Molecular Docking in Structure-Based Design

Trevor W. Heritage
Tripos Inc., St. Louis, Missouri, U.S.A.

1 INTRODUCTION

The design of novel therapeutic agents based on knowledge of the three-dimensional structure of target proteins has increased significantly in recent years, driven by advances in 3D protein structure determination by high-resolution X-ray crystallography and NMR. Moreover, the possibility of linking computational structure-based design technologies (1–3) with functional genomics via threading and homology modeling is a tantalizing prospect. With the 3D protein structure in hand, regardless of how it is determined, there are essentially three structure-based design approaches via which we may exploit it. *Geometric searching* (4,5) finds molecules that match a set of distance and angular relationships between specific molecular features (a pharmacophore). *De novo design* (6,7) constructs molecules directly within the receptor site, either by combining and linking separately docked fragments or by "growing" molecules from a docked anchor fragment. *Docking* methods fit a small molecule (ligand) into the binding site by optimization of steric, hydrophobic, and electrostatic complementarity in conjunction with an estimate of the corresponding binding free energy (scoring).

This chapter focuses on the various techniques available for molecular docking and assumes at its outset that the 3D protein structure is already established. The discussion within this chapter is also restricted to small-molecule docking, and thus macromolecular docking methods that are reviewed elsewhere (8,9) are not considered herein. The following sections describe each of the fundamental steps involved in docking a small molecule into a 3D protein structure—receptor site identification and characterization; determination of optimal placement, orientation, and conformation of a small molecule at the receptor site; and scoring functions to evaluate the fit or complementarity of the resulting receptor–ligand complex. The subsequent two sections discuss extensions of docking technologies that enable large numbers of small molecules to be computationally screened against the 3D protein structure—virtual screening and combinatorial library docking. The chapter concludes with some example applications and a brief discussion of the most current trends in docking and future directions.

2   RECEPTOR SITE IDENTIFICATION AND CHARACTERIZATION

The first step in molecular docking is to identify those regions on the protein structure that upon binding a ligand would interfere with normal function, such as an enzyme active site, the binding site of a receptor, or an allosteric site. These regions are typically determined by mutation experiments or are known through cocrystallization and X-ray structure determination of an inhibitor–receptor complex. In the absence of this information, automated methods exist for identification and characterization of "interesting" regions. A site is "characterized" by different descriptors that can subsequently be used to orient a ligand within the site. Many site characterization methods have been developed, all of which can broadly be divided into two classes based on their use of either geometric features of the site or chemical functionality.

The SPHGEN algorithm available within the well-known DOCK suite of programs (10) computes a set of spheres that correspond to the shape of the receptor site. Initially a set of overlapping spheres is generated over the entire receptor surface; spheres with varying radii are generated analytically in such a way that they touch the surface of the receptor at two points and do not penetrate any receptor atom. The spheres are then separated into clusters, based on radial overlap, and typically the largest cluster of spheres is assumed to be the ligand-binding site. The cluster of spheres at the binding site form a "negative image" of the receptor site. Concepts such as *anchor points*, regions where specific functional groups or atoms are known to bind within the receptor, and *colored spheres*, spheres that contain specific types of functional groups, e.g., hydrogen bond donors, can also be introduced to guide the docking algorithm (11).

The PASS (putative active sites with spheres) algorithm (12) program fills the cavities in a protein structure with spheres and identifies those spheres (ASPs—active site points) located at likely binding pockets. Initially the protein surface is coated with spherical probes; probes that clash with the protein, are insufficiently buried, or lie within 1 Å of a more buried probe are eliminated. A second layer of spheres is accreted onto those spheres remaining from the previous step, and again spheres are eliminated based on the aforementioned criteria. This process is continued until no newly added probes "survive" the subsequent filtering step. Potential binding sites are then identified as invaginations in the protein surface that are large enough to accommodate a ligand and possess solvent-excluded volume in which hydrophobic ligand moieties may be buried.

The GRIN and GRID programs (13–15) calculate regions within the binding site that show high affinity for different kinds of "probe." The probes can be single atoms or functional groups (e.g., methyl, hydroxyl), and the energy is calculated using a semiempirical potential. This approach was successfully used in the design of potent sialidase inhibitors of influenza virus replication (16) and thymidylate synthase inhibitors (17).

In the MCSS (multiple-copy simultaneous search) approach (18), energetically favorable orientations and positions of functional groups (e.g., acetonitrile, methanol) are computed using a CHARMm potential (19). Thousands of copies of a molecular fragment are distributed in the target region of the protein, and energy minimization is performed to yield distinct local minima for each functional group. A feature of the method is that the functional groups do not "see" each other, and their interactions with the protein do not impact each other.

Besides computational approaches to binding site characterization, there are also several empirical approaches (20–22) that rely on rules derived from analysis of the Cambridge Structural Database (23) (CSD) to determine favorable interaction geometries between ligand and protein functional groups. Such empirical methods implicitly encode information pertaining to atom–atom interactions in proteins that is difficult to represent within force field–based approaches (24). The X-SITE program (25) is based on analysis of 3D packing geometries observed within the Protein Data Bank[26] (PDB). Each protein side chain and main chain is broken down into overlapping three atom fragments, and the observed spatial distributions of various probe atoms are used to predict favorable interaction sites.

3 LIGAND DOCKING

After the receptor binding region has been identified and characterized, we are ready to address the basic problem of molecular docking, namely finding the binding mode of a ligand within a receptor site. This is achieved by searching the conformational and orientational space of the ligand and receptor for a geometry that exhibits a favorable binding energy. Unfortunately this represents an enormous search space and a systematic "brute-force" approach that checks all possible configurations of the ligand within the binding site is not practical. Many of the early docking methods reduced the search space by docking a single, fixed conformer of the ligand into a rigid binding site model. This approach, which also ensures that only low-energy conformations are considered in the search, has been surprisingly successful in finding highly active molecules (1), but of course it has the drawback that potential "hits" can be missed due to unfortunate choice of ligand conformation or the inability of the binding site to adjust its conformation to accommodate the ligand. Table 1 summarizes the most well-known docking algorithms that are discussed in the following text.

The DOCK algorithm (10) performs rigid-body docking by comparing the sphere centers representing the binding site "negative image" (output from the SPHGEN program) with ligand atom centers. Sets of sphere centers "match" sets of ligand atoms if the intersphere distances are roughly equal to the corresponding interatomic distances within the ligand. A fitting procedure (27) is used to determine the rotation-translation matrix that best overlaps matched pairs of atoms and spheres. Multiple orientations are generated by this procedure and evaluated using force-field terms (28). An additional optimization procedure has been added that adjusts each orientation to improve the intermolecular interactions (29,30). Techniques that require ligand atoms to match so-called "colored spheres" that represent the location of a ligand atom if it were to form an idealized hydrogen-bonding interaction geometry with the protein can further optimize this process by limiting the search space (31,32). Several other groups have developed docking procedures that use the general superpositioning approach pioneered in DOCK, including CLIX (33), which uses two-point ligand superpositioning followed by rotation, FLOG (34); which includes an efficient matching algorithm, grid-based scoring, and rigid-body minimization; and the rigid-body docking capabilities in LUDI (35). The geometric fit between the ligand and receptor is optimal when the molecular surfaces come into contact over a large region. One approach for trying to try to optimize the surface contact between receptor and ligand calculates a spiral path over the surface of the binding site and a separate spiral path over the surface of the ligand (36). The spiral paths effectively order the surface points enabling corresponding points on the surface of the protein and ligand to be identified and superimposed. Alternatively, the molecular surface can be represented as a sparse set of critical surface points that are then matched using geometric hashing schemes (37–39).

Table 1 Summary of Rigid-Body and Flexible Docking Algorithms

Program	Year	Refs.	Algorithm	Author(s)	Time[a]
DOCK	1982	10	Rigid-body[b]	Kuntz et al.	F
CLIX	1992	33	Rigid-body	Lawrence and Davis	
FLOG	1994	34	Rigid-body	Kearsley et al.	
LUDI	1994	35	Rigid-body	Böhm	
	1992	36	Rigid-body	Bacon and Moult	M
AutoDock	1993	61,62	Metropolis	Goodsell and Olsen	S
	1995	66,67	Metropolis	Hart et al.	
Directed DOCK	1992	31	Systematic	Leach and Kuntz	M
FlexX	1996	43	Incremental	Rarey et al.	F
	1996	49	Incremental	Jain et al.	M
ADAM	1994	52–54	Incremental	Itai et al.	M
DIVALI	1995	75,76	Genetic	Judson et al.	VS
	1995	77	Genetic	Clark and Ajay	
	1994	75	Genetic	Oshiro and Kuntz	S
	1995	82	Evolutionary	Gelhaar et al.	S
GOLD	1995	78,79	Genetic	Jones et al.	M[c]
	1994	84		Leach	VS[c]

[a]The time column gives a qualitative estimate of the run time for the various methods listed, *F* = fast (< 2–3 min), M = medium (~ 5 min), S = slow (10 + min), VS = very slow (30 + min).
[b]All methods in the table treat both the ligands as flexible, with the exception of those marked "rigid-body" in this column.
[c]These methods have the option to also treat the protein side chains flexibly.

The superpositioning approach just outlined is well suited to docking of rigid molecules, but it is more problematic if conformational flexibility of the ligand is to be considered. However, incorporation of ligand flexibility is a critical issue since it is generally accepted that correct docking modes cannot be obtained using rigid-body methods unless the starting conformation is close to the active conformation. One approach to this problem is to generate multiple, diverse conformations for each ligand molecule, and then to dock each conformation into the binding site using rigid-body docking (40,41). These approaches have successfully identified inhibitors of human immunodeficiency virus (HIV) protease (42), collagenase, and cyclin-dependent kinase 2 (41).

Another approach to addressing conformational flexibility of the ligand is the so-called incremental construction approach. This approach forms the basis of de novo design programs, although it is only discussed herein as a docking tool. The original idea was developed by DesJarlais et al. (180), who broke flexible molecules into rigid fragments, each of which was independently docked into the binding site. High-scoring fragment positions and orientations were then recombined using energy minimization. In a related approach Leach and Kuntz (31) docked a single rigid "anchor" fragment into the binding site and then attached the remainder of the ligand using systematic conformational searching to find low-energy conformers.

The FlexX program (43) uses an incremental construction approach that combines the ligand placement ideas of the LUDI program (35) with an enhanced version of the Böhm scoring function (35). Conformational flexibility of the ligand is handled based on conformational preferences observed in the Cambridge Structural Database (23) of up to 12 discrete torsion angle values derived from the MIMUMBA program (44) for each acyclic single bond. The initial base fragment is placed using a technique known as pose clustering (45,46). A greedy strategy (47,48) is used for incremental construction; i.e., a fragment is added in all possible conformations to all placements identified in the previous iteration and the n best placements are taken on to the next iteration (Fig. 1). Figure 2 shows the top-ranked FlexX solution from docking methotrexate into dihydrofolate reductase (DFR). In this case the highest-ranked solution is extremely close to the crystal structure of the ligand, although in some cases it is necessary to process lower-ranking solutions to find the best solution.

FlexX and other incremental construction programs, such as HAMMERHEAD (49), rely on the assumption that all partial structures should have near-optimum energies. In a related approach (50), a variant on the backtrack algorithm (51) is used that limits the sampling of similar conformations without reducing sampling of distinct conformations. Partial energy calculations are used within the backtrack algorithm but

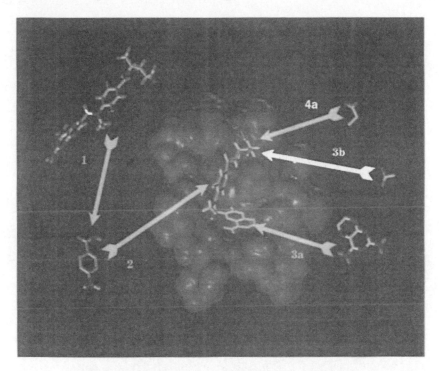

Figure 1 FlexX docking procedure: (1) Select base fragment. (2) Dock base fragment into binding site in multiple placements. (3) Attach remaining ligand fragments at favorable torsion angles. (4) Eliminate branches of search tree where attachment is impossible.

only to reduce computational time rather than as a partial solution selection criterion. Although the backtrack algorithm can rapidly explore many conformations, the number of conformations to be searched grows rapidly as the flexibility of the ligand increases, and incremental construction approaches have the advantage that they avoid this explosion in conformational search space.

Incremental construction approaches assume that it is possible to identify a rigid anchor fragment, which may not always be possible. The ADAM program (52–54) uses energy minimization to adjust the conformation of the anchor fragment to obtain a better fit to the site points prior to placement within the binding site. Side chains are appended to the docked anchor fragment using systematic search to find low-energy conformers. The optimization procedure in ADAM seeks to maximize hydrogen-bonding interactions rather than the shape complementarity used by DOCK.

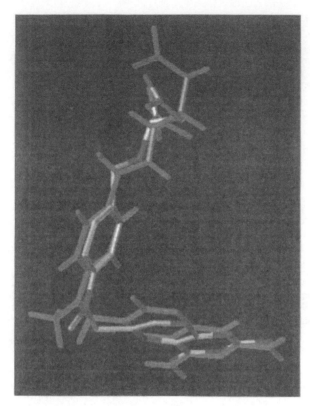

Figure 2 Highest-ranked solution for docking methotrexate to dihydrofolate reductase with the FlexX program. The crystal structure orientation and conformation of methotrexate is shown by atom type for reference. The energy of the highest-ranked solution is −64.8 kcal/mol, with an RMSD from the crystal structure of 1.2 Å. The run time was 120 seconds on an SGI R10K.

Other docking methods sample the orientational and conformational space using efficient search engines such as molecular dynamics (55), the metropolis Monte Carlo algorithm, and evolutionary and genetic algorithms. These methods have the advantage that they can more naturally include conformational flexibility of the protein, but they are correspondingly slower than the preceeding approaches. All of these approaches optimize an objective function that is either entirely or in part the scoring function described in the following section.

Molecular dynamics simulations cannot currently be run for long enough to simulate protein–ligand docking. It is, however, possible to generate alternative ligand orientations and conformations within the binding site using modified molecular dynamics procedures, such as the SHAKE algorithm, that hold bond lengths and bond angles fixed (56,57). High-temperature dynamics may also be used to ensure more thorough exploration of the available search space and avoid the problem of being stuck in local minima (58). In an alternative approach, the metropolis Monte Carlo algorithm (59,60), also known as simulated annealing, generates a sequence of structures that initially identify low-energy regions of search space, and then randomly explores the surrounding vicinity. Metropolis Monte Carlo procedures make small adjustments to a starting ligand conformation and orientation, evaluate the energy of the new configuration, and accept it based on the *metropolis criterion*, or probability function $p = e^{-\Delta E/kT}$, where ΔE is the difference in energy between the starting and new configurations. If the new configuration has lower energy than the initial configuration, then it is always accepted. The metropolis Monte Carlo approach is implemented within the AutoDock program (61,62) that docks flexible molecules into rigid protein binding sites using a grid-based energy evaluation function. This approach has been used successfully in several studies (63–65). A multiple-start Monte Carlo method that uses a two-step process to generate multiple binding modes has been proposed by Hart (66,67). Flexible ligands are broken into rigid fragments that are then docked individually. In the first step of the process, the metropolis energy function is replaced by a measure of the distance of the fragment to the protein surface; the second step uses a traditional grid-based energy evaluation function. The procedure is repeated multiple times to identify all favorable binding modes. A similar procedure is used by Wang (68) in MCDOCK, which employs a three-stage process involving geometry-based Monte Carlo docking, energy-based Monte Carlo docking, and a final force-field-based energy minimization. Another Monte Carlo–based approach intended to generate multiple binding modes is the multiple-copy simultaneous search (MCSS) approach (18). Multiple starting positions are generated for the ligand, each of which is simultaneously minimized, with each copy "feeling" the interaction with the protein but not the other ligand copies. Duplicate minimizations that are converging to the same minimum are periodically eliminated.

Genetic algorithms (GAs) borrow ideas from genetics and natural selection (69,70). A population of "chromosomes" encodes solutions that "evolve" through a series of genetic operations, including crossover and mutation. Simplified natural selection is simulated using a "fitness" function, with the fittest members of the population "surviving" to "reproduce" and generate child chromosomes in successive generations. Genetic algorithms are ideally suited to problems that require optimization of a large and diverse set of variables. Genetic algorithms have been used in numerous chemical applications, including conformational searching of small molecules (71) and pharmacophore determination (72,73), and the method appears to be faster than simulated annealing approaches. In the case of molecular docking, the chromosomes generally encode the ligand rotational and translational degress of freedom and the torsion angles of the ligand, and thus each chromosome represents a potential solution to the problem. Kuntz et al. have examined the utility of GAs for molecular docking as an alternative to the sphere-atom mapping technique used for rigid-body docking in DOCK and for flexible ligand docking (74).

Judson and coworkers (75,76) were among the first to attempt molecular docking using a genetic algorithm. They adapted their GA for conformational searching (71) and made several other adjustments to their algorithm to render it more suitable to molecular docking. The ligand is translated and rotated around a pivot atom of the ligand, and a fast "bump count" potential function is used to eliminate all configurations in which a ligand atom overlaps with the protein. As in incremental construction approaches, they use a "growing" algorithm that initially docks only a substructure of the ligand containing the pivot atom and its neighbors, the remainder of the ligand being added as the search proceeds. Other genetic algorithm–driven docking methods include DIVALI (Docking with eVolutionary ALgorIthms) (77), which uses a grid-based AMBER potential function, and GOLD (Genetic algOrithm for Ligand Docking) (78,79). The latter algorithm, probably the best-known GA for docking, explores full conformational flexibility of the ligand as well partial flexibility of the protein. A comparison of GAs (GOLD) and incremental construction (FlexX (43)) is shown in Table 2. As is true for all GAs, GOLD's use of a nondeterministic optimization technique can lead to long computation times—much longer than the geometric matching and incremental construction approaches described earlier. More recently, the DARWIN program has been described (80). It uses a genetic algorithm to dock large molecules into proteins and a parallel interface to CHARMm for energy evaluations.

A related approach to molecular docking uses the concept of *evolutionary programming* (81). This approach attempts to overcome the possible drawback that genetic algorithms generally require a binary encoding of the solution space within chromosomes that may lead to overly complex evaluation functions; evolutionary programming approaches employ real-valued representations. The algorithm itself proceeds by comparing the "score" of each population member with a number of randomly selected opponents, with the number of "wins" determining whether or not the population member survives. All surviving members generate offspring by self-adaptive Gaussian mutation so as to maintain a constant population size. The work of Gehlaar (82) and coworkers uses this approach, with chromosomes encoding the six rigid-body coordinates of the ligand and

Table 2 GOLD[a] and FlexX[b], Two of the Most Widely Used Docking Programs, Along with DOCK[c]

	Top-ranked by energy		Best RMS	
	FlexX	GOLD	FlexX	GOLD
4dfr	0.89	1.44	0.61	0.80
6rsa	0.39	4.42	0.39	4.29
3cpa	3.34	1.58	0.67	0.90
1tmn	0.83	1.68	0.62	1.46
1ldm	0.62	1.00	0.62	1.00
1dwd	0.99	1.71	0.74	1.71
3ptb	0.54	0.96	0.54	0.64
2phh	0.61	0.72	0.35	0.63
2ctc	0.56	0.32	0.43	0.24
1ulb	0.40	0.32	0.40	0.32
1stp	0.52	0.69	0.45	0.56
4phv	1.09	1.11	1.09	1.02

This table compares the two algorithms for a variety of test cases selected from the PDB. The first two columns show the RMSD of the highest-ranked solution from FlexX and GOLD, respectively. The last two columns show the lowest RMS solution found by the same two programs.
[a] From Ref. 78
[b] From Ref. 43
[c] From Ref. 10.

the dihedral angles around its rotatable bonds. A drawback of this approach is that the Gaussian mutation operations tend to leave solutions trapped near local minima, and thus it seems appropriate to combine the global searching property of genetic or evolutionary algorithms with local search techniques to improve the quality of the generated solutions. Recently, the FCEA (family competitive evolutionary algorithm) has been proposed for docking conformationally flexible ligands (83). The FCEA approach combines three mutation operators intended to provide a balance between global exploration and local optimization, family competition, and adaptive rules for controlling probability of each mutation operator.

Leach described an approach that explored the conformational degrees of freedom of the protein side chains and the ligand in which the side chains were allowed to adopt different discrete conformations during the run (84). The MSNI/MCM (minimization with shifted nonbonded interactions/Monte Carlo minimization) procedure developed by Caflisch et al. (85) can in principle model the entire protein and ligand flexibility. The ligand is initially located near the binding site, allowing configurations to occur in which ligand atoms overlap with the protein. Minimization is performed initially using modified nonbonded terms that avoid high-energy gradients, which are adjusted back to their original form during the course of the process. Bumps between ligands and protein atoms are eliminated either by displacement of the ligand or, if the ligand has moved into a favorable binding pocket, by conformational change in the protein. The CHARMm (19) force field is used for energy evaluations, finite difference Poisson-Boltzmann (86) calculations are used to model the electrostatic energy of the complexes, and non-polar solvation free energy is approximated based on solvent-accessible surface area. Monte Carlo minimization (87,88) was then applied to the best structures, allowing random perturbation of the conformation of the binding site as well as the conformation and orientation of the ligand.

Multistep approaches to the docking problem have been investigated by several groups, with encouraging results (89,90). Hoffman and coworkers describe a two-stage procedure in which a large number of ligand conformations are generated within the binding site using the FlexX program (43), and in a second step these conformations are minimized and reranked using the CHARMm force field. Kuntz and coworkers use a divide-and-conquer based approach (89) in which they divide the search space into so-called *conformation space* and *orientation space*. A systematic scan of the conformational space of the ligand is used to select an ensemble of low-energy conformers. Geometric complementarity is used to search the orientation space at the binding site of each selected conformer, and scoring is performed based on the AMBER force field. The low-quality solutions generated by this coarse searching protocol are then subjected to molecular mechanics minimization, torsional optimization of the ligand fixed in a given orientation at the binding site, and a short simulated annealing run to shake the structures near their local minimum.

4 SCORING FUNCTIONS

Once docking has occurred, we are faced with the problem of evaluating the quality of those docked solutions. Currently, scoring is the weakest link in the docking process, since small differences in free energy correspond to much larger differences in binding affinity—each order of magnitude change in binding affinity is equivalent to only about 1.4 kcal/mol in free energy, while the energy of a single hydrogen bond is about 4 kcal/mol (91).

Ligand–receptor binding is controlled by electrostatic and hydrophobic interactions, hydrogen bonding, and dispersion or van der Waals forces (92,93). Binding itself is driven primarily by the hydrophobic interactions, while electrostatics and hydrogen bonding govern specificity (94). During binding, ligand–water and receptor–water hydrogen bonds are broken and replaced by ligand–receptor hydrogen bonds, with only a small change in overall free energy (95). Estimation of the free energy of binding is ideally the quantity of interest and, although it can be computed using methods such as FEP (96,97), these methods are extremely time consuming (98), forcing docking methods to employ a variety of simplifications. Empirical schemes (99) that emphasize computational efficiency and qualitative or rank order accuracy are generally used as so-called *scoring functions*. Such scoring functions are useful primarily for screening out those compounds that are unlikely to bind, allowing the researcher to focus on a smaller set of potentially active candidates (100).

Before entering a discussion of the various empirical scoring schemes available to us, it is important to note that there are two types of function: *tailored* and *generalized*. A tailored function is derived by parameterization that is specifically aimed at reproducing as closely as possible the experimental binding affinities for a known set of inhibitors acting at a particular site (101–103). Such functions may yield very impressive results within the domain in which they were developed but are not generally useful as docking scoring functions. A docking scoring function must have properties that enable it to be transferable between systems and must thus be parameterized using as wide a range of experimental data as possible. Generalized scoring functions are usually energetic in nature, although the DOCK program (10,27,104,180) includes a shape-based scoring function that counts the number of receptor atoms within a specified distance of each ligand atom. Other examples of geometric or shape-based scoring functions are the complementarity function of the LIGIN algorithm (105,106), which is based on "legitimate" and "illegitimate" contacts between chemical types, buried and exposed hydrophobic and hydrophilic surfaces (107), the extension of the latter proposed by Wallqvist that includes interactions between buried atoms (108,109), and approaches based on spatial correlation theory (110,111).

One type of empirical energetic scoring function is based on force-field energy terms. The DOCK program (27) approximates the receptor–ligand binding energy using AMBER (112,113) interaction energies, and GRID (13,14) uses interaction energies computed between small chemical probes (e.g., methyl, hydroxyl, amino) and receptor surface atoms using a 6–12 vdW function, a coulombic potential, and an angle-dependent hydrogen-bonding term. Force-field energy evaluations are usually approximated using precalculated scoring grids, since otherwise the nonbonded interaction terms cause the computational effort to grow enormously as the size of the system increases (28). Further scoring function terms implemented in the DOCK program are chemical scoring (11) and empirical hydrophobicities (114).

The second type of energetic scoring function is based on a weighted sum of interaction energies (115). The VALIDATE[116] scoring function was based on analysis of 51 complexes and derived 12 terms in which the coefficients were determined using partial least squares (PLS). An excellent cross-validated estimate of error of 6.5 kJ/mol was obtained as well as good predictions for test complexes. The best-known function of this type, and the first attempt at extremely fast evaluation, is the Böhm (35,117) scoring function that was derived by regression analysis of data from 45 protein-ligand complexes available in the PDB, with binding affinities spanning 12 orders of magnitude. The function takes the following form and includes terms for hydrogen bonding, entropy based on the number of rotatable bonds frozen during binding, and desolvation based on hydrophobic complementarity; $f(\Delta R, \Delta \alpha)$ is a penalty function that accounts for deviations from ideal hydrogen bond lengths and angles:

$$\Delta G_{\text{binding}} = \Delta G_0 + \Delta G_{\text{hb}_{\text{bonds}}} f(\Delta R, \Delta \alpha) + \Delta G_{\text{ionic}_{\text{ionic\_int}}} f(\Delta R, \Delta \alpha)$$

$$+ \Delta G_{\text{lipo}} |A_{\text{lipo}}| + \Delta G_{\text{rot}} \cdot \text{NROT}$$

An enhanced version of the Böhm function is implemented within the FlexX docking program (43). The ChemScore (118) function, today considered one of the most reliable scoring functions (119), builds on the concept of Böhm. The function reproduces the binding affinity of a set of 82 ligand–receptor complexes with a cross-validated error of 8.68 kJ/mol, and external validation tests suggest this result is transferable to other complexes. The equation itself consists of only four terms, each of which is intended to be physically interpretable:

$$\Delta G_{\text{binding}} = \Delta G_0 + \Delta G_{\text{hbond}}{}_{il} g_1(\Delta r) g_2(\Delta \alpha) + \Delta G_{\text{metal}}{}_{aM} f(r_{aM})$$

$$+ \Delta G_{\text{lipo}}{}_{1L} f(r_{1L}) + \Delta G_{\text{rot}} H_{\text{rot}}$$

The second term scores the number and quality of the hydrogen bonds in a similar way to Böhm, although no distinction is made between charged and uncharged interactions, and water-mediated hydrogen bonds are also considered. The third term scores contacts between metals and heteroatoms in the ligand. The fourth term is a contact term that provides an estimate of the interations between lipophilic atoms in the ligand and receptor. The final term scores those rotatable bonds that are frozen during ligand binding.

The regression-based functions proposed by Jain (120) and Rose (121) are designed to overcome problems associated with incorrect orientation of the ligand within the binding site and may be well suited to virtual high-throughput screening applications, where the goal is to evaluate more than

100,000 per day, and to select those with high binding affinity from an approximate docking run.

Although empirical scoring functions have performed remarkably well, most of them omit ligand internal strain energy, which causes problems during flexible docking. Another major factor in scoring that is often completely ignored by scoring functions is desolvation. This is the most difficult part of scoring, since force-field methods are known to overestimate the importance of hydrogen bonds (122), and the AMSOL program (123), which combines a semiempirical molecular orbital approach with a continuum solvation model to calculate solvation free energies, is too computationally expensive for docking. Empirical solvation models estimate solvation free energy as a function of solvent-accessible surface area and produce qualitatively reasonable results (124–127), but few docking methods use this approach. Alternatively, it may be possible to penalize configurations that position lipophilic groups in solvent (128,129). Recently, several groups have included desolvation terms within docking scoring functions (130,131).

Unlike empirical functions, which attempt to define binding based on intuitively important terms, such as hydrogen bonding, surface contacts, and entropic considerations, recently published knowledge-based potential functions (132–134) are derived from statistical analysis of protein–ligand atom pair distances in X-ray structures. The potential of mean force (PMF) function (132) has been implemented within DOCK4 (135) and has been shown to outperform empirical and force-field-based scoring functions (136,137). The DrugScore (134) scoring function has been implemented within FlexX (43).

Other concepts that can be used as scoring function components include overlap with predefined site or anchor points and so-called "themes": structural motifs that are prevalent among high-scoring docking solutions (138,139). Two concepts that attempt to address the imperfect nature of scoring functions are those of *diversity* and *consensus scoring*. The diversity-based approach is most suitable when presented with too many good-scoring candidates. Since the errors within scoring functions are not distributed uniformly, some compound types will be affected more significantly than others, so taking a diverse sampling of hits reduces our vulnerability to this phenomenon. Consensus scoring (119,140,141) acknowledges at its outset that scoring functions are imperfect and that we cannot reliably discriminate between small differences in score. Consensus scoring makes use of several scoring functions, usually of varying type, and accepts only those compounds that attain a certain threshold score in several functions. Tripos' CScore program (142) uses this approach and includes several scoring functions, including FlexX (43), ChemScore (118), and PMF (132) as well as functions similar in nature to the GOLD (131) and DOCK (27) scoring functions. CScore also performs torsional minimization of the ligand within the binding site prior to scoring, since small displacements of the ligand can dramatically affect the score (29). In a recently published study, Rarey demonstrated that an optimized combination of the piecewise linear potential (PLP) function (143,144) and FlexX scoring functions leads to significantly improved performance when evaluated against a set of seven receptor–ligand complexes of pharmaceutical relevance (145).

5   VIRTUAL SCREENING

The preceeding sections reviewed the process of docking small molecules into protein binding sites and the various algorithms and scoring functions available for achieving that objective. Up until now we have focused the discussion on "getting the right answer," i.e., accurate prediction of binding mode and a scoring function that has reasonable correlation with experimentally observed binding affinities. However, techniques such as combinatorial chemistry and high-throughput screening have made it possible to synthesize large numbers of compounds, and the question of which subset of a huge "virtual chemistry space" should actually be synthesized and tested needs to be addressed. A variety of so-called "virtual screening" techniques are now being investigated that make it possible to reduce an enormous virtual chemistry space or virtual library down to a more manageable subset. Docking is one of the main techniques, along with 2D and 3D database searching (5), being investigated and adapted for this purpose.

With a practical or synthesizable virtual chemistry space that may exceed as many as 10 (15) possible compounds it is not possible to directly apply docking methodologies. Instead a multistep approach is taken in which a series of 1D (e.g., molecular weight, lipophilicity, floppiness) and 2D (substructural or similarity searching) filters are applied in sequence to limit the search space, as described in an excellent review by Walters et al. (146). In the context of virtual screening we are looking for docking technologies with two key properties: extremely rapid placement of the ligand within the binding site, and a scoring function that is fast and able to distinguish good from bad dockings. Typically in virtual screening a large number of molecules will successfully dock to the receptor's binding site, and so it is vital that the scoring function be able to prioritize those dockings and guide selection toward the most promising candidates for further analysis.

The rigid-body docking approach used by the DOCK program (10) is extremely fast, about 1–2 seconds per conformer, and appears quite attractive for virtual screening purposes. Recently, Kuntz and coworkers described the use of rigid-body DOCK and an extension that docks ensembles of rigid conformers for each compound for database screening (147). In an interesting variant using rigid-body DOCK, the database of ligands was presolvated, resulting in an improvement in the ranking of known ligands and elimination of molecules within inappropriate charge states and sizes in comparison to screening in the absence of solvation (148). However, the generation of conformers to feed into rigid-body docking can be the rate-limiting step, and this must be addressed properly to reduce the chance of missing hits simply due to sampling poor conformations. DOCK has also been extended for flexible ligand docking and database screening, and was able to screen 10% of the Available Chemicals Directory (ACD) against dihydrofolate reductase (DHFR), finding 7 out of the top 13 hits to be dihydrofolate or methotrexate derivatives (50).

The HAMMERHEAD program (49) was used to screen 80,000 compounds from the ACD in a "few days" for binding to streptavidin, with the natural inhibitor biotin ranked as the top scoring hit. HAMMERHEAD uses up to 300 hydrogen-bonding and van der Waals interaction points to define a template. An incremental construction algorithm is used in which fragments are docked by matching ligand atoms to template points with compatible internal distances in a similar approach to the matching algorithm in DOCK.

The PRO_LEADS program (149) docks flexible ligands into a rigid receptor using a tabu search algorithm (150) and the ChemScore scoring function (118). The tabu search algorithm has the property that it avoids revisiting previous solutions and thus encourages wider exploration of the available search space (151). In a recent study, PRO_LEADS was used to dock a screening set of 10,000 compounds plus small sets of known inhibitors into thrombin, factor Xa, and estrogen receptor binding sites (152). It was found that the ChemScore scoring function was able to distinguish between the known inhibitors and the remaining compounds, and enrichment factors

$$Ef = N_{\text{actives\_found}} / \left(N_{\text{actives\_in\_databases}} \cdot \%_{\text{database\_screened}} \right)$$

of about 14 were obtained with 5% of the dataset screened (Fig. 3). The run time itself was slower than that of other methods, such as FlexX (43), Hammerhead (49), and FLOG (34), with a docking time averaging 6 minutes per structure; thus it is possible to dock 100,000 structures in about 9 days on a 48-processor SGI Origin machine.

The FlexX (43) program described previously has been developed with the problem of virtual screening in mind, and with typical run times of the

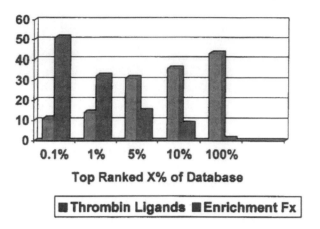

Figure 3   Enrichment factors obtained in virtual screening using PRO_LEADS to screen a set of 10,000 compounds for thrombin inhibitors.

order of 1–2 minutes per structure it is reasonable to expect to dock around a million structures per month on a 48-processor SGI Origin machine.

The SLIDE program (179) uses a template consisting of hydrogen bond and hydrophobic interaction points. Critical solvent is included based on predictions from the Consolv program (153) or by bound water molecules conserved in a series of crystal structures. Docking proceeds by matching dynamically chosen anchor points onto triangles of template points; full ligand flexibility and protein side-chain flexibility is also taken into account. The program is able to screen over 67,000 small molecules within a "few hours."

Virtual screening of a molecular database usually results in a small number, say less than 1%, of the best-fitting molecules from the original database being retained for further evaluation. Depending on the database screened, it is often the case that the resulting hit list contains molecules that are very reminiscent of each other. This phenomenon arises from the fact that most databases are generated by chemical analoging, and it's generally true that if a molecule fits the binding site well, then its analogs are also likely to fit well. Thus, screening a database containing many analog series may result in loss of some interesting hits, simply because they were not analogs of a better-scoring series and ranked below the desired threshold of hits. In a simple approach (154) Shoichet and coworkers used a strategy to increase the diversity of hits from virtual screening that involved clustering the original database, docking every compound, but only assigning a rank to the highest-scoring member of each cluster. The remaining molecules in a cluster can, if desired, be evaluated in a subsequent lead explosion step.

6 COMBINATORIAL DOCKING

In the general case of virtual screening, we are faced with analyzing large collections of arbitrary chemical structures, but the advent of combinatorial chemistry introduces a special case to the problem of virtual screening. The structure of combinatorial libraries can be exploited in such a way that considerable savings in computation time can be achieved when analyzing virtual combinatorial libraries.

In the pioneering work at combining structure-based design and combinatorial chemistry (155), calculations were based on fixed scaffold orientations, with fragments scored independently for each attachment site. The fixed scaffold orientations used were justified based on experimental evidence of limited orientational and conformational freedom for the scaffold. However, in the general case it will be necessary to take into account the interdependency of fragments without prior knowledge of the scaffold orientation; and in the traditional approach to screening, all possible reagent combinations are enumerated and evaluated individually. In the case of virtual combinatorial libraries this might result in billions of compounds to be screened, a number that is far beyond our computational resources. The CombiDOCK algorithm (156) is an extension of the DOCK approach, in which the sphere-matching step is performed using only the combinatorial library scaffold instead of the entire ligand. Once a scaffold is matched onto the active site, each reagent group is attached individually and scored, with the best-scoring fragments combined and checked for intramolecular clashes.

An approach based on the FlexX (43) program attempts to overcome the limitation of the CombiDOCK (156) and PRO_SELECT (157) approaches, which place the combinatorial library scaffold in the binding site in the absence of the substituent groups. This approach, known as CombiFlexX (158), uses the OptiSim algorithm (159,160) to select a diverse, representative subset of the library without enumeration and flexibly docks those molecules using FlexX. The scaffold orientations and conformations are extracted from the docked products and clustered. These unique scaffolds are then used as the base fragment to which each reagent is individually attached using the standard incremental construction algorithm in FlexX. A postdocking processing step is then performed that "builds" and scores the library products using only those docked reagent combinations that do not contain side-chain overlap. For a two-component library, the computational complexity of the CombiFlexX algorithm is $(N + M)$ × *unique_scaffolds* rather than $N \times M$ for full library enumeration. Additionally, the number of unique scaffolds necessary to represent the scaffold diversity does not grow linearly with library size, but in fact reaches a saturation point where it is not necessary to use any more scaffolds to represent a 1 million–compound library than a 100,000-compound library. In test cases the overall run time for all steps in the CombiFlexX process, including initial subset selection, scaffold clustering, docking, and postprocessing, averages about 2–3 seconds per library member. This represents a considerable saving over fully enumerated docking, which averages about 120 seconds per structure using FlexX.

In some cases reagents are joined consecutively, and thus it is difficult to define a meaningful scaffold for the combinatorial library. The DREAM++ algorithm (161) positions the anchor fragments of a basis set of molecules (reagents) into the active site using the DOCK approach. This set of molecules is then virtually "reacted" with another set of "reagents" to yield "products"; a conformational search is performed as each incremental reagent is added. This process is repeated until the entire product is constructed in the binding site.

The de novo approach used by Böhm in the LUDI (35) program is readily extended to combinatorial chemistry; fragments are read from a combinatorial library and docked onto interaction sites within the binding site (162). A set of rules is then applied that determines which so-called link sites (163), e.g. $-NH_2$, $-CHO$, CO_2H, CH_2Br, and $-OH$, may be connected together. In a similar approach (164), Jones and coworkers have extended the GOLD program (78,79) to combinatorial docking, in which each reagent is docked individually, thereby reducing the combinatorial problem from $N \times M$ (for a two component library) to a considerably more computationally feasible $N + M$ problem. The basic assumption underlying this method is that the binding mode of the product is unaffected when that product is partitioned into fragments and those are docked individually and relinked in a subsequent postdocking step that retains only those docked fragment combinations with overlap at the reaction center.

An incremental construction approach to combinatorial docking based on FlexX (43) and called FlexX^c has been developed by Rarey and Lengauer (165). This method recursively adds and removes substituent R-group instances, allowing their interdependencies to be taken into account during docking. The first library member is docked using the standard FlexX approach, with several hundred favorable orientations being retained. Thereafter these orientations are used as the base placement for docking of the next-in-sequence library member, again using the incremental construction algorithm (Fig. 4). This approach offers vast savings in computation time, since the time-consuming steps of base fragment selection and placement within the binding site are eliminated. Drawbacks of this approach are that there is an implicit assumption that all library members

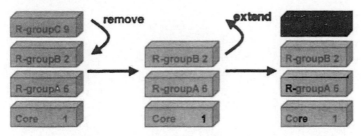

Figure 4 Recursive combinatorial docking algorithm used by FlexX^C.

interact with the receptor in basically the same way, and the outcome is dependent on the order in which substituent groups are considered (Table 3).

7 APPLICATIONS

The accuracy with which docking programs can regenerate receptor–ligand geometries observed in X-ray crystal structures was discussed previously in this chapter and is also discussed as a function of the validation work performed for each of the docking methods discussed herein. Docking is today in routine and growing use as a vital technology for many drug discovery projects. The purpose of this section is to highlight some of the examples that have been reported where docking played a role in the discovery of a compound of significant pharmaceutical interest.

The first experimental test of docking was performed by DesJarlais and coworkers using the DOCK program (10) to search a diverse subset of the Cambridge Structural Database (23) for molecules that might bind to HIV-1 protease (166). One of the hits from the DOCK search was bromoperidol, a close analog of which, haloperidol (Fig. 5a), was tested and found to be a 100 μM inhibitor, and subsequent analog synthesis yielded a thioketal derivative with 15 μM inhibition (Fig. 5b). In addition, Merck's HIV protease inhibitor Indinavir sulfate (Fig. 6) (marketed under the brand name Crixivan®) was developed in part using docking.

Oxalic bis(2-hydroxyl-1-naphthyl-methylene) hydrazide was identified as a 6 μM inhibitor of malarial cysteine protease (167). In this example, 55,000 compounds from the Fine Chemicals Directory were screened using the DOCK program, with the top-ranking 4,400 retained for subsequent evaluation. Following on from this lead, other potent bisarylacylhydrazides and chalcones have been found to be active against chloroquinine-sensitive and -resistant strains of malaria (168).

Table 3 Comparison of Sequential (FlexX[a]) and Combinatorial (FlexX[b]) Library Docking for Three Libraries

Library	No. of strucs	Sequential docking		Buildup order	Combinatorial docking	
		Total	Per structure		Total	Per structure
Benzamidine	92	5 h 4 min	3:18 min	1	11 min	7.2 s
Pyridine	3,864	3 days	6:42 min	4-3-5	4 h 13 min	3.9 s
				3-4-5	4 h 18 min	4.0 s
				5-4-3	8 h 27 min	7.9 s
Ugi-160	160			3-0-1-2-4	24 min	9.0 s
Ugi-20000	20,000			3-0-1-2-4	25 h 42 min	4.6 s

Significant computation time can be saved using the combinatorial algorithm, although the R-group order dependency is shown in the pyridine library. The increase in computation time for the 5-4-3 variant is probably an indication that the algorithm has difficulty placing the final substituent.
[a] From Ref. 43.
[b] From Ref. 165.

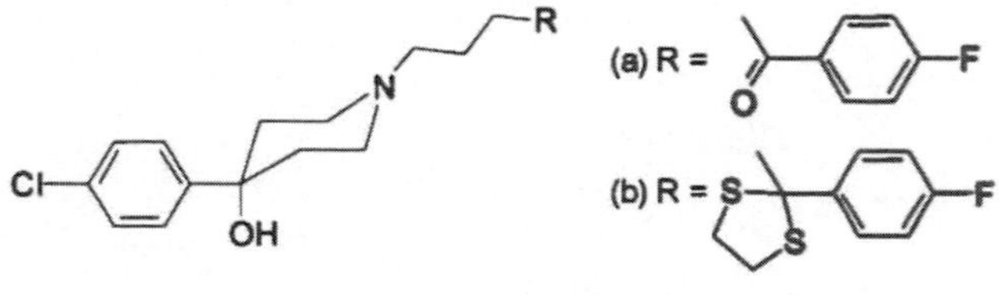

Figure 5 (a) Haloperidol and (b) thioketal derivative.

Kick and coworkers used docking techniques to select side chains in a combinatorial library design to search for inhibitors of the aspartyl protease cathepsin D. Ten side chains were selected at each of three positions on the scaffold, yielding a 1,000-compound library. The library was synthesized and assayed at 1 μM, 330 nM, and 100 nM, with 67, 23, and 7 compounds showing greater than 50% inhibition at each the respective concentrations (155). The CombiDOCK program (156) generated enrichment factors of 2.5 and 4 at the 1 μM and 330 nM levels, respectively.

Böhm and coworkers identified the first noncovalent thrombin inhibitor with Mw < 400 and K_i < 100 nM using an extension of the LUDI (35) de novo design approach (162). In this study, 5,300 amines were initially docked into the thrombin-binding site, and only those with predicted K_i less than 1 mM were retained. A set of 540 substituted benzaldehydes was then attached to the top-ranking amines in the binding site. Based on the predicted K_i and availability of synthetic building blocks, 10 compounds were selected for synthesis. The best compound (Fig. 7) was found to have $K_i = 0.095 \, \mu$M.

8 CONCLUSION AND FUTURE DIRECTIONS

This chapter is intended to give the reader an overall understanding of the fundamental steps involved in molecular docking, and a broad overview of the array of techniques and programs that have been developed to address the various aspects of this problem. However, the reader should by no

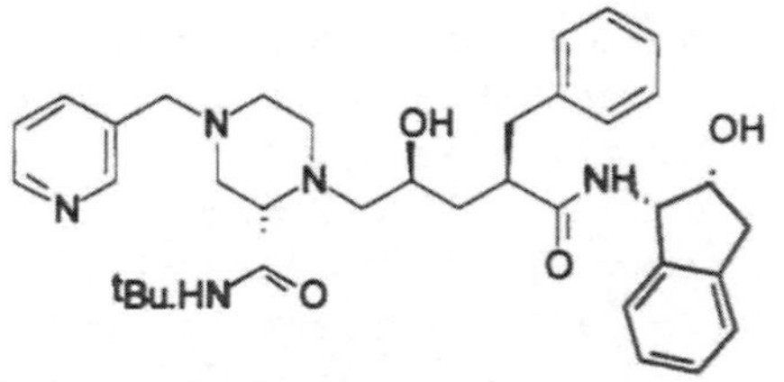

Figure 6 Indinavir sulfate, marketed by Merck as Crixivan®.

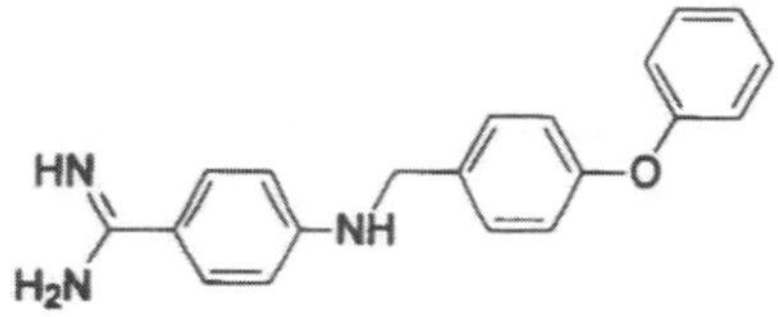

Figure 7   Compound with $K_i = 0.095\,\mu$M.

means be tempted to conclude that this area of science is completely understood. There is in fact a significant amount of work to be done and challenges to be overcome. On the one hand there remain challenges to be addressed in order to accurately predict the binding mode and affinity of conformationally flexible ligands and binding sites. Success in this area will be crucial for molecular docking to expand its horizons beyond identification of inhibitors and antagonists to the more challenging task of identification of agonists that act by very specific mechanisms. On the other hand, there is the somewhat orthogonal and growing need for faster, more approximate methods that can reliably screen tens or even hundreds of thousands of compounds per day.

The fundamental premise underlying all docking calculations is that the free energy of binding a ligand to a receptor can be computationally determined. However, in practice this can be very difficult, and various efforts are under way to improve the ability of force fields to accurately model the enthalpy of binding (169). Concurrent with these efforts are ongoing attempts to improve scoring functions, which have the more modest goal of ranking ligands in order of their complementarity to a particular target.

Another significant challenge in docking and scoring is that of predicting the locations of conserved water molecules and prediction of water-mediated ligand-binding interactions. A step toward achieving this has been described by Kuhn and coworkers (153). Their Consolv program employs a hybrid *k*-nearest-neighbors classifier and genetic algorithm to predict bound water molecules conserved between free and ligand-bound protein structures. The approach is based on the water molecule's crystallographic temperature factor, the number of hydrogen bonds between the water molecule and protein, and the density and hydrophilicity of neighboring protein atoms. The method was trained using a data set of 13 nonhomologous proteins and was able to predict conserved active-site water molecules for seven test proteins with 75% accuracy. In another approach, Rarey and coworkers introduced the particle concept (170) into the FlexX program (43) that adds water molecules at favorable positions during the incremental construction of the ligand in the binding site. This approach was tested for 200 receptor–ligand complexes, with improved accuracy in some cases.

With more and more protein sequences becoming available through the Human Genome Project and crystallization still a difficult and time-consuming task, structure determination by NMR is increasing. NMR, however, does not produce a single structure, but rather an ensemble of structures each of which is in agreement with the experimental data. Although it is possible to derive an averaged structure, it has been shown (171) that the entire ensemble provides a more complete description of the system and new docking methods are being developed to handle this circumstance (172). A promising new method for docking flexible ligands into ensembles of protein structures is under development at GMD (173). This method, called FlexE, is based on efficient docking into ensembles of protein structures. These methods go a step further toward docking into flexible protein structures than attempts that consider only rotational flexibility of hydrogen bonding groups (78,79) or the use of rotamer libraries (84) while adopting a computationally more conservative approach than methods that explicitly treat protein flexibility or domain movements (174,175).

Finally, it is interesting to contrast the structure-based approach to compound design with the more traditional ligand-based approaches. Ligand-based approaches, based on the *similar structure–similar property* principle (176), have in the past tended to dominate our discovery efforts, since 3D protein structures were often not available at the outset of a project. In general, structure-based and ligand-based approaches have focused only on the piece of information in their own domain—docking methods focus on the protein without consideration of the ligand, while similarity methods focus on ligand superpositioning and/or QSAR approaches, without consideration of the receptor structure. However, with the increase in availability of target information it now seems appropriate to develop protocols that combine these two approaches, either within a single step or as pre- or postprocessing steps. Procedures of this type have recently been described (177) that are based on the combination of the DOCK (10) and MIMIC (178) programs. The so-called *similarity-guided* approach incorporates the similarity of the target ligand to a reference structure or pharmacophore structure within the docking score.

REFERENCES

1. ID Kuntz. Science 257:1078–1082, 1992.
2. ID Kuntz et al. Acc Chem Res 27:117–123, 1994.
3. GV Nikiforovich. Int J Peptide Protein Res 44:513–531, 1994.

4. YC Martin, MG Bures, P Willett. In: KB Lipkowitz, DB Boyd (eds.). Reviews in Computational Chemistry, Vol. 1. VCH, New York, 1990, pp. 213–263.
5. T Hurst. Flexible 3D searching: the directed tweak technique. J Chem Inf Comput Sci 34:190–196, 1994.
6. H-J Böhm. Current computational tools for de novo ligand design. Curr Opin Biotech 7:433–436, 1996.
7. RA Lewis, AR Leach. Current methods for site-directed structure generation. J Comput Aided Mol Design 8:467–475, 1994.
8. J Cherfils, J Janin. Protein docking algorithms: simulating molecular recognition. Curr Opin Struct Biol. 3:265–269, 1993.
9. NC Strynadka, M Eisenstein, E Katchalski-Katzir, BK Shoichet, ID Kuntz, R Abagyan, M Totrov, J Janin, J Cherfils, F Zimmerman, A Olson, B Duncan, M Rao, R Jackson, M Sternberg, MN James. Molecular docking programs successfully predict the binding of a beta-lactamase inhibitory protein to TEM-1 beta-lactamase. Nature Struct Biol 3:233–239, 1996.
10. ID Kuntz, JM Blaney, SJ Oatley, R Langridge, TE Ferrin. A geometric approach to macromolecule–ligand interactions. J Mol Biol 161:269–288, 1982.
11. BK Shoichet, ID Kuntz. Matching chemistry and shape in molecular docking. Protein Eng 6:723–732, 1993.
12. GP Brady Jr, PFW Stouten. Fast prediction and visualization of protein binding pockets with PASS. J Comput Aided Mol Design 14:383–401, 2000.
13. PJ Goodford. A computational procedure for determining energetically favorable binding sites on biologically important macromolecules. J Med Chem 28:849–857, 1985.
14. DN Boobbyer, PJ Goodford, PM McWhinnie, RC Wade. New hydrogen-bond potentials for use in determining energetically favorable binding sites on molecules of known structure. J Med Chem 32:1083–1094, 1989.
15. PJ Goodford, RC Wade. Further development of hydrogen bond functions for use in determining energetically favorable binding sites on molecules of known structure. 2. Ligand probe groups with the ability to form more than two hydrogen bonds. J Med Chem 36:148–156, 1993.
16. M von Itzstein, WY Wu, GB Kok, MS Pegg, JC Dyason, B Jin, T Van Phan, ML Smythe, HF White, SW Oliver. Rational design of potent sialidase-based inhibitors of influenza virus replication. Nature 363 (6428):418–423, 1993.
17. K Appelt, RJ Bacquet, CA Bartlett, CL Booth, ST Freer, MA Fuhry, MR Gehring, SM Herrmann, EF Howland, CA Janson. Design of enzyme inhibitors using iterative protein crystallographic analysis. J Med Chem 34:1925–1934, 1991.
18. A. Miranker, M. Karplus. Functionality maps of binding sites: a multiple-copy simultaneous search method. Proteins: Struct Funct Genet 11:29–34, 1991.
19. BR Brooks, RE Bruccoleri, BD Olafson, DJ States, S Swaminathan, M Karplus. CHARMM: a program for macromolecular energy, minimization, and dynamics calculations. J Comp Chem 4:187–217, 1983.

20. DJ Danziger, PM Dean. Automated site-directed drug design: the prediction and observation of ligand point positions at hydrogen-bonding regions on protein surfaces. Proc Roy Soc Ser B 236:115–124, 1989.

21. G. Klebe. The use of composite crystal-field environments in molecular recognition and the de novo design of protein ligands. J Mol Biol 237:212–235, 1994.

22. DE Clark. PRO-LIGAND: an approach to de novo molecular design. 1. Application to the design of organic molecules. J Comput Aided Mol Design 9:13–32, 1995.

23. FH Allen, S Bellard, MD Brice, BA Cartwright, A Doubleday, H Higgs, T Hummelink, BG Hummelink-Peters, O Kennard. The Cambridge Crystallographic Data Center: computer-based search, retrieval, analysis and display of information. Acta Crystallog Sect B 35:2331–2339, 1979.

24. JBO Mitchell, RA Laskowski, A Alex, JM Thornton. BLEEP—potential of mean force describing protein–ligand interactions: I. Generating potential. J Chem Soc Farad Trans 89:2619–2630, 1993.

25. RA Laskowski, JM Thornton, C Humblet, J Singh. X-SITE: use of empirically derived atomic packing preferences to identify favorable interaction regions in the binding sites of proteins. J Mol Biol 259:175–201, 1996.

26. FC Bernstein, TF Koetzle, GJ Williams, EE Meyer Jr, MD Brice, JR Rodgers, O Kennard, T Shimanouchi, M Tasumi. The Protein Data Bank: a computer-based archival file for macromolecular structures. J Mol Biol 112:535–542, 1977.

27. BK Shoichet, DL Bodian, ID Kuntz. Molecular docking using shape descriptors. J Comput Chem 13:380–397, 1992.

28. EC Meng, BK Shoichet, ID Kuntz. Automated docking with grid-based energy evaluation. J Comput Chem 13:505–524, 1992.

29. EC Meng, DA Gschwend, JM Blaney, ID Kuntz. Orientational sampling and rigid-body minimization in molecular docking. Proteins: Struct Funct Genet 17:266–278, 1993.

30. DA Gschwend, ID Kuntz. Orientational sampling and rigid-body minimization in molecular docking revisited: on-the-fly optimization and degeneracy removal. J Comput Aided Mol Design 10:123–132, 1996.

31. AR Leach, ID Kuntz, Conformational analysis of flexible ligands in macromolecular receptor sites. J Comput Chem 13:730–748, 1992.

32. RL DesJarlais, JS Dixon. A shape- and chemistry-based docking method and its use in the design of HIV-1 protease inhibitors. J Comput Aided Mol Design 8:231–242, 1994.

33. MC Lawrence, PC Davis. CLIX: a search algorithm for finding novel ligands capable of binding proteins of known three-dimensional structure. Proteins: Struct Funct Genet 12:31–41, 1992.

34. MD Miller, SK Kearsley, DJ Underwood, RP Sheridan. FLOG: a system to select "quasi-flexible" ligands complementary to a receptor of known three-dimensional structure. J Comput Aided Mol Design 8:153–174, 1994.

35. H-J Böhm. The computer program LUDI: a new method for the de novo design of enzyme inhibitors. J Comput Aided Mol Design 6:61–78, 1992.

36. DJ Bacon, J Moult. Docking by least-squares fitting of molecular surface patterns. J Mol Biol 225:849–858, 1992.

37. SL Lin, R Nussinov, D Fischer, HJ Wolfson. Molecular surface representations by sparse critical points. Proteins: Struct Funct Genet 18:94–101, 1994.

38. R Norel, D Fischer, HJ Wolfson, R Nussinov. Molecular surface recognition by a computer vision-based technique. Prot Eng 7:39–46, 1994.

39. D Fischer, SL Lin, HL Wolfson, R Nussinov. A geometry-based suite of molecular docking processes. J Mol Biol 248:459–477, 1995.

40. SK Kearsley, DJ Underwood, RP Sheridan, MD Miller. Flexibases: a way to enhance the use of molecular docking methods. J Comput Aided Mol Design 8:565–582, 1994.

41. PS Charifson, AR Leach, A Rusinko III. The generation and use of large 3D databases in drug discovery. Network Sci 1, Sept 1995.

42. MD Miller, RP Sheridan, SK Kearsley, DJ Underwood. Advances in automated docking applied to human immunodeficiency virus type 1 protease. Methods Enzymol 241:354–370, 1994.

43. M Rarey, B Kramer, T Lengauer, G Klebe. A fast flexible docking method using an incremental construction algorithm. J Mol Biol 261:470–489, 1996.

44. G Klebe, T Mietzner. A fast and efficient method to generate biologically relevant conformations. J Comput Aided Mol Design 8:583–606, 1994.

45. S Linnainmaa, D Harwood, LS Davis. Pose determination of a 3-D object using triangle pairs. IEEE Trans Pattern Anal Machine Intell 10:636–646, 1988.

46. M Rarey, S Wefing, T Lengauer. Placement of medium-sized molecular fragments into active sites of proteins. J Comput Aided Mol Design 10:41–54, 1996.

47. M Gondran, M Minoux. Graphs and Algorithms. Wiley, New York, 1984.

48. JB Moon, WJ Howe. Computer design of bioactive molecules: a method for receptor-based de novo ligand design. Proteins: Struct Funct Genet 11:314–328, 1991

49. W Welch, J Ruppert, AN Jain. Hammerhead: fast, fully automated docking of flexible ligands to protein binding sites. Chem Biology 3:449–462, 1996.

50. S Makino, ID Kuntz. Automated flexible ligand docking method and its application for database search. J Comput Chem 18:1812–1825, 1997

51. RM Karp, Y Zhang. Randomized parallel algorithms for backtrack search and branch-and-bound computation. J ACM 40:765–789, 1993.

52. M Yamada, A Itai. Development of an efficient automated docking method. Chem Pharm Bull 41:1200–1202, 1993.

53. M Yamada, A Itai. Application and evaluation of the automated docking method. Chem Pharm Bull 41:1203–1205, 1993.

54. MY Mizutani, N Tomioka, A Itai. Rational automatic search method for stable docking models of protein and ligand. J Mol Biol 243:310–326, 1994.

55. H Grubmuller, B Heymann, P Tavan. Ligand binding: molecular mechanics calculation of the streptavidin-biotin rupture force. Science 271:997–999, 1996.

56. JP Ryckaert, G Ciccotti, HJC Berendsen. Numerical integration of the Cartesian equations of motion of a system with constraints: molecular dynamics of *n*-alkanes. J Comput Phys 23:327–341, 1977.

57. KD Gibson, HA Scheraga. Variable-step molecular dynamics: an exploratory technique for peptides with fixed geometry. J Comput Chem 11:468–486, 1990.

58. RE Bruccoleri, M Karplus. Conformational sampling using high-temperature molecular dynamics. Biopolymers 29:1847–1862, 1990.

59. N Metropolis, AW Rosenbluth, MN Rosenbluth, AH Teller, E Teller. Equation of state calculations by fast computing machines. J Chem Phys 21:1087–1092, 1953.

60. S Kirkpatrick, CD Gelatt, MP Vecchi. Optimization by simulated annealing. Science 220:671–680, 1983.

61. DS Goodsell, AJ Olsen. Automated docking of substrates to proteins by simulated annealing. Proteins 8:195–202, 1990.

62. DS Goodsell, H Lauble, CD Stout, AJ Olson. Automated docking in crystallography: analysis of the substrates of aconitase. Proteins: Struct Funct Genet 17:1–10, 1993.

63. BL Stoddard, DE Koshland Jr. Prediction of the structure of a receptor–protein complex using a binary docking method. Nature 358:774–776, 1992.

64. BL Stoddard, DE Koshland Jr. Molecular recognition analyzed by docking simulations: the aspartate receptor and isocitrate dehydrogenase from *Escherichia coli*. Proc Natl Acad Sci USA 90:1146–1153, 1993.

65. AR Friedman, VA Roberts, JA Tainer. Predicting molecular interactions and inducible complementarity: fragment docking of Fab–peptide complexes. Proteins: Struct Funct Genet 20:15–24, 1994.

66. TN Hart, RJ Read. A multiple-start Monte Carlo docking method. Proteins: Struct Funct Genet 13:206–222, 1992.

67. RJ Read, TN Hart, MD Cummings, SR Ness. Monte Carlo algorithms for docking to proteins. Supramol Chem 6:135–140, 1995.

68. M Liu, S Wang. MCDOCK: a Monte Carlo simulation approach to the molecular docking problem. J Comput Aided Mol Design 13:435–451, 1999.

69. JH Holland. Adaption in Natural and Artificial Systems. University of Michigan Press, Ann Arbor, 1975.

70. D Goldberg. Genetic Algorithms in Search, Optimization and Machine Learning. Addison-Wesley, Reading, MA, 1989.

71. RS Judson, EP Jaeger, AM. Treasurywala, ML Peterson. J Comput Chem 14:1407–1414, 1993.

72. AWR Payne, RC Glen. Molecular recognition using a binary genetic search algorithm. J Mol Graph 11:74–91, 1993.

73. G Jones, P Willett, RC Glen. A genetic algorithm for flexible molecular overlay and pharmacophore elucidation. J Comput Aided Mol Design 9:532–549, 1995.

74. CM Oshiro, ID Kuntz, JS Dixon. Flexible ligand docking using a genetic algorithm. J Comput Aided Mol Design 9:113–130, 1995.

75. RS Judson, EP Jaeger, AM Treasurywala. A genetic algorithm–based method for docking flexible molecules. Theochem 114:191–206, 1994.

76. RS Judson, YT Tan, E Mori, C Melius, EP Jaeger, AM Treasurywala, A Mathiowetz. Docking flexible molecules: a case study of three proteins. J Comput Chem 16:1405–1419, 1995.

77. KP Clark, Ajay. Flexible ligand docking without parameter adjustment across four ligand–receptor complexes. J Comput Chem 16:1210–1226, 1995.

78. G Jones, P Willett, RC Glen. Molecular recognition of receptor sites using a genetic algorithm with a description of desolvation. J Mol Biol 245:43–53, 1995.

79. G Jones, P Willett, RC Glen, AR Leach, R Taylor. Development and validation of a genetic algorithm for flexible docking. J Mol Biol 267:727–748, 1997.

80. JS Taylor, RM Burnett. DARWIN: a program for docking flexible molecules. Proteins: Struct Funct Genet 41:173–191, 2000.

81. DB Fogel. Evolutionary Computation: Toward a New Philosophy of Machine Intelligence. IEEE Press, Piscataway, NJ, 1995.

82. DK Gehlhaar, GM Verkhivker, PA Rejto, CJ Sherman, DB Fogel, LJ Fogel, ST Freer. Molecular recognition of the inhibitor AG-1343 by HIV-1 protease: conformationally flexible docking by evolutionary programming. Chem Biol 2:317–324, 1995.

83. J Yang, C Kao. Flexible ligand docking using a robust evolutionary algorithm. J Comput Chem 21:988–998, 2000.

84. AR Leach. Ligand docking to proteins with discrete side-chain flexibility. J Mol Biol 235:345–356, 1994.

85. J Apostolakis, A Plückthun, A Caflisch. Docking small ligands in flexible binding sites. J Comput Chem 19:21–37, 1998.

86. ME Davis, JA McCammon. Dielectric boundary smoothing in finite difference solutions of the Poisson equation: an approach to improve accuracy and convergence. J Comput Chem 12:909–912, 1991.

87. Z Li, HA Scheraga. Monte Carlo minimization approach to the multiple-minima problem in protein folding. Proc Natl Acad Sci USA 84:6611–6615, 1987.

88. A Caflisch, S Fischer, M Karplus. Docking by Monte Carlo minimization with a solvation correction: application to an FKBP–substrate complex. J Comput Chem 18:723–743, 1997.

89. J Wang, PA Kollman, ID Kuntz. Flexible ligand docking: a multistep strategy approach. Proteins: Struct Funct Genet 36:1–19, 1999.

90. D Hoffmann, B Kramer, T Washio, T Steinmetzer, M Rarey, T Lengauer. Two-stage method for protein–ligand docking. J Med Chem 42:4422–4433, 1999.

91. PA Bartlett, CK Marlowe. Evaluation of intrinsic binding energy from a hydrogen bonding group in an enzyme inhibitor. Science 235:569–571, 1987.

92. PM Dean. Molecular Foundations of Drug–Receptor Interaction. Cambridge University Press, Cambridge, UK, 1987.
93. PR Andrews, M Tintelnot. In: C Hansch, Ed., Quantitative Drug Design, Vol. 4. Pergamon Press, New York, 1990, pp 321–347.
94. A Fersht. The hydrogen bond in molecular recognition. Trends Biochem Sci 12:3214–3219, 1987.
95. D Sali, M Bycroft, A Fersht. In: JJ Villafranca, Ed. Techniques in Protein Chemistry, Vol. II. Academic Press, New York, 1991, pp 295–303.
96. AE Mark, WF van Gunsteren. In: PM Dean, G Jolles, CG Newton, Eds. New Perspectives in Drug Design. Academic Press, London, 1995, pp 185–200.
97. PA Kollman. Free-energy calculations—applications to chemical and biochemical phenomena. Chem Rev 93:2395–2417, 1993.
98. PR Gerber, AE Mark, WF van Gunsteren. An approximate but efficient method to calculate free-energy trends by computer simulation: application to dihydrofolate reductase–inhibitor complexes. J Comput Aided Mol Design 7:305–323, 1993.
99. H-J Böhm, M Stahl. Rapid empirical scoring functions in virtual screening applications. Med Chem Res 9:445–462, 1999.
100. CS Ring, E Sun, JH McKerrow, GK Lee, PJ Rosenthal, ID Kuntz, FE Cohen. Structure-based inhibitor design by using protein models for the development of antiparasitic agents. Proc Natl Acad Sci USA 90:3583–3587, 1993.
101. RS Bohacek, C McMartin. Multiple highly diverse structures complementary to enzyme binding sites: results of extensive application of a de novo design method incorporating combinatorial growth. J Am Chem Soc 116:5560–5571, 1994
102. MK Holloway, JM Wai, TA Halgren, PM Fitzgerald, JP Vacca, BD Dorsey, RB Levin, WJ Thompson, LJ Chen, SJ deSolms. A priori prediction of activity for HIV-1 protease inhibitors employing energy minimization in the active site. J Med Chem 38:305–317, 1995.
103. G Verkhivker, K Appelt, ST Freer, JE Villafranca. Empirical free-energy calculations of ligand–protein crystallographic complexes. I. Knowledge-based ligand–protein interaction potentials applied to the prediction of human immunodeficiency virus 1 protease binding affinity. Protein Eng 8:677–691, 1995.
104. RL DesJarlais, RP Sheridan, GL Seibel, JS Dixon, ID Kuntz, R Venkataraghavan. Using shape complementarity as an initial screen in designing ligands for a receptor binding site of known three-dimensional structure. J Med Chem 31:722–729, 1988.
105. V Sobolev, M Edelman. Modeling the quinone-B binding site of the photosystem-II reaction center using notions of complementarity and contact-surface between atoms. Proteins 21:214–225, 1995.
106. V Sobolev, RC Wade, G Vriend, M Edelman. Molecular docking using surface complementarity. Proteins: Struct Funct Genet 25:120–129, 1996.
107. N Horton, M Lewis. Calculation of the free energy of association for protein complexes. Protein Sci 1:169–181, 1992.

108. A Wallqvist, DG Covell. Docking enzyme–inhibitor complexes using a preference-based free-energy surface. Proteins: Struct Funct Genet 25:403–419, 1996.

109. A Wallqvist, RL Jernigan, DG Covell. A preference-based free-energy parameterization of enzyme–inhibitor binding. Applications to HIV-1-protease inhibitor design. Protein Sci 4:1881–1903, 1995.

110. E Katchalski-Katzir, I Shariv, M Eisenstein, AA Friesem, C Aflalo, IA Vakser. Molecular surface recognition: determination of geometric fit between proteins and their ligands by correlation techniques. Proc Natl Acad Sci USA 89:2195–2199, 1992.

111. HA Gabb, RM Jackson, MJ Sternberg. Modelling protein docking using shape complementarity, electrostatics and biochemical information. J Mol Biol 272:106–120, 1997.

112. SJ Weiner, PA Kollman, DA Case, UC Singh, C Ghio, G Alagona, S Profeta Jr, P Weiner. A new force field for molecular mechanical simulation of nucleic acids and proteins. J Am Chem Soc 106:765–784, 1984.

113. SJ Weiner, PA Kollman, DT Nguyen, DA Case. An all-atom force field for simulations of proteins and nucleic acids. J Comput Chem 7:230–252, 1986.

114. EC Meng, ID Kuntz, DJ Abraham, GE Kellogg. Evaluating docked complexes with the HINT exponential function and empirical atomic hydrophobicities. J Comput Aided Mol Design 8:299–306, 1994.

115. RS DeWitte, EI Shakhnovich. SMoG: de novo design method based on simple, fast, and accurate free-energy estimates. 1. Methodology and supporting evidence. J Am Chem Soc 118:11733–11744, 1996.

116. RD Head, ML Smythe, TI Oprea, CL Waller, SM Green, GR Marshall. VALIDATE: a new method for the receptor-based prediction of binding affinities of novel ligands. J Am Chem Soc 118:3959–3969, 1996.

117. H-J Böhm. LUDI: rule-based automatic design of new substituents for enzyme inhibitor leads. J Comput Aided Mol Design 6:593–606, 1992.

118. MD Eldridge, CW Murray, TR Auton, GV Paolini, RP Mee. Empirical scoring functions: I. The development of a fast empirical scoring function to estimate the binding affinity of ligands in receptor complexes. J Comput Aided Mol Design 11:425–445, 1997.

119. PS Charifson, JJ Corkery, MA Murcko, WP Walters. Consensus scoring: a method for obtaining improved hit rates from docking databases of three-dimensional structures into proteins. J Med Chem 42:5100–5109, 1999.

120. A Jain. Scoring noncovalent protein–ligand interactions: a continuous differentiable function tuned to compute binding affinities. J Comput Aided Mol Design 10:427–440, 1996.

121. PW Rose. Scoring Methods in Ligand Design. 2nd USCF Course in Computer-Aided Molecular Design, San Francisco, 1977.

122. JM Blaney, PK Weiner, A Dearing, PA Kollman, EC Jorgensen, SJ Oatley, JM Burridge, CCF Blake. Molecular mechanics simulation of protein–ligand interactions: binding of thyroid hormone analogs to prealbumin. J Am Chem Soc 104:6424–6434, 1982.

123. CJ Cramer, DG Truhlar. An SCF solvation model for the hydrophobic effect and absolute free energies of aqueous solvation. Science 256:213–217, 1992.
124. D Eisenberg, AD McLachlan. Solvation energy in protein folding and binding. Nature 319:199–203, 1986.
125. T Ooi, M Oobatake, G Nemethy, HA Scheraga. Accessible surface areas as a measure of the thermodynamic parameters of hydration of peptides. Proc Natl Acad Sci USA 84:3086–3090. 1987.
126. L Wesson, D Eisenberg. Atomic solvation parameters applied to molecular dynamics of proteins in solution. Protein Sci 1:227–235, 1992.
127. WC Still, A Tenpczyk, RC Hawley, T Hendrickson. Semi-analytical treatment of solvation for molecular mechanics and dynamics. J Am Chem Soc 112:6127–6129, 1990.
128. PFW Stouten, C Froemmel, H Nakamura, C Sander. An effective solvation term based on atomic occupancies for use in protein simulations. Mol Simul 10:97–120, 1993.
129. M Hahn. Receptor surface models. 1. Definition and construction. J Med Chem 38:2080–2090, 1995.
130. BA Luty, ZR Wasserman, PFW Stouten, CN Hodge, M Zacharias, JA McCammon. A molecular mechanics/grid method for evaluation of ligand–receptor interactions. J Comput Chem 16:454–464, 1995.
131. G Jones, P Willett, RC Glen. Molecular recognition of receptor sites using a genetic algorithm with a description of desolvation. J Mol Biol 245:43–53, 1995.
132. I Muegge, YC Martin, A general and fast-scoring function for protein–ligand interactions: a simplified potential approach. J Med Chem 42:791–804, 1999.
133. JBO Mitchell, RA Laskowski, A Alex, JM Thornton. BLEEP—potential of mean force describing protein–ligand interactions: I. Generating potential. J Comput Chem 20:1165–1177, 1999.
134. H Gohlke, M Hendlich, G Klebe. Knowledge-based scoring function to predict protein–ligand interactions. J Mol Biol 295:337–356, 2000.
135. T Ewing, ID Kuntz. Critical evaluation of search algorithms for automated molecular docking and database screening. J Comput Chem 18:1175–1189, 1997.
136. I Muegge, YC Martin, PJ Hajduk, SW Fesik. Evaluation of PMF scoring in docking weak ligands to the FK506 binding protein. J Med Chem 42:2498–2503, 1999.
137. S Ha, R Andreani, A Robbins, I Muegge. Evaluation of docking/scoring approaches: a comparative study based on MMP3 inhibitors. J Comput Aided Mol Design 14:435–448, 2000.
138. VJ Gillet, W Newell, P Mata, G Myatt, S Sike, Z Zsoldos, AP Johnson. SPROUT: recent developments in the de novo design of molecules. J Chem Inf Comput Sci 34:207–217, 1994.
139. DE Clark, CW Murray. J Chem Inf Comput Sci 37:914–923, 1995.

140. C Bissantz, G Folkers, D Rognan. Protein-based virtual screening of chemical databases. 1. Evaluation of different docking/scoring combinations. J Med Chem 43:4759–4767, 2000.

141. B. Clark. J Mol Graph, 2001, in press.

142. Tripos Inc., St. Louis, Missouri.

143. DK Gehlhaar, GM Verkhivker, PA Rejto, CJ Sherman, DB Fogel, LJ Fogel, ST Freer. Molecular recognition of the inhibitor AG-1343 by HIV-1 protease: conformationally flexible docking by evolutionary programming. Chem Biol 2:317–324, 1995.

144. GM Verkhivker, D Bouzida, DK Gehlhaar, PA Rejto, S Arthurs, AB Colson, ST Freer, V Larson, BA Luty, T Marrone, PW Rose. Deciphering common failures in molecular docking of ligand–protein complexes. J Comput Aided Mol Design 14:731–751, 2000.

145. M Stahl, M Rarey. Detailed analysis of scoring functions for virtual screening. J Med Chem 44:1035–1042, 2001.

146. WP Walters, MT Stahl, MA Murcko. Virtual screening—an overview. Drug Discovery Today 3:160–178, 1998.

147. DM Lorber, BK Shoichet. Flexible ligand docking using conformational ensembles. Protein Science 7:938–950, 1998.

148. BK Shoichet, AR Leach, ID Kuntz. Ligand solvation in molecular docking. Proteins: Struct Funct Genet 34:4–16, 1999.

149. CA Baxter, CW Murray, DE Clark, DR Westhead, MD Eldridge. Flexible docking using Tabu search and an empirical estimate of binding affinity. Proteins 33:367–382, 1998.

150. DR Westhead, DE Clark, CW Murray. A comparison of heuristic search algorithms for molecular docking. J Comput Aided Mol Design 11:209–228, 1997.

151. F Glover, M Laguna. In: CR Reeves, Ed. Modern Heuristic Techniques for Combinatorial Problems. Blackwell Scientific Publications, Oxford, UK, 1993, p 70.

152. CA Baxter, CW Murray, B Waszkowycz, J Li, RA Sykes, RG Bone, TD Perkins, W Wylie. New approach to molecular docking and its application to virtual screening of chemical databases. J Chem Inf Comput Sci 40:254–262, 2000.

153. ML Raymer, PC Sanschagrin, WF Punch, S Venkataraman, ED Goodman, LA Kuhn. Predicting conserved water-mediated and polar ligand interactions in proteins using a K-nearest-neighbors genetic algorithm. J Mol Biol 265:445–464, 1997.

154. AI Su, DM Lorber, GS Weston, WA Baase, BW Matthews, BK Shoichet. Docking molecules by families to increase the diversity of hits in database screens: computational strategy and experimental evaluation. Proteins: Struct Funct Genet 42:279–293, 2001.

155. EK Kick, DC Roe, AG Skillman, G Liu, TJ Ewing, Y Sun, ID Kuntz, JA Ellman. Structure-based design and combinatorial chemistry yield low nanomolar inhibitors of cathepsin D. Chem Biol 4:297–307, 1997.

156. Y Sun, TJ Ewing, AG Skillman, ID Kuntz. CombiDOCK: structure-based combinatorial docking and library design. J Comput Aided Mol Design 12:597–604, 1998.

157. CW Murray, DE Clark, TR Auton, MA Firth, J Li, RA Sykes, B Waszkowycz, DR Westhead, SC Young. PRO_SELECT: combining structure-based drug design and combinatorial chemistry for rapid lead discovery. 1. Technology. J Comput Aided Mol Design 11:193–207, 1997.

158. D Lowis, T Heritage, S Burkett, J Bikker, M Snow. Manuscript in preparation.

159. RD Clark. OptiSim: an extended dissimilarity selection method for finding diverse representative subsets. J Chem Inf Comput Sci 37:1181–1188, 1997.

160. RD Clark, WJ Langton. Balancing representativeness against diversity using optimizable K-dissimilarity and hierarchical clustering. J Chem Inf Comput Sci 38:1079–1086, 1998.

161. S Makino, TJ Ewing, ID Kuntz. DREAM++: flexible docking program for virtual combinatorial libraries. J Comput Aided Mol Design 13:513–532, 1999.

162. H-J Böhm, DW Banner, L Weber. Combinatorial docking and combinatorial chemistry: design of potent nonpeptide thrombin inhibitors. J Comput Aided Mol Design 13:51–56, 1999.

163. H-J Böhm. Towards the automatic design of synthetically accessible protein ligands: peptides, amides and peptidomimetics. J Comput Aided Mol Design 10:265–272, 1996.

164. G Jones, P Willett. In: AL Parrill, MR Reddy, Eds. Rational Drug Design: Novel Methodology and Practical Applications. ACS Symposium Series 719, American Chemical Society, 1999, pp 271–291.

165. M Rarey, T Lengauer. A recursive algorithm for efficient combinatorial library docking. Perspectives Drug Discovery Design 20:63–81, 2000.

166. RL DesJarlais, GL Seibel, ID Kuntz, PS Furth, JC Alvarez, PR Ortiz de Montellano, DL DeCamp, LM Babe, CS Craik. Structure-based design of nonpeptide inhibitors specific for the human immunodeficiency virus 1 protease. Proc Natl Acad Sci USA 87:6644–6648, 1990.

167. CS Ring, E Sun, JH McKerrow, GK Lee, PJ Rosenthal, ID Kuntz, FE Cohen. Structure-based inhibitor design by using protein models for the development of antiparasitic agents. Proc Natl Acad Sci USA 90:3583–3587, 1993.

168. R Li, X Chen, B Gong, PM Selzer, Z Li, E Davidson, G Kurzban, RE Miller, EO Nuzum, JH McKerrow, RJ Fletterick, SA Gillmor, CS Craik, ID Kuntz, FE Cohen, GL Kenyon. Structure-based design of parasitic protease inhibitors. Bioorg Med Chem 4:1421–1427, 1996.

169. PA Kollman. Advances and continuing challenges in achieving realistic and predictive simulations of the properties of organic and biological molecules. Acc Chem Res 29:461–469, 1996.

170. M Rarey, B Kramer, T Lengauer. The particle concept: placing discrete water molecules during protein–ligand docking predictions. Proteins: Struct Funct Genet 34:17–28, 1999.

171. MJ Sutcliffe. Representing an ensemble of NMR-derived protein structures by a single structure. Protein Sci 2:936–944, 1993.
172. R Knegtel, C Oshiro, ID Kuntz. Molecular docking to ensembles of protein structures. J Mol Biol 266:424–440, 1997.
173. German National Research Center for Information Technology, Institute for Algorithms and Scientific Computing (GMD-SCAI), Schloss Birlinghoven, D53754 Sankt Augustin, Germany.
174. M Totrov, R Abagyan. Flexible protein–ligand docking by global energy optimization in internal coordinates. Proteins: Struct Funct Genet Supplement 1:215–220, 1997.
175. B Sandak, HJ Wolfson, R Nussinov. Flexible docking allowing induced fit in proteins: insights from an open to closed conformational isomers. Proteins: Struct Funct Genet 32:159–174, 1998.
176. MA Johnson, GM Maggiora, Eds. Concepts and Applications of Molecular Similarity. Wiley, New York, 1990.
177. X Fradera, RM Knegtel, J Mestres. Similarity-driven flexible ligand docking. Proteins: Struct Funct Genet 40:623–636, 2000.
178. J Mestres, DC Rohrer, GM Maggiora. MIMIC: A molecular-field matching program. Exploiting applicability of molecular similarity approaches. J Comput Chem 18:934–954, 1997.
179. V Schnecke, LA Kuhn. Database screening for HIV protease ligands: the influence of binding-site conformation and representation on ligand selectivity. Pro Int Conf Intell Syst Mol Biol pp 242–251, 1999.
180. RL DesJarlais, RP Sheridan, JS Dixon, ID Kuntz, R Venkataraghavan. Docking flexible ligands to macromolecular receptors by molecular shape. J Med Chem 29:2149–2153, 1986.

17

Use of Pharmacophores in Structure-Based Drug Design

Omoshile Clement and Adrea T. Mehl
Accelrys, San Diego, California, U.S.A.

1 BACKGROUND

A *pharmacophore* can be defined as a three-dimensional configuration of
chemical features that is necessary for binding or modulating biological
activity at a given receptor site (1). Feature-based pharmacophores are useful search queries for mining databases for new leads (2,3) or predicting
activities of proposed structures (4–6). Feature definitions are not limited
to descriptions of specific chemical topology. Rather, they describe the kinds
of interactions important for ligand–receptor binding. They generally
include hydrogen bond acceptors, hydrogen bond donors, and hydrophobes
but have also been defined for positive and negative charge centers and
extended to other custom definitions (7,8). This allows for a broad range
of topologies to be considered as drug candidates. Substitution of one chemical moiety for another while still maintaining the same overall chemical
functionality can be an effective means of circumventing unwanted side
effects inherent to a particular class of molecules.

Traditionally, the approach to pharmacophore model development
has been based on known active ligands. Lacking a known receptor structure, a variety of analog-based methods can be applied to the design of new
therapeutics. Among these are the active analog approach (9), de novo
methods such as Ludi (10–12) and TOPAS (13), 3D quantitative struc-

ture–activity relationship (QSAR) methods (14–16), and the generation of 3D pharmacophore hypotheses (17). Regression analyses from 3D QSAR and automatic pharmacophore perception techniques can suffer from data overfitting since they are biased toward compounds in the training set (18). In many cases, the training set compounds lack enough diversity to capture the key interactions that come into play at the receptor binding site.

A second approach, which will be the subject of this chapter, involves pharmacophores derived from a known or putative receptor structure and bound ligands. This approach is referred to as *structure-based drug design*. Once the structure of the receptor target is known, pharmacophore-based queries can be derived from the shape of the binding cavity, the bound ligand, bound water molecules, computationally derived interactions from GRID maps (19), and multiple-copy similarity search (MCSS) minima (20,21), plus any known positions of the residues involved in ligand binding. This chapter will *not* cover the general topic of structure-based drug design, but rather those studies involving pharmacophore modeling of the receptor active site in identifying important ligand–receptor binding features.

Structures of receptors and drug targets are often determined from experimental [X-ray crystallography and nuclear magnetic resonance (NMR) spectroscopy] and theoretical (homology modeling) studies. The most optimal situation occurs when the structure of both the receptor and the bound ligand are known. For example, structure-based design methodologies have been used to generate analogs of bound inhibitors with known binding modes (22). Using information derived from high-resolution NMR structure determination of an inhibitor bound to MMP-13, a potent hybrid inhibitor was synthesized (23) and found to exhibit a high degree of specificity for MMP-13, relative to other closely related enzymes.

In the absence of a known crystal structure, homology models can be useful for further study. For example, information from SAR data of a set of oxysterols and the crystal structure of RARγ were used to generate a homology model of the binding domain of the orphan nuclear receptor LXRRα (24). A pharmacophore model constructed from the binding domain was shown to incorporate the structural requirements necessary to activate the receptor. This model can then be used in a ligand-based approach to design inhibitors of the LXRRα receptor.

2 EARLY SUCCESSES OF STRUCTURE-BASED PHARMACOPHORE MODELING

The application of pharmacophore perception techniques in structure-based design of new drugs has been well described in a recent book on pharmacophores and their use in drug design (25). An early approach that applied pattern recognition to the design and development of a drug was reported about 25 years ago by Cushman and coworkers (26) and by Patchett et al. (27). These studies represent the first reports of successful pharmacophore-based design that produced commercially viable drugs—inhibitors of the angiotensin-converting enzyme (ACE).

In 1977, despite the lack of a 3D structure of the ACE, Cushman and coworkers (26) reported the first rationally designed inhibitor for this receptor. Postulating that since the catalytic properties of ACE resembles those of two other zinc proteinases—carboxypeptidase A and thermolysin—whose structures are known, these workers inferred that the receptor active site in ACE must be ca. 3.4 Å larger than that of carboxypeptidase A. From this postulate, they were able to design successive succinyl-proline derivatives, including the potent inhibitor 3-mercapto-2-methylpropanoyl-L-proline, which became a commercial success under the market name Captopril® (Fig. 1a). A few years after this discovery, Patchett and coworkers (27), at Merck, replaced a cystenyl group in Captopril with phenylalanine, to produce Enalapril® (Fig. 1b), a drug with significantly reduced side effects relative to Captopril.

In a related study using the active analog approach (9), Henry and Güner (28) used structural information derived from inhibitors of carboxypeptidase A as well as the active site of this enzyme in building a receptor-based pharmacophore query for inhibitors of angiotensin converting enzymes. A pharmacophore query was derived from the bound conformations of three different inhibitors of carboxypeptidase A and some of the amino acid residues in the active site. The model contained two lipophilic groups, a ring aromatic and a carbonyl functional group with distance constraints representing coverage of the binding features in the three carboxypeptidase A–bound inhibitors (Fig. 2a). The pharmacophore thus derived was used as a search query in database-mining experiments.

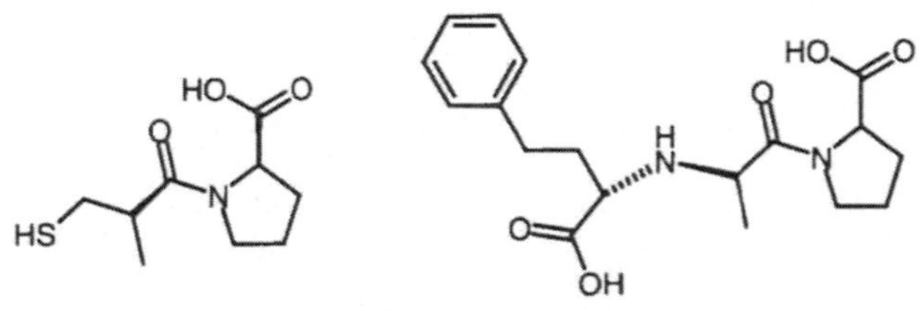

(a) CAPTOPRIL   (b) ENALAPRIL

Figure 1 Known ACE inhibitors (a) Captopril® (from Ref. 26), and (b) Enalapril® (from Ref. 27).

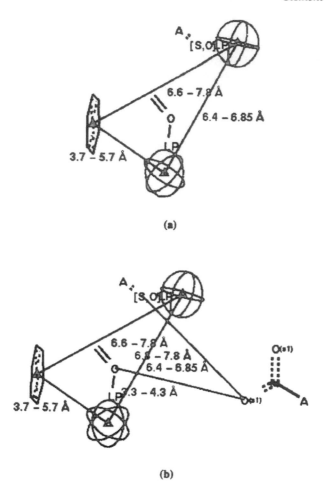

Figure 2 (a) Receptor-based query derived for ACE. (b) Final composite ACE inhibitor query. (From Ref. 27.)

In a search of MDLs drug database—MDDR-3D (29)—containing 209 angiotensinase inhibitors, the derived pharmacophore model returned a total of 17,091 "hits." The hit list contained all of the 209 angiotensinase inhibitors, along with 3,438 compounds listed as antihypertensives. A modified form of the search query (Fig. 2b) was used to search the same database (MDDR-3D Version 94.1). The results showed that of the 5,041 compounds in MDDR-3D that contain the substructural fragments of this query, 713 were antihypertensive compounds and 193 were angiotensinase inhibitors.

3 PHARMACOPHORE DESIGN

Knowledge of protein structure can be incorporated into a pharmacophore model that describes the generalized interactions that are important for ligand–receptor binding. The pharmacophore components, or features, are defined by general chemical functions, such as hydrogen bond acceptors, hydrogen bond donors, and hydrophobes. Ludi, a de novo design approach to generating new potential ligands (10,30), can be used when the structure of the protein-bound ligand is unknown. Based solely on the structure of the target receptor, Ludi will locate potential binding interaction sites. These suggested binding interactions are characterized by the ability of the ligand and receptor to participate in hydrogen bonding (both donor and acceptor) and hydrophobic interactions. Ludi then searches a fragment library for small molecules that will complement the functionalities at the active site.

When information is available about how the ligand binds to the receptor, the receptor structure, and ligand-binding mode, these essential receptor–ligand interactions can be described by 3D pharmacophores. Even without a bound ligand, the active site of a protein can be characterized by a map of possible interaction sites. The shape and feature types in the interaction map (hydrogen bond donors, hydrogen bond acceptors, and hydrophobes) represent the complement of the functionality at the binding site. Further processing of this interaction map, as described later, allows one to generate sets of pharmacophore models that are suitable for searching 3D databases. The proposed pharmacophore is made up of the features necessary for the ligand to bind to the receptor. This technique of generating a pharmacophore from the active site is automated through the Cerius2 (31) interface and is known as *structure-based focusing* (SBF).

4 STRUCTURE-BASED FOCUSING

In C2·SBF (31) (see Scheme 1), the interaction site is defined by a sphere. The location of the sphere center and the radius of the sphere are user defined. The sphere should include the key residues of the protein that are involved in ligand binding. SBF then calls LUDI to define hydrogen bond acceptors, hydrogen bond donors, and hydrophobic sites on the protein. Although all interactions in the active site are identified, only subsets of these sites are actually involved in the ligand–receptor interaction. Clustering techniques within the Cerius2 package can be applied to cluster similar pharmacophore types to reduce the overall number of interaction sites. When the ultimate goal is to formulate queries for database searching, those queries must be limited by the number of pharmacophore features they contain in order to successfully mine databases for new leads. In

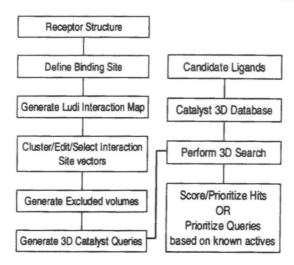

Scheme 1 Flowchart for Accelrys's Cerius2 structure-based focusing methodology. (From Ref. 31.)

general, queries containing three to seven features are suitable for database mining (2).

In limiting the number of features in the model, one can come up with many pharmacophore models based on the original interaction map. The key task is to decipher which patterns are biologically significant and to allow for the possibility that there are multiple modes of binding. The SBF technique has been used to generate pharmacophore models derived from the dihydrofolate reductase/MTX complex (32) as well as for the estrogen receptor (33,34).

In a study of structure-based design of estrogen receptor agonists, Venkatachalam and coworkers (33) applied the C2·SBF algorithm to the development and analyses of receptor-based pharmacophore models based on the flowchart shown in Scheme 1. The target receptor structure used in the study was 1ERE (35). A LUDI interaction map of the residues within 9 Å of the bound estradiol (E2) agonist was generated (see Fig. 3) consisting of hydrogen bond donors, hydrogen bond acceptors, and hydrophobes. These features were clustered via a complete linkage hierachical clustering method, and a representative member of each cluster closest to the centroid was retained (see Fig. 4). Multiple queries containing three-, four-, five-, and six-feature combinations were generated from the cluster centroids. A total of 228 exclusion spheres with a radius of 1.3 Å (derived for all nonhydrogen atoms within 9 Å of the Ludi radius) were added to each pharmacophore model. Validation of these models was performed via database mining using the models as search queries to mine a database collection of 31 estrogen ligands. Ligands encoding the features in the models that most approximates the ligand-binding requirements for estrogen agonists were retrieved. Examples are shown in Figure 5. Model quality was evaluated using the methodology described by Güner and Henry (36) (see Sec. 5).

5 EVALUATION OF PHARMACOPHORE MODELS

Once pharmacophore models are derived, their utility must still be evaluated. Although they can be used to search a database of small druglike molecules to give hit lists of potential ligands, this does not address the quality of the hits. Güner and Henry (36) have proposed a metric that analyzes database search hit lists based on both the percent actives in the hit list (% *Y*) and the percent of all actives in the entire database that were retrieved by the query (% *A*) (see Scheme 2).

Taken together, these terms can define a "goodness of hit" score (GH). In its most functional form, the formula can be expressed as:

$$GH = \frac{H_a(3A + H_t)}{4H_tA} \times \left(1 - \frac{H_t - H_a}{D - A}\right)$$

where *D* is the number of compounds in the database, *A* is the number of active compounds in the database, H_t is the number of compounds in a

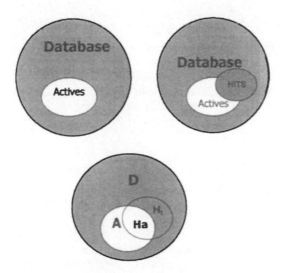

Scheme 2 Schematic description of database analysis as a metric for analyzing pharmacophore models. (From Ref. 36.)

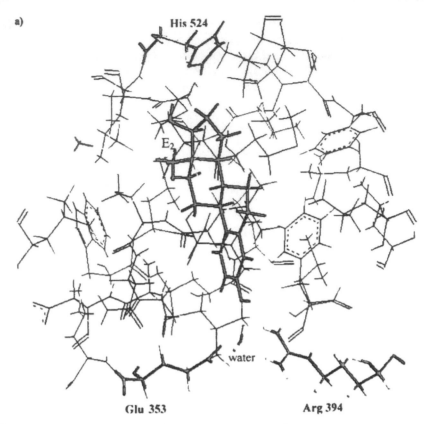

a)

His 524

E₂

water

Glu 353   Arg 394

Figure 3 (a) Binding site of ERα. Residues within 9 Å of the bound E2 ligand's geometric center are shown. Three residues and a crystallographic water molecule thought to be important for hydrogen bonding are labeled and displayed with heavier lines. The bound E2 ligand drawn with heavier lines is also displayed. (b) Ludi interaction model for the ERα binding site. Donor and acceptor features are displayed as rays, and lipophilic features are displayed as spheres. (From Ref. 33.)

search hit list, and H_a is the number of active compounds in the hit list. % Y is defined as $(H_t/D) \times 100$, and % A is defined as $(H_a/A) \times 100$.

In cases where multiple binding modes are known, a single pharmacophore model can account for only one of these modes. In such cases, the % Y component should carry more weight than % A because some actives in the database are associated with alternative binding modes. The GH formula can account for variable weightings of % Y and % A, and is a useful tool for evaluating hit lists as pharmacophore models are modified. This approach was recently applied to evaluate the effectiveness of similarity

b)

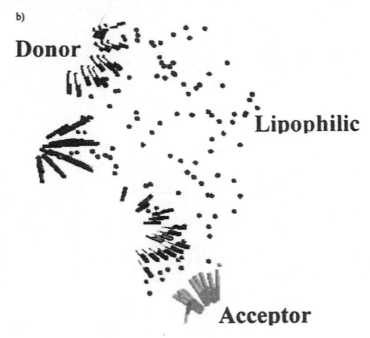

Donor

Lipophilic

Acceptor

Figure 3 Continued

searches in databases containing both structural and biological activity data (37). The study found the GH score as most useful in quantifying the effectiveness of 2D fragment-based similarity searching of databases.

6 STERIC CONSIDERATIONS

Quite often, the hit list contains the specified features from the search query, yet the ligands have shapes that are incongruous with the receptor cavity. Queries can be augmented with additional features that indicate the positions that make up the binding cavity itself. These ligand-inaccessible features, termed *excluded volumes*, can be added during structure-based focusing by the appropriate placement of small spheres inside the sphere that defines the active site (4).

A recent study of a structure-based design of inhibitors of the thyroid hormone receptor (THR) ligands has been described by Greenidge and coworkers (38). As a starting point, structural information from the two natural thyroid hormones, $3,3',5$-triiodo-L-thyronine (T_3 (1), Fig. 6) and $3,3'5, 5'$-tetraiodo-L-thyronine (T_4), were identified. These natural hormone ligands are known to exert primary physiological effects associated with

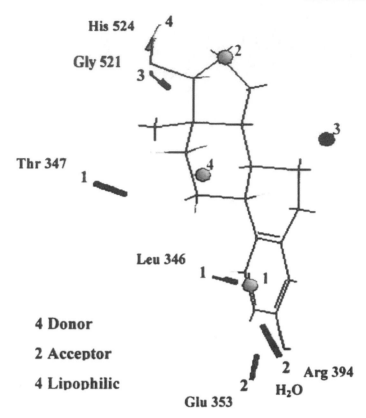

His 524

Gly 521

Thr 347

Leu 346

4 Donor

2 Acceptor

4 Lipophilic

Arg 394

H₂O

Glu 353

Figure 4 Cluster centers of the interaction model overlaid on the bound E2 ligand. The same feature types are numbered consecutively and labeled with the receptor residue number that produced that feature. (From Ref. 33.)

energy metabolism, the cardiovascular system, and lipid metabolism (39). Mimics of these natural hormones are of increasing therapeutic importance in the treatment of obesity, hypercholesterolemia, cardiac arrythmia, etc. Against the THR-α receptor, T_4's activity is only ca. 10% of T_3's; the latter has an IC_{50} of ca. 200 μM. The crystal structure of the rat THR-α-T_3 complex has been described by Wagner et al. (40), providing important information for structure-based design of mimics of the natural thyroid hormones. Using this information, Greenidge and coworkers (38) built pharmacophore models from the active site residues of THR-α, the bound T_3 ligand, and the addition of ligand-inaccessible regions, or excluded volume spheres using the CATALYST® program (31) [see, e.g., Fig. 7 (41)]. These models were used as search queries against a commercial database [Catalyst-formatted, Maybridge (42)], and compounds found to map to these models were

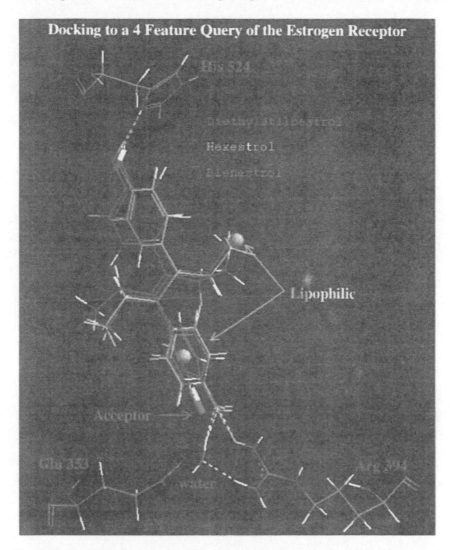

Figure 5 Example of hits obtained for a four-feature query. Docked conformations of the three most active ligands examined in the study are shown with the features of the query that retrieved them. Also shown, with dashed lines, are the hydrogen bonds formed between the docked conformations and several receptor residues.

assayed. Several micromolar-active thyroid hormonal ligands were identified in the process.

In the study, crystallographic structure-based pharmacophores were derived based on the active site of the THR–T$_3$ complex. These pharmacophore models were constructed with hydrophobic features from the receptor site, hydrogen bond donors and acceptors from the T_3 ligand, and, for the first time, the inclusion of excluded volumes for ligand-inaccessible regions in the binding site of the receptor. In building these pharmacophore models, hydrophobic features were placed at centroids of the phenyl rings and the three iodine atoms of the receptor-bound geometry of T_3, while the 4'-phenolic oxygen of T_3 and imidaole N $\in$ 2 atom of His-381 in the receptor active site were populated by hydrogen bond acceptors and donors, respectively. The sizes of the exclusion volume spheres were scaled between 25% and 50% of their respective van der Waals radii and centered within 6–8 Å of any T_3 hormone atom.

It is important to keep in mind that both the ligand and the receptor may make conformational adjustments to induce binding in the active site (43). Excluded volumes cannot accommodate the binding cavity flexibility, for they do not allow for any protrusions of the ligand into the hard exclusion spheres. To partially compensate for this limitation, the radii of the spherical exclusion spheres can be reduced.

The major findings of the study using steric considerations in pharmacophore models for THR ligands are:

> Model specificity was assessed via database searching. At the minimum, models must retrieve the T_3 ligand from a search of the database containing this hormone. Testing against an in-house database containing 18 agonists, 1 partial agonist, and 32 antagonists of the thyroid hormone receptor found that models without excluded volumes retrieved most of the agonists in the database, confirming the higher activity of agonists against this receptor.

> With the addition of ligand-forbidden exclusion spheres, database retrieval was modulated by different van der Waal sizes of the exclusion spheres. Hit lists were always significantly smaller for models with excluded volumes than for those without exclusion spheres.

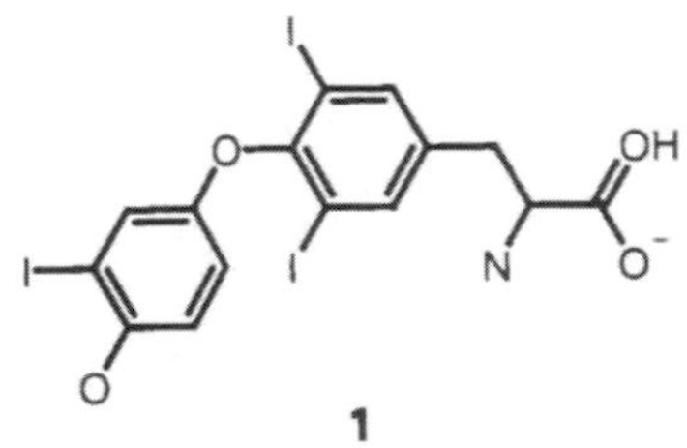

1

Figure 6 Structure of the natural thyroid hormone ligand, 3,3',5-triiodo-L-thyronine, T_3. (From Ref. 38.)

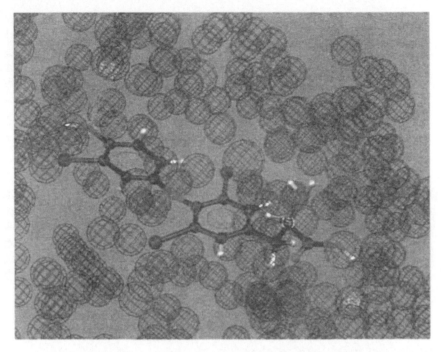

Figure 7 Overlay of T_3 onto the receptor-based pharmacophore model with exclusion spheres. The model contained five hydrophobes and two hydrogen bond acceptors. (From Ref. 41.)

The number of actives ($IC_{50} \leq 1 \mu M$ and ≤ 10 nM) retrieved by models with excluded spheres was about half the number returned by those without exclusion spheres. Correspondingly, the number of false positives and false negatives retrieved by models with and without exclusion spheres differed significantly. Models with excluded volumes generally had a greater number of false negatives (compounds active but predicted inactive) than those without excluded volumes; however, false-positive (compounds inactive but predicted active) rates were reduced by a factor of 2–5 times among those with excluded volumes.

Inclusion of excluded volumes to pharmacophore models increased database search times by ca. 70%; this was offset by significant reduction in the number of false positives retrieved.

Experimental validation of the ability of these models to identify potent thyroid hormone-α receptor ligands were performed via 3D database searching. Several "hits" retrieved from a search of the

47,000-compound Maybridge database were assayed. The most selective of these models returned a single hit, which was assayed and found to have an IC_{50} of 69 μM (2). Another of these models returned 52 hits with 12 confirmed active leads. Of these, four had IC_{50} values that ranged from 0.93 to 39 μM (3–4, Fig. 8). These findings confirmed the success of these models to identify potent new thyroid hormone receptor ligands.

In summary, information from the X-ray crystallographic structure of the THR-α–T_3 complex (40) was employed in the manual building of pharmacophore models (38) using the CATALYST program (31). Addition of ~ 200–300 ligand-inaccessible regions (excluded volumes) to these models were found to lead to a significantly reduced number of false positives (database hits that are inactive) when used as search queries in database mining. However, although the queries with excluded volumes did have fewer false positives, they also increased the number of false negatives (active compounds missed by the query) in the hit lists.

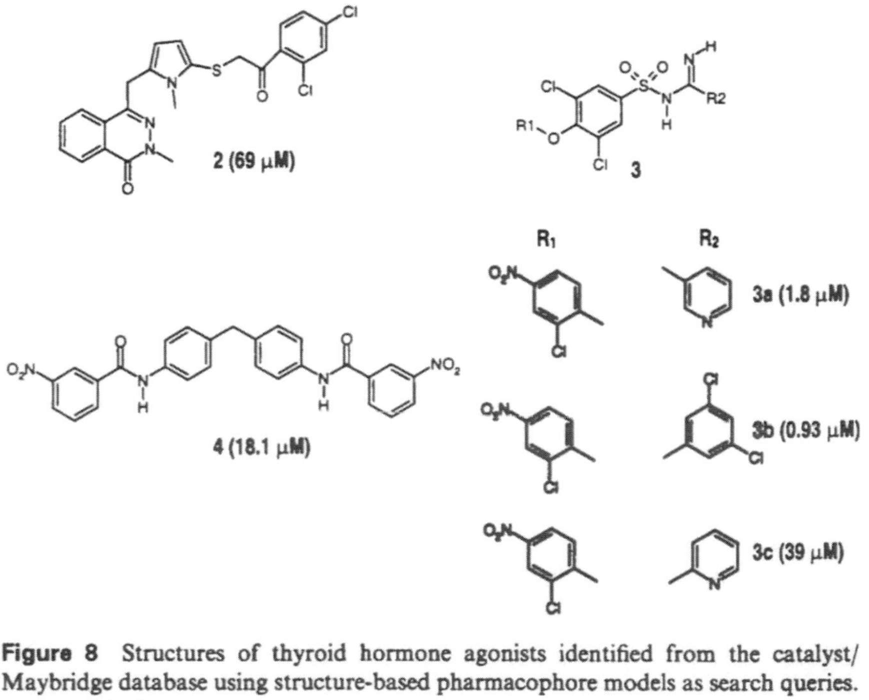

Figure 8 Structures of thyroid hormone agonists identified from the catalyst/ Maybridge database using structure-based pharmacophore models as search queries. (From Ref. 38.)

7 DOCKING-DERIVED PHARMACOPHORES

The G-protein-coupled receptors (GPCRs) constitute one of the largest groups of biological targets for drug design. Historically, proteins in this class of receptors have been difficult to crystalize for high-resolution structural studies, but recent success with crystallography of a few members of the family (44–48) has provided new structural insights for pharmacophore descriptions of ligand binding. Griffith et al. (49) conducted a receptor-based pharmacophore modeling of the α_{1A} and α_{1B} subtypes of the adrenergic receptor (AR), a member of the GPCR superfamily. These workers constructed models of the α_{1A} and α_{1B} subtypes based on a template model for the 3D arrangement of the transmembrane helices and of the alpha-carbon positions in the helices of the rhodopsin family of GPCRs described by Baldwin et al. (48).

Rigid, α_{1A}-selective isoquinolinocarbazide (IQC) ligands (Fig. 9) were rigidly docked into the adrenaline-binding domain of this receptor. The

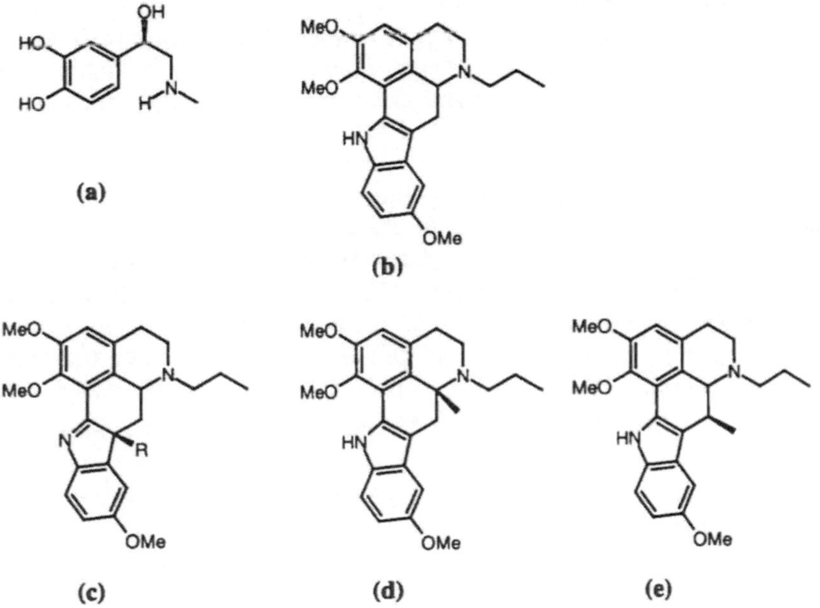

R = CH_3, CH_2CH_3, $CH_2CH_2CH_3$, $CH_2CH_2CH_2CH_3$, $CH(CH_3)_3$, $CH_2CH(CH_3)_2$,

$CH_2C_6H_5$, $CH_2CH_2CH_2CH_2CH_3$

Figure 9 Structures of (a) adrenaline, (b) IQC, (c)–(e) α_{1B}-selective target compounds. (From Ref. 48.)

resulting ligand–receptor complexes were minimized using the InsightII/ Discover energy minimization program (31). Calculated binding energies for both the natural ligand (adrenaline) and the rigid antagonists (IQC) compared favorably with experimental binding studies. This afforded structures where specific interactions between ligands and receptors could be used as templates for creating pharmacophore models.

Using information derived from the manual docking of IQC to the α_{1A} and α_{1B} receptors, chemical features in residues located within a 9-Å radius of the bound IQC were selected as ensembles of pharmacophoric features. The resulting "docking-derived pharmacophores," including Cartesian coordinates, location constraints, and excluded volume spheres (80–100), were created using Catalyst/HypoEdit and the feature-editing utility program (Exclude/OR) within the Catalyst user interface. A proposed advantage of creating pharmacophores using this approach is the simplification of the analysis of steric requirements in the docking of a ligand to two different protein receptors (49). An example of a docking-derived pharmacophore model is shown in Figure 10.

The pharmacophores were able to express the different π–π interactions in α_{1A} and α_{1B} by incorporating the more stringent ring-aromatic vectored function in the former and the single-point aromatic hydrophobic function in the latter (7). Ligand candidates can be screened based on how well they "fit" to the pharmacophore model. Theoretically, those ligands with the highest-scoring fits would be targeted for further study as potentially selective therapeutic agents. In this study, it was found that the flexibility of the α_{1A} site accommodates some of the ligands that were hypothesized to be less active based on their diminished fit to the pharmacophore. As described previously by Greenidge and coworkers (38), one way to offset this effect in the pharmacophore model is to reduce the size of excluded volumes. This can help prevent active molecules from being dismissed as false negatives.

8 PHARMACOPHORE MODELS FROM MOLECULAR DYNAMICS

The issue of flexibility in the protein active site was addressed by Carlson and coworkers (50) in their recent application of molecular dynamics (MD) and Monte Carlo (MC) simulations to derive "dynamic" as well as "static" pharmacophore models for the HIV-1 integrase. Surface-accessible binding regions were identified using the MUSIC (multiunit search for interacting conformers) program. MUSIC simulations use probe molecules to locate the binding positions and orientations for various functional groups that complement the functionality on the active site. By overlaying configura-

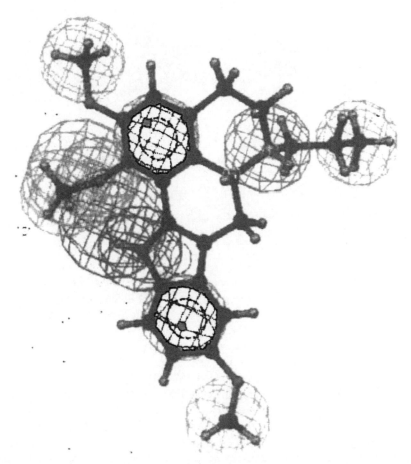

Figure 10 The docking-derived α_{1B} pharmacophore with IQC mapped (without excluded volumes). (From Ref. 48.)

tions extracted from a molecular dynamics simulation of the active site (Fig. 11), binding regions that remain occupied during the simulation were identified. In principle, these conserved regions should also allow an active ligand to bind while still maintaining the same flexibility.

In the study of HIV-1 integrase, a pharmacophore model was created based on the averaged positions of six conserved regions. A "dynamic" pharmacophore model was created from the ensemble of MD configurations using the Catalyst program (31). This model contained six hydrogen bond donor sites and three excluded-volume spheres that define part of the binding cavity. The tolerance sizes of these features varied from ca. 0.4 to 1.5 Å.

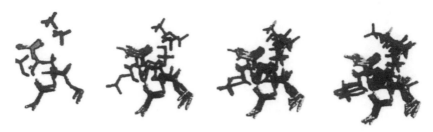

Figure 11 Process for overlaying the binding sites from the MUSIC studies using methanol molecules to determine the binding sites for hydroxyl groups within the active site of HIV-1 integrase. Each cluster from the MUSIC simulation is represented by its probe with the most favorable interaction energy. (From Ref. 49.)

As comparisons, "static" models were constructed using information from the crystal structure of the protein template used to initiate the MD study. These models typically contained four to five hydrogen bond donors and three exclusion spheres (see Table 1).

Testing of the pharmacophore models was performed by using them as search queries against a collection of literature compounds previously screened as HIV-1 integrase inhibitors (53–58). Excellent fits between the dynamically derived pharmacophore model and the most active (lowest IC_{50}) HIV-1 integrase inhibitors were found. In contrast, the static models performed poorly in fitting to the same active ligands. These results are shown in Table 2. Since the nine-featured hypothesis was too limiting to produce any hits, subsets containing five hydrogen donor sites and three excluded volumes were used to search the ACD (59) database, retrieving novel compounds for further in vitro testing. Overall, the dynamic model, though obtained using incomplete crystal structure, was found to closely approximate the pharmacophoric features important in HIV-1 integrase inhibition.

9   USING PHARMACOPHORE-BASED DOCKING IN DATABASE MINING

An alternative approach to database mining focuses on the fit of the ligand in the binding cavity rather than the fit of the ligand to predefined pharmacophoric features. Molecular docking algorithms (60–65) have been developed that aim to accommodate both the flexibility of the ligands and their orientations in the binding cavity. Although the structure of the protein target must be known, the conformational model of the ligands can be either generated on the fly or stored in a database. Precomputed conformations are advantageous in cases where docking is used to virtually screen large libraries, affording much faster search times.

A recent report of pharmacophore-based docking (64) uses the 3D fingerprints of a conformationally expanded database to describe the ligands. This implementation uses four types of pharmacophore features: hydrogen bond donor, hydrogen bond acceptor, dual hydrogen bond donor/acceptor (capable as acting as both), and a five- or six-membered ring centroid. Each conformer is stored as the coordinates of its pharmacophore features to allow for simultaneous, rapid matching to selected points on the target site. The basic DOCK (60) methodology is followed to identify hits. When a match between the distances in a single four-point pharmacophore and those in the active site is found, all conformers that share that four-point pharmacophore are scored on the basis of how well they fit the receptor site in a variety of orientations. The process continues until all possible orientations are exhausted for all four-point 3D fingerprints in the database that meet the initial distance criteria.

Docking methodologies and scoring functions have been evaluated for their ability to rank hits from a database search (66). Since no single scoring method consistently outperformed another for all target sites, it was proposed that for each target, a docking method and consensus scoring function be optimized for a small dataset (1000 compounds comprising 10% known actives) before being applied to a large database.

10 CONCLUDING REMARKS

Pharmacophore perception is the most important first step toward the understanding of drug–receptor interactions. The combination of pharmacophore perception with advances in 3D database-searching methodologies has propelled the use of this approach in the design and discovery of new drug candidates. Whereas pharmacophores are most often derived from ligand information, the increase in crystallographic structures of drug targets has led to a concomitant increase in receptor-based pharmacophore modeling. This, in turn, has produced some notable successes in the development of new drugs via this approach. Two direct examples of this has have been shown for the ACE drugs—Captopril and Enalapril. Computation algorithms that apply protein structure data in modeling ligand–receptor interactions via pharmacophores are coming into common use today as this approach grows in popularity within drug discovery teams

Table 1 Characteristics of the Dynamic Pharmacophore Model based on MD Simulations and the Static Pharmacophore Models Based on Three Crystal Structures

	Radius (Å)	X (Å)	Y (Å)	Z (Å)
Dynamic Model				
HBdonor1	1.316	7.249	4.783	2.405
HBdonor2	1.088	9.543	4.462	1.849
HBdonor3	0.388	11.037	3.382	1.497
HBdonor4	1.106	10.877	1.845	-2.410
HBdonor5	1.088	8.232	7.622	-1.851
HBdonor6	1.494	9.072	8.404	-4.178
Q62	1.5	5.842	4.291	-3.330
D64	1.5	7.819	2.218	0.311
D116	1.5	10.461	5.219	-2.795
Static Model 1 from Crystal Structure in the MD Study				
HBdonor1	0.364	5.127	-1.955	-2.406
HBdonor2	0.748	7.612	-2.655	-2.819
HBdonor3	0.534	9.487	-2.311	-3.876
HBdonor4	0.250	11.464	-0.353	1.304
HBdonor5	0.692	12.149	-0.340	-0.079
Q62	1.5	6.573	0.345	2.229
D64	1.5	4.765	1.167	-1.907
D116	1.5	9.278	0.472	-1.425

Static Model 2 from Crystal Structure of Maignan et al.[a]				
HBdonor1	0.464	6.346	-4.762	10.626
HBdonor2	0.590	9.455	-4.219	14.306
HBdonor3	1.510	11.052	-2.038	9.695
HBdonor4	0.804	11.056	1.222	9.286
O of L63[b]	1.5	7.763	0.359	16.393
D64	1.5	7.409	-2.046	12.892
D116	1.5	12.001	0.425	12.406
Static Model 3 from Crystal Structure of Goldgur et al.[c]				
HBdonor1	0.920	-7.970	2.051	-3.353
HBdonor2	0.470	-9.712	-0.847	-4.840
HBdonor3	0.740	-9.794	-2.587	0.591
HBdonor4	1.008	-10.858	-6.280	-5.223
Q62	1.5	-8.909	-0.797	4.047
D64	1.5	-8.019	-1.392	-1.845
D116	1.5	-11.446	-5.914	-1.851

Atoms with gray spheres are hydrogen bond donors; the black spheres are excluded volumes based on active site residues.

[a] Ref. 51.

[b] The side chain of Q62 is in an orientation away from D64 and D116 in the structure by Maignan et al. (Ref. 51). For this structure, the carbonyl oxygen of L63 was chosen to represent the bottom of the active site (Ref. 49.).

[c] Ref. 52.

Source: Ref. 49.

Table 2 Performance of the Pharmacophore Models Tested Against Compounds from the Literature That Have Been Tested for Inhibitory Activity

Compound	IC_{50}s 3'/ST	Dynamic		Static 1		Doubled radii		Static 2 Maignan et al.[a]		Static 3 Goldgur et al.[a]	
		Fast	Best	Fast	Best	Fast	Best	Fast	Best	Fast	Best
Chichoric Acid[c]	0.15/0.13	✓									
107[c]	0.23/0.11	✓									
4.5-DCQA[c]	0.25/0.46	✓									
81[c]	0.4/0.2	✓	X			✓	X		X		
67[c]	0.5										
71[c]	0.5										
85[c]	0.5/0.2	✓	X		X	✓	X		X		
3.5-DCQA[c]	0.64/0.66	✓	X								
3.4-DCQA[c]	0.79/0.54	✓	X					✓			
1.5-DCQA[c]	0.68/1.08	✓	X								
NSC 118695[d]	0.9/0.3	✓	X						X		
Quercetegetin[e]	1.3/0.6	✓	X						X		
105[c]	0.98/0.81	✓	X					✓	X		
NSC 64205[d]	1.1/0.5	✓	X						X		
NSC 158383[f]	15/0.8										
NSC 607319[d]	1/4/1.0	✓	X			✓	X	✓	X		X
NSC 309121[d]	1.7/1.0	✓	X				X		X		
68[c]	1.7	✓	X								
Myricetin[a]	2/0.6		X								
Doxorubicin[c]	0.9/2.4	✓	X						X		

Very Active Compounds

Active Compounds

Compound	3'/ST	Fast	Best	Fast	Best	Fast	Best	Fast	Best	Fast	Best	Fast	Best
Purpurogallin[g]	2.1												
111[c]	2.3/1.1												
NSC 310217[f]	2/1.5												
NSC 64452[d]	1.2/3.6	✓	X										
Quinalizarin[a]	4.1												
83[c]	3.3/1.9	✓	X										
NSC 261045[d]	2.3/4.1	✓	X								X		
90[c]	1.38/4.71	✓	X								X		
NSC 642710[f]	5.3/5.0									✓			
NSC 115290[b]	5	✓	X										
Eliagic Acid[g]	5.1												
115[c]	6.7/5.2												
Mitoxantrone[c]	3.8/8.0	✓	X			✓	X			✓	X		X
89[c]	9/4	✓	X										
Tyrophostin A51[c]	10.3												
110[c]	9.1/5.8												
92[c]	9.5/7.8	✓	X										
141[c]	11.6/7.9		X										
Hypericin[g]	10												
UCSD1[g]	17/5												
NSC 318213[d]	23.9/14.0	✓	X										
66[c]	21.4/5.4		X										
NSC 233026[d]	20.6/19.7	✓	X							✓			
NSC 371056[f]	29.9/16.5	✓	X			✓	X				X		X
NSC 48240[f]	26/20.6	✓	X										
97[c]	33/33	✓	X								X		X

Active Compounds

Table 2 Continued

Compound	IC_{50} 3'/ST	Dynamic Fast	Dynamic Best	Static 1 Fast	Static 1 Best	Doubled radii Fast	Doubled radii Best	Static 2 Maignan et al.[a] Fast	Static 2 Maignan et al.[a] Best	Static 3 Goldgur et al.[a] Fast	Static 3 Goldgur et al.[a] Best
Chlorogenic Acid[c]	87.8/45.8		X	Ineffective Compounds							
13[b]	120/96										
NSC 641547[f]	224/134		X				X				
NSC 674503[d]		✓									
NSC 635971[f]		✓	X								
NSC 642651[d]		✓	X								
112[c]		✓	X						X		
9[h]		✓	X					✓	X		
52[h]		✓	X			✓		✓	X	✓	X
NSC 281311[d]		✓	X			✓	X	✓	X		
103[c]		✓	X				X		X		
5[f]											X
NDGA[g]		✓	X								

Compounds ordered by inhibitory activity.

[a] Ref. 51.
[b] Ref. 52.
[c] Ref. 56.
[d] Ref. 55.
[e] Ref. 57.
[f] Ref. 54.
[g] Ref. 58.
[h] Ref. 53.

Source: Ref. 49.

in the pharmaceutical and biotechnology industries. Issues of conformational flexibility at the active site of the receptor and ligand binding can be accounted for using molecular dynamics/Monte Carlo simulations. Steric considerations have been tackled by including exclusion spheres to represent ligand-inaccessible regions in the active site of the receptor. As the examples in this report demonstrate, the methodologies for the use of pharmacophores continue to improve and will increasingly enhance the ability to design new and potent lead compounds for drug discovery.

REFERENCES

1. P Gund. Three-dimensional pharmacophoric pattern searching. In: FE Hahn, ed. Progress in Molecular and Subcellular Biology. New York: Springer Verlag, 1977, pp 117–143.
2. PW Sprague, R Hoffmann. Catalyst pharmacophore models and their utility as queries for searching 3D databases. In: H Van de Waterbeemd, B Testa, G Folkers, eds. Computer-Assisted Lead Finding and Optimization—Current Tools for Medicinal Chemistry. Basel, Switzerland: VHCA, 1997, pp 230–240.
3. JJ Kaminski, DF Rane, ML Rothofsky. Database mining using pharmacophore models to discover novel structural prototypes. In: O Güner, ed. Pharmacophore Perception, Development, and Use in Drug Design. La Jolla, CA: International University Line, 2000, pp 251–268.
4. U Norinder. Refinement of catalyst hypotheses using simplex optimization. J Comp Aided Molec Design 14:545–557, 2000.
5. A Palomer, J Pascual, F Cabré, ML García, D Mauleón. Derivation of pharmacophore and CoMFA models for leukotriene D4 receptor antagonists of the quinolinyl(bridged)aryl series. J Med Chem 43:392–400, 2000.
6. C Daveu, R Bureau, I Baglin, H Prunier, J-C Lancelot, S Rault. Definition of a pharmacophore for partial agonists of serotonin 5-HT$_3$ receptors. J Chem Inf Comput Sci 39:362–369, 1999.
7. J Greene, S Kahn, H Savoj, P Sprague, S Teig. Chemical function queries for 3D database search. J Chem Inf Comput Sci 34:1297–1308, 1994.
8. S Berezin, J Greene, S Kahn, S Ku, S Teig. CHM: a chemically expressive database query language. Noordwijkerhout Camerino Medicinal Chemistry Symposium. Noordwijkerhout, Netherlands, 1993.
9. GR Marshal. Binding-site modeling of unknown receptor. In H Kubinyi, ed. 3D QSAR in Drug Design: Theory, Methods and Applications. Leiden, Netherlands: ESCOM Scientific, 1993, pp 80–116.
10. H-J Böhm. The computer program Ludi: a new method for the de novo design of enzyme inhibitors. J Comp Aided Molec Design 6:61–78, 1992
11. J Grembecka, WA Sokalski, P Kafarski. Computer-aided design and activity prediction of leucine aminopeptidase inhibitors. J Comp Aided Molec Design 14:531–544, 2000.

12. A Lew, AR Chamberlain. Blockers of human T-cell KV1.3 potassium channels using de novo ligand design and solid-phase parallel combinatorial chemistry. Bioorg Med Chem Lett 9:3267–3272, 1999.

13. G Schneider, O Clément-Chomienne, L Hilfiger, P Schneider, S Kirsch, H-J Böhm, W Neidhart. Virtual screening for bioactive molecules by evolutionary de novo design. Angew Chem Int Ed 39:4130–4133, 2000.

14. RD Cramer III, DE Patterson, JD Bunce. Comparative molecular field analysis (CoMFA). 1. Effect of shape on binding of steroids to carrier proteins. J Am Chem Soc 110:5959–5967, 1988.

15. M Recanatini, A Bisi, A Cavalli, F Belluti, S Gobbi, A Rampa, P Valenti, M Palzer, A Palusczak, RW Hartmann. A new class of nonsteroidal aromatase inhibitors: design and synthesis of chromone and xanthone derivatives and inhibition of the P450 enzymes aromatase and 17α-Hydroxylase/C17,20-lyase. J Med Chem 44:672–680, 2001.

16. LM Shi, H Fang, W Tong, J Wu, R Perkins, RM Blair, WS Branham, SL Dial, CL Moland, DM Sheehan. QSAR models using a large diverse set of estrogens. J Chem Inf Comput Sci 41:186–195, 2001.

17. RD Hoffmann, JJ Bourguignon. Building a hypothesis for CCK-B antagonists using the catalyst program. In: F Sanz, J Giraldo, F Manaut, eds. QSAR and Molecular Modeling: Concepts, Computational Tools and Biological Applications. Barcelona: Prous Science, 1995, pp 298–300.

18. M Gillner, P Greenidge. The use of multiple excluded volumes derived from X-ray crystallographic structures in 3D database searching and 3D QSAR. In: O Güner, ed. Pharmacophore Perception, Development, and Use in Drug Design. La Jolla, CA: International University Line, 2000, pp 371–384.

19. P Goodford. A computational procedure for determining energetically favorable binding sites on biologically important macromolecules. J Med Chem 28:849–857, 1985.

20. A Miranker, M Karplus. Functionality maps of binding sites: a multiple-copy simultaneous search method. Proteins 11:29–34, 1991.

21. E Evensen, D Joseph-McCarthy, M Karplus. MCSS Version 2.1. Cambridge, MA: Harvard University, 1997.

22. JC Bressi, J Choe, MT Hough, FS Buckner, WC Van Voorhis, CLMJ Verlinde, WGJ Hol, MH Gelb. Adenosine analogues as inhibitors of *Trypanosoma brucei* phosphoglycerate kinase: elucidation of a novel binding mode for a 2-amino-N^6-substituted adenosine. J Med Chem 43:4135–4150, 2000.

23. JM Chen, FC Nelson, JI Levin, D Mobilio, FJ Moy, R Nilakantan, A Zask, R Powers. Structure-based design of a novel, potent, and selective inhibitor for MMP-13 utilizing NMR spectroscopy and computer-aided molecular design. J Am Chem Soc 122:9648–9654, 2000.

24. TA Spencer, D Li, JS Russel, JL Collins, RK Bledsoe, TG Consler, LB Moore, CM Galardi, DD McKee, JT Moore, MA Watson, DJ Parks, MH Lambert, TM Wilson. Pharmacophore analysis of the nuclear oxysterol receptor LXRα. J Med Chem 44:886–897, 2001.

25. OF Güner, ed. Pharmacophore Perception, Development, and Use in Drug Design. La Jolla, CA: IUL Biotechnology, 2000.

26. DW Cushman, HS Cheung, EF Sabo, MA Ondetti. Biochemistry 16: 5484–5491, 1977.

27. AA Patchett, E Harris, EW Tristram, MJ Wyvratt, MT Wu, D Taub, ER Peterson, TJ Ikeler, J Ten Broeke, LG Payne, DL Ondeyka, ED Thorsett, WJ Greenlee, NS Lohr, RD Hoffsomer, H Joshua, WV Ruyle, JW Rothrock, SD Aster, AL Maycock, FM Robinson, R Hirschmann. A new class of angiotensin-converting enzyme inhibitors. Nature 288:280–283, 1980.

28. DR Henry, OF Güner. Techniques for searching databases of three-dimensional (3D) structures with receptor-based queries. HS Rzepa, JM Goodman, eds. In: Electronic Conference on Trends in Organic Chemistry (ECTOC-1). Royal Society of Chemistry Publications, 1995. http://www.ch.ic.ac.uk/ectoc/papers/guner/

29. MACCS Drug Data Report (MDDR) is a drug database available from MDL Information Systems, Inc., San Leandro, CA.

30. H-J Boehm, G Klebe. What can we learn from molecular recognition in protein–ligand complexes for the design of new drugs? Angew Chem Int Ed Engl 35:2588–2614, 1996.

31. Cerius2, Catalyst and InsightII/Discover are distributed by Accelrys, 9685 Scranton Road, San Diego, CA 92121.

32. R Hoffmann, H Li, T Langer. Feature-based pharmacophores: application to some biological systems. In: O Güner, ed. Pharmacophore Perception, Development, and Use in Drug Design. La Jolla, CA: International University Line, 2000, pp 303–318.

33. CM Venkatachalam, P Kirchhoff, M Waldman. Receptor-based pharmacophore perceptions and modeling. In: O Güner, ed. Pharmacophore Perception, Development, and Use in Drug Design. La Jolla, CA: International University Line, 2000, pp 339–350.

33a. PD Kirchhoff, R Brown, S Kahn, M Waldman, CM Venkatachalam. Application of Structure-Based Focusing to the Estrogen Receptor. J Comp Chem, 2001, 22, 993–1003.

34. O Clement, C Freeman, J Wang. Structure-based design of estrogen agonists. Manuscript in preparation.

35. AM Brzozowski, AC Pike, Z Dauter, RE Hubbard, T Bonn, O Engstrom, L Ohman, GL Greene, JA Gustafsson, M Carlquist. Molecular basis of agonism and antagonism in the oestrogen receptor. Nature 389:753–760, 1997.

36. OF Güner, DR Henry. Metric for analyzing hit lists and pharmacophores. In: O Güner, ed. Pharmacophore Perception, Development, and Use in Drug Design. La Jolla, CA: International University Line, 2000, pp 193–212.

37. SJ Edgar, JD Holliday, P Willett. Effectiveness of retrieval in similarity searches of chemical databases: a review of performance measures. J Mol Graph Model 18:343–375, 2000.

38. PA Greenidge, B Carlsson, L-G Bladh, M Gillner. Pharmacophore incorporating numerous excluded volumes defined by X-ray crystallographic structure

in three-dimensional database searching: application to the thyroid hormone receptor. J Med Chem 41:2503–2512, 1998.

39. PD Leeson, AH Underwood. Thyroid hormone receptors. In: JC Emmet, ed. Comprehensive Medicinal Chemistry. New York: Pergamon, 1991, pp 1145–1173.

40. RL Wagner, JW Apriletti, ME McGrath, BL West, JD Baxter, RJ Fletterick. A structural role for hormone in the thyroid hormone receptor. Nature 378:690–697, 1995.

41. PA Greenidge, M Gillner. Database Searching Using Structure-Based Pharmacophores that Include Many Excluded Volumes. http://www.accelrys.com/cases/greenidge.html.

42. Maybridge Database is a product of Maybridge Plc. Trevillett, Tintagel, Cornwall PL34 OHW, England.

43. BP Klaholz, J-P Renaud, A Mitschler, C Zusi, P Chambon, H Gronemeyer, D Moras. Conformational adaptation of agonists to the human nuclear receptor RARg. Nature Struct Biol 5:199–202, 1998.

44. M Pellegrini, DF Mierke. Molecular complex of cholecystokinin-8 and N-terminus of the cholecystokinin-A receptor by NMR spectorscopy. Biochemistry 38:14775, 1999.

45. MM Teeter, MF Froimowitz, B Stec, CJ Durand. Homology modeling of dopamine D2 receptor and its testing by docking of agonists and tricylic antagonists. J Med Chem 37:2874, 1994.

46. TM Savarese, CM Fraser. In vitro mutagenesis and research for structure–function relationships among GPCRs. Biochem J 283:1–19, 1992.

47. A Beck-Sickinger. Structural characterization and binding sites of GPCRs. Drug Discovery Today 1:502–513, 1996.

48. JM Baldwin, GFX Schertler, VM Unger. An alpha-carbon template for the transmembrane helices in the rhodopsin family of G-protein-coupled receptors. J Mol Biol 272:144–164, 1997.

49. R Griffith, JB Bremner, B Coban. Docking-derived pharmacophores from models of receptor–ligand Complexes. In: O Güner, ed. Pharmacophore Perception, Development, and Use in Drug Design. La Jolla, CA: International University Line, 2000, pp 385–408.

50. HA Carlson, KM Masukawa, K Rubins, FD Bushman, WL Jorgensen, RD Lins, JM Briggs, JA McCammon. Developing a dynamic pharmacophore model for HIV-1 integrase. J Med Chem 43:2100–2114, 2000.

51. S Maignan, J-P Guilloteau, Q Zhou-liu, C Clement-Mella, V Mikol. Crystal structures of the catalytic domain of HIV-1 integrase free and complexed with its metal cofactor: high level of similarity of the active site with other viral integrases. J Mol Biol 282:359-368, 1998.

52. Y Goldgur, F Dyda, AB Hickman, TM Jenkins, R Craigie, DR Davies. Three new structures of the core domain of HIV-1 integrase: an active site that binds magnesium. Proc Natl Acad Sci USA 95:9150–9154, 1998.

53. MC Nicklaus, N Neamati, H Hong, A Mazumder, S Sunder, J Chen, GWA Milne, Y Pommier. HIV-1 integrase pharmacophore: discovery of inhibitors

through three-dimensional database searching. J Med Chem 40:920–929, 1997.

54. H Hong, N Neamati, S Wang, MC Nicklaus, A Mazumder, H Zhao, TR Burke Jr, Y Pommier, GWA Milne. Discovery of HIV-1 integrase inhibitors by pharmacophore searching. J Med Chem 40:930–936, 1997.

55. N Neamati, H Hong, S Sunder, GWA Milne, Y Pommier. Potent inhibitors of human immunodeficiency virus type-1 integrase: identification of a novel four-point pharmacophore and tetracyclines as novel inhibitors. Mol Pharmacol 52:1041–1055, 1997.

56. N Neamati, S Sunder, Y Pommier. Design and Discovery of HIV-1 integrase inhibitors. DDT 2:487–498, 1997.

57. CM Farnet, B Wang, JR Lipford, FD Bushman. Differential inhibition of HIV-1 preintegration complexes and purified integrase protein by small molecules. Proc Natl Acad Sci USA 93:9742–9747, 1996.

58. CM Farnet, B Wang, M Hansen, JR Lipford, L Zalkow, WE Robinson Jr, J Siegel, FD Bushman. Human immunodeficiency virus type-1 cDNA integration: new aromatic hydroxylated inhibitors and studies of the inhibition mechanism. Antimicrob Agents Chemother 42:2245–2253, 1998.

59. The Available Chemical Directory (ACD) is a database available from MDL Information Systems, Inc., San Leandro, CA.

60. ID Kuntz, JM Blaney, SJ Oatley, R Langridge, TE Ferrin. A geometric approach to macromolecule–ligand interactions. J Mol Biol 161:269–288, 1982.

61. M Rarey, B Kramer, T Lengauer, G Klebe. A fast flexible docking method using an incremental construction algorithm. J Mol Biol 261:470–489, 1996.

62. G Jones, P Willet, RC Glen, AR Leach, R Taylor. Development and validation of a genetic algorithm for flexible docking. J Mol Biol 267:727–748, 1997.

63. GM Morris, DS Goodsell, R Halliday, R Huey, WE Hart, RK Belew, AS Olson. Automated docking using a Lamarckian genetic algorithm and an empirical binding free-energy function. J Comp Chem 19:1139–1162, 1998.

64. DS Goodsell, AJ Olson. Automated docking of substrates to proteins by simulated annealing. Proteins 8:195–202, 1990.

65. BE Thomas IV, D Joseph-McCarthy, JC Alvarez. Pharmacophore-based molecular docking. In: O Güner, ed. Pharmacophore Perception, Development, and Use in Drug Design. La Jolla, CA: International University Line, 2000, pp 351–367.

66. C Bissantz, G Folkers, D Rognan. Protein-based virtual screening of chemical databases. 1. Evaluation of different docking/scoring combinations. J Med Chem 43:4759–4767, 2000.

18

The Structure of Human Interferon-β-1a (Avonex®) and its Relation to Activity: A Case Study of the Use of Structural Data in the Arena of Protein Pharmaceuticals

Adrian Whitty
Biogen, Inc., Cambridge, Massachusetts, U.S.A.

Michael Karpusas
University of Crete Medical School, Heraklion, Crete, Greece

1 INTRODUCTION

The usefulness of high-resolution protein structural data in the development of small-molecule drugs is well established. In contrast, the role of structural information in the development of protein pharmaceuticals may not initially be so apparent. This chapter describes the determination of the X-ray crystal structure of human interferon-β-1a (IFN-β-1a), the active ingredient in Avonex®, the leading treatment worldwide for relapsing forms of multiple sclerosis. We review several ways in which this structure has been used to help address the biochemical and biological properties of this important cytokine and also its use in the design of second-generation drugs. In so doing, we illustrate some of the ways in which protein structure determination can be integrated with biochemical studies to elucidate the biochemical and biological properties of cytokines and how such work can have an impact on drug development in the biopharmaceutical industry.

Human IFN-β is a member of the Type I interferon (IFN) family, a group of homologous four-helix-bundle cytokines that in humans comprises at least 12 isotypes of IFN-α, one IFN-β, one IFN-ω, and possibly other members (1–4). The Type I IFNs display broad biological activity, including control of cell proliferation, induction of genes responsible for protecting cells against the effects of viral infection, and regulation of the differentiation state of immune cells and modulation of their function (5). IFN-β itself comprises a single polypeptide chain of 166 amino acids, with a disulfide bond between residues Cys31 and Cys141 and an additional, free cysteine at position 17. Unlike most other Type I IFNs, IFN-β is a glycoprotein; it contains a single N-linked glycosylation site at Asn 80 (6). All Type I IFNs signal through a common receptor, the Type I IFN receptor, comprising two distinct receptor chains, IFNAR1 (7) and IFNAR2 (8). IFNAR1 and IFNAR2 are single-pass transmembrane proteins, which belong to the family of Class II cytokine receptors that also includes the alpha and beta chains of the Type II IFN receptor (i.e., the receptor for IFN-γ) and the IL-10 receptor (9). Like other Class I and Class II cytokine receptors, the Type I IFN receptor signals through the JAK/STAT pathway and also activates other signaling pathways (10,11).

The Type I IFN receptor is unique among cytokine receptors; there is no other example of such a large number of cytokines acting through a common receptor. Although there is evidence to suggest that different Type I IFNs engage the receptor in distinct ways (12–19) and in certain experimental systems can be shown to bring about the transduction of distinct signals (20–25), the extent to which the biological functions of these proteins are truly nonredundent remains unclear. Available data suggest that the mechanism by which Type I IFNs bind to and activate their receptor is complex compared to some of the well-studied cytokine receptors, such as the receptors for human growth hormone (hGH) or erythropoietin. The mechanism of Type I IFN receptor activation remains incompletely understood.

1.1 Recombinant IFN-β as a Drug

Before discussing the three-dimensional structure of the protein and how this information has been employed to understand the biochemistry of the molecule, it is worthwhile to briefly review the discovery of IFN-β and its development as a drug. In particular, it is useful to highlight some of the differences in properties that have been observed in vivo between structurally different forms of the protein, because the desire to understand the biochemical origins of these functional differences was one of the motivations for the work described herein. The cloning of human IFN-β was first reported in 1980 (26). Although the therapeutic potential of IFN-β was recognized early on, it was another 13 years before a form of recombinant IFN-β was first introduced as a drug. In the mid-1990s, two different forms of recombinant IFN-β, Avonex® (IFN-β-1a) and Betaseron® (IFN-β-1b), were approved for sale in the United States, Europe, and elsewhere for the treatment of relapsing-remitting multiple sclerosis (RRMS), a serious neurodegenerative disorder for which there previously existed no chronic treatment (27,28). IFN-β-1b is expressed in *E. coli*, and as such it lacks the glycosylation at Asn 80 that exists in the natural protein. Moreover, IFN-β-1b is one amino acid shorter than the natural protein, lacking the N-terminal methionine residue, and also differs from the natural sequence at position 17, which has been mutated from a Cys to a Ser to facilitate correct disulfide bond formation during refolding (29). In contrast, IFN-β-1a, which is expressed in mammalian cells and is secreted as a fully folded protein, contains the full natural sequence, including a cysteine at position 17, and is glycosylated at Asn 80. A third recombinant IFN-β drug, Rebif®, also a version of IFN-β-1a, has more recently been approved for the treatment of RRMS. The utility of recombinant IFN-β in disease settings other than RRMS has been established, and additional new indications are being tested.

Several important differences between the biological activities of IFN-β-1a and IFN-β-1b have been established. IFN-β-1a has a specific antiviral activity of 2×10^8 IU/mg, 10-fold higher than that of IFN-β-1b, and also shows higher activity than IFN-β-1b in assays measuring the antiproliferative and immunomodulatory activities of IFN-β (30). Moreover, Avonex® is administered by intramuscular rather than subcutaneous injection. As a result of these factors, full therapeutic activity with Avonex® is achieved by giving 30 µg of protein once weekly, instead of the 250 µg every second day (amounting to 875 µg weekly) that is required with Betaseron®. Several differences between the in vivo effects of IFN-β-1a and IFN-β-1b have also been shown. For example, clinical results indicate that the drugs differ greatly in immunogenicity, i.e., in the frequency with which treated patients develop antibodies that are specific for the IFN-β component of the drug. Published data indicate that 81–97% of RRMS patients receiving Betaseron® raise antidrug antibodies, including 35–44% of patients who develop a substantial level of so-called neutralizing antibodies (i.e., antibodies that block the ability of the drug to elicit a response in functional assays) (31–34). In contrast, only about 20–30% of RRMS patients receiving Avonex® raised binding antibodies against the drug, and in only 3–6% of patients was a significant neutralizing titer observed (34,35). This large difference in immunogenicity likely is clinically important; it has been reported that patients who raise significant levels of such neutralizing antibodies lose responsiveness to the drug therapy (31,32,36). Understanding the origin of the activity differences between IFN-β-1a and IFN-β-1b that are observed in vitro and in vivo, and particularly the extent to which they result from the distinct structures of the two molecules, was one of the aims that drove interest in elucidating the relationship between structure and function in IFN-β-1a.

2 DETERMINATION OF THE IFN-β-1a CRYSTAL STRUCTURE

The structure determination of IFN-β-1a was prompted by several factors. Firstly, we wished to gain a better understanding of the role of the covalently attached sugar in IFN-β-1a and particularly the extent to which it contributes to the significantly higher in vitro activity of this protein compared to the nonglycosylated mutant IFN-β-1b (30). A high-resolution structure of IFN-β-1a was also desired to guide subsequent studies involving the mutagenesis of IFN-β-1a and potentially to assist in the design of forms of the molecule possessing altered properties. Also, it was recognized that the successful crystallization and structure solution of a protein pharmaceutical such as Avonex® provides the ultimate level of confidence concerning the proper folding and general high quality of the protein preparation. Several structural studies on various Type I IFNs preceded our work on IFN-β-1a. The first report of crystallization of a Type I interferon (IFN-αA) appeared in 1982 (37). However, the crystals were of low quality and no successful structure determination was reported. A three-year effort to crystallize *E. coli*–expressed, nonglycosylated human IFN-β, either with or without the Cys17Ser modification, was not successful, due to the tendency of the protein to aggregate (38). The same group switched their efforts to murine IFN-β expressed in *E. coli*, and succeeded in crystallizing it and determining its structure to 2.15-Å resolution (39). While the structural work on IFN-β-1a was in progress, the crystal structure of human IFN-α2b at 2.9-Å resolution was reported (40), followed soon after by the NMR structure of human IFN-α2a (41). The structure of IFN-β-1a thus enabled a detailed comparison of its three-dimensional structure with that of IFN-α2, as well as providing the first look at the structure of a glycosylated Type I IFN. Subsequent to the publication of the IFN-β-1a structure in 1998, a crystal structure was reported for ovine IFN-τ (42).

Our attempts to crystallize human IFN-β were initiated in 1996. The material used for the crystallization attempts was recombinant human IFN-β-1a (Avonex®, Biogen Inc., Cambridge, MA) expressed and secreted from Chinese hamster ovary (CHO) cells. This material, like the natural protein, is characterized by the presence of a carbohydrate chain covalently attached via Asn80 (6). As a biopharmaceutical product the protein was available in large quantities, which allowed extensive screening of a large number of crystallization conditions. Also, due to the stringent characterization that is required for a protein that is intended for use in humans, the protein preparation available to us was of high purity (a necessary factor for crystallization) and had been extensively characterized by a variety of biochemical, biophysical, and other analytical techniques. To further increase the chances of crystallization, we improved the homogeneity of the material in terms of glycosylation by performing an additional fractionation step using Zn-chelating sepharose chromatography. Standard crystallization screening produced crystals by hanging-drop vapor diffusion using PEG 4000 as a precipitant. The crystals were small and diffracted X-rays only weakly. The size of the crystals was improved considerably by growing them in hanging drops containing silica hydrogel (Hampton Research). X-ray diffraction data were collected to 2.2-Å resolution from frozen crystals using Cu Kα radiation. Data processing indicated that the unit cell was orthorhombic, with cell dimensions $a = 55.3$, $b = 65.91$, $c = 121.51$ Å. The systematic absences in the unit cell suggested a space group of $P2_12_12_1$. The asymmetric unit was found to contain two molecules, designated A and B.

Phase information was obtained by molecular replacement. The search probe used was a polyalanine model based on the Cα coordinates available for murine IFN-β. Rotation and translation searches revealed the locations of the two IFN-β molecules in the asymmetric unit, the positions of which were optimized by rigid-body refinement. A partial initial model was used for calculation of electron density maps. Subsequent iterative cycles of model building and positional and temperature factor refinement resulted in the final structure of human IFN-β-1a (Protein Data Bank entry code 1au1) (43). The structure has a crystallographic R-factor of 22.3% and an R-free of 28.3% for data in the range of 100–2.2 Å. The stereochemistry of the structure is good, with 92.9% of all amino acid residues in the most favored regions of the Ramachandran diagram and only one residue in the disallowed regions.

2.1 Structure of Human IFN-β-1a

The structure shows that IFN-β has the typical, simple fold of Type I IFNs (Fig. 1a,b) characterized by the presence of five α-helices that are connected by loops and form a left-handed, type II bundle (44). The Type I IFN fold constitutes a structural subfamily of the helical, or hematopoietic, cytokines (45). This family also includes, among other members, human growth hormone (hGH), erythropoietin, granulocyte colony-stimulating factor (G-CSF) and several interleukins, all characterized by the presence of a bundle of four α-helices. The helices of IFN-β are designated A, B, C, D and E (Fig. 1a,b) (39). Helix A runs parallel to helix B and D and antiparallel to helices

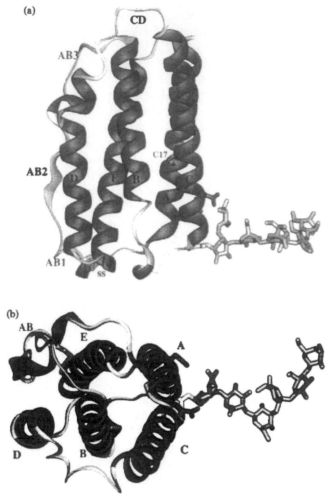

Figure 1 Structure of human IFN-β-1a. The molecule shown is molecule A of the two noncrystallographically related molecules in the unit cell. The protein backbone is shown in ribbon representation and the observed portion of the carbohydrate in stick representation. Additional sugar residues that are present in the molecule are not visible in the crystal structure due to disorder. (a) and (b) views are "side" and "top", respectively.

C and E. The corresponding loops that connect the helices are termed the AB (subdivided to AB1, AB2, and AB3), BC, CD (subdivided to CD1 and CD2), and DE loops (Fig. 1a). Short sections of 3_{10} or α-helix are present within some of the loops. The AB and CD loops are highly flexible, as

(c)

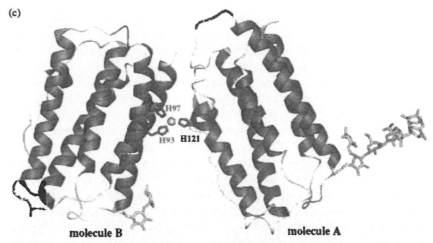

molecule B   molecule A

Figure 1 (c) Crystallographic dimer of human IFN-β. The zinc ion is shown as a sphere. The coordinating histidines and the observed portion of the carbohydrates are also shown. (Based on the coordinates from Ref. 43.)

evinced by their high temperature factors and by the fact that they occupy different conformations in the noncrystallographically related molecules A and B in the crystal (Fig. 1c). The N- and C-termini of the protein lie close together, toward the upper end of the molecule as it is represented in Figure 1a. A disulfide bridge interconnects the AB1 and DE loops and may play a role in stabilizing the structure of this region. In addition, the free cysteine residue (Cys17) is located on helix A, proximal to the surface but buried. The single glycosylation site, at Asn80, lies toward the C-terminal end of helix C. The carbohydrate is biantennary; only a portion of it was sufficiently ordered to be well defined in the crystal structure. The observed electron density allowed only seven of the ten hexose rings typically found in a biantennary complex carbohydrate (4 GlcNAc, 3 mannose, 2 galactose, and 1 fucose) to be modeled for molecule A, and only two rings could be modeled for molecule B (Figs. 1, 3).

A zinc ion was observed to mediate a contact between molecules A and B in the asymmetric unit of the crystal. This cation was coordinated by the side chains of three histidine residues: His121 of molecule A and His 93 and His 97 of molecule B (Fig. 1c). A water molecule occupies the fourth tetrahedral Zn^{2+} coordination site. Although we now know the observation of an apparent Zn^{2+}-bridged dimer to be a crystallization artifact, this observation was initially interesting due to the fact that the determination of the IFN-α2b structure also showed the presence of a zinc-mediated dimer, albeit with different relative orientation of the monomers (40). Because dimerization has been documented for other helical cytokines, such as ciliary neuro-trophic factor (CNTF) (46) and hGH (47), it was decided to examine the role of the zinc binding site in IFN-β function. Two mutants, H121A and H93A/H97A, were made in which one or two of the Zn^{2+}-chelating histidines were mutated to alanine residues, thus presumably disrupting the Zn^{2+}-mediated interaction between neighboring IFN-β molecules that was observed in the crystal structure. These mutants were compared to wild-type IFN-β-1a in standard assays measuring their antiviral activity, their affinity for binding to the Type I IFN receptor on cells, and their ability to bind to a soluble IFNAR2-Fc fusion protein (48). The assays indicated that the activity of each of these mutants was comparable to that of the wild-type protein. Additional mutations at sites on IFN-β that were seen to be in direct contact in molecules A and B in the crystallographic unit cell also had no effect on the activity of the molecule in a panel of functional and receptor binding assays (48). In addition, using biophysical methods we could find no convincing evidence for the existence of Zn^{2+}-mediated IFN-β dimers in solution. Taken together, these results indicated that the Zn^{2+}-mediated dimers that are observed in the crystal structure of IFN-β-1a are most likely functionally irrelevant.

2.2   Comparison to the Structure of IFN-α2b

Human IFN-β has ~35% sequence identity to the consensus sequence of IFN-α (1,49). Comparison of the high-resolution structures of human IFN-β and human IFN-α2b shows that the backbone folds are very similar (Fig. 2). The root mean square (rms) difference between the positions of structurally homologous residues of human IFN-β and IFN-α2b is 1.25 Å. Major differences are observed, however, in the structures of certain loops, such as the CD and AB1 loops. These differences in conformation not only reflect intrinsic structural differences of the two IFN molecules but are also dependent on the particular crystal contacts formed. In Type I IFNs these loops are very flexible, as confirmed by the NMR structure of IFN-α2a (41). Because of their flexibility, these loops are susceptible to deformation, as indicated by the presence of different conformations for these regions in molecules A and B in the asymmetric unit of the IFN-β-1a crystal structure (Fig. 1c). In addition to the differences in backbone structure described earlier, the many sequence differences that exist between IFN-β and IFN-α2 mean that there are significant differences in the surface structures of the two molecules due to differences in the structure and conformation of surface-exposed side chains. Despite the common tendency to focus on differences in backbone structure as being the most important causes of functional differences between structurally related molecules, it is the surface

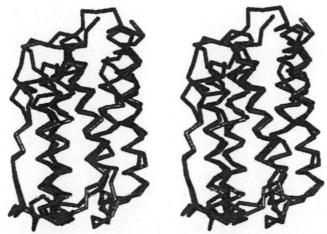

Figure 2 Stereo diagram of superimposed human IFN-β and human IFN-α2b Cα-backbone structures. Several regions of IFN-α2b are missing from the model, due to disorder.

of the IFN molecule that interacts with the receptor. Therefore, differences in surface structure potentially can also contribute to differences in receptor binding and activity, even in regions where the underlying backbone structures are similar (50,51).

3 STRUCTURAL AND FUNCTIONAL DIFFERENCES BETWEEN IFN-β-1a AND IFN-β-1b: THE ROLE OF GLYCOSYLATION

For many glycoproteins the role of the glycan is poorly understood. The relevance of glycosylation to the functional activity of human IFN-β was suggested by the significant biochemical and pharmacological differences that are observed between two different forms of recombinant IFN-β that are used clinically, IFN-β-1a and IFN-β-1b (see Sec. 1.1). A detailed comparison of these two proteins (30) showed that the specific antiviral activity of IFN-β-1a, at 2×10^8 IU/mg, was 10-fold higher than that of IFN-β-1b. A similar activity difference was seen in assays measuring the antiproliferative and immunomodulatory activities of IFN-β. The three principal structural differences between IFN-β-1a and IFN-β-1b—the presence or absence of glycosylation at Asn 80, a cysteine versus a serine at position 17, and the presence or absence of Met 1—were evaluated separately by preparing three different protein constructs in which each of these structural differences was introduced individually (30). It was found that removal of Met1 or the mutation of Cys17 to Ser had no apparent effect on the in vitro activity of the protein. These results can be understood by reference to the structure of the protein; the N-terminus of IFN-β is now known not to be involved in interactions with the receptor (48), and neither the loss of Met1 nor the Cys17Ser mutation would be expected to introduce significant perturbations to the structure of the protein. However, removal of the carbohydrate resulted in a substantial reduction in in vitro activity that was due primarily to a decrease in the solubility of the protein. This change resulted in the formation of an insoluble IFN-β precipitate that could be separated out by centrifugation (30). The precipitate was analyzed by SDS-PAGE under reducing and nonreducing conditions. Under reducing conditions the precipitate migrated with the predicted mass of nonglycosylated IFN-β. However, under nonreducing conditions the precipitate migrated as multiple bands corresponding to disulfide-linked IFN-β multimers. Size exclusion chromatography (SEC) experiments provided additional evidence for this aggregation effect. When Betaseron® was subjected to SEC under physiological buffer conditions, 40% of the material eluted as monomer and 60% as a multimolecular complex with an apparent molecular weight above 600 kDa. In contrast, 98% of IFN-β-1a, subjected to SEC under the same conditions, eluted as a monomer (30). Similar results were obtained using a variety of different chromatography media and buffer conditions. These results show that the tendency of nonglycosylated IFN-β to aggregate is independent of the existence of a free cysteine at position 17 and thus does not require the formation of intermolecular disulfide bonds. Since all of the cysteine residues in IFN-β are buried (43,52), the formation of intermolecular disulfide bonds by the deglycosylated IFN-β-1a indicated that at least partial unfolding occurs in the absence of the attached carbohydrate. Indeed, thermal denaturation measurements showed that the melting temperature of IFN-β was lowered by 4–5°C after the molecule was deglycosylated by PNGase F treatment (30), indicating that the structure of the molecule was significantly destabilized when its carbohydrate was removed.

Inspection of the crystal structure of IFN-β provides a possible explanation for the stabilizing effect of the carbohydrate. For example, the structure shows that the α1-6 fucose residue of the carbohydrate forms hydrogen bond contacts with the side chains of Gln 23 (helix A) and Asn 86 (helix C) (Fig. 3a). These observations indicate that the carbohydrate of IFN-β is closely integrated with the tertiary structure of this protein. The carbohydrate increases the number of interactions between the A and C helices and might play a role in preventing partial unfolding events that expose Cys17 of helix A to the solvent and thus promote intermolecular disulfide bond formation. Stabilization of protein structure by glycosylation has been

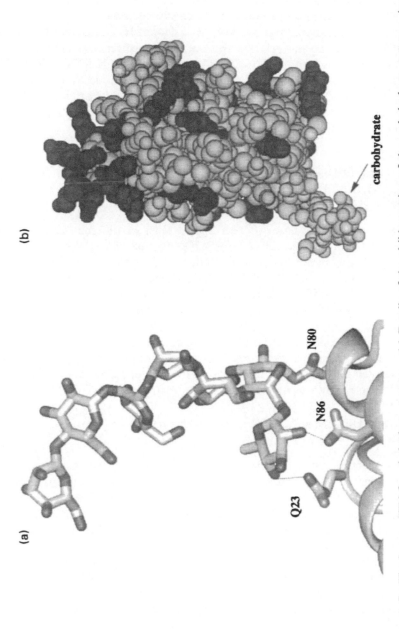

Figure 3 The human IFN-β carbohydrate structure. (a) Details of the visible portion of the carbohydrate structure, including hydrogen bonds (dotted lines) formed with protein residues. Additional sugar residues that are present in the molecule are not visible in the crystal structure, due to disorder. (b) Space-filling representation of the human IFN-β-1a molecule in the vicinity of the glycosylation site. Charged residues are colored dark gray, while uncharged residues are colored light gray.

studied in the case of ribonuclease, for which it was shown that stabilization resulted from a dampening of conformational fluctuations in the protein backbone (53). In addition, inspection of the surface of IFN-β in the vicinity of the carbohydrate shows a relative absence of charged residues (Fig. 3b). The corresponding surface of IFN-α2b, which contains no N-linked glycosylation site, possesses a substantial number of charged residues (30). Thus, another role of the carbohydrate in IFN-β may be to shield from solvent a relatively uncharged surface of the molecule that, if exposed, might make the molecule susceptible to aggregation.

4 USE OF STRUCTURAL DATA IN EXPLORATIONS OF THE MECHANISM OF RECEPTOR ENGAGEMENT AND ACTIVATION BY IFN-β-1a

Central to understanding how different Type I IFNs or different forms of IFN-β perform their biological functions is the question of how these molecules engage their common receptor on cells to induce the various cellular responses that have been shown to result. In particular, it was of interest to know which regions of IFN-β-1a interact directly with which components of the receptor and whether it was possible to learn anything about how interactions between specific regions of the IFN molecule and their complementary sites on the receptor contribute to bringing about receptor activation and downstream functional responses. The question of how these properties differed between IFN-β-1a and other Type I IFNs or other members of the helical cytokine family was also of interest.

4.1 Structural Aspects of the Interaction of the Type I Interferon Receptor with Type I IFNs

No crystal structure has yet been determined for the complex of a Type I IFN with either of its receptor chains. However, the crystal structures of several other helical cytokines in complex with the extracellular domains of their receptors have been determined and may serve as models for understanding the interaction of Type I IFNs with their receptor (54,55). These structures include hGH (56), erythropoietin (57), and granulocyte colony-stimulating factor (58). The structure of the homodimeric cytokine IFN-γ in complex with one of its receptor chains (59), which like IFNAR1 and IFNAR2 is a Class 2 cytokine receptor, is also potentially relevant to ligand–receptor binding in the Type I IFN receptor system (60). All of these cytokine receptors have extracellular domains that contain tandem fibronectin type III-related (FNIII) repeats. Typically the receptor chains interact with the cytokine through residues close to the junction between

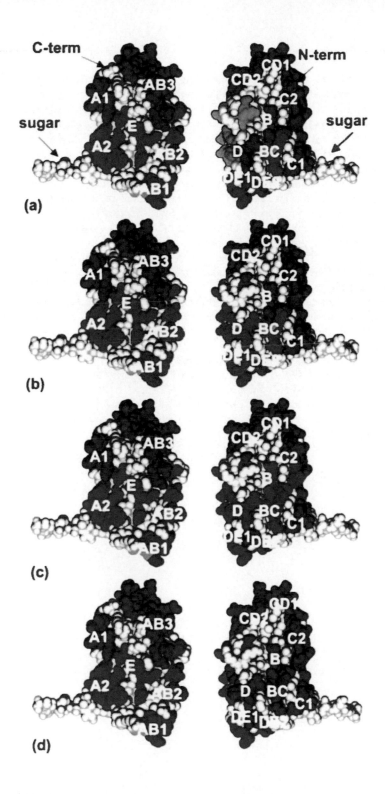

Figure 18.5 Mutational effects on binding and functional activity mapped onto the three-dimensional structure of IFN-β. Front and back views of a space-filling representation of the crystal structure of IFN-β, color-coded to summarize the effects of the mutations on the activity of the mutants in assays measuring (a) antiviral activity on A549 cells, (b) antiproliferation assay using Daudi cells, (c) affinity for binding to the receptor on Daudi cells, and (d) ability to bind to a fusion construct, IFNAR2-Fc, comprising the extracellular domain of IFNAR2 fused to the hinge, CH2 and CH3 domains of human IgG1 Fc. The magnitude of the mutational effect on activity in a given assay is color-coded as follows: For panels (a)–(c), residues that, when mutated, resulted in no loss of activity (i.e., less than twofold reduction) in a given assay are colored green; residues that, when mutated, caused a reduction in activity of two- to fivefold are colored blue; residues that, when mutated, caused a fivefold or greater loss in activity are colored red. In panel (d), mutations that caused a complete loss of IFNAR2-Fc binding in the assay are colored red; mutations that caused no detectable effect on IFNAR2-Fc binding are colored green. In all four panels, portions of the molecule colored yellow were not altered by the mutations (see Fig. 18.4). All of the mutant proteins tested contained an identical His-tag N-terminal extension. The positions of the protein's N- and C-termini are indicated by arrows, as is the position of the carbohydrate on Asn 80. In addition to the 15 alanine-substitution mutants A1–E, the effects of mutating residues R27, R35, and K123 on the antiviral activity of IFN-β have been reported previously (42) and are included in (a). Two additional his-IFN-β mutants, H93A/H97A and H121, were analyzed in three of the four assays and in all cases gave wild-type activity. These three histidine residues are therefore colored green in panels (a), (c), and (d). (From Ref. 48, Ⓒ Biochemistry 2000.)

two such repeats. In the case of the hGH–receptor complex as well as the erythropoietin–receptor complex, a cytokine molecule is observed to be "cradled" between two identical receptor molecules (56,57). Mutagenesis experiments combined with binding measurements have shown that one hGH receptor chain interacts with hGH through a high-affinity binding site ("Site 1") while the second chain interacts with a low-affinity site ("Site 2") on the opposite face of the hGH molecule (50,56,61). An analogous situation may exist for the complex of IFN-β with IFNAR1 and IFNAR2. Cells transfected with the IFNAR2 chain alone have been shown to bind IFNs with moderate affinity (62,63). In contrast, when cells were transfected with the IFNAR1 chain alone, no binding to IFNs was detected. However, cotransfection of IFNAR1 with IFNAR2 increased the affinity of IFN binding by ~10-fold compared with cells transfected with IFNAR2 alone (62–64). These experiments established that the IFN-β interaction with IFNAR2 alone is of relatively high affinity, while binding to IFNAR1 alone is not detectable. One significant structural difference between the Type I IFN receptor and the other cytokine receptors described earlier is that the extracellular domain of IFNAR1 contains four FNIII repeats, as opposed to IFNAR2, which, like the extracellular domains of the hGH and erythropoietin receptors, contains only two such repeats. This structural feature suggests that the binding geometry between IFN and IFNAR1 may differ from that seen for the hGH–low-affinity receptor interaction (25,65).

4.2 Systematic Mutational Mapping of the IFNAR1 and IFNAR2 Binding Sites on IFN-β-1a

A number of previous studies had employed various strategies to probe the effects on activity of modifying the amino acid sequence of Type I IFNs, including IFN-β, at different sites within the primary sequence. The results of these studies suggested that, for IFN-α, sites within the AB loop, the DE loop, and the B, C, and E helices are important for function (38) and that, in IFN-β, regions lying within the AB loop and the C and D helices were important (43,66). However, these previous mutagenesis studies were necessarily performed without the aid of a high-resolution crystal structure to guide the design of the mutated proteins and the interpretation of the results obtained therefrom. Consequently, certain mutations that in the original studies were interpreted to directly affect IFN–receptor binding have been shown, upon reanalysis in light of subsequent high-resolution crystal structures, to be buried in the protein's core and thus presumably to exert their effect through long-range perturbation of the IFN structure rather than though direct interaction with the receptor (43).

The availability of the high-resolution crystal structure of IFN-β-1a made possible a systematic approach to mapping the surface interactions of the molecule with its receptor (48). The crystal structure was used to identify those residues that, because they possessed surface-exposed side chains, were 1) candidates to interact directly with the receptor and 2) likely, if mutated to a different amino acid, to affect any such interactions in which they were involved. Residues with side chains that were substantially buried or that appeared to be involved in structurally important interactions with other residues in the IFN-β structure were not altered, to avoid causing any global or long-range disruption of the molecule's structure. In most cases mutations were to alanine, so the resulting truncation of the side chains to a simple methyl group would remove any favorable binding interaction between the side chain of the mutated residue and the receptor without introducing any increased steric bulk that might additionally perturb the free energy of interaction with the receptor (61). Thus, the magnitude of the resulting effect on the protein's activity could, at least to a first approximation, be quantitatively interpreted in terms of the energetic contributions that the mutated residues make to the stability of the activated receptor complex. The importance of the glycan at position Asn 80 in IFN-β-1a had previously been established (30). Consequently, the mutant proteins used in the structure–activity analysis were expressed in mammalian cells, to ensure that they were produced as glycosylated proteins. The additional difficulty of generating mutant proteins in mammalian cells, compared to a simpler bacterial expression system, made it necessary to mutate the residues in groups rather than individually, to limit the number of separate mutant proteins required for a comprehensive mutational scan of the protein's surface to a manageable number. A panel of 15 different IFN-β-1a mutants was therefore made, in each of which a contiguous group of two to eight surface-exposed residues was altered (Fig. 4). Collectively, this set of mutant proteins covered essentially the entire surface of the molecule, systematically denuding successive regions of the molecular surface of potential receptor-binding side chains. The structural integrity of the mutant proteins was assessed using antibodies known to be specific for natively folded protein (48).

The mutants were tested in four different binding or activity assays measuring (a) the ability to induce an antiviral response in A549 human lung carcinoma cells challenged with encaphalomyocarditis virus, (b) the ability to inhibit the proliferation of human Daudi Burkitt's lymphoma cells in culture, (c) binding affinity for the Type I IFN receptor on similar Daudi cells, and (d) the ability to bind to a soluble form of the IFNAR2 extracellular domain. Two different binding assays were used to establish whether a reduction in binding affinity for the intact receptor on Daudi cells,

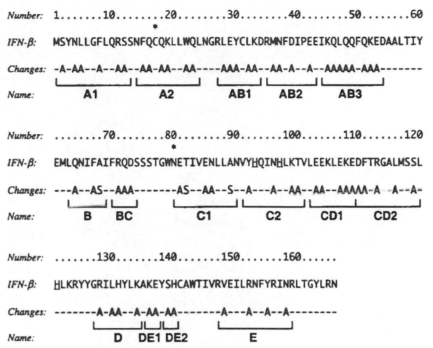

Figure 4 Locations of the mutations introduced into the primary sequence of human IFN-β in the systematic mutational mapping of receptor interaction sites reported in Ref. 48. The sequence of each mutant, A1–E, is shown below the section of wt IFN-β sequence in which the mutations occur. The individual mutants A1–E are named according to the secondary structural element (helix or loop) in which the amino acid substitutions occur.

seen with a given IFN-β-1a mutant, was due to disruption of binding to IFNAR2 or to IFNAR1, by determining whether binding was affected in the assay containing IFNAR2 only. The mutants were evaluated in both antiviral and antiproliferation activity assays to address the possibility that these distinct functional activities might derive from distinct interactions with the receptor. If so, mutations of specific receptor-binding residues on IFN-β might differentially affect these two activities, as has been shown to result from certain mutations in the receptor (16). The results of the structure-based mapping of the receptor binding sites on IFN-β-1a are summarized in Figure 5, which shows the effect of each set of mutations in each of the four assays (a)–(d) just listed, color-coded and mapped onto the appropriate region of the IFN-β-1a molecular structure.

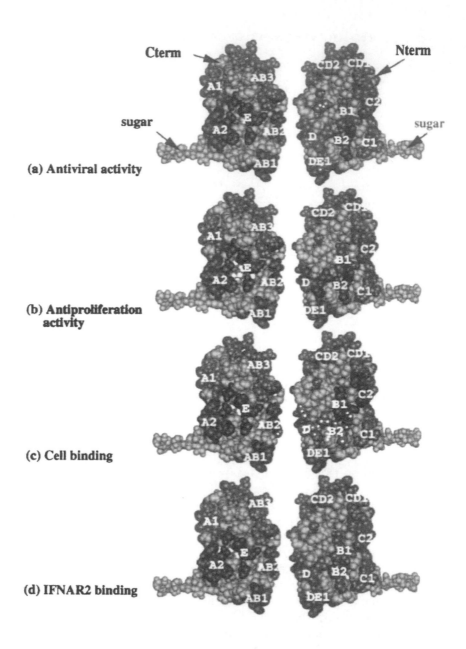

(a) Antiviral activity

(b) Antiproliferation activity

(c) Cell binding

(d) IFNAR2 binding

4.2.1 Locations of the IFNAR1- and IFNAR2-Binding Sites on IFN-β.

The locations of the IFNAR1- and IFNAR2-binding sites were inferred from the results shown in Figure 5 (48). Examination of Figure 5d shows that only four of the mutants displayed any substantial decrease in their ability to bind to the extracellular domain of IFNAR2. Moreover, although the modifications in these four mutant proteins involve two widely separated regions of the protein sequence (Fig. 4), Figure 5d shows that in the folded protein these mutations define a contiguous patch of the molecular surface. Thus, the IFNAR2-binding site was concluded to comprise regions of the A helix, AB loop, and E helix (i.e., the regions colored red in Figure 5d). Figure 5a–c shows that, in addition to the mutations that affected binding to IFNAR2, a separate set of mutations led to a substantial reduction in activity in the antiviral and antiproliferation assays and/or reduced the ability of the protein to bind to the intact receptor on Daudi cells without showing any effect on IFNAR2 binding. This separate set of activity-altering mutations define a second contiguous patch on the surface of the folded

---

Figure 5 Mutational effects on binding and functional activity mapped onto the three-dimensional structure of IFN-β. Front and back views of a space-filling representation of the crystal structure of IFN-β, color-coded to summarize the effects of the mutations on the activity of the mutants in assays measuring (a) antiviral activity on A549 cells, (b) antiproliferation assay using Daudi cells, (c) affinity for binding to the receptor on Daudi cells, and (d) ability to bind to a fusion construct, IFNAR2-Fc, comprising the extracellular domain of IFNAR2 fused to the hinge, CH2 and CH3 domains of human IgG1 Fc. The magnitude of the mutational effect on activity in a given assay is color-coded as follows: For panels (a)–(c), residues that, when mutated, resulted in no loss of activity (i.e., less than twofold reduction) in a given assay are colored green; residues that, when mutated, caused a reduction in activity of two- to fivefold are colored blue; residues that, when mutated, caused a fivefold or greater loss in activity are colored red. In panel (d), mutations that caused a complete loss of IFNAR2-Fc binding in the assay are colored red; mutations that caused no detectable effect on IFNAR2-Fc binding are colored green. In all four panels, portions of the molecule colored yellow were not altered by the mutations (see Fig. 4). All of the mutant proteins tested contained an identical His-tag N-terminal extension. The positions of the protein's N- and C-termini are indicated by arrows, as is the position of the carbohydrate on Asn 80. In addition to the 15 alanine-substitution mutants A1–E, the effects of mutating residues R27, R35, and K123 on the antiviral activity of IFN-β have been reported previously (42) and are included in (a). Two additional his-IFN-β mutants, H93A/H97A and H121, were analyzed in three of the four assays and in all cases gave wild-type activity. These three histidine residues are therefore colored green in panels (a), (c), and (d). (From Ref. 48, © Biochemistry 2000.) (See color insert.)

protein, on the opposite face from the IFNAR2 binding site. Since mutations in this region did not affect binding to soluble IFNAR2, they presumably exert their effects by disrupting the ability of the protein to interact with IFNAR1. The IFNAR1-binding site on IFN-β was thus concluded to encompass the regions colored red or blue in the right-hand panels of Figures 5a–c, involving parts of the B, C, and D helices and of the BC and DE loops.

4.2.2 Comparison to Human Growth Hormone/Human Growth Hormone Receptor System

Biochemical studies have shown that the interaction of IFN-β with IFNAR2 is a relatively high-affinity binding event, compared to the much weaker binding to IFNAR1 (62,63). Thus, the interactions of IFN with IFNAR2 and IFNAR1 have typically been considered as functionally analogous to the interactions of hGH with its receptor through the high-affinity receptor-binding site ("Site 1") and the low-affinity site ("Site 2") on hGH, respectively. Interestingly, an alignment of the three-dimensional structure of IFN-β-1a with that of hGH, available in the FSSP database (67), revealed that the region comprising the IFNAR2-binding site on IFN-β coincides with the location of Site 1 on hGH (Fig. 6). In contrast, the region comprising the IFNAR1-binding site did not correspond to the location of Site 2 on hGH (48). The locations of the receptor-binding sites on IFN-β thus shed new light on the analogy with the hGH/hGH-R system by showing that, at a structural level, the interaction of IFN-β with IFNAR2 resembles the interaction of hGH with its receptor through Site 1 but that the structural details of the interaction with IFNAR1 differ radically from the way in which hGH interacts with its second receptor chain via Site 2. As noted in Sec. 4.1, the notion that the way in which Type I IFNs interact with IFNAR1 differs from how prototypical helical cytokines, such as hGH and erythropoietin, interact with their receptors is also suggested by the additional pair of FNIII domains that are present in the extracellular portion of IFNAR1 (25,65).

4.3 Insights into the Activation Mechanism of the Type I IFN Receptor Derived from the Mutational Analysis of IFN-β-1a

Despite extensive study, key elements of the Type I IFN receptor activation mechanism remain poorly understood. Though IFNAR2 alone is able to bind IFN with relatively high affinity (62,63,68), both IFNAR1 and IFNAR2 are required for a functional response to IFN stimulation (7,69–73). Binding of IFNAR1 alone to IFN cannot, in general, be detected,

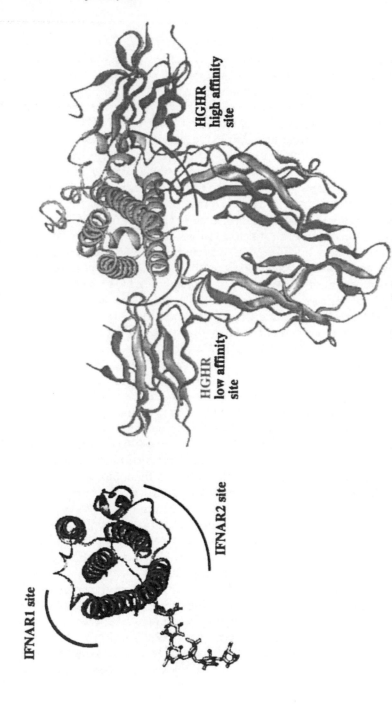

Figure 6 Locations of the high-affinity (IFNAR2) and low-affinity (IFNAR1) binding sites on human IFN-β-1a compared to the corresponding high- and low-affinity sites through which hGH interacts with its two identical receptor chains. It can be seen that the IFNAR2-binding site on IFN-β coincides with the high-affinity receptor-binding site ("site 1'') of hGH but that the putative IFNAR1-binding site on IFN-β does not coincide with the low-affinity "site 2'' on hGH.

though its coexpression with IFNAR2 increases the affinity of IFN binding to the receptor by ~10-fold (62,63). Several studies have shown that the binding of IFN can induce a close association between IFNAR1 and IFNAR2 (12,19,62,74). These observations have led to the proposal that the Type I IFN receptor becomes activated by a mechanism of ligand-induced receptor association in which IFN first binds to IFNAR2 followed by recruitment into the complex of IFNAR1 (62), analogous to the activation mechanism proposed for numerous other cytokine receptors (75–77). However, there are a number of indications that the activation mechanism of the Type I IFN receptor is more complex than a simple ligand-induced association of IFNAR1 with IFNAR2. First, the structure of the Type I IFN receptor differs from that of the some other cytokine receptors for which ligand-induced receptor association is believed to occur in that IFNAR1 contains four FNIII repeats, double the number found in prototypical cytokine receptors such as the receptors for hGH or erythropoietin. The gp130 component of the receptor for interleukin-6, which also contains additional FNIII repeats in its extracellular domain, has been shown to engage in additional binding interactions that stabilize a higher-order complex containing two molecules of bound cytokine and two molecules of each receptor chain (78). As an additional element of structural complexity, IFNAR2 is typically expressed on the cell surface as a disulfide-linked homodimer rather than as a monomer (8) and exists in full-length and truncated forms. Both of these observations suggest the possibility, so far unproven, that the activated receptor complex may contain more than one molecule each of bound IFN and of IFNAR2 (though a thorough examination of the interactions of IFN-β with the soluble IFNAR1 and IFNAR2 ectodomains (74) showed no evidence for complexes of higher order than 1:1:1). Second, published data imply that there is functionally important allosteric communication between IFN binding to the receptor ectodomain and the binding of the Janus-family kinase Tyk2 to the IFNAR1 cytoplasmic domain (79,80). Moreover, in the murine system a naturally occurring soluble form of the IFNAR2 extracellular domain has been shown to restore partial IFN sensitivity to cells that express IFNAR1 but not IFNAR2 on their surface (81), an observation that appears to imply either the involvement of multiple receptor chains in addition to IFNAR2 or the existence of an allosteric component to IFNAR1 signaling or both. Finally, there is the issue of whether the receptor functionally discriminates between different Type I IFNs, as numerous reports suggest (12–25,82,83) and, if so, how this discrimination might be achieved. All of these considerations suggest that IFN-induced association of IFNAR1 and IFNAR2 may be necessary, but probably is not sufficient, to fully account for activation of the Type I IFN receptor.

The results of the systematic mutational analysis of IFN-β-1a, described earlier (48), were used to address a number of questions concerning how the binding of IFN-β is coupled to activation of the Type I IFN receptor. Because the antiviral and antiproliferation activities of IFN-β-1a could be measured in separate assays, it was possible to quantitatively compare the effect of each IFN-β-1a mutation on these two distinct activities. The ability to separate these activities by demonstrating that a mutational change had disparate effects on the activities of IFN-β-1a in these two assays would have been strong evidence that these two different cellular responses to IFN arise from distinct effects of IFN binding to the receptor. In fact, the effects of mutations in IFN-β on the activity of the molecule in the antiviral assay correlated quite well with the effects of the same mutations on antiproliferation activity, though the existence of small deviations from proportionality could not be ruled out (48). Similar correlations have been observed between the antiviral and antiproliferation activities of a series of IFN-α mutants (60), though other studies have reported no correlation between antiviral and antiproliferation activities for different IFN-α subtypes (83,84). While the inability to separate these two activities to any great degree by mutating the structure of IFN-β in this study is not conclusive, it nevertheless argues that the changes in receptor structure and conformation that are required for IFN-β to trigger these two distinct activities are broadly similar.

Additional insights into the receptor activation mechanism were gained by quantitatively correlating each mutation's effects on receptor-binding affinity with its effects on functional activity (48). This analysis exploited the fact that both the receptor-binding assay and the antiproliferation activity assay were performed using Daudi cells. Thus, it was possible to calculate the fraction of receptors occupied at any given IFN-β concentration tested in the antiproliferation assay from the affinity of each mutant for binding to the receptor measured under similar conditions and using the same cell type. Several interesting points emerged from this analysis, which is illustrated in Figure 7 for w.t. his-IFN-β and for two of the mutants. Figure 7 shows that 50% inhibition of cell proliferation is achieved at a concentration of w.t. his-IFN-β that is sufficient to occupy only 0.3% of the receptors present on the cell. Virtually complete inhibition of proliferation is achieved at only ~2% receptor occupancy. This finding suggests that only a few receptors are required to become activated by IFN-β in order to maximally block proliferation of the cells, though the possibility that the transient, low-level engagement of the receptor might cause a long-lived activated form of the receptor to accumulate over time was not explicitly ruled out in this study. Surprisingly, the IFN-β mutant A2, with its cluster of six surface mutations on helix A (Fig. 4) that disrupt the interaction with

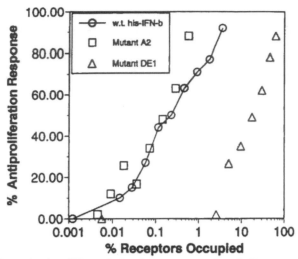

Figure 7 Quantitative differentiation between mutational effects on receptor binding and on antiproliferation activity. Dose-response data from representative antiproliferation assays performed with w.t. his-IFN-β (circles) and mutants A2 (squares) and DE1 (triangles), in which the concentration axis is expressed in terms of % receptors occupied. Both mutant and "wild-type" proteins contained an identical His-tag N-terminal extension. The percentage of receptors occupied at each concentration of wild-type or mutant his-IFN-β was calculated using a single site (i.e., hyperbolic) binding equation and the appropriate receptor-binding affinity measured for each mutant. Both antiproliferation activity and receptor binding were measured using Daudi cells. (From Ref. 48, © Biochemistry 2000.)

IFNAR2 and cause a tenfold reduction in specific activity in the antiproliferation assay (Fig. 5b), was nevertheless effective in eliciting the wild-type level of antiproliferation response at each level of receptor occupancy (Fig. 7). The essentially identical results for w.t. his-IFN-β-1a and mutant A2 seen in Figure 7, despite the substantial difference in their specific activities, indicates that although its 20-fold reduced affinity for the receptor requires substantially higher concentrations for receptor occupancy compared to wild-type his-IFN-β, the A2 mutant displays the full wild-type ability to induce an antiproliferative response once it has engaged the receptor. Two of the three other mutants that disrupted binding to IFNAR2 similarly showed proportionate effects on receptor binding and on antiproliferative activity. This result implies that the binding energy that is generated through interactions of the cytokine with IFNAR2 is used to stabilize the bound complex rather than to bring about any change in energetic state of the receptor that is linked to signaling (48).

In contrast, mutations at the IFNAR1-binding site on IFN-β appeared to show disproportionate effects on binding affinity versus activity (c.f. Fig. 5a and b versus 5c). Mutant DE1 in particular showed a substantially reduced activity in the antiproliferation assay that was not accompanied by any decrease in receptor binding affinity (Fig. 7), which suggests it must occupy a substantially higher number of receptors on Daudi cells in order to achieve a given level of functional response. This result implies that the binding energy derived from interaction of the DE loop residues K135 and E136 with the IFNAR1 chain may not be expressed as an increase in the stability of the bound complex but may be used instead to bring about receptor activation, presumably by stabilizing an energetically unfavorable activated state of the receptor (48). Overall, the analysis indicates that the two receptor-binding sites on IFN-β possess somewhat distinct functional roles. Interactions with IFNAR2 serve to bind the IFN-β to the cell surface; once bound, IFN-β can interact with and probably induce a conformational change in IFNAR1 to achieve an activated state that triggers signaling (48). The cytoplasmic domain of IFNAR2 is also known to be involved in signaling (72,73). However, the analysis suggests that IFN-β interaction with IFNAR2 likely serves only to bring it into the complex with IFNAR1, while the IFN-β interaction with IFNAR1 causes more elaborate molecular transformations. The view that signaling by IFNAR1 involves something other than simply bringing this molecule into proximity with IFNAR2 is supported by 1) the partial restoration of signaling in mouse cells lacking IFNAR2 by supplying a soluble form of the IFNAR2 intracellular domain together with IFN-β (mentioned earlier and in Ref. 81) and 2) the allosteric communication between the extracellular and cytoplasmic protions of IFNAR1 (79,80).

4.4 Comparison of Receptor Engagement by IFN-β versus IFN-α2

As was described in Sec. 1, Type I IFNs all act through a common receptor that consists of the protein chains IFNAR1 and IFNAR2. However, there is a significant amount of evidence to suggest that different Type I IFNs may engage the receptor differently (12–19,25) and may even induce somewhat different biological activities (20–24,82,83). Some reports suggest that the gene expression profiles induced upon treatment of cells with IFN-α or IFN-β are distinct, with certain genes being uniquely induced by one or other interferon subtype (84a–85). However, most of these studies compared gene expression profiles at a single concentration of each IFN, making it difficult to distinguish whether the observed differences reflect distinct gene expression patterns that are intrinsic to the IFNs themselves or instead result from differences in potency and thus would disappear if different doses of IFN had been used (86). It is therefore of some interest to understand the structural basis for this putative ability of the receptor to functionally discriminate between the Type I IFN subtypes. A systematic mutational analysis of the IFNAR2-binding site on IFN-α2 has recently been published (18,60). In this study, the authors introduced point mutations covering a region of the IFN-α2 surface that had previously been implicated in the binding of this molecule to IFNAR2. They assessed the binding of these mutants to a soluble form of the IFNAR2 extracellular domain attached to a solid surface. A comparison of the results of this study on IFN-α2 with those described earlier for IFN-β highlights some interesting similarities and differences between how these two cytokines engage and activate the Type I IFN receptor. The IFNAR2-binding site on IFN-α2 was found to involve the same regions of the protein, on the AB loop and the A and E helices, that were shown to comprise the IFNAR2-binding site on IFN-β (Figs. 5d, 6). However, comparison of the energetic contributions made by individual residues in the IFNAR2-binding site on IFN-α2, with the contributions made by groups of residues in IFN-β, suggested that the atomic details of the interactions of the receptor with these two proteins, which have many differences in their surface structures, may be quite different (60). Interestingly, individual mutations in the IFNAR2-binding site on IFN-α2 tended to have proportionate effects on IFNAR2-binding affinity and on functional activity in cell-based antiviral and antiproliferation assays (60). This result mirrors the observation made for the IFNAR2 site in IFN-β (Sec. 4.3). Overall, these findings indicate that IFN-α2 and IFN-β bind to IFNAR2 via very similar regions on their surfaces, though the interactions differ at the atomic level, as expected given the requirement to achieve complementarity with the different amino acids that define the surface structures of the two IFNs. Moreover, for both IFNs, binding to IFNAR2 appears to serve a similar function in the activation of the receptor, i.e., to bind the IFN to the cell surface and present it to IFNAR1 while bringing the cytoplasmic domain of the IFNAR2 chain and its associated signaling molecules into productive interaction with the IFNAR1 cytoplasmic domain. A mutational analysis of IFNAR2 has shown that the interaction sites for IFN-α2 and for IFN-β on this receptor component are overlapping but may not be identical (18), and thus some difference in the orientation with which IFNAR2 binds to these two IFNs may exist that might affect function. No systematic mutational analysis of the IFNAR1-binding site on IFN-α2 has yet been performed. It therefore remains unknown whether the IFNAR1-binding sites on these two IFNs occupy similar locations on the surfaces of the molecules or whether the way in which IFN-α2 engages this component of the receptor differs from the fairly complex activation mechanism that was proposed for IFN-β (48).

5 USE OF STRUCTURAL DATA TO PROBE THE FUNCTIONS OF BLOCKING AND NONBLOCKING ANTIBODIES TO IFN-β

A number of monoclonal antibodies (mAbs) directed against IFN-β have been generated as laboratory reagents, some of which are able to block the activity of IFN-β in cell-based functional assays (87). Moreover, patients treated with IFN-β in various disease settings have been found to raise antibodies against the drug (32,34,35,88,89), and in some studies the generation of neutralizing antibodies against IFN-β has been shown to diminish the drug's treatment effect (31,32,36,90). Interestingly, as described in Sec. 1.1, the incidence of antidrug antibodies is much higher in patients treated with Betaseron® (IFN-β-1b; nonglycosylated ΔMet1, Cys17Ser IFN-β expressed in *E. coli*) than in those treated with Avonex® (IFN-β-1a; glycosylated, full length, natural sequence IFN-β expressed in mammalian cells) (34,35,91), though the extent to which this difference in immunogenicity arises from the structural differences between the two drugs, versus other differences, such as dosing, route of administration, formulation, and aggregation state (92), has not yet been definitively established. A small pilot study, using a small number of serum samples from MS patients treated with Betaseron® or with Avonex®, suggested that the characteristics of the antidrug antibody response, including the epitope specificities of the antibodies it comprises, can vary significantly from one patient to another (93). Understanding where on the IFN-β molecule different antibodies bind and how their binding affects the biological activities of the protein is important for several reasons. First, it can potentially provide information on what regions of the molecule are important for its function and thus can provide a complementary perspective to that obtained in the alanine scanning mutagenesis study described in Sec. 4.2. Secondly, such information can provide insight into the different mechanisms by which antibodies can interfere with IFN-β signaling. Finally, studies with antibodies from the serum of patients treated with drug can potentially provide information about what regions of the IFN-β molecule are recognized by antibodies that might affect treatment outcome in these patients.

A peptide-scanning approach was used to show that two different neutralizing mAbs recognized epitopes encompassing IFN-β residues in the C-terminal (AB3) region of the AB loop and in the C helix (87).

Examination of the locations of these regions on the three-dimensional structure of IFN-β-1a shows that they lie on the edge of the IFNAR2-binding site that was identified by alanine scanning mutagenesis (Fig. 5d,6). The availability of the high-resolution crystal structure of IFN-β-1a enabled the epitopes for a larger group of anti-IFN-β mAbs to be mapped onto the surface of the molecule (48,94), using as probes the set of alanine mutants described in Figure 4. The locations of these epitopes were correlated with the ability of each mAb to block the activity of IFN-β in an antiviral assay and its ability to block the binding of IFN-β-1a to a soluble form of the IFNAR2 extracellular domain. Interestingly, the results of this analysis suggest that some mAbs can inhibit IFNAR2 binding and block the antiviral activity of IFN-β even though they bind to epitopes that are not close to receptor-binding sites on the IFN-β molecule (94). While the explanation for this surprising finding remains uncertain, it is possible that it reflects an ability of certain mAbs, upon binding to IFN-β, to cause long-range perturbations in the structure of the molecule that interfere with its ability to bind to and activate the receptor (94).

No comprehensive study has been performed to identify the locations of neutralizing epitopes that are recognized by antibodies occurring in the serum of patients treated with recombinant IFN-β. In a small pilot study, aimed primarily at developing methods for analyzing patient antibody responses, antibodies from a small number of patient serum samples were analyzed using a panel of ELISA assays based on their ability to recognize intact IFN-β-1a presented in different ways or to bind peptides derived from the amino acid sequence of IFN-β (93). Epitope locations were determined only for the subset of antibodies, found in some of the serum samples, that were able to recognize linear peptides from the IFN-β sequence. In the small number of samples that were included in this study, antibodies capable of binding to linear IFN-β-derived peptides recognized epitopes at the N-terminus of the protein, in the AB loop, the CD loop, or the D helix. Examination of the X-ray crystal structure of IFN-β shows that the first three of these regions exist in an extended conformation in the folded protein. In the case of the relevant part of the D helix, the region containing the antibody-binding sites, though helical in one of the two molecules that comprises the crystallographic unit cell, exists as an extended loop in the other, indicating that this region of the protein can adopt an extended conformation in the folded molecule without undue energetic cost. Thus, at least in this limited number of serum samples, no antibodies were found that recognized peptide antigens corresponding to regions of the structure that are part of the organized secondary structure of IFN-β. Although these findings are suggestive, it will be necessary to study a much larger collection of serum samples in order to draw any general conclusions about the epitope specificities of antidrug antibodies that occur in patients treated with recombinant IFN-β.

6 USE OF STRUCTURAL DATA IN THE DESIGN OF SECOND-GENERATION RECOMBINANT IFN-β DRUGS

A strategy that has been employed to improve the pharmacokinetic properties of protein drugs is to chemically modify the protein by covalently attaching one or more polyethylene glycol (PEG) molecules (95–97). The PEG preparations used for this purpose comprise linear or branched polymeric chains with molecular weights typically in the range of 5–50 kDa. In addition to its effects on clearance rates, "pegylation" can also alter the bioavailability and biodistribution of a protein and can potentially reduce its immunogenicity if the attached PEG groups mask immunodominant epitopes on the protein's surface. A variety of strategies have been employed when modifying therapeutic proteins with PEG, using a number of different modification chemistries and linker groups to attach the PEG to the protein and varying the size and the number of PEG groups attached. Attachment of more or larger PEG groups typically results in larger effects on clearance rates but also increases the likelihood that the modification will interfere with the activity of the cytokine. So, for example, in the successful development of a pegylated form of IFN-α2b (PEG-INTRON™) a relatively nonspecific chemistry was used to attach 12-kDa PEG to the cytokine, resulting in a heterogeneous product that contained PEG groups attached at various sites on the IFN molecule (98). The heterogeneously pegylated material was shown to be fourfold less active than unmodified IFN-α2b in in vitro activity assays, but its serum half-life was increased by ~sixfold, allowing less frequent dosing of the drug and thereby resulting in an overall improvement in the pharmaceutical properties of the protein as a treatment for hepatitis C (99,100). Pegylated IFN-α2a nonspecifically modified with single linear 5-kDa PEG (101) or a branched 40-kDa PEG (102) have been tested in healthy volunteers and in patients suffering from advanced renal cell carcinoma, respectively. These preparations too comprised multiple species containing a PEG group attached at different sites around the surface of the molecule (103). A form of IFN-β that was selectively modified by the attachment of a PEG group via the free cysteine at position 17 has been reported in a patent application (104).

A rational, structure-based approach to optimizing the trade-off between biological activity and pharmacokinetic properties has recently been described for the development of a pegylated form of IFN-β-1a (105). The mutational analysis of IFN-β-1a, described in Sec. 4.2, established that the solvent-exposed N- and C-termini of the protein are both fairly remote from the IFNAR1- and IFNAR2-binding sites and that mutations over a large fraction of the protein's surface in the vicinity of the two termini have no measurable effect on the functional activity of the cytokine in vitro [(48); Figure 5a, b]. Therefore, the N-terminal amine of IFN-β-1a was used as the attachment site for a PEG molecule with the expectation that it would provide maximal scope for attaching a PEG molecule large enough to achieve the desired change in the pharmacokinetic properties of the cytokine without compromising its activity. The selective coupling chemistry that was employed resulted in the formation of IFN-β-1a that was uniformly modified at the N-terminal methionine residue by a single 20-kDa PEG molecule, with no evidence for contamination by unmodified or multiply modified forms of the protein (105). The activity of this material in an antiviral assay was shown to be indistinguishable from that of unmodified IFN-β-1a. Pharmacokinetic studies showed that the systemic clearance rates for this preparation in monkeys, rats, and mice were decreased by ca. 8-, 14- and 13-fold, respectively (105). Thus, by employing a detailed knowledge of the relationship of structure to activity in IFN-β-1a and an appropriately chosen selective coupling chemistry, it was possible to substantially improve the pharmacokinetic properties of the cytokine without deleteriously affecting its activity.

A detailed knowledge of the structure of a protein and its relation to activity has utility in many other types of modifications that are relevant to the development of protein drugs. For example, the design of fusion proteins such as immunoadhesins (106), constructed by fusion of a protein of interest to a second protein to render it multivalent or hetero- or bifunctional or to alter its pharmakokinetics, benefits greatly from detailed structural information. Similarly, structural information can help guide the identification and removal, by mutagenesis, of immunodominant epitopes in the protein, with the goal of reducing the protein's immunogenicity in patients (107–109). Other mutations or chemical modifications can be envisioned, with the goal of enhancing the potency, selectivity, or pharmacokinetics of a protein therapeutic (110,111), of converting an agonist into an antagonist (112), or of generating multivalent forms of a protein for increased avidity (113–115). In all of these cases, detailed structural information facilitates design of the engineered proteins. Many of these approaches are relatively new, and in most cases validation in the clinic has yet to be achieved. Nevertheless, it is clear that progress in these areas is rapid and in some cases has already resulted in new drug approvals (116,117). It is equally clear that a sound and detailed knowledge of structure and its relation to activity will play a prominent part in achieving additional successes in the future.

7 CONCLUSIONS CONCERNING THE ROLE OF STRUCTURAL WORK IN THE DEVELOPMENT OF PROTEIN PHARMACEUTICALS

Although important insights can sometimes be inferred directly from the experimental protein structure itself, more often the value of structural data can only be fully exploited when used in conjunction with other biochemical, biophysical, and molecular and cell biological approaches. The work described in this chapter illustrates some of the ways in which structure determination can be employed, as part of an integrated multidisciplinary approach, to elucidate the biochemical and biological properties of proteins of pharmaceutical interest or to directly aid in the design of protein drugs. A common role of the crystal structure in the studies on IFN-β was to allow a general question to be reformulated as a specific hypothesis and to point the way to how this hypothesis could be definitively tested. For example, detailed information concerning which residues in the IFN-β-1a are exposed to solvent and thus are candidates to come into direct contact with the receptor allowed a specific set of mutant proteins to be designed to experimentally define the regions of the protein that participate in receptor binding. A detailed knowledge of the structure can also help improve experimental design. For example, structural information can help avoid mutations that are likely to result in global disruption of the protein's structure, giving results that might be misinterpreted as local effects on binding or activity. Knowledge of the structure can also help in the interpretation of experimental data, as was the case in interpreting the effects of glycosylation on the biochemical and functional properties of IFN-β-1a. There are other activities that can proceed in the absence of detailed structural information but that knowledge of the structure makes much easier or improves the likelihood of a successful outcome. Into this category falls the IFN-β-1a pegylation work as well as other protein engineering or design activities, such as antibody humanization, fusion protein design, design of other engineered constructs, and other structure–function work aimed at engineering forms of the protein with improved properties. Finally, notwithstanding all of these practical uses of structural information in the design and development of protein drugs, it is important to emphasize the value of working to achieve a thorough, molecular-level understanding of how a protein of interest performs its biological function. Its role in enabling basic investigations of this kind, such as some of those described in this chapter, represents one of the major values delivered by the structural work on IFN-β.

ACKNOWLEDGEMENTS

We thank Paula Hochman, Susan Goelz, Laura Runkel, Joe Rosa, and Blake Pepinsky for their valuable comments on the manuscript.

REFERENCES

1. Weissmann, C., and H. Weber. The interferon genes. Prog Nucleic Acid Res 33: 251–300, 1986.
2. Allen, G., and M.O. Diaz. Nomenclature of the human interferon proteins. J Interferon Cytokine Res 16(2):181–184, 1996.
3. Roberts, R.M., et al. Trophoblast interferons. Placenta 20(4):259–264, 1999.
4. Nardelli, B. IFN-κ, a novel type I interferon. European Cytokine Network 11S:539, 2000.
5. Tyring, S.K. Interferons: biochemistry and mechanisms of action. Am J Obstet Gynecol. 172:1350–1353, 1995.
6. Kagawa, Y., et al. Comparative study of the asparagine-linked sugar chains of natural human interferon-beta 1 and recombinant human interferon-beta 1 produced by three different mammalian cells. J Biol Chem 263(33):17508–17515, 1988.
7. Uze, G., G. Lutfalla, and I. Gresser. Genetic transfer of a functional human interferon α receptor into mouse cells: cloning and expression of its cDNA. Cell 60:225–234, 1990.
8. Novick, D., B. Cohen, and M. Rubinstein. The human interferon α/β receptor: characterization and molecular cloning. Cell 77:391–400, 1994.
9. Bazan, J.F. Structural design and molecular evolution of a cytokine receptor superfamily. Proc Natl Acad Sci USA 87:6934–6938, 1990.
10. Stark, G.R., et al. How cells respond to interferons. Annu Rev Biochem 67:227–264, 1998.
11. Platanias, L.C. and E.N. Fish. Signaling pathways activated by interferons. Exp Hematol 27(11):1583–1592, 1999.
12. Croze, E., et al. The human type I interferon receptor. Identification of the interferon beta–specific receptor-associated phosphoprotein. J Biol Chem 271(52):33165–33168, 1996.
13. Platanias, L.C., et al. Differences in interferon alpha and beta signaling. Interferon beta selectively induces the interaction of the alpha and betaL subunits of the type I interferon receptor. J Biol Chem 271(39):23630–23633, 1996.
14. Domanski, P., et al. Differential use of the betaL subunit of the type I interferon (IFN) receptor determines signaling specificity for IFN alpha2 and IFN beta. J Biol Chem 273(6):3144–3147, 1998.
15. Lu, J., et al. Structure–function study of the extracellular domain of the human IFN-α receptor (hIFNAR1) using blocking monoclonal antibodies: the role of domains 1 and 2. J Immunol 160:1782–1788, 1998.

16. Lewerenz, M., K.E. Mogensen, and G. Uze. Shared receptor components but distinct complexes for α and β interferons. J Mol Biol 1998.

17. Chuntharapai, A., et al. Determination of residues involved in ligand binding and signal transmission in the human IFN-alpha receptor 2. J Immunol 163(2):766–773, 1999.

18. Piehler, J. and G. Schreiber. Mutational and structural analysis of the binding interface between type I interferons and their receptor Ifnar2. J Mol Biol 294(1):223–237, 1999.

19. Russell-Harde, D., et al. Formation of a uniquely stable type I interferon receptor complex by interferon beta is dependent upon particular interactions between interferon beta and its receptor and independent of tyrosine phosphorylation. Biochem Biophys Res Commun 255(2):539–544, 1999.

20. Pellegrini, S., et al. Use of a selectable marker regulated by alpha interferon to obtain mutations in the signaling pathway. Mol Cell Biol 9:4605–4612, 1989.

21. Rosenblum, M.G., et al. Growth inhibitory effects of interferon-beta but not interferon-alpha on human glioma cells: correlation of receptor binding, 2′,5′-oligoadenylate synthetase and protein kinase activity. J Interferon Res 10(2):141–151, 1990.

22. Abramovitch, C., et al. Differential tyrosine phosphorylation of the IFNAR chain of the Type I interferon receptor and of an associated surface protein in response to IFN-α and IFN-β. Embo J 13:5871–5877, 1994.

23. Platanias, L.C., S. Uddin, and O.R. Colamonici. Tyrosine phosphorylation of the α and β subunits of the type I interferon receptor. J Biol Chem 269:17761–17764, 1994.

24. Constantinescu, S.N., et al. Expression and signaling specificity of the IFNAR chain of the type I interferon receptor complex. Proc Natl Acad Sci USA 92(23):10487–10491, 1995.

25. Mogensen, K.E., et al. The type I interferon receptor: structure, function, and evolution of a family business. J Interferon Cytokine Res 19(10):1069–1098, 1999.

26. Derynck, R., et al. Isolation and structure of a human fibroblast interferon gene. Nature 285(5766):542–547, 1980.

27. Jacobs, L.D., et al. Intramuscular interferon beta-1a for disease progression in relapsing multiple sclerosis. The Multiple Sclerosis Collaborative Research Group (MSCRG). Ann Neurol 39(3):285–294, 1996.

28. Interferon beta-1b is effective in relapsing-remitting multiple sclerosis. I. Clinical results of a multicenter, randomized, double-blind, placebo-controlled trial. The IFNB Multiple Sclerosis Study Group. Neurology 43(4):655–661, 1993.

29. Mark, D.F., et al. Site-specific mutagenesis of the human fibroblast interferon gene. Proc Natl Acad Sci USA 81(18):5662–5666, 1984.

30. Runkel, L., et al. Structural and functional differences between glycosylated and nonglycosylated forms of human interferon-beta (IFN-beta). Pharm Res 15(4):641–649, 1998.

31. Interferon beta-1b in the treatment of multiple sclerosis: final outcome of the randomized controlled trial. The IFNB Multiple Sclerosis Study Group and The University of British Columbia MS/MRI Analysis Group. Neurology 45(7):1277–1285, 1995.

32. Neutralizing antibodies during treatment of multiple sclerosis with interferon beta-1b: experience during the first three years. The IFNB Multiple Sclerosis Study Group and the University of British Columbia MS/MRI Analysis Group. Neurology 47(4):889–894, 1996.

33. Kivisakk, P., et al. Neutralizing and binding anti-interferon-beta-I b (IFN-beta-I b) antibodies during IFN-beta-I b treatment of multiple sclerosis. Mult Scler 3(3):184–190, 1997.

34. Kivisakk, P., et al. Neutralizing and binding anti-interferon-beta (IFN-beta) antibodies. A comparison between IFN-beta-1a and IFN-beta-1b treatment in multiple sclerosis. Eur J Neurol 7(1):27–34, 2000.

35. Rudick, R.A., et al. Incidence and significance of neutralizing antibodies to interferon beta-1a in multiple sclerosis. Multiple Sclerosis Collaborative Research Group (MSCRG). Neurology 50(5):1266–1272, 1998.

36. Panitch, H.S. Early treatment trials with interferon-beta in multiple sclerosis. Mult Scler 1(Suppl 1):S17–S21, 1995.

37. Miller, D.L., H.F. Kung, and S. Pestka. Crystallization of recombinant human leukocyte interferon A. Science 215(4533):689–690, 1982.

38. Mitsui, Y., et al. Structural, functional and evolutionary implications of the three- dimensional crystal structure of murine interferon-beta. Pharmacol Ther 58(1):93–132, 1993.

39. Senda, T., S. Saitoh, and Y. Mitsui. Refined crystal structure of recombinant murine interferon-beta at 2.15-Å resolution. J Mol Biol 253(1):187–207, 1995.

40. Radhakrishnan, R., et al. Zinc-mediated dimer of human interferon-alpha 2b revealed by X-ray crystallography. Structure 4(12):1453–1463, 1996.

41. Klaus, W., et al. The three-dimensional high-resolution structure of human interferon alpha-2a determined by heteronuclear NMR spectroscopy in solution. J Mol Biol 274(4):661–675, 1997.

42. Radhakrishnan, R., et al. Crystal structure of ovine interferon-tau at 2.1-Å resolution. J Mol Biol 286(1):151–162, 1999.

43. Karpusas, M., et al. The crystal structure of human interferon beta at 2.2-Å resolution. Proc Natl Acad Sci USA 94(22):11813–11818, 1997.

44. Presnell, S.R., and F.E. Cohen. Topological distribution of four-alpha-helix bundles. Proc Natl Acad Sci USA 86(17):6592–6596, 1989.

45. Sprang, S.R., and J.F. Bazan. Cytokine structural taxonomy and mechanisms of receptor engagement. Curr Opin Struct Biol 3:815–827, 1993.

46. McDonald, N.Q., N. Panayotatos, and W.A. Hendrickson. Crystal structure of dimeric human ciliary neurotrophic factor determined by MAD phasing. Embo J 14(12):2689–2699, 1995.

47. Cunningham, B.C., M.G. Mulkerrin, and J.A. Wells. Dimerization of human growth hormone by zinc. Science 253(5019):545–548, 1991.

48. Runkel, L., et al. Systematic mutational mapping of sites on human interferon-beta-1a that are important for receptor binding and functional activity. Biochemistry 39(10):2538–2551, 2000.

49. Pestka, S., et al. Interferons and their actions. Annu Rev Biochem 56:727–777, 1987.

50. Clackson, T., et al. Structural and functional analysis of the 1:1 growth hormone: receptor complex reveals the molecular basis for receptor affinity. J Mol Biol 277(5):1111–1128, 1998.

51. DeLano, W.L., et al. Convergent solutions to binding at a protein–protein interface. Science 287(5456):1279–1283, 2000.

52. Conradt, H.S., et al. Structure of the carbohydrate moiety of human interferon-beta secreted by a recombinant Chinese hamster ovary cell line. J Biol Chem 262(30):14600–14605, 1987.

53. Wormald, M.R., and R.A. Dwek. Glycoproteins: glycan presentation and protein-fold stability. Structure Fold Des 7(7):R155–R160, 1999.

54. Seto, M.H., et al. Homology model of human interferon-α8 and its receptor complex. Protein Sci 4:655–670, 1995.

55. Uze, G., G. Lutfalla, and K.E. Mogensen. α and β interferons and their receptors and their friends and relations. J. Interferon Cytokine Res 15:3–26, 1995.

56. de Vos, A.M., M. Ultsch, and A.A. Kossiakoff. Human growth hormone and extracellular domain of its receptor: crystal structure of the complex. Science 255(5042):306–312, 1992.

57. Syed, R.S., et al. Efficiency of signalling through cytokine receptors depends critically on receptor orientation. Nature 395(6701):511–516, 1998.

58. Aritomi, M., et al. Atomic structure of the GCSF–receptor complex showing a new cytokine-receptor recognition scheme. Nature 401(6754):713–717, 1999.

59. Walter, M.R., et al. Crystal structure of a complex between interferon-γ and its soluble high-affinity receptor. Nature 376:230–235, 1995.

60. Piehler, J., L.C. Roisman, and G. Schreiber. New structural and functional aspects of the type I interferon–receptor interaction revealed by comprehensive mutational analysis of the binding interface. J Biol Chem 275(51):40425–40433, 2000.

61. Cunningham, B.C., et al. Receptor and antibody epitopes in human growth hormone identified by homolog-scanning mutagenesis. Science 243(4896):1330–1336, 1989.

62. Cohen, B., et al. Ligand-induced association of the type I interferon receptor components. Mol Cell Biol 15:4208–4214, 1995.

63. Cutrone, E.C., and J.A. Langer. Contributions of cloned type I interferon receptor subunits to differential ligand binding. FEBS Lett 404(2–3):197–202, 1997.

64. Lim, J.-K., et al. Intrinsic ligand-binding properties of the human and bovine α-interferon receptors. FEBS Lett 350:281–286, 1994.

65. Goldman, L.A., et al. Characterization of antihuman IFNAR-1 monoclonal antibodies: epitope localization and functional analysis. J Interferon Cytokine Res 19(1):15–26, 1999.

66. Runkel, L., et al. Differences in activity between alpha and beta type I interferons explored by mutational analysis. J Biol Chem 273(14):8003–8008, 1998.

67. Holm, L. and C. Sander. The FSSP database: fold classification based on structure–structure alignment of proteins. Nucleic Acids Res 24(1):206–209, 1996.

68. Piehler, J., and G. Schreiber. Biophysical analysis of the interaction of human ifnar2 expressed in *E. coli* with IFN-alpha2. J Mol Biol 289(1):57–67, 1999.

69. Cleary, C.M., et al. Knockout and reconstitution of a functional human type I interferon receptor complex. J Biol Chem 269:18747–18749, 1994.

70. Muller, U., et al. Functional role of type I and type II interferons in antiviral defense. Science 264(5167):1918–1921, 1994.

71. Hwang, S.Y., et al. A null mutation in the gene encoding a type I interferon receptor component eliminates antiproliferative and antiviral responses to interferons alpha and beta and alters macrophage responses. Proc Natl Acad Sci USA 92(24):11284–11288, 1995.

72. Lutfalla, G., et al. Mutant U5A cells are complemented by an interferon-αβ receptor subunit generated by alternative processing of a new member of a cytokine receptor gene cluster. Embo J 14:5100–5108, 1995.

73. Domanski, P., et al. Cloning and expression of a long form of the β subunit of the interferon αβ receptor that is required for signaling. J Biol Chem 270:21606–21611, 1995.

74. Arduini, R.M., et al. Characterization of a soluble ternary complex formed between human interferon-beta-1a and its receptor chains. Protein Sci 8(9):1867–1877, 1999.

75. Wells, J.A. Structural and functional basis for hormone binding and receptor oligomerization. Curr Opin Cell Biol 6(2):163–173, 1994.

76. Stahl, N., and G.D. Yancopoulos. The alphas, betas, and kinases of cytokine receptor complexes. Cell 74(4):587–590, 1993.

77. Heldin, C.H. Dimerization of cell surface receptors in signal transduction. Cell 80(2):213–223, 1995.

78. Chow, D., et al. Structure of an extracellular gp130 cytokine receptor signaling complex. Science 291(5511):2150–2155, 2001.

79. Gauzzi, M.C., et al. The amino-terminal region of Tyk2 sustains the level of interferon alpha receptor 1, a component of the interferon-alpha/-beta receptor. Proc Natl Acad Sci USA 94(22):11839–11844, 1997.

80. Yeh, T.C., et al. A dual role for the kinase-like domain of the tyrosine kinase Tyk2 in interferon-alpha signaling. Proc Natl Acad Sci USA 97(16):8991–8996, 2000.

81. Hardy, M.P., et al. The soluble murine type I interferon receptor Ifnar-2 is present in serum, is independently regulated, and has both agonistic and antagonistic properties. Blood 97(2):473–482, 2001.

82. Einhorn, S., and H. Strander. Is interferon tissue specific? Effect of human leukocyte and fibroblast interferons on the growth of lymphoblastoid and osteosarcoma cell lines. J Gen Virol 35(3):573–577, 1977.

83. Fish, E.N., K. Banerjee, and N. Stebbing. Human leukocyte interferon subtypes have different antiproliferative and antiviral activities on human cells. Biochem Biophys Res Commun 112(2):537–546, 1983.

84. Hu, R., et al. Evidence for multiple binding sites for several components of human lymphoblastoid interferon-alpha. J Biol Chem 268(17):12591–12595, 1993.

84a. Rani, M.R., Foster, G.R., Leung, S., Leaman, D., Stark, G.R., Ransohoff, R.M. Characterization of beta-R1, a gene that is selectively induced by interferon beta (IFN-beta) compared with IFN-alpha. J Biol Chem. 13;271(37):22878–84, 1996.

84b. Arany, I., Arany, M., Brysk, H., Tyring, S.K., Brysk, M.M. Interferons alpha, beta and gamma induce different patterns of gene expression in cultured human epidermal keratinocytes. In Vivo. 11(2):157–61, 1997.

85. Der, S.D., et al. Identification of genes differentially regulated by interferon-α, -β, or -γ using oliginucleotide arrays. Proc Natl Acad Sci USA 95:15623–15628, 1998.

86. da Silva, A., et al. Comparison of gene expression patterns induced by treatment of human umbilical vein endothelial cells with IFN-α 2b vs. IFN-β1a: understanding the functional relationship between distinct Type 1 interferons that act through a common receptor. J Interferon Cytokine Res 22(2):173–88, 2002.

87. Redlich, P.N., et al. Antibodies that neutralize human beta interferon biologic activity recognize a linear epitope: analysis by synthetic peptide mapping. Proc Natl Acad Sci USA 88(9):4040–4044, 1991.

88. Konrad, M.W., et al. Assessment of the antigenic response in humans to a recombinant mutant interferon-beta. J Clin Immunol 7(5):365–375, 1987.

89. Fierlbeck, G., et al. Neutralizing interferon-beta antibodies in melanoma patients treated with recombinant and natural interferon beta. Cancer Immunol Immunother 39(4):263–268, 1994.

90. Dummer, R., et al. Formation of neutralizing antibodies against natural interferon-beta, but not against recombinant interferon-gamma during adjuvant therapy for high-risk malignant melanoma patients. Cancer 67(9):2300–2304, 1991.

91. Jacobs, L.D., et al. Intramuscular interferon beta-1a therapy initiated during a first demyelinating event in multiple sclerosis. CHAMPS Study Group. N Engl J Med 343(13):898–904, 2000.

92. Perini, P., et al. Interferon-beta (INF-beta) antibodies in interferon-beta1a- and interferon-beta1b-treated multiple sclerosis patients. Prevalence, kinetics, cross-reactivity, and factors enhancing interferon-beta immunogenicity in vivo. European Cytokine Network 12(1):56–61, 2001.

93. Brickelmaier, M., et al. ELISA methods for the analysis of antibody responses induced in multiple sclerosis patients treated with recombinant interferon-beta. J Immunol Methods 227(1–2):121–135, 1999.

94. Runkel, L., et al. Mapping of IFN-β epitopes important for receptor binding and biologic activation: comparison of results achieved using antibody-based methods and alanine substitution mutagenesis. J Interferon Cytokine Res 21(11):931–941, 2001.

95. Delgado, C., G.E. Francis, and D. Fisher. The uses and properties of PEG-linked proteins. Crit Rev Ther Drug Carrier Syst 9(3–4):249–304, 1992.

96. Delgado, C., M. Malmsten, and J.M. Van Alstine. Analytical partitioning of poly(ethylene glycol)-modified proteins. J Chromatogr B Biomed Sci Appl 692(2):263–272, 1997.

97. Francis, G.E., et al. PEGylation of cytokines and other therapeutic proteins and peptides: the importance of biological optimization of coupling techniques. Int J Hematol 68(1):1–18, 1998.

98. Grace, M. et al. Structural and biologic characterization of pegylated recombinant IFN-α2b. J Interferon Cytokine Res 21(12):1103–1115, 2001.

99. Glue, P., et al. Pegylated interferon-alpha2b: pharmacokinetics, pharmacodynamics, safety, and preliminary efficacy data. Hepatitis C Intervention Therapy Group. Clin Pharmacol Ther 68(5):556–567, 2000.

100. Glue, P., et al. A dose-ranging study of pegylated interferon alfa-2b and ribavirin in chronic hepatitis C. The Hepatitis C Intervention Therapy Group. Hepatology 32(3):647–653, 2000.

101. Nieforth, K.A., et al. Use of an indirect pharmacodynamic stimulation model of MX protein induction to compare in vivo activity of interferon alfa-2a and a polyethylene glycol-modified derivative in healthy subjects. Clin Pharmacol Ther 59(6):636–646, 1996.

102. Motzer, R.J., et al. Phase I trial of 40-kd branched pegylated interferon alfa-2a for patients with advanced renal cell carcinoma. J Clin Oncol 19(5):1312–1319, 2001.

103. Monkarsh, S.P., et al. Positional isomers of monopegylated interferon alpha-2a: isolation, characterization, and biological activity. Anal Biochem 247(2):434–440, 1997.

104. El Tayar, N., et al. Polyol-IFN-beta Conjugates. Patent application WO99/55377, 1999.

105. Pepinsky, R.B., et al. Improved pharmacokinetic properties of a pegylated form of interferon-β-1a with preserved in vitro bioactivity. J Pharmacol Exper Therapeutics. 297(3):1059–1066.

106. Ashkenazi, A. and S.M. Chamow. Immunoadhesins as research tools and therapeutic agents. Curr Opin Immunol 9(2):195–200, 1997.

107. Jolliffe, L.K. Humanized antibodies: enhancing therapeutic utility through antibody engineering. Int Rev Immunol 10(2–3):241–250, 1993.

108. Hurle, M.R., and M. Gross. Protein engineering techniques for antibody humanization. Curr Opin Biotechnol, 5(4):428–433, 1993.

109. Sturniolo, T., et al. Generation of tissue-specific and promiscuous HLA ligand databases using DNA microarrays and virtual HLA class II matrices. Nat Biotechnol 17(6):555–561, 1999.

110. Keyt, B.A., et al. A faster-acting and more potent form of tissue plasminogen activator. Proc Natl Acad Sci USA 91(9):3670–3674, 1994.
111. Modi, N.B., et al. Pharmacokinetics of a slower-clearing tissue plasminogen activator variant, TNK-tPA, in patients with acute myocardial infarction. Thromb Haemost 79(1):134–139, 1998.
112. Fuh, G., et al. Rational design of potent antagonists to the human growth hormone receptor. Science 256:1677–1680, 1992.
113. Kipriyanov, S.M., et al. Affinity enhancement of a recombinant antibody: formation of complexes with multiple valency by a single-chain Fv fragment-core streptavidin fusion. Protein Eng 9(2):203–211, 1996.
114. Terskikh, A.V., et al. "Peptabody": a new type of high avidity binding protein. Proc Natl Acad Sci USA 94(5):1663–1668, 1997.
115. Christiansen, D., et al. Octamerization enables soluble CD46 receptor to neutralize measles virus in vitro and in vivo. J Virol 74(10):4672–4678, 2000.
116. Moreland, L.W., et al. Etanercept therapy in rheumatoid arthritis. A randomized, controlled trial. Ann Intern Med 130(6):478–486, 1999.
117. Pislaru, S.V., and F. Van de Werf. TNK-tPA for acute myocardial infarction: the clinical experience. Thromb Haemost 82 Suppl 1:117–120, 1999.

19

G-Protein-Coupled Receptors: Diverse Functions and Shared Mechanisms of Action Interpreted Through the Structure of Rhodopsin

S. Roy Kimura and Daniel I. Chasman
Variagenics, Inc., Cambridge, Massachusetts, U.S.A.

1 INTRODUCTION

The precise response of a cellular physiology to specific agents in the environment is mediated by transduction of signals across the plasma membrane. The specific signals are ligands of a variety of types—small chemical entities, peptides, or proteins—and their presence in the extracellular environment is recognized by their binding to highly specialized receptor proteins embedded in the membrane. Receptors in one superfamily, the G-protein-coupled receptors (GPCRs), respond to a very wide diversity of signaling agents. Through the binding of the signal on the extracellular side of the membrane, GPCRs undergo a conformational change that modifies their interaction with intracellular G-proteins at the membrane and leads to a cascade of additional signaling events within the cell.

Although all GPCRs share a characteristic pattern of seven transmembrane helices, the whole GPCR family is naturally divided into five classes (A–E) on the basis of functional properties and sequence similarity of their members, and exemplified by rhodopsin, calcitonin or secretin receptors, metabotropic receptors, fungal pheromone receptors, and dictyostelium

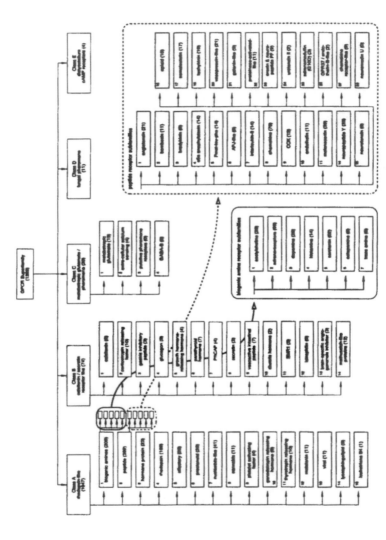

Figure 1 Hierarchical functional classification of GPCRs in the GPCRDB database. In parentheses are the numbers of full (i.e., nonfragment) SwissProt sequences. Boxes on the lower right show the subfamilies of the biogenic-amine (A-1) and peptide (A-2) receptor families. The GPCRDB further subdivides some of these families into finer subclassifications. Not all subclassifications are shown. (Data from Refs. 1 and 2.)

cAMP receptors, respectively (Fig. 1). According to the GPCRDB (Ref. 1, see also http://www.cmbi.kun.nl/7tm), the largest comprehensive online repository of GPCR-related information, 4660 GPCR sequences from 609 different species have been identified and characterized to varying degrees so far. These 4660 sequences include 1283 full-length SwissProt (2) sequences, of which 306 are human, 85 olfactory receptors, and 38 orphan GPCRs.

The rhodopsin class (A) is by far the largest (> 80% of the full-length SwissProt GPCR sequences); in humans it represents perhaps as much as 1–3% of the coding potential of the human genome, or at least 300 genes and encoded proteins (3,4). Families in class A include biogenic amine- (206 sequences) and peptide- (369) receptors and the rhodopsin family (166). In addition to their essential roles in physiology, GPCRs are a major class of pharmaceutical targets, with about half of all drugs today serving either as antagonists or agonists of normal receptor function. Pharmaceutical development efforts continue to recognize the central role of GPCRs by devoting substantial research to discovering the vital physiological functions of new GPCR family members (orphan receptors) identified on the basis of sequence alone by the Human Genome Project (4,5).

The patterns of sequence similarity in the rhodopsin-like class A reflect both the conserved aspects and the diversity of GPCR structure and function. At first hypothesized and later shown, the most conserved part of the sequence corresponds to helical elements of secondary structure—seven in all—that traverse the membrane. The structural transitions accompanying their rearrangement upon receptor activation are also believed to be widely shared among family members. Peptide segments at the amino terminus, at the carboxy terminus, and connecting the helices are much more variable both in length and sequence. These regions form subdomains that provide the ligand-binding specificity on the extracellular side of the membrane and the selection of the correct G-protein α subunit on the intracellular side of the membrane from among a number of basic types, including $G\alpha_i$, $G\alpha_o$, $G\alpha_q$, $G\alpha_{11-16}$, and $G\alpha_t$, themselves constituting a superfamily that includes the Ras oncoprotein (6). The interaction of all GPCRs with the G-protein causes the displacement of GDP by GTP and its ultimate hydrolysis back to GDP. But the subsequent functions of the activated GTP·G-protein complexes are again diverse and can include stimulation of enzymes to generate inositol phosphate or hydrolyze cyclic nucleotides, activation of the JAK2 kinase, activation of protein kinase C (PKC), or many other signaling cascades (6).

Due to the comparative ease of isolating rhodopsin concentrated in disc membranes from retina rod outer segment, rhodopsin is among the best-characterized class A GPCRs, and its biochemical and genetic properties have served as the basis for understanding many shared aspects of the

GPCR mechanism of action. Rhodopsin transduces energy from visible light (498 nM optimum; see Ref. 7) into a cellular response. It is exquisitely sensitive, requiring only a single photon for excitation. It is also selective, remaining stably unactivated in the absence of light for very long periods of time, and uses much of the energy in a photon (about 32 kcal/mole) for activation (8–11). Rhodopsin's ligand, 11-*cis*-retinal, is covalently bound to the protein through a Schiff's base and is converted to the all-trans form by light (12–14). This ligand mediated transition between unactivated and activated forms is found in all GPCRs, and its molecular mechanism involves a rearrangement of their characteristic seven transmembrane helices. Rhodopsin's coupled G-protein, transducin, is a member of the G_t class.

Until very recently, the structural analysis of GPCRs lagged behind biochemical and genetic analysis because of the difficulties in expressing, purifying, and crystallizing membrane proteins. Early models for GPCR structure and activation were based on medium-resolution structures (~3.5 Å) from electron crystallography of bacteriorhodopsin, a seven-transmembrane helix protein from halobacteria that harvests light energy with retinal for transporting hydrogen ions across the membrane (15,16). More recently, models have been derived from a GPCR α-carbon trace inferred from analysis of patterns of GPCR sequence conservation and constraints imposed by the helical density seen in a 9-Å reconstruction of rhodopsin by electron diffraction of 2D crystals (Refs. 17–20; and see http://www.gpcr.org/7tm/models/vriend2/index.html). Among class B receptors, crystal structures of the extracellular amino terminal-ligand binding domains of the metabotropic glutamate receptor from human (21) and the Methuselah receptor from *Drosophilia* (22) revealed the details of ligand-binding interactions. And crystal structures of several representatives of the G-protein superfamily have been solved, including transducin (23), the rhodopsin coupled G-protein, and Ras, one of the first identified members of the family (24).

For rhodopsin, incremental advances from low-resolution electron diffraction of two-dimensional crystals and early attempts at X-ray diffraction of three-dimensional crystals of detergent-solubilized protein have led very recently to an X-ray crystal structure of the unactivated form of rhodopsin at 2.8 Å (25). This landmark study provides the first detailed views of both the transmembrane helices and the G-protein interacting surface that are common to all class A GPCRs. It provides an excellent framework for modeling other class A GPCRs and anticipates the structural transition associated with receptor activation.

Many excellent reviews appeared a few years before and immediately after the publication of the 2.8-Å rhodopsin structure, with the goal of interpreting the body of knowledge about GPCR biochemistry, mutations, and sequence with increasing structural precision (e.g., Refs. 22, 26–29). The new structure has reinvigorated efforts to understand the transition of GPCRs from their unactivated state to their activated state and their inter-actions with G-proteins at the highest level of detail. This chapter will draw on some of the analysis in the recent reviews as well as on our own analysis of class A GPCR sequences and on some of the experiments that reveal the salient features of GPCR function. It hopes to show how the structure of rhodopsin advances our understanding of GPCRs and our ability to spec-ulate about the structural transition that accompanies receptor activation.

2 RHODOPSIN: PURIFICATION, CRYSTALLIZATION, AND STRUCTURAL CHARACTERIZATION

The first structural information for rhodopsin was derived from electron microscopy of two-dimensional crystals grown in reconstituted lipid bilayers or in detergent-extracted rod outer-segment disc membranes. Images of these crystalline specimens confirmed the presence and general arrangement of the seven transmembrane helices inferred from analysis of the amino acid sequence of the first cloned rhodopsin gene and biochemical studies (30,31). In addition, the reconstruction of electron density was good enough to estimate the tilt angles of the rhodopsin transmembrane helices, measured as their deviation from a perpendicular to the membrane. Close scrutiny of sequence conservation and covariant relationships among a large number of rhodopsin-like sequences further corroborated and extended the structural picture for rhodopsin and other members of the class A GPCR family (18,32). Three-dimensional crystallization of rhodopsin was hampered by the usual difficulties with membrane proteins (see Chapter 3, Crystallization of Membrane Proteins).

The situation changed abruptly with the discovery that the combina-tion of neutral detergents (e.g., allylthioglycosides) and divalent cations from the II-B series (e.g., Zn^{2+} and Cd^{2+}) could be used to extract rhodop-sin selectively from a precipitate containing other disc membrane proteins and residual lipid to yield a nearly homogeneous preparation in a single step (33). Handled entirely in the dark or under dimmed light, the soluble rho-dopsin could be induced to form crystals as well. Refinements to the extrac-tion procedure, including the switch to the detergent nonylglyucoside and the inclusion of heptane-1,2,3,-triol during the crystallization, led to crystals grown over a period of a few weeks with an ammonium sulfate precipitant and yielding diffraction first to 3.5 Å (34) and later to atomic resolution, about 2.8 Å (25). After soaking the crystals in mercury acetate for about two months, the crystals were sufficiently derivatized to enable a MAD solution at 3.3 Å using the mercury signal with synchrotron radiation in the wavelength range 0.96–1.04 Å. Thought initially to belong to the $P4_{1or3}22$ space group (34), the crystals instead belong to $P4_1$ but are merohedrally twinned at a fraction of about 0.3 (25). The initial trace for the model was refined against a second data set from a mercury derivative diffracting to 2.8 Å (PDB Id 1F88). This first model contained the helices and some of the loops between the helices but none of the posttranslational modifications or detergent molecules. Additional refinements of the first model implementing improved protocols for addressing the twinning allowed the second and current model, which includes the covalently bound palmitoyl groups and N-acetyl glucosamine carbohydrate as well as some detergent and heptanetriol molecules and slightly lower R factor values than the first model (R_{free} = 0.212, R_{cryst} = 0.175, PDB Id 1HZX) (8).

3 RHODOPSIN STRUCTURE

As anticipated by the biochemical studies, the sequence analysis, and the low-resolution structural models, the structure of rhodopsin is dominated by the seven transmembrane helices, numbered in order of sequence from I to VII (Fig. 2a). The amino terminus precedes helix I on the extracellular (interdisc) side of the membrane, and the carboxy terminus follows helix VII on the cytoplasmic side. Viewed from the extracellular side of the membrane, the helices form a bundle ordered by number in a counterclockwise arrangement. The axes of helices I–III and V are notably tilted away from a perpendicular to the membrane (25°, 25°, 33°, and 26°, respectively) (8). In particular, the tilted disposition of helix III is part of a geometry that allows it to extend across the center of the bundle contacting the other helices and forcing helix IV to the periphery, where it makes extensive contact with lipid, as predicted in earlier models (18,32). The axes of the other helices are near the perpendicular. Within the bundle, bends in all but two of the helices account for the detailed packing; the most significant bends occur in helices II (30°), IV (30°), V (25° and 15°), VI (30°), and VII (24° and 21°). The most tilted helix, III, is relatively free of bends.

The helical bundle is decorated on the extracellular side of the membrane by the amino terminal peptide and loops E-I through E-III between the helices and on the intracellular side by loops C-I through C-III and the carboxy terminal peptide (Fig. 2a). While not entirely resolved in the crystal structure, the loops do reveal some important structural features. A disulfide bridge, which is highly conserved among class A GPCRs, connects the E-II loop to the amino terminal end of helix III. Part of loop E-II also forms a two-stranded antiparallel β-loop that dips into the retinal-binding pocket, and residues (Glu[181], Cys[187], Gly[188], Ile[189], Tyr[191]) on this segment contact the chromophore retinal directly. The amino terminal peptide reaches across the extracellular face of rhodopsin, occluding much of antiparallel β-loop from solvent and burying the retinal more deeply in the core of the receptor. On the cytoplasmic side, the loops present an overall basic surface (25,26), with notable isolated acidic interruptions due to Glu[134] from the end of helix III and Glu[247] from the end of helix VI. The carboxy terminal peptide forms an unanticipated α-helix oriented entirely parallel to the membrane (tilt angle 90°). This helical segment is flanked on its amino terminal end by a few residues connecting it to the end of transmembrane helix VII and on its carboxy terminal end by the dipeptide Cys[322]-Cys[323], which are clearly modified by palmitoyl moieties in the more highly refined structure. The helical segment is amphipathic (8), and this structure is likely formed also in the membrane-bound form of the rhodopsin, where it is suspected of playing a role in the interaction with the G-protein (35,36). It could be kept in place parallel to the membrane by the palmitoyl moieties embedded in the membrane and by hydrophobic interactions between its hydrophobic face (residues Phe[313], Met[317], and Leu[321]) and a complementary hydrophobic environment on rhodopsin. Charged residues (Asn[310], Lys[311], Arg[314], Asn[315]) on the other face of the helix might then be accessible for interactions with the G-protein (see also Sec. 5.4, GPCR Activation and G-Protein Coupling).

The structural transition from unactivated to activated receptor is thought to involve ligand-mediated structural changes that originate in the ligand-binding pocket (Fig. 2b). In the rhodopsin structure, the retinal ligand in rhodopsin is covalently linked to the protein, through a Schiff's base, with Lys[296] from helix VII, which is stabilized by Glu[113] from helix III, as had been deduced previously (12–14). In close contact with the chromophore are residues from helices I, II, III, VI, and VII, including Trp[265] from helix VI, whose indole ring packs against the β-ionone ring of the retinal. In part, the multiplicity of contacts to the ligand is facilitated by the bends in helix VI. Isomerization of retinal by light would be expected to affect the disposition of all five helices directly. The transition to the activated form is likely also to involve polar, ionic, and hydrogen-bonding contacts between the helices and two predominant clusters of interacting residues; both involve helix II. Hydrogen bonds connect helices I, II, and VII through Asn[55] and Asp[83], both conserved among GPCRs, and a backbone carbonyl group from helix VII. Two-thirds of a helical turn away, Asn[78] on helix II is critical to contacts among Ser[127] (helix III), Thr[160] (helix IV), and Trp[161] (Helix VI).

The authors of the rhodopsin structure report also note significant cavities within the seven-transmembrane helical bundle, as expected in the packing of divergent (tilted) and bent helices (8). In the case of rhodopsin, the functional roles of the cavities in the transition from the unactivated to the activated state may involve serving as reservoirs for water in the hydro-

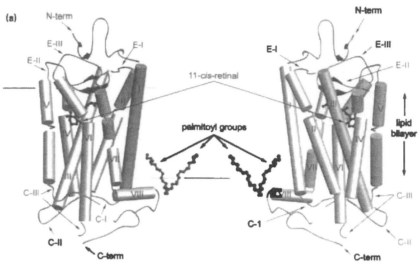

Figure 2 Overview of the crystal structure of bovine rhodopsin (PDB ID 1HZX; Ref. 8). (a) These two views of rhodopsin (left and right) can be related to each other by a 180° rotation around an axis perpindicular to the membrane. For both views, the extracellular (interdisc) and intracellular (intradisc) environments are at the top and the bottom of the image, respectively. The helices (gray cylinders, designation indicated by Roman numerals) are almost entirely embedded within the lipid bilayer, leaving their ends, the loops, and the amino and carboxy termini of rhodopsin exposed to the aqueous environment. The aliphatic tails of palmitoyl groups are expected to be anchored in the membrane. 11-*cis*-Retinal is buried toward the extracellular side of the helical bundle by an antiparallel β-sheet (black ribbon) formed by loop E-II. The cytoplasmic loops and helix VIII on the intracellular of the membrane interact with the G-protein. This figure and all of the other molecular images were made with the program RIBBONS (Ref. 87). (b) The ligand-binding pocket in the helical bundle viewed from the extracellular side of the membrane. Key contacts to the retinal are made by Lys[296] from helix VII, which forms a Schiff's base with the retinal amino group, and Glu[113] from helix III, which forms a salt bridge with the positively charged Schiff's base. The β-sheet of the E-II loop is held in place by a disulfide bond between its conserved Cys[187] and the conserved Cys[110] in helix III. The indole ring of Trp[265] packs against the β-ionone ring of retinal and likely helps transmit the light-induced isomerization of retinal to the helical bundle initiating the large conformational change associated with the activation of rhodopsin. The amino terminal peptide [see (a)], which rests against the extracellular side of the E-II loop, has been omitted for a clearer view of the retinal-binding pocket.

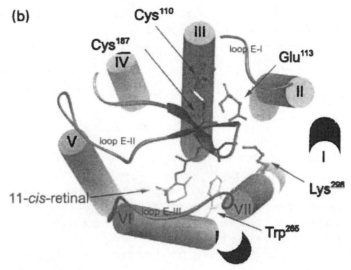

Figure 2 Continued

lysis of the Schiff's base that accompanies retinal isomerization and restoring the 11-*cis*-retinal to the binding pocket once the all-trans form has diffused away and the activated state has decayed. This last function for the cavities may be analogous to their role in ligand binding in other GPCRs, where occupancy of the pocket regulates a dynamic equilibrium between unactivated and activated states.

Some have asked if the existence of the seven-transmembrane-helix bundle reflects a fundamental principle of membrane protein architecture. One suggestion is that seven helices provide a minimum-sized core for functions requiring more specificity than simple membrane protein functions like the selective traffic of ions across the cell membrane (37).

A more concrete issue is whether all of the known seven-transmembrane-helix proteins have a similar arrangements of helices. The comparison of the structure of rhodopsin to the structure of bacteriorhodopsin (PDB Id 1C3W) emphasizes the similarities and differences. The two proteins have essentially no sequence similarity but share the same overall fold and topology. A structural superposition of the two identifies 79 (out of about 350) residues with structurally related Cα atoms, an rms spatial difference of 2.13 Å, and an intermediate z-score in FSSP (38) of 13.5. But the helices of rhodopsin are longer, and their bends cause substantial displacements from some of the bacteriorhodopsin helices in the superposition. In particular, helices II and IV overlap quite poorly; and although the retinal β-ionone rings in the two aligned structures overlap, the Schiff's base attachment sites on helix III are entirely different (8).

4 DIVERSITY OF GPCR FUNCTION AND SEQUENCE

4.1 Overall Sequence Diversity

Despite sharing a common seven-transmembrane-helix bundle architecture and virtually the same signal transduction mechanism, GPCR sequences are highly diverse. This dichotomy may reflect the robust nature of evolutionarily selected protein topologies in general (39), the stable and versatile seven-transmembrane-helix architecture in particular (37), and the large number of specific adaptations that occurred to allow for the variety of signaling modalities exhibited by these proteins (37).

A natural way to characterize the diversity of GPCRs is to compare sequences according the amino acid identity for aligned pairs of sequences both within (intra) and between (inter) family functional classifications (Fig. 3). The broadest functional classes (A, B, C, D) correspond well with the hierarchy derived from sequence similarity analysis. Although this may be a trivial observation of the very design of the classification scheme, it is worth restating that sequences from different classes usually have no detectable similarity, in spite of their similar functional and structural characteristics and a likely common evolutionary origin. Because of this, some authors prefer to use the term *clan* instead of *family* or *superfamily* to describe GPCRs, since *family* usually implies detectable homology among their member sequences, whereas *superfamily* often implies structural or functional similarities without regard to a possible evolutionary relationship.

The rhodopsin family sequences (A-4) are intermediate in their similarity to other class A GPCRs, sharing greater than 20% sequence identity with many other families but less than 20% sequence identity with the prostaglandin (A-6), olfactory (A-5), lysosphyngolipid (A-14), cannabis (A-8), and hormone protein (A-3) receptors. The nearest neighbor to the rhodopsin family (A-4) is the melatonin family (A-12), with an average of 24% sequence identity (ID) (data not shown), although these sequences have very long C-terminal domains unlike the rhodopsins (see Fig. 5). The average similarity between the bovine rhodopsin sequence (SwissProt ID: OPSD_BOVIN) and all sequences within the subfamilies of the biogenic amine- and peptide-receptor families is relatively low (Table 1), ranging from 10% (GPR37/endothelin-like receptors) to 27% (somatostatin receptors). The distant relationship of GPCRs to bacteriorhodopsins (BRs) that is suggested by the rhodopsin structure is clear from this analysis as well.

As expected, sequences within the same family are quite similar to each other, with the majority of the pairwise IDs exceeding 30% identity (Fig. 3, right). Exceptions are the class A orphans and viral GPCR sequences (A-13), both of which are expected to contain a diverse set of sequences, by definition. Several families contain highly similar sequences, such as the thyrotropin-releasing hormone (A-11), gonadotropin-releasing hormone (A-10), pituitary adenylate cyclase–activating peptide (PACAP) (B-7), lysosphingolipid (A-14), and GABA (C-4) receptors, each containing sequence pairs greater than 95% identity; these are likely to be pairs of the same functional proteins in closely related species or from fine subtype classifications. The rhodopsin (A-4) family spans a fairly wide range of identity, from 25% to 65%. These similarity distributions, however, should be interpreted with caution, for they may largely be influenced by the nonuniform representation of receptor subtypes and species, especially for the families with a small number of sequences.

4.2 Other Systematic GPCR Classifications

The functional assignments and categorization of sequences in the GPCRDB are based mainly on the SwissProt database (2), whose annotations are extracted from published studies, usually involving the isolation and characterization of specific gene sequences through biochemical as well as computational techniques. Many other specialized biological databases also exist that can provide useful resources for the characterization and annotation of GPCRs. For example, some databases either directly or indirectly cluster GPCRs into families or groups based on conserved features occurring in multiple alignments, such as recurrent motifs, regular expressions, homologous domains, or groups of sequence signatures. These databases include Pfam (40), PROSITE (41), PRINTS (42), and E-motif (43). Hypertext links between sequences in these databases may be useful for uncovering previously unnoticed GPCR functions or involvement in alternative biochemical pathways.

The Pfam database (40) identifies six families of GPCRs, 7tm_1 through 7tm_6, from a total of 4569 SwissProt and TrEMBL sequences. The first three of the Pfam families appear to correspond directly to classes A, B, and C of the GPCRDB and contain 3561, 233, and 138 sequences, respectively. 7tm_4 and 7tm_5 are two distinct families of nematode chemoreceptors containing a total of 574 sequences. Sequences in 7tm_6 form a family of 63 putative odorant receptor sequences from *Drosophila*. Pfam families are clustered according to conserved domains identified by specific hidden Markov models (HMMs) trained on hand-adjusted seed alignments constructed for each family. These specific HMMs are highly sensitive for

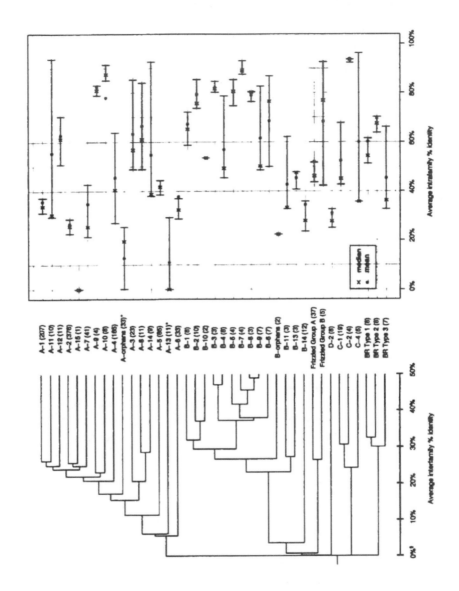

Figure 3 Average sequence similarities between and within GPCRDB families. (*left*): Hierarchical clustering of sequence families constructed from the average percent amino acid identities of all sequence pairs from different GPCRDB families aligned using BLAST (Ref. 88). Families are numbered according to Figure 1. In parentheses are the number of full-length SwissProt sequences in each family used in the calculation. 0% identity (§) indicates that there were no significant BLAST hits between any of the sequences in the two involved families, with a BLAST E-value threshold of 1×10^{-3}. Families whose members had no significant BLAST hits with those in all other families are not shown. (*right*): Distribution of intrafamily sequence similarity. The mean and median of the percent IDs for all pairs of sequences within each family are shown. The bars indicate the first-to-third-quartile range of the all-pair comparison, except for the sequences marked with astersisks, for which the ranges shown are $+/-$ one standard deviation from the mean (lower limit truncated at 0); for these families, a large number of nonhomologous (0% ID) pairs resulted in meaningless (0) quartiles.

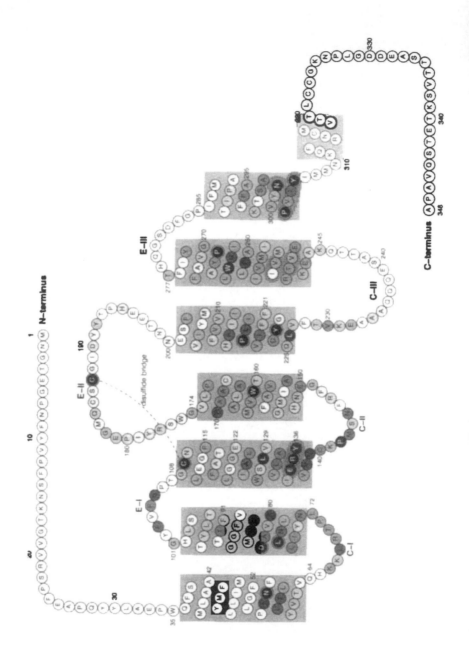

Figure 4 Conservation of residue positions in the Pfam (Ref. 40) 7tm_1 alignment (class A GPCRs) mapped onto the bovine rhodopsin sequence. Darker shades indicate more conservation. Doubly circled residues are those that showed greater than 70% conservation in the equivalent position of the 7tm_1 alignment. Horizontal hashes indicate regions of well-known GPCR sequence motifs. The vertically hashed region shows residues near the D/ERY motif in the structure that may be involved in the interaction with the G-protein. Much of the N- and C-terminal portions are left blank, since Pfam alignments usually do not contain these variable regions.

Table 1 Average* Percent Amino Acid Identity Between Bovine Rhodopsin and All Full SwissProt Sequences in the Biogenic Name (A-1) and Peptide Receptor (A-2) Subfamilies

Class-family-subfamily	Subfamily name	% Id with rhodopsin
A-1-1	Acetylcholine (muscarinic)	24.7
A-1-2	Adrenoceptors	22.6
A-1-3	Dopamine	23.2
A-1-4	Histamine	22.3
A-1-5	Serotonin	21.6
A-1-6	Octopamine	24.0
A-2-1	Angiotensin	22.1
A-2-2	Bombesin	22.1
A-2-3	Bradykinin	23.9
A-2-4	C5Anaphylatoxin	25.9
A-2-5	fmet-leu-phe	22.9
A-2-6	APJ-like	22.8
A-2-7	Interleukin-8	24.4
A-2-8	Chemokine	22.7
A-2-9	CCK	26.6
A-2-10	Endothelin	21.7
A-2-11	Melanocortin	13.2
A-2-14	Neuropeptide Y	23.4
A-2-15	Neurotensin	23.0
A-2-16	Opioid	23.7
A-2-17	Somatostatin	27.2
A-2-18	Tachykinin	24.9
A-2-20	Vasopressin-like	20.5
A-2-21	Galanin-like	23.4
A-2-22	Proteinase-activated-like	21.8
A-2-23	Orexin/neuropeptideFF	18.6
A-2-24	UrotensinII	20.4
A-2-25	Adrenomedullin(G10D)	21.4
A-2-26	GPR37/endothelinB-like	9.5
A-2-27	Chemokinereceptor-like	20.2

*Averages were calculated from BLAST alignments of all pairs of sequences included in the SwissProt (Ref. 2) GPCR list (http://www.expasy.org/cgi-bin/lists?7tmrlist.txt).

detecting remote homology and are thus well suited for clustering of widely divergent protein families such as GPCRs.

Rather than classifying sequences through global similarity, the E-motif (43) and PROSITE (41) patterns databases collect short sequence motifs that frequently occur in blocks of aligned sequence constructed from large numbers of distantly related sequences. Such short motifs that occur in GPCRs can be used to identify functionally or structurally significant "micro-domains" that are often the signatures of different classes or families. The PRINTS (42) database further clusters sequences according to combinations of recurrent short motifs appearing within each individual sequence. By identifying groups of sequences that share specific combinations of motifs ("fingerprints"), the database not only identifies the broadest GPCR classes, but also distinguishes finer hierarchical subtypes, depending on how many and which motifs are shared among sequences (44). Knowledge of these subtle differences is critical for the development of drugs specifically targeted to a single receptor subtype, for example, to reduce the possibility of cross-reactivity.

Recently, a new method for automated GPCR classification, based on a learning algorithm, has been described (45). The method uses support vector machines (SVMs), a classification algorithm that was originally developed by Vapnik (46) and is now gaining popularity due to its demonstrated low misclassification rate. Although the method is relatively computationally expensive compared to traditional methods for biological sequence comparison, its superior performance has been demonstrated in a twofold cross-validation experiment involving classification of subfamily memberships for class A and class C GPCRs: low error rates (13.7% errors per sequence compared to 25.5% for a BLAST-based nearest-neighbor method) and improved receiver operating characteristics (i.e., high number of true positives in the group of test sequences containing the first false-positive classification).

With the availability of genome-wide sequence information, GPCR deorphaning is thus now receiving widespread attention from the pharmaceutical industry as a key strategy in a "reverse pharmacology" approach to drug discovery (47). Here, the identification of cognate ligands and corresponding drug candidates for large numbers of GPCRs is attempted even before the biological principles of the possibly associated disease states are thoroughly known. All of the resources cited earlier for classifications of receptors with known function may also play an important role in the identification of endogenous ligands for the large number of human orphan GPCRs, some of which may be potential drug targets (47).

4.3 General Sequence Conservation Among GPCRs

The large number of sequences in class A GPCRs provides an opportunity to infer functional significance for residues based on their level of evolutionary conservation (Fig. 4). Most of the highly conserved residues map to positions within the helical domains of bovine rhodopsin, with some exceptions, including Cys^{187} in the E-II loop, which forms a disulfide bridge with Cys^{110} of Helix III. The locations of these highly conserved residues also appear to be biased toward the cytosolic ends of the helices, especially in helices I, II, III, IV, and VII. Some of these conserved positions lie within well-known motifs in class A GPCRs, such as the D/ERY motif (positions 134 to 136 in bovine rhodopsin; see Sec. 5.3.4 for details) and NPXXY motif (positions 302–306), whose function is not well understood. Almost all of the other highly conserved positions are known to play significant functional or structural roles common to most GPCRs, including involvement in inter-helical contacts required for structural stability and the activation of signal transduction mechanisms. A detailed structural interpretation of these con-served sites is described in Sec. 5.3.

Among the cytoplasmic loops, C-III appears to be relatively more variable in sequence than the others. This observation is consistent with evidence suggesting that residues in this loop may be responsible for Gα-subunit specificity (48). On the extracellular side, loops E-II and E-III appear to have more residue diversity than E-I, with the exception of the aforementioned Cys^{187} of E-II.

The length distributions among the loops of sequences in class A families also suggest functional constraints (Fig. 5). As with the residue conservation patterns, the C-III and E-II loops show the most variability, apart from the N- and C-terminal domains. E-I, E-III, and C-I loops, on the other hand, show relatively tight and shorter length distributions, suggesting that these loops perform functions conserved throughout class A. The C- and N-terminal domains both have wide length distributions. They are less likely to affect the arrangement and flexibility of the transmembrane helices responsible for the shared signal transduction mechanism of GPCRs. The N-terminal length diversity is also consistent with evidence suggesting its involvement in the ligand recognition and binding processes for some GPCR families (37).

4.4 Correlated Positions: Functional Specificity

A few authors have demonstrated the utility of correlation analysis (corre-lated mutational analysis, CMA) applied to positions in GPCR sequences (49–51). In its most basic form, the degree of correlation between two col-umns in a multiple alignment (i.e., two residue positions) is calculated using correlation formulas for discrete functions. The hope is that a high degree of correlation will indicate some functional relationship between the two posi-tions, the most likely one being spatial proximity or contact (50).

A useful extension of this approach is to calculate the correlation between each residue position in an alignment and a "pseudo-residue" consisting of a column of letters representing different functional characteristics of each aligned sequence (51). For example, Horn et al. (52) have shown that residue positions that are highly correlated with a pseudo-residue representing Gα-subunit specificity correspond well with experimentally verified specificity determining residues. In another study (51) correlation analysis was applied to the identification of residues important for the spectral tuning of retinal in opsins and residues that are responsible for the specificity of ligand binding in biogenic amine receptors.

Applying CMA to a class A GPCR alignment (GPCRDB, 1047 SwissProt sequences) with pseudo-residues reflecting each receptors' family classification reveals some functionally important positions (Fig. 6). When mapped to the structure of rhodopsin, the residues most highly correlated with family function (Fig. 6, darker shades of gray) correspond surprisingly well to residues that are in close proximity to the retinal molecule in rhodopsin (Fig. 6, doubly circled residues). In the class A GPCRs, these residue positions likely interact with a wide variety of ligands and possibly contribute to binding specificity.

5 THE RHODOPSIN STRUCTURE AS A MODEL FOR UNDERSTANDING GPCR FUNCTION

5.1 Introduction

The crystal structure of rhodopsin provides an opportunity to reinterpret the sequence and biochemical analysis of GPCRs toward a structural explanation of their functional properties. The basic approach involves mapping the sequence of a GPCR onto the rhodopsin structure through the residue correspondence established by a sequence alignment and then examining the structural context of important residues. The models can illuminate the functional roles of residues conserved in sequence throughout the class A GPCR family, e.g., the activation process or the interaction with G-protein. When further refined by molecular modeling techniques (53), they can allow interpretation of subfamily-specific properties, e.g., ligand binding.

5.2 Structural Similarity Among GPCRs

Although the class A GPCRs are defined by sequence homology, many of the member sequences are only remotely related to rhodopsin (e.g., having undetectable sequence similarity or as little as 16.7% minimum detectable amino acid identity for the case of the mouse adrenocorticoid receptor) and might be expected to share only some of rhodopsin's structural features. One experimental approach for understanding the degree of structural conservation among the class A receptors involves mutating residues

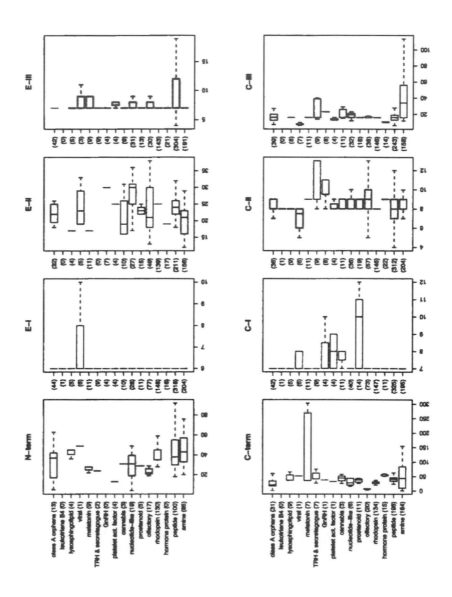

Figure 5 Distribution of loop lengths among sequences in each class A GPCR family. Shown are box plots in which each box indicates the range of the central two quartiles for the distribution of loop lengths in each family. The line in the box indicates the median length. Whiskers around each box indicate the most extreme data point that is within 1.5 times the box width. Loop lengths were computed by mapping the loop boundaries of bovine rhodopsin to all class A SwissProt sequences using BLAST. In parentheses are the number of sequences analyzed for each case. These vary from loop to loop, due to the occasional lack of a correspondence between boundary positions in bovine rhodopsin and each subject sequence.

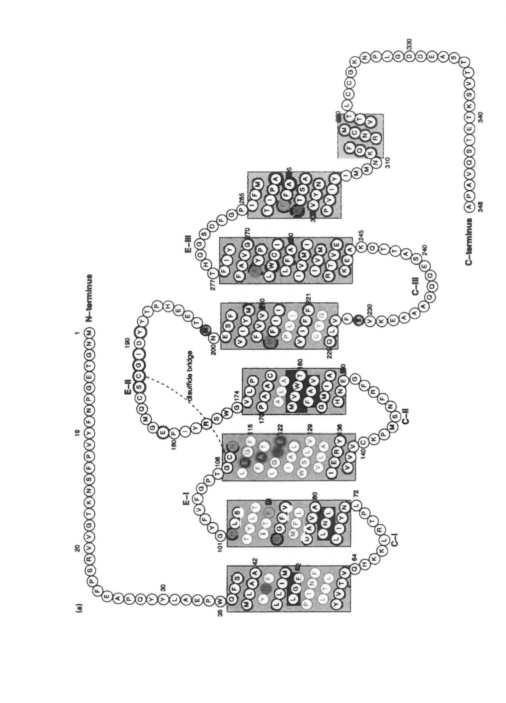

(b)

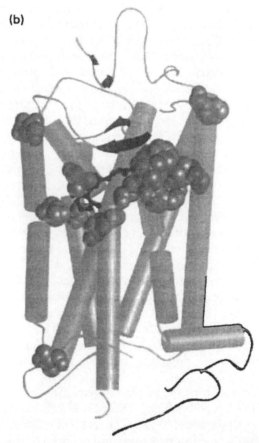

Figure 6 Correlation of residues with the different class A families based on Pfam 7tm_1 alignment (class A GPCRs) mapped onto bovine rhodopsin. (a) Correlated positions mapped onto a helical net representation of the rhodopsin sequence. Darker shades indicate higher correlation with the class A family classification. Doubly circled residues are within 5 Å of the retinal molecule in the rhodopsin binding site. (b) Structural disposition of correlated residues. The darkened residues in (a) are located in the bovine rhodopsin structure oriented as in Figure 2a, left. All but three of the most correlated residues line the ligand-binding pocket, and most make direct contact to 11-*cis*-retinal (black ball-and-stick representation). One of the remaining correlated residues is on the cytosolic end of helix V, at the boundary with loop C-III, and may be involved in an interaction with G-protein. The other two are at the boundary between extracellular ends of helices II and V and the loops.

in the seven-transmembrane helices to cysteine and determining the accessibility of the introduced thiols to solvent by their reactivity with charged and therefore lipid-insoluble sulfhydryl reagents. The method, called the *substituted-cysteine accessibility method*, or SCAM, distinguishes between cysteine substituted at residues that are accessible to the extracellular solvent, which will be derivatized, and those packed within the protein or at the interface with lipid, which will not (28). Applied to the dopamine D_2 receptor sharing 26% amino acid identity with rhodopsin within the transmembrane helical segments and less overall, the method shows a very high degree of correspondence with solvent-accessible surface area (SASA) computed from the rhodopsin structure. The SCAM approach suggests that the helices of the dopamine D_2 receptor are between a half and one turn more extensive than suggested by the SASA of corresponding residues in the rhodopsin structure, but the results could equally reflect a high degree of mobility of the helix terminal residues in solution or an increased accessibility of residues juxtaposed with the charged lipid head group than the aliphatic lipid tails. The greatest disparity in the comparison occurs in helix IV, where three residues, Tyr^{192}, Ile^{195}, and Val^{196}, are predicted from rhodopsin to be packed against the helical bundle in dopamine D_2 receptor but are instead exposed to solvent. These residues may be extremely flexible, or they may adopt a different conformation from the corresponding residues in rhodopsin, facing away from the helical bundle in the dopamine D_2 receptor to interact with other proteins in the membrane, possibly including other dopamine receptor molecules, to form a dimer (28,54).

A high degree of correspondence between the retinal-binding pocket of rhodopsin and the ligand-binding pockets of GPCRs can be inferred as well. In the SCAM analysis, about 79% of the residues inferred to contact ligand in the dopamine D_2 receptor correspond to residues in the rhodopsin structure that are inaccessible to solvent (< 10% SASA) in the presence of the retinal. From the perspective of sequence analysis, nearly all of the residues that show the greatest correlation with receptor family correspond with retinal-contacting residues in rhodopsin (Fig. 6a; see also Ref. 51) Remarkably, these covarying residues include the Lys^{296} that forms the highly specific Schiff's base with retinal in rhodopsin and its ion pair, Glu^{113} (Figs. 2 and 6).

The crystal structure also confirms the mutational analysis that has been used to probe rhodopsin and other GPCR helix–helix interactions in solution. These experimental approaches are diverse and include: examining the formation of disulfide or Zn^{2+} bridges between pairs of introduced cysteine or histidine residues, measuring distances between residues by attaching spin labels to introduced cysteine residues, and introducing second-site mutations that restore function to primary mutations (see Ref. 28 for a summary). Summarizing for rhodopsin, these studies infer close contact between residue helices VII and I-III, III and V-VI, and V and VI, all of which are observed in the rhodopsin structure. For other GPCRs, second-site reverting mutations in the gonadotropin-releasing hormone receptor (GRHR, releasing hormone subfamily, 19.5% identity with rhodopsin) the serotonin receptor (5H2A, serotonin receptor subfamily, 20.8% identity), and the muscarinic M2 (ACM2, acetylcholine (muscarinic) subfamily, 26.4% identity) suggest interactions between helices I and VII, II and VII, and II and VII, respectively, all observed for corresponding residues in the rhodopsin structure. Disulfide bridge formation between introduced cysteine residues in the muscarinic M2 and M3 receptors is consistent with the proximity of helices III and VI in the rhodopsin structure. Zn^{2+} bridges between residues mutated to histidine or cysteine in the substance K receptor (NK1R, tachykinin receptor subfamily, 24.2% identity), the muscarinic M1 receptor (ACM1, acetylcholine (muscarinic) subfamily, 25.9% identity), and the β_2 adrenergic receptor (B2AR, adrenergic receptor subfamily, 21.4% identity) all validate the interpretation of the rhodopsin structure as a model for these GPCRs. One Zn^{2+} bridge between helices III and VII in the β_2 adrenergic receptor would be expected to span a distance (15.5 Å) measured between corresponding residues in the rhodopsin structure that exceeds the maximum reach of this type of cross-link (14.0 Å). Instead of implying a structural discrepancy with rhodopsin, this cross-link is found only in the ligand-activated form of the receptor, consistent with the anticipated structural rearrangement. Another Zn^{2+}-bridging cross-link between helices was engineered successfully in the parathyroid hormone receptor, a secretin-like class B GPCR, on the basis of its extremely remote homology to rhodopsin, suggesting that many of the structural features identified in rhodopsin exist in the distantly related class B GPCRs (55).

5.3 Residues Conserved Among Class-A GPCRs

It has long been recognized that some residues in the rhodopsin-like GPCRs are almost completely conserved; their function in rhodopsin would be expected to be representative of the whole class. At the very least, roles in ligand binding, stabilization of the unactivated form of the receptor, the transition to and stabilization of the activated form of the receptor, and the interactions with G-protein might all be attributed to these residues by examination for their disposition in rhodopsin. Following are the relevant observations for these most conserved residues (Table 2).

Table 2   Most Conserved Residues Among Class A
GPCRs

Amino acid	Position in rhodopsin	Conservation[a]
Asn	55	1.00
Leu	79	0.98
Asp	83	0.93
Cys	110	0.92
Arg	135	1.00
Trp	161	0.98
Cys	187	0.91[b]
Pro	215	0.91
Pro	267	0.99
Asn	302	0.85
Pro	303	0.98
Tyr	306	0.93

[a]Conservation is calculated as the fraction of sequences
containing the most prevalent amino acid at the expected
position in the GPCRDB alignment of helical regions from class
A GPCR sequences in SwissProt.
[b]Cys[187] is in the E-II loop and therefore not represented in the
GPCRDB alignment. Instead, conservation for this residue is
calculated as the fraction of sequences containing the E-II loop
cysteine in the Pfam alignment of class A GPCR sequences
with the TrEMBL sequences removed.

5.3.1   Disulfide Bridge Between Conserved Cysteine Residues in Helix III and Extracellular Loop II

A cysteine residue (position 110 in rhodopsin) one turn from the amino
terminal (extracellular) end of helix III forms a disulfide bond with a
cysteine residue (position 187 in rhodopsin), the E-II loop of the class A
GPCRs (see Fig. 5 for a summary of the loops). In rhodopsin, this second
cysteine is located a few amino acids toward the carboxy terminus from the
β-hairpin structure (Fig. 2b) that covers the retinal chromophore on the
extracellular face of the molecule, and it anchors the second strand of the
hairpin within van der Waals contact of the retinal. The E-II loop is one of
the most variable in length among class A GPCRs (Fig. 5), presumably
reflecting different modes of access and specificity of the ligand-binding
pocket. In spite of this variation, the disulfide bridge is believed to be present
throughout class A and may serve roles in regulating access to the ligand-
binding pocket, sensing the occupancy of the pocket, transmitting the occupancy to the transmembrane helices, or coordinating a change in accessi-

bility to the pocket associated with the structural transition between the unactivated and activated forms of the receptor.

5.3.2 Conserved Residues in the Helices

In contrast to the residues correlated with receptor family that line the ligand-binding pocket on the extracellular side of GPCRs, many of the residues that are conserved within class A map toward the cytoplasmic side of the GPCR helices (Fig. 7 inset). Some of the residues are involved in helix–helix contacts and must be critical for the reversible transitions between the receptors' unactivated and activated forms (Fig. 7). The contacts between helices I and VII involve an absolutely conserved asparagine residue (Asn[55] in rhodopsin) that forms a hydrogen bond with a carbonyl oxygen (residue Ala[299] in rhodopsin). Slightly less conserved, an aspartate residue in helix II (Asp[83] in rhodopsin) is poised to make a second hydrogen bond to the same carbonyl on helix VII as the conserved asparagine. This aspartic acid is the only potentially charged residue in the core of rhodopsin that is not paired with an amino acid of opposite charge, although in the

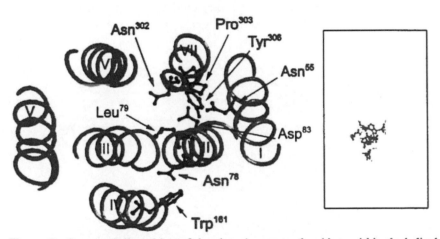

Figure 7 Structural disposition of the class A conserved residues within the helical bundle of rhodospin. The view in the main part of the figure is from the cytoplasmic side of the membrane, with the helices designated by Roman numerals. Residues Asn[55] and Asp[83] form hydrogen bonds with a carbonyl on Ala[299] in helix VII. Asn[78] is not conserved but forms a hydrogen bond with Trp[161]. None of the other residues make particularly conserved contacts in this unactivated form of rhodopsin. The most striking feature of the conserved residues within the helical bundle is that they are clustered together toward the cytoplasmic side of the structure, as shown in the inset (same view as Fig. 2a, right).

unactivated receptor it is likely protonated to serve as a hydrogen bond donor to the carbonyl of Ala[299] (25). It may become solvent accessible and perform other functions in the activated form of the receptor. These two residues appear to be stabilizing helical contacts in the unactivated form of the receptor.

Nearby in the helical bundle, forming a group together with Asn[55] and Asp[83], a cluster of two conserved residues and a conserved motif makes an assortment of contacts in the unactivated rhodopsin structure that do not fully justify their functional importance inferred from their conservation (Fig. 8). A highly conserved leucine in helix II (Leu[79] in rhodopsin) is just over one turn away from the conserved Asp[83]. Its side chain points toward helices III and VII but does not make highly specific contacts, except perhaps a van der Waals interaction between its Cγ and the Cγ of an asparagine (Asn[302] in rhodopsin) that is part of the conserved NPXXY motif (residues 302–306 in rhodopsin). In spite of its own conservation across class A GPCRs, NPXXY motif makes no other conserved contacts. One residue away from the conserved leucine, an asparagine residue (Asn[78] in rhodopsin) forms a hydrogen bond with a conserved tryptophan (Trp[161] in rhodopsin), but the asparagine is not especially conserved among GPCRs. In other respects, the tryptophan also does not make specific contacts: One face of the ring is positioned to interact only with lipid in the membrane at the

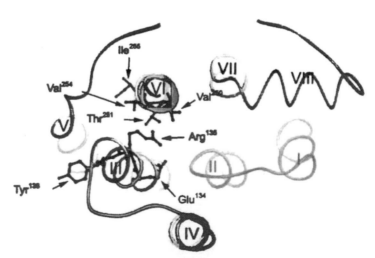

Figure 8 Structural disposition of the ERY motif in rhodopsin and its proximity to residues in helix VI that are important in the interaction of some class A GPCRs with the G-protein. The view is from the cytoplasm. The indicated residues are within a turn or two of the cytoplasmic ends of helices III and VI.

interface with the receptor. It is tempting to speculate that these two conserved residues and the conserved motif engage in conserved interhelical interactions in the activated state of the receptor, possibly with each other or with other conserved residues in the GPCR. Alternatively, they may engage in a conserved dynamic behavior during the activation of the receptor, with functional constraints reflected in their extreme conservation.

5.3.3 Proline Residues in the Helices

One of the structural features of the helices identified by the crystal structure is their disruption by bends. These distortions play important roles in the packing of the helices (8,25) and are likely involved in receptor activation, as are some helical distortions in other membrane proteins (56). The sources of the bends are varied but involve both proline and glycine residues. Two of the proline residues are among the most conserved in class A GPCRs (Table 2). The proline (Pro^{267} in rhodopsin) in helix VI is extremely conserved, and it accounts for the largest helical bend (36°) in the whole structure (8). In the yeast α-factor pheromone GPCR, mutation of this conserved proline to leucine caused constitutive receptor activation (8,57). A proline (Pro^{215} in rhodopsin) residue in helix V is nearly as conserved. Helix V has two bends (25° and 15°), but the conserved proline does not appear to be responsible for either. Instead, they can be attributed to much less conserved residues (Phe^{203} and His^{211} in rhodopsin), and the conserved proline is part of a stretch of regular helical geometry roughly one turn away from the smaller bend, i.e., the 15° one. Like the conserved residues elsewhere in the helical bundle that do not make conserved contacts, this proline may be involved in the activation of the receptor, possibly by seeding a bend in helix V in the activated state of rhodopsin and the other class A GPCRs.

5.3.4 The D/ERY Motif

Near the carboxy terminus of helix III at the interface with the cytoplasm, the amino acid triplet ERY in rhodopsin is part of a highly conserved motif with the sequence apartate or glutamate–arginine–tyrosine (D/ERY), the arginine of which is found in 99.7% of the known full-length GPCRs in SwissProt (2) (Table 2). The motif almost surely participates in the activation of rhodopsin, since mutation of the arginine causes the transition to the activated metarhodopsin II form but eliminates its ability to activate rhodopsin's G-protein, transducin. In the rhodopsin structure, the motif resides in a very hydrophobic environment formed by residues from helices III (Val^{133}, Val^{137}, Val^{138}, Val^{139}), V (Leu^{226}), and VI (Val^{250}) and cytoplasmic loops C-I (Pro^{71}) and C-II (Pro^{142}, Phe^{148}) (8). The guanidinium group of the arginine in the structure forms a salt bridge with the glutamate.

Moreover, the triplet of residues have some of the highest B-factors in the entire structure, hinting at a potential dynamic role in the transition between unactivated and activated forms of rhodopsin (25). This interaction may be more critical for regulation than for activation, since some substitutions at the equivalent aspartate in the α_{1B} adrenergic receptor lead to constitutive activation of the receptor. Nevertheless, protonation of the glutamate and the corresponding aspartate is observed in rhodopsin and in the α_{1B} adrenergic receptor, respectively, upon activation, and the arginine becomes solvent exposed (58–60). In a model of the serotonin 2A receptor based on the rhodopsin structure, the arginine is poised to form a salt bridge with a glutamate (Glu^{318}) on helix VI. Mutation of this glutamate to alanine also causes constitutive activation of the receptor (61). In the class A GPCRs, the structural transition associated with activation seems likely to unmask the arginine and allow an activating interaction with residues on the surface of the G-protein.

5.4 GPCR Activation and G-Protein Coupling

One could hope that inspection of the rhodopsin and transducin structures (25,26,56) would reveal surfaces that are sufficiently complementary to explain their mode of interaction. This hope is partly fulfilled. The cytoplasmic surface of rhodopsin is largely basic, while the surface of transducin thought to interact with rhodopsin is largely acidic. To some degree, acidic patches punctuating the basic surface on rhodopsin can be structurally aligned with basic patches on the transducin surface. A cleft between the α-subunit of transducin and the $\beta\gamma$ subunits can crudely accommodate ridges on the cytoplasmic surface of rhodopsin. But there are serious discrepancies in addition to the overall imprecise nature of the complementarity. For example, the critical arginine in the E/DRY motif at the end of helix III is not solvent accessible in the rhodopsin structure, and some of the mutational data are inconsistent with a simple docking model for activation and formation of the complex with the G-protein. At least part of the discrepancy can be resolved by invoking the conformational changes accompanying rhodopsin activation.

Much of our understanding of the structural transitions that characterize receptor activation comes from chemical probes introduced into residues in rhodopsin and other receptors (55,62–68). Measuring distances between spin labels introduced through cysteine-substituted residues at a single reference position near the cytoplasmic end of helix III and a series of consecutive test positions at the cytoplasmic end of helix VI, Farrens et al. inferred that rhodopsin activation involves a compound motion of helix VI. When viewed from the cytoplasm, this structural change can be described as a rigid body motion of helix VI away from the helical bundle together with a clockwise rotation (32,53,62,64,69). Consistent with this picture, disulfide cross-links between the same pairs of cysteine residues in helices III and VI that were used for the spin labeling inhibit activation, and a wealth of mutations in other GPCRs at the predicted interface between helices III and VI affect the activation process (Refs. 62,64, and, for example, 28 and 61). The activation model has been supported by additional spin-labeling experiments (see Refs. 70–73) and suggests an "opening" of the helical bundle on the cytoplasmic face, causing increased solvent accessibility of residues near the center of the bundle. The transformation initiated by the isomerization of retinal may be propagated through direct contacts with Trp^{265} in helix VI, a position that is in contact with ligand both in rhodopsin and in many other receptors (see earlier). Consistent with this mechanism involving large conformational changes, the ring of a photoreactive derivative of retinal forms cross-links to Trp^{265} in the unactivated rhodopsin but to Ala^{169} in helix IV in the activated state (74). Measured on the unactivated rhodopsin structure, the cross-linking sites are 14 Å apart.

Once activated, the GPCR can bind a trimeric G-protein and stimulate the exchange of GDP for GTP, but the details of this interaction on the GPCR side have been only partly resolved. Inspection of GPCR sequences for candidate conserved residues interacting with the G-protein reveals little except the D/ERY motif and a concentration of basic residues in the C-II and C-III loops. Horn et al. used CMA to find (see Sec. 4.4) weak correspondence of sequence and G-protein specificity that included residues predominantly in the C-II and C-III loops as well as scattered throughout helices I–IV and VI (49). Biochemical and mutational studies have focused on the C-II and C-III loops (48) and for the case of rhodopsin have suggested separate interactions responsible for binding the G-protein transducin and stimulating the guanine nucleotide exchange.

Biochemical and mutational analyses suggest that the GPCR interaction with G-protein is multivalent. Mutant rhodopsin molecules with a substitution for loop C-II residues 140–152 or a deletion of loop C-III residues 237–249 were capable of binding transducin but not affecting the GDP–GTP exchange (48,75). Reversing the order of glutamate and arginine in rhodopsin's D/ERY motif eliminated binding of transducin (76). One study mutated basic residues in loop C-I, C-II, and C-III of the α_{1b}-adrenergic receptor but found only mutations at two, Arg^{254} and Lys^{258}, that impaired receptor-mediated signaling (77). The "fourth" intracellular loop between the carboxy terminal end of transmembrane helix VII and the palmitoyl anchors to the membrane at Cys^{322} and Cys^{323} also appear to be a contact site (35). Peptides derived from loop C-II or C-III or the carboxy terminal region can all inhibit rhodopsin activation of transducin, and mutations at the amino terminus of the carboxy terminal region disrupt rhodopsin's interaction with transducin (36).

Residues at the amino terminal (cytoplasmic) end of transmembrane helix VI have been inferred to be especially important for determining the specficity of G-protein interactions. These residues (Val[250], Thr[251], Val[254], Ile[255] in rhodopsin; Fig. 8) provide part of the hydrophobic environment packing against the aliphatic portion of arginine in the helix III D/ERY motif and are likely exposed to solvent during activation. Swapping helix VI residues Val[385], Thr[386], Ile[389], and Leu[390] (VTIL) from the muscarinic M2 receptor for the corresponding muscarinic M3 receptor's AALS sequence allows reciprocal changes in their selectivity for binding different subtypes of G-proteins (48,78). Adding another dimension to the complexity of these interactions, bifunctional receptors activated by both peptide and biogenic amines exhibit different G-protein subtype selectivity and presumably different binding modes, depending on the identity of their bound ligand (Ref. 79 and references therein).

Some of the contacts on the G-protein have been mapped more precisely. Evolutionary trace sequence analysis methods suggested 17 residues in the G-protein that are important for the interaction with receptor, including four at the carboxy terminus with suspected importance from alanine scanning mutagenesis (80). More directly, Itoh, Cai, and Khorana used two different reagents to cross-link rhodopsin to transducin through derivatized cysteine mutations in rhodopsin's loops C-I (R69C), C-II (K141C), and C-III (S240C, T243C, K245C, K248C; Refs. 67 and 68). The targets on transducin for the derivatized S240C rhodopsin variant could be identified by mass spectrometry after affinity purification, and they corresponded in transducin to an amino terminal peptide (residues 19–28) for one reagent and two carboxy terminal peptides (residues 310–313 RDVK, 347–345 ENLK) for the other. This last peptide is only five residues from the carboxy terminus of transducin and had previously been recognized as a target of rhodopsin (35,81–84). Although none of the amino terminal residues was identified by the sequence analysis methods (80), the different cross-linked peptides can be reconciled by appreciating that the amino and carboxy termini of transducin are very near each other in the structure (Ref. 26; PDB Id 1TND, < 15 Å). Transducin's γ subunit also appears to have a contact site, since peptides spanning its residues 50–71 inhibit the interaction with rhodopsin, apparently through contacts with the stretch of peptide between the end of helix VII (Tyr[306]) and the palmitoyl anchors at Cys[322] and Cys[323] (85).

6 CONCLUSIONS

In addition to representing a tremendous achievement in membrane protein crystallography, the new structure of rhodopsin provides a framework for interpreting a large amount of data toward a mechanistic understanding of class A GPCRs. The structure reveals the detailed packing of the transmembrane helices, including their tilt angles and their bent regions. It shows that the packing is not optimized for density but allows for cavities that may facilitate the structural rearrangements that have been inferred to occur upon activation. It reveals the geometry of residue interactions with retinal and the access to the retinal- (ligand-) binding pocket. Completely unanticipated by the previous low-resolution models, an eighth helical segment with amphipathic character lying parallel to the membrane on the cytoplasmic side of the molecule was found by the structure. Mapping the most highly conserved residues among GPCRs, residues that are correlated with class A GPCR family assignment, and the functional mutations for individual receptors onto the rhodopsin structure dramatically refines our hypotheses about GPCR function.

It now seems more possible than ever to understand GPCRs at a level of detail that would address remaining questions about the structural diversity of the ligand-binding pockets, the conformation of the activated receptors, and the determinants of the interactions with G-proteins. Resolving these issues will require more structures of other GPCRs and of an activated rhodopsin, possibly in a complex with transducin. The experience with isolating and crystallizing the unactivated rhodopsin will help with these difficult problems, and there may be ways to use disulfide bridges between introduced cysteine residues to trap a rhodopsin in an activated state for crystallization (86). The rewards for trying are potentially great, not only for drug discovery but also for understanding some of the most basic and widespread mechanisms of signal transduction in biology.

ACKNOWLEDGEMENTS

We are grateful to Al Lau for a critical reading of the manuscript.

REFERENCES

1. F Horn, G Vriend, FE Cohen. Collecting and harvesting biological data: the GPCRDB and NucleaRDB information systems. Nucleic Acids Res 29:346–349, 2001.
2. E Gasteiger, E Jung, A Bairoch. SWISS-PROT: connecting biomolecular knowledge via a protein database. Curr Issues Mol Biol 3:47–55, 2001.

3. T Gudermann, B Nurnberg, G Schultz. Receptors and G proteins as primary components of transmembrane signal transduction. Part 1. G-protein-coupled receptors: structure and function. J Mol Med 73:51–63, 1995.

4. JC Venter, MD Adams, EW Myers, PW Li, RJ Mural, et al. The sequence of the human genome. Science 291:1304–1351, 2001.

5. ES Lander, LM Linton, B Birren, C Nusbaum, MC Zody, et al. Initial sequencing and analysis of the human genome. Nature 409:860–921, 2001.

6. AJ Morris, CC Malbon. Physiological regulation of G-protein-linked signaling. Physiol Rev 79:1373–1430, 1999.

7. SJ Hug, JW Lewis, CM Einterz, TE Thorgeirsson, DS Kliger. Nanosecond photolysis of rhodopsin: evidence for a new, blue-shifted intermediate. Biochemistry 29:1475–1485, 1990.

8. DC Teller, T Okada, CA Behnke, K Palczewski, RE Stenkamp. Advances in determination of a high-resolution three-dimensional structure of rhodopsin, a model of G-protein-coupled receptors (GPCRs). Biochemistry 40:7761–7772, 2001.

9. A Cooper. Energy uptake in the first step of visual excitation. Nature 282:531–533, 1979.

10. GA Schick, TM Cooper, RA Holloway, LP Murray, RR Birge. Energy storage in the primary photochemical events of rhodopsin and isorhodopsin. Biochemistry 26:2556–2562, 1987.

11. A Cooper, CA Converse. Energetics of primary processes in visula escitation: photocalorimetry of rhodopsin in rod outer segment membranes. Biochemistry 15:2970–2978, 1976.

12. PA Hargrave, D Bownds, JK Wang, JH McDowell. Retinyl peptide isolation and characterization. Methods Enzymol 81:211–214, 1982.

13. D Bownds. Site of attachment of retinal in rhodopsin. Nature 216:1178–1181, 1967.

14. G Wald. The molecular basis of visual excitation. Nature 219:800–807, 1968.

15. N Grigorieff, TA Ceska, KH Downing, JM Baldwin, R Henderson. Electron-crystallographic refinement of the structure of bacteriorhodopsin. J Mol Biol 259:393–421, 1996.

16. R Henderson, JM Baldwin, TA Ceska, F Zemlin, E Beckmann, KH Downing. Model for the structure of bacteriorhodopsin based on high-resolution electron cryomicroscopy. J Mol Biol 213:899–929, 1990.

17. U Gether, BK Kobilka. G-protein-coupled receptors. II. Mechanism of agonist activation. J Biol Chem 273:17979–17982, 1998.

18. JM Baldwin, GF Schertler, VM Unger. An alpha-carbon template for the transmembrane helices in the rhodopsin family of G-protein-coupled receptors. J Mol Biol 272:144–164, 1997.

19. VM Unger, PA Hargrave, JM Baldwin, GF Schertler. Arrangement of rhodopsin transmembrane alpha-helices. Nature 389:203–206, 1997.

20. VM Unger, GF Schertler. Low-resolution structure of bovine rhodopsin determined by electron cryomicroscopy. Biophys J 68:1776–1786, 1995.

21. N Kunishima, Y Shimada, Y Tsuji, T Sato, M Yamamoto, T Kumasaka, S Nakanishi, H Jingami, K Morikawa. Structural basis of glutamate recognition by a dimeric metabotropic glutamate receptor. Nature 407:971–977, 2000.

22. AP West, Jr., LL Llamas, PM Snow, S Benzer, PJ Bjorkman. Crystal structure of the ectodomain of Methuselah, a *Drosophila* G-protein-coupled receptor associated with extended lifespan. Proc Natl Acad Sci USA 98:3744–3749, 2001.

23. JP Noel, HE Hamm, PB Sigler. The 2.2-Å crystal structure of transducin-alpha complexed with GTP gamma S. Nature 366:654–663, 1993.

24. LA Tong, AM de Vos, MV Milburn, SH Kim. Crystal structures at 2.2-Å resolution of the catalytic domains of normal ras protein and an oncogenic mutant complexed with GDP. J Mol Biol 217:503–516, 1991.

25. K Palczewski et al. Crystal structure of rhodopsin: A G-protein-coupled receptor. Science 289:739–745, 2000.

26. HE Hamm. How activated receptors couple to G-proteins. Proc Natl Acad Sci USA 98:4819–4821, 2001.

27. EC Meng, HR Bourne. Receptor activation: what does the rhodopsin structure tell us? Trends Pharmacol Sci 22:587–593, 2001.

28. JA Ballesteros, L Shi, JA Javitch. Structural mimicry in G-protein-coupled receptors: implications of the high-resolution structure of rhodopsin for structure–function analysis of rhodopsin-like receptors. Mol Pharmacol 60:1–19, 2001.

29. ST Menon, M Han, TP Sakmar. Rhodopsin: structural basis of molecular physiology. Physiol Rev 81:1659–1688, 2001.

30. J Nathans, DS Hogness. Isolation, sequence analysis, and intron-exon arrangement of the gene encoding bovine rhodopsin. Cell 34:807–814, 1983.

31. J Nathans, DS Hogness. Isolation and nucleotide sequence of the gene encoding human rhodopsin. Proc Natl Acad Sci USA 81:4851–4855, 1984.

32. JM Baldwin. The probable arrangement of the helices in G-protein-coupled receptors. Embo J 12:1693–1703, 1993.

33. T Okada, K Takeda, T Kouyama. Highly selective separation of rhodopsin from bovine rod outer segment membranes using combination of divalent cation and alkyl(thio)glucoside. Photochem Photobiol 67:495–499, 1998.

34. T Okada, I Le Trong, BA Fox, CA Behnke, RE Stenkamp, K Palczewski. X-Ray diffraction analysis of three-dimensional crystals of bovine rhodopsin obtained from mixed micelles. J Struct Biol 130:73–80, 2000.

35. OP Ernst, CK Meyer, EP Marin, P Henklein, WY Fu, TP Sakmar, KP Hofmann. Mutation of the fourth cytoplasmic loop of rhodopsin affects binding of transducin and peptides derived from the carboxyl-terminal sequences of transducin alpha and gamma subunits. J Biol Chem 275:1937–1943, 2000.

36. EP Marin, AG Krishna, TA Zvyaga, J Isele, F Siebert, TP Sakmar. The amino terminus of the fourth cytoplasmic loop of rhodopsin modulates rhodopsin–transducin interaction. J Biol Chem 275:1930–1936, 2000.

37. TH Ji, M Grossmann, I Ji. G-protein-coupled receptors. I. Diversity of receptor–ligand interactions. J Biol Chem 273:17299–17302, 1998.

38. L Holm, C Sander. Mapping the protein universe. Science 273:595–603, 1996.
39. DM Taverna, RA Goldstein. Why are proteins so robust to site mutations? J Mol Biol 315:479–484, 2002.
40. A Bateman et al. The Pfam protein families database. Nucleic Acids Res 30:276–280, 2002.
41. L Falquet, M Pagni, P Bucher, N Hulo, CJ Sigrist, K Hofmann, A Bairoch. The PROSITE database, its status in 2002. Nucleic Acids Res 30:235–238, 2002.
42. TK Attwood et al. PRINTS and PRINTS-S shed light on protein ancestry. Nucleic Acids Res 30:239–241, 2002.
43. JY Huang, DL Brutlag. The EMOTIF database. Nucleic Acids Res 29:202–204, 2001.
44. TK Attwood. A compendium of specific motifs for diagnosing GPCR subtypes. Trends Pharmacol Sci 22:162–165, 2001.
45. R Karchin, K Karplus, D Haussler. Classifying G-protein-coupled receptors with support vector machines. Bioinformatics 18:147–159, 2002.
46. VN Vapnik. Estimation of dependencies based on empirical data. Springer series in statistics. New York: Springer-Verlag, 1982, pp 399.
47. AD Howard, G McAllister, SD Feighner, Q Liu, RP Nargund, LH Van der Ploeg, AA Patchett. Orphan G-protein-coupled receptors and natural ligand discovery. Trends Pharmacol Sci 22:132–140, 2001.
48. J Wess. G-protein-coupled receptors: molecular mechanisms involved in receptor activation and selectivity of G-protein recognition. Faseb J 11:346–354, 1997.
49. F Horn, EM van der Wenden, L Oliveira, IJ AP, G Vriend. Receptors coupling to G proteins: Is there a signal behind the sequence? Proteins 41:448–459, 2000.
50. U Gobel, C Sander, R Schneider, A Valencia. Correlated mutations and residue contacts in proteins. Proteins 18:309–317, 1994.
51. W Kuipers, L Oliveira, A Paiva, F Rippman, C Sander, G Vriend, A IJzerman. Sequence–function correlation in G-protein-coupled receptors. In: J. Findally, ed. Membrane Protein Models. Oxford, UK: BIOS Scientific, 1996, pp 27–45.
52. H Luecke, B Schobert, HT Richter, JP Cartailler, JK Lanyi. Structure of bacteriorhodopsin at 1.55-Å resolution. J Mol Biol 291:899–911, 1999.
53. I Visiers, JA Ballesteros, H Weinstein. Three-dimensional representations of G-protein-coupled receptor structures and mechanisms. Methods Enzymol 343:329–371, 2002.
54. MK Dean, C Higgs, RE Smith, RP Bywater, CR Snell, PD Scott, GJ Upton, TJ Howe, CA Reynolds. Dimerization of G-protein-coupled receptors. J Med Chem 44:4595–4614, 2001.
55. SP Sheikh, JP Vilardarga, TJ Baranski, O Lichtarge, T Iiri, EC Meng, RA Nissenson, HR Bourne. Similar structures and shared switch mechanisms of the beta2-adrenoceptor and the parathyroid hormone receptor. Zn(II) bridges

between helices III and VI block activation. J Biol Chem 274:17033–17041, 1999.

56. RP Riek, I Rigoutsos, J Novotny, RM Graham. Non-alpha-helical elements modulate polytopic membrane protein architecture. J Mol Biol 306:349–362, 2001.

57. JB Konopka, SM Margarit, P Dube. Mutation of Pro–258 in transmembrane domain 6 constitutively activates the G-protein-coupled alpha-factor receptor. Proc Natl Acad Sci USA 93:6764–6769, 1996.

58. S Arnis, K Fahmy, KP Hofmann, TP Sakmar. A conserved carboxylic acid group mediates light-dependent proton uptake and signaling by rhodopsin. J Biol Chem 269:23879–23881, 1994.

59. K Fahmy, TP Sakmar. Regulation of the rhodopsin–transducin interaction by a highly conserved carboxylic acid group. Biochemistry 32:7229–7236, 1993.

60. A Scheer, F Fanelli, T Costa, PG De Benedetti, S Cotecchia. The activation process of the alpha1B-adrenergic receptor: potential role of protonation and hydrophobicity of a highly conserved aspartate. Proc Natl Acad Sci USA 94:808–813, 1997.

61. DA Shapiro, K Kristiansen, DM Weiner, WK Kroeze, BL Roth. Evidence for a model of agonist-induced activation of 5-hydroxytryptamine 2A serotonin receptors that involves the disruption of a strong ionic interaction between helices 3 and 6. J Biol Chem 277:11441–11449, 2002.

62. DL Farrens, C Altenbach, K Yang, WL Hubbell, HG Khorana. Requirement of rigid-body motion of transmembrane helices for light activation of rhodopsin. Science 274:768–770, 1996.

63. C Altenbach, K Yang, DL Farrens, ZT Farahbakhsh, HG Khorana, WL Hubbell. Structural features and light-dependent changes in the cytoplasmic interhelical E-F loop region of rhodopsin: a site-directed spin-labeling study. Biochemistry 35:12470–12478, 1996.

64. TD Dunham, DL Farrens. Conformational changes in rhodopsin. Movement of helix F detected by site-specific chemical labeling and fluorescence spectroscopy. J Biol Chem 274:1683–1690, 1999.

65. AS Yang, B Honig. An integrated approach to the analysis and modeling of protein sequences and structures. II. On the relationship between sequence and structural similarity for proteins that are not obviously related in sequence. J Mol Biol 301:679–689, 2000.

66. SP Sheikh, TA Zvyaga, O Lichtarge, TP Sakmar, HR Bourne. Rhodopsin activation blocked by metal-ion-binding sites linking transmembrane helices C and F. Nature 383:347–350, 1996.

67. Y Itoh, K Cai, HG Khorana. Mapping of contact sites in complex formation between light-activated rhodopsin and transducin by covalent cross-linking: use of a chemically preactivated reagent. Proc Natl Acad Sci USA 98:4883–4887, 2001.

68. K Cai, Y Itoh, HG Khorana. Mapping of contact sites in complex formation between transducin and light-activated rhodopsin by covalent cross-linking:

use of a photoactivatable reagent. Proc Natl Acad Sci USA 98:4877–4882, 2001.

69. JA Javitch, L Shi, MM Simpson, J Chen, V Chiappa, I Visiers, H Weinstein, JA Ballesteros. The fourth transmembrane segment of the dopamine D2 receptor: accessibility in the binding-site crevice and position in the transmembrane bundle. Biochemistry 39:12190–12199, 2000.

70. C Altenbach, J Klein-Seetharaman, K Cai, HG Khorana, WL Hubbell. Structure and function in rhodopsin: mapping light-dependent changes in distance between residue 316 in helix 8 and residues in the sequence 60–75, covering the cytoplasmic end of helices TM1 and TM2 and their connection loop CL1. Biochemistry 40:15493–15500, 2001.

71. C Altenbach, K Cai, J Klein-Seetharaman, HG Khorana, WL Hubbell. Structure and function in rhodopsin: mapping light-dependent changes in distance between residue 65 in helix TM1 and residues in the sequence 306–319 at the cytoplasmic end of helix TM7 and in helix H8. Biochemistry 40:15483–15492, 2001.

72. C Altenbach, K Cai, HG Khorana, WL Hubbell. Structural features and light-dependent changes in the sequence 306–322 extending from helix VII to the palmitoylation sites in rhodopsin: a site-directed spin-labeling study. Biochemistry 38:7931–7937, 1999.

73. C Altenbach, J Klein-Seetharaman, J Hwa, HG Khorana, WL Hubbell. Structural features and light-dependent changes in the sequence 59–75 connecting helices I and II in rhodopsin: a site-directed spin-labeling study. Biochemistry 38:7945–7949, 1999.

74. B Borhan, ML Souto, H Imai, Y Shichida, K Nakanishi. Movement of retinal along the visual transduction path. Science 288:2209–2212, 2000.

75. OP Ernst, KP Hofmann, TP Sakmar. Characterization of rhodopsin mutants that bind transducin but fail to induce GTP nucleotide uptake. Classification of mutant pigments by fluorescence, nucleotide release, and flash-induced light-scattering assays. J Biol Chem 270:10580–10586, 1995.

76. RR Franke, B Konig, TP Sakmar, HG Khorana, KP Hofmann. Rhodopsin mutants that bind but fail to activate transducin. Science 250:123–125, 1990.

77. PJ Greasley, F Fanelli, A Scheer, L Abuin, M Nenniger-Tosato, PG DeBenedetti, S Cotecchia. Mutational and computational analysis of the alpha(1b)-adrenergic receptor. Involvement of basic and hydrophobic residues in receptor activation and G-protein coupling. J Biol Chem 276:46485–46494, 2001.

78. J Liu, BR Conklin, N Blin, J Yun, J Wess. Identification of a receptor/G-protein contact site critical for signaling specificity and G-protein activation. Proc Natl Acad Sci USA 92:11642–11646, 1995.

79. PD Evans, S Robb, TR Cheek, V Reale, FL Hannan, LS Swales, LM Hall, JM Midgley. Agonist-specific coupling of G-protein-coupled receptors to second-messenger systems. Prog Brain Res 106:259–268, 1995.

80. O Lichtarge, HR Bourne, FE Cohen. An evolutionary trace method defines binding surfaces common to protein families. J Mol Biol 257:342–358, 1996.

81. MR Mazzoni, HE Hamm. Interaction of transducin with light-activated rhodopsin protects It from proteolytic digestion by trypsin. J Biol Chem 271:30034–30040, 1996.
82. M Natochin, AE Granovsky, KG Muradov, NO Artemyev. Roles of the transducin alpha-subunit alpha4-helix/alpha4-beta6 loop in the receptor and effector interactions. J Biol Chem 274:7865–7869, 1999.
83. M Natochin, KG Muradov, RL McEntaffer, NO Artemyev. Rhodopsin recognition by mutant G(s)alpha containing C-terminal residues of transducin. J Biol Chem 275:2669–2675, 2000.
84. R Onrust, P Herzmark, P Chi, PD Garcia, O Lichtarge, C Kingsley, HR Bourne. Receptor and betagamma binding sites in the alpha subunit of the retinal G protein transducin. Science 275:381–384, 1997.
85. O Lichtarge, HR Bourne, FE Cohen. Evolutionarily conserved Galphabetagamma binding surfaces support a model of the G protein-receptor complex. Proc Natl Acad Sci USA 93:7507–7511, 1996.
86. M Struthers, H Yu, DD Oprian. G protein-coupled receptor activation: analysis of a highly constrained, "straitjacketed" rhodopsin. Biochemistry 39:7938–7942, 2000.
87. M Carson. Ribbons. In: RM Sweet, CW Carter, eds. Methods in Enzymology. Orlando, FL: Academic Press, 1997, pp 493–505.
88. SF Altschul, W Gish, W Miller, EW Myers, DJ Lipman. Basic local alignment search tool. J Mol Biol 215:403–410, 1990.

20

Functional Assessment of Amino Acid Variation Caused by Single-Nucleotide Polymorphisms: A Structural View

Daniel I. Chasman
Variagenics, Inc., Cambridge, Massachusetts, U.S.A.

1 INTRODUCTION

If the draft of the human genome sequence marks the establishment of genomic technologies in biology, it also ushers in the analysis of human genetic variation in unprecedented detail (1–3). Even as these studies have begun, common genetic variation in humans ($>1\%$ allele frequency) is already recognized as taking the predominant form of single-nucleotide polymorphisms (SNPs) and one large collaborative initiative has already identified millions of these small elements of genetic diversity (4,5). While SNPs in any part of the genome can potentially affect biological function, it seems likely that the ones with the most profound effects will map to the coding sequences of genes and to the sequences that control gene expression, e.g., promoters, enhancers, and sequences important for pre-mRNA splicing. Of the millions of SNPs in the population, perhaps 250,000–400,000 map to coding sequences (6,7). Both synonymous cSNPs, which do not alter the amino acid sequence of proteins, and nonsynonymous cSNPs (nsSNPs), which do, can have effects on biological function, but genetic arguments favor greater functional consequences for nsSNPs on average (6–8). This difference is due to the more direct impact of nsSNPs on protein stability and biological activity. In turn, nsSNPs are obvious candidates for analysis in the study of fundamental processes in human evolution, of the genetic basis of disease, and—in applied research—of the influence of genetics on drug response, also known as pharmacogenomics (9). A major challenge for research in the post–human genome sequence world is to find links between SNPs and their effects on biological function as rapidly and accurately as possible.

Foreshadowing the current explosion in genomic information, computational tools have been developed since the early 1990s for inferring biological properties directly from protein sequence and structure (see, for example, Refs. 10–13). To this end, derived databases and computational methods exist for classifying proteins into fold families (14–16), identifying sequence patterns that signify structural and functional motifs (17–21) and understanding patterns of sequence conservation in the context of protein structure (15,22). At the same time, there are increasing opportunities for examining protein structure directly that complement the new sequences of complete genomes. High-throughput structure determination methods (see Chapter 4) are maturing and are being used to populate the "universe of protein folds" (23,24), while computational homology modeling technologies increasingly allow the construction of precise structural models for new sequences from the experimentally determined structures of related proteins (25–29). Together, the increased information and advances in analysis for both protein sequence and structure are providing ways to annotate the features of proteins with respect to function. The annotations, in turn, can guide hypotheses about the effects on function caused by genetics.

This chapter will describe computational approaches to the functional analysis of nsSNPs, emphasizing the use of protein structure. It will first briefly review the prevailing sequence-based methods for inferring functional effects of nsSNPs and then demonstrate the advantages of recent structure-based methods. Many of the ideas relating structure to the potential functional effects of amino acid polymorphisms have been distilled from the existing structural biology literature (see Ref. 30 for an early example and Ref. 31 for a review). The novel aspect is their application through computational methods to large numbers of amino acid polymorphisms derived from nsSNPs in the human population (32). Three groups—ourselves (33), Sunyaev et al. (34), and Wang and Moult (35)—have recently published preliminary analyses of the structural contexts of amino acid polymorphisms encoded by nsSNPs in clinically important genes. All three groups largely agree that an appreciable fraction of nsSNPs in the human population can be expected to have an effect on function. There is further agreement between predictions of effects on function for particular nsSNPs and the literature. The conclusions pertaining to statistical aspects of nsSNPs in human populations have been corroborated by a recent and purely genetic study (36).

2 NsSNPs AND EVOLUTION

The origins of most SNPs are usually explained by one of two competing genetic mechanisms. According to the neutral theory of evolution, common alleles will have become established through mutation processes followed by stochastic genetic drift (37); this view contrasts with the class of explanations that recognize functional selection as the primary mechanism for establishing genetic variation in the population, especially in coding sequences, transcription control regions, and sequences involved in mRNA processing. There are now many examples of mutations that appear to have been established through functional selection, and the neutral theory provides a null hypothesis against which to quantify the extent of functional changes in evolution (for some examples, see Refs. 36, and 38–42). In this framework, estimates of the heterozygosity of nsSNPs derived from sets of clinically important genes range from $2.8–6.3 \times 10^{-4}$ (SNPs/diploid base pair) compared with about $9.0–16.9 \times 10^{-4}$ for cSNPs with no effect on amino acid sequence and $5.2–10.9 \times 10^{-4}$ for noncoding SNPs revealing a clear selection against nucleotide polymorphisms that change protein sequence (6,7) (Table 1). The normalized rate of occurrence of nsSNPs, a second measure of this same effect, is 39% the rate of synonymous SNPs in coding regions. Moreover, in the population, nsSNPs are disproportionately rare compared with synonymous SNPs (36). Together, these observations suggest that many nsSNPs have deleterious effects on function in the current population. They may have become established through their offsetting potential benefit in some (historical) circumstance but are found only at low frequency now because of their deleterious side effects on protein function. Whatever the detailed mechanism, the evolutionary processes controlling their establishment are almost certainly nonneutral. On the Y chromosome, where mutation is more frequent than elsewhere, a different kind of nonneutral selection is observed. In this region of the genome, nsSNPs occur at a higher rate than predicted by neutral theory, but the discrepancy can be understood by the strong preference for chemically conservative amino acid changes encoded by the excess of nsSNPs (40). Again the hypothesis under the neutral theory is rejected for nsSNPs, and the evidence suggests a functional basis for the establishment of amino acid altering alleles.

Table 1 Estimates of Some Genetic Properties of SNPs in Clinically Important Genes

	Coding synonymous[a]			Coding nonsynonymous[b]			Nodcoding		
	$\hat{\theta}^c$	π^d	Frequency[e]	$\hat{\theta}^c$	π^d	Frequency[e]	$\hat{\theta}^c$	π^d	Frequency[e]
Cargill et al. (Ref. 6)	10.0	10.7	1/187	3.6	2.8	1/523	5.3	5.1	1/354
Haluska et al. (Ref. 7)	9.0–16.5			3.0–6.3			8.2–8.5		

All decimal values are reported $\times 10^{-4}$.

[a]The number of synonymous sites was the sum of the number of fourfold degenerate sites and half the number of twofold degenerate sites.

[b]The number of nonsynonymous sites was the sum of the number of nondegenerate sites and half the number of twofold degenerate sites.

[c]$\hat{\theta}$ = estimator of the population genetic parameter, θ, under the neutral theory model with infinite sites.

[d]π = heterozygosity per base pair, estimated from allele frequency values.

[e]Frequency = number of SNPs of each type per base pair in the sample (average 114 and 148 chromosomes/gene for Cargill et al. (Ref. 6) and Haluska et al. (Ref. 7), respectively).

What does it mean to talk about an nsSNP's "effect on protein function"? One definition involves an evolutionary context, in which the functional properties of a protein with respect to its environment are altered due to the mutation. In their discussion of mutations associated with molecular (genetic) diseases, Zuckerland and Pauling emphasize that the concept of biological function for a protein is inextricable from a description of its environment (43). For example, *function* for them can refer to protein stability in the cytoplasm, the interaction of amino acid side chains with cofactors, the interaction of a protein with other molecules, and properties deriving from the ionic and oxidative environment within the cell or the presence of exogenous agents. In their now-classic example, the alanine-to-serine mutation in beta-globin that causes globin polymerization and the resulting sickle cell disorder simultaneously offers a protective adaptation against the parasite that causes malaria. The biological environment in this case includes both the high concentration of globin molecules in a red cell and the malarial parasite itself. For Zuckerland and Pauling, the environment and the functional changes caused by mutation are so tightly interwoven in a molecular description of life that they state "at the limit, life itself is a molecular disease, which it overcomes temporarily by depending on its environment." To be sure, this is an extreme reduction; but it provides a context for thinking about protein function and suggests that assessing the effects of amino acid substitutions due to nsSNPs must acknowledge simultaneously a multitude of aspects of the normal cellular environment.

3 INFERRING FUNCTIONAL EFFECTS FROM SEQUENCE ALONE

One could hope to infer the consequences of nsSNPs on protein function using sequence data alone. The different amino acids are well known to have distinct chemical properties that allow their exchange in some structural contexts (environments) but not in others. The chemical similarities can be expressed as values indicating the average likelihood that one amino acid will be exchanged for another without a serious effect on function. In practice, the values are log-odds ratios of the likelihood of exchange, determined empirically from sequences of related proteins, compared with a likelihood determined from amino acid abundance estimates alone. Two popular families of amino acid exchange tables are the BLOSUM and PAM series. Through the tables, an observed amino acid polymorphism resulting from an underlying nsSNP can be assessed as being common or rare on average within the probabilistic framework of the log-odds formalism. In addition to the groupings of similar amino acids types implicit in the substitution tables, many other amino acid classifications exist, and these alternatives can be based on hydropathy, amino acid size, charge, polar character, etc. (see Refs. 44–46) and http://www.genome.ad.jp/dbget/aaindex.html). While a good start, approaches based solely on a single amino acid exchange table, without consideration of the biological context, are not very accurate for predicting effects on function (47).

A recent extension of these ideas combines both a comparison of amino acid chemical and biological properties with sequence relationships implicit in the genetic code. Two approaches have been described. Wyckoff and Wu start with the Grantham distances between amino acids that measure the ratios of the weights of side-chain noncarbon to carbon atoms (48). This value is then adjusted according to the likelihood of an exchange between the two amino acids based on their codons' nucleotide sequences, transition and transversion nucleotide exchange rates, and the possible mutation paths through the genetic code between codons encoding each amino acid pair (49). The result is an "exchangeability index" that reflects both a measure of the chemical differences for pairs of amino acids and the likelihood of their exchange by mutational processes. In a second approach, Goldman and others enumerate quantitative exchangeability for all pairs of codons explicitly, again using empirically determined transition and transversion rates as well as Grantham distances (50–52). Both of these methods can be tailored for nucleotide prevalence and mutation rates at individual loci or in particular organisms. As with the purely amino acid–based substitution tables, the determined exchangeability values in both approaches reflect average or typical behavior for each of the amino acids or codons, irrespective of context or environment. These approaches may be particularly useful for an evolutionary description of some nsSNPs.

Another approach for evaluating the functional significance of an nsSNP compares the alternative amino acids at a polymorphic residue in a test protein to the set or profile of amino acids tolerated at the equivalent residues in the family of proteins homologous to the test protein. With so much sequence information available today, a majority of polymorphic residues can be examined this way. The analysis of the family of sequences related to the test protein sequence can provide more insight than is gained by the average likelihood of amino acid exchange for all proteins represented in substitution tables. nsSNP's encoding amino acids that are observed at the corresponding residue in the related sequences are assumed to be tolerated without substantial effects on function, and may even be interpreted to be adaptive, reflecting "positive" selection (40). Encoded amino acids not found at the corresponding residue in the related sequences are inferred to be deleterious to function. In addition, polymorphisms occurring at sites that are relatively conserved are more likely to affect function than those occurring at variable residues. Methods for individualized assessment of amino acid variation can be discrete: Either the amino acids encoded by the nsSNP are represented at the corresponding residue in a family of related sequences or they are not (for example, Ref. 53). Alternatively, the methods can be probabilistic and estimate quantitatively the tolerance of the test protein to substitution at a particular residue by each of the 20 amino acids (11,17). When just a few homologous sequences are available, these approaches can be elaborated with phylogenetic constructs and Bayesian statistical arguments (54,55) to infer the set of tolerated amino acids (11,17). One recent probabilistic method, SIFT, holds great promise (47).

4 INFERRING FUNCTIONAL EFFECTS FROM STRUCTURE: A MULTITUDE OF STRUCTURE-BASED EXPLANATIONS

If the most comprehensive definition of biological function involves interactions with the environment defined as broadly as possible, then the information in the protein sequence alone will only provide an incomplete picture. Interactions with biological function occur in three dimensions with defined chemistry and high degrees of specificity that may not be revealed by inference from sequence analysis alone. Instead, models of protein structure from X-ray crystallography, NMR, or computational modeling can provide crucial insights into the functional roles performed by polymorphic residues, by providing a three-dimensional representation of their critical interactions. For example, in both the lac repressor (LacI) and the λ repressor, a few structure-based rules combining solvent-accessible context and amino acid type can account for much of the observed effects of mutations on function (31,56–58). Similarly, first Matthews and colleagues and later Rennell et al. succeeded in explaining effects on function of mutations in T4 lysozyme with a related set of purely structural features that include the crystallographic B-factor in addition to the commonly recognized features (59–62).

Since the solution of the first structures of hemoglobin, it has been recognized that there are a large number of structure-based features of polymorphic residues that can suggest their effects on function (30,43). A structural model can reveal the chemical nature of the contacts made by a polymorphic residue, for example, whether they are hydrophobic, polar, or charged in character, whether they involve many other residues or simply solvent molecules, or whether they include interactions with other subunits, ligands, or cofactor molecules. It can reveal whether a polymorphic residue coincides with a region of special secondary structure (a turn, a β-sheet, or an α-helix) or a region with a recognized functional property, e.g., an enzyme-active site. In combination with phylogenetic analysis, a structural model can indicate whether the polymorphic residue is part of a highly conserved region of the protein or one that carries a particular charge combination. All of these three-dimensional structural features (and more; see Tables 2–4 and later) are useful for identifying links to function that may not be made with sequence information alone.

For a protein structure that can be represented by a very precise three-dimensional model, it is possible to make correspondingly precise predictions about the effects on function caused by amino acid substitutions. Wang and Moult have devised a set of categorically valued features that can be used to detect structural model interactions that signify effects on function caused by reduced thermodynamic stability (35). Evaluated on both experimentally and computationally derived structural models of a protein with the two alternative amino acids encoded by an nsSNP, these categorically valued features include the loss of stabilizing hydrogen bonding or hydrophobic interactions, over- or underpacking of a protein's hydrophobic core, loss of stabilizing salt bridge interactions, and introduction of strain into the polypeptide backbone (Table 2). All of these features are defined in terms of amino acid side-chain chemical properties (e.g., charge, hydrophobicity, volume, geometry) embedded in a particular structural context. Furthermore, the penalty to protein stability for amino acid substitutions meeting the criteria of these features can be estimated in a semiquantitative way. A vast literature of extensive mutagenesis of T4 lysozyme, bacterial repressors, and other proteins combined with high-resolution crystallography and biophysical measurements of protein stability serve as empirical guides (31,61,63,64) for the loss of free energy (in these cases about 1–3 kcal/mol) that can be explained by these precise structural perturbations.

Other structural features may be more suitable for inferring effects on function with models of proteins structure that are less precisely defined. We suggested that the use of continuously valued parameters, termed *environment features*, can be used to measure the intrinsic local tolerance to amino acid variation within a relatively crude protein structural model (33) (Table 3). For evaluating some of the environment features, we also suggested the construction of a structural neighborhood around the model for a polymorphic residue, defined as the collection of residues in the model having at least one atom within approximate van der Waals contact of the model for the polymorphic residue. The environment features are divided into three classes, representing different explanations for effects on function caused by amino acid substitution: (1) residue accessibility to solvent, measured directly or on a relative basis (65), summarizes the degree to which the polymorphic residue interacts with the solvent or other residues; (2) phylogenetic entropy or multiple alignment information content (11,66) of the

Table 2 Categorically Valued (Binary) Features for Structure-Based Analysis of nsSNPs—Wang and Moult[a]

Feature name	Description
Effects on stability	The models show significant changes in the intramoelcular interactions caused by the nsSNP due to: 1. Loss of one or more hydrogen bonds 2. Reduced hydrophobic interaction measured as a loss burial of $>50\text{-Å}^2$ nonpolar area 3. Loss of a salt bridge 4. Burying a charged residue in the hydrophobic core 5. Overpacking of the hydrophobic core 6. Generation of an internal cavity 7. Causing electrostatic repulsion by introducing charged residue within 4.5 Å of a like charged residue 8. Burying a polar residue 9. Loss of coordination to a metal ligand 10. Breaking a disulfide bond 11. Straining the backbone by substitution for glycine or introduction of proline into regions with secondary structure geometry that is unfavorable for the substitution 12. Any of the foregoing criteria involving residues in a neighboring subunit
Change in ligand binding	Any of the rules defining effects on stability involving the polymorphic residue and a ligand in the model
Catalysis	The polymorphic residue is known to be involved in catalysis
Allosteric regulation	The polymorphic residue is known to be involved in an allosteric mechanism
Postranslational modification	An N-X-S/T sequence pattern for N-glycosylation is disrupted (X = any residue but proline)

[a] Ref. 35.

Table 3 Continuously Valued Environment Features and Categorically Valued (Binary) Features for Structure-Based Analysis of nsSNPs—Chasman and Adams[a]

Feature name	Description
Continuously valued environment features	
Residue accessibility	Solvent-accessible area of model residue
Residue relative accessibility	Accessibility relative to maximum accessibility for model residue
Residue relative phylogenetic entropy	Phylogenetic entropy of model residue normalized to average and S.D. in phylogenetic entropy for other residues in the same PDB chain
Neighborhood relative phylogenetic entropy	Phylogenetic entropy of model residue's structural neighborhood relative to average phylogenetic entropy of other collections of the same number of residues from the same PDB chain
Residue relative B-factor	B-factor of model residue normalized to average and S.D. in B-factor for other residues in the same chain
Neighborhood relative B-factor	B-factor of model residue's structural neighborhood relative to average B-factor of other collections of the same number of residues from the same chain
Categorically valued (binary) features	
Unusual amino acid	One of the amino acids in the polymorphism is not in the phylogenetic profile
Unusual amino acid by class	One of the amino acids in the polymorphism is not in the smallest amino acid class that includes the phylogenetic profile
Rare amino acid	The polymorphism includes an amino acid that occurs less than 10% of the time in phylogeny
Buried charge	The model residue is bruied and the polymorphism includes a charged amino acid; often a special case of unusual amino acid
Turn breaking	The polymorphism occurs at a glycine or proline in a turn; often a special case of unusual amino acid

Helix breaking	The polymorphism occurs in a helical region of the model and includes a glycine or proline; often a special case of unusual amino acid
Conserved position	The polymorphism occurs at an absolutely conserved position in phylogeny; always a special case of unusual amino acid
Near conserved position	The polymorphism occurs in a structural neighborhood that includes a conserved position
Near heterogen atom	The model for the polymorphism occurs near a ligand (heterogen atom) for the model
Near interface	The model for the polymorphism occurs near a subunit interface in the model

[a] Ref. 33.

Table 4 Categorically Valued (Binary) Features for Structure-Based Analysis of nsSNPs—Sunyaev, et al.[a]

Feature name	Description
Important site	The polymorphic residue coincides with a biologically important site defined in the SWISS-PROT database (ACT_SITE, BINDING, MOD_RES, SITE, LIPID, METAL, DISULFID)
Unlikely amino acid	Variant amino acid is incompatible with the amino context (profile) at the corresponding position among sequences homologous to the polymorphic sequence. The likelihood of each amino acid is estimated using PSIC, and nsSNPs encoding amino acids with an absolute profile score difference > 1.7 were considered significant
Buried charge	The relative solvent accessibility of the model residue < 0.25, and the nsSNP encodes amino acids with an absolute difference in their accessibility surface propensity > 0.75
Change in solubility	The model residue relative accessibility is > 0.5, and the nsSNP encodes amino acids with an absolute difference in their accessibility surface propensity > 2.0
Proline in a helix	The polymorphism introduces a proline residue into a region of helical secondary structure
Ligand interacting	The polymorphic residue has an atom within 6 Å of a ligand atom in the model, and the difference in the PSIC profile scores of the alternative amino acids is > 1.0

[a] Ref. 34.

model for the polymorphic residue or its structural neighborhood summarizes the observed mutability of the local structure among proteins
related to the polymorphic protein; and (3) the crystallographic B-factor
of the model for the polymorphic residue or its structural neighborhood
serves as experimental evidence of the rigidity of the local structure and,
by inference, its tolerance to the structural changes caused by mutation. All
of these features can be evaluated on the basis of relatively low-resolution
crystallographic models or from structural models of homologous proteins
that may deviate from the protein of interest by as much as 1–3 Å rms (25,
33). Models derived from NMR and homology modeling can also provide
the accessibility features for residues and the phylogenetic entropy features
for residues and structural neighborhoods. There may be modeling-specific
parameters for these two structure determination methods that could sub-
stitute for the crystallographic B-factor in representing model rigidity (see
Chapter 5). In general, a crudely defined likelihood of an effect on function
varies monotonically with each of the environment features, making them
particularly useful for ranking polymorphisms for further inspection by
some of the other criteria or by experimentation.

Features in a third class lend predictive insights into functional perturbations for models spanning a range of structural precision (Tables 3 and
4). These features include designations for polymorphisms that occur in
proximity to structural elements with clear biological function. For example,
nsSNPs that encode substitutions in a residue that is near a ligand molecule,
a structural motif with recognized biological role (18,21,67), the interface
with other protein subunits, or residues that are conserved in phylogeny will
all be likely to affect biological function. Other features can reflect the
differences in side-chain chemistry introduced by the polymorphism combined with the solvent accessibility from the structural model. These indicate
reduced stability due to burying charged or polar amino acids in the protein's hydrophobic core or altering its solubility (34,35,68). Still others try to
anticipate effects on stability by identifying polymorphisms that disrupt
secondary structure in the model (33,35). Finally, even in imprecise structural models, the presence of disulfide bonds can be accurately determined,
and nsSNPs that replace one of the paired cysteine residues in a disulfide
bond can be expected to affect stability and function (34,35) (Tables 2–4).

Of course, the existence of a structural model does not obviate the
insight from the purely sequence-based approaches described earlier, and
two of the groups exploring the functional consequences of nsSNPs included
sequence-based as well as structure-based features in their analysis.
Polymorphisms in residues that are entirely conserved in phylogeny can
be considered likely to affect function, especially if the conservation extends
among all members of a large family of related sequences from diverse

species. Similarly, polymorphisms that introduce an amino acid not found at the corresponding residue in related sequences can be considered an "unusual amino acid" or an "unlikely amino acid" (Tables 3 and 4), and will likely affect function. As already mentioned, phylogenetic comparisons of small families of related sequences can be extended through the use of Bayesian arguments and prior distributions of amino acid likelihoods (11) or through the implementation of amino acid classes as we have done (33); for example, see Ref. 53 for methodology. The work by Sunyaev et al. used these approaches also and considered a quantitative and continuous measure of amino acid functional fitness in position-specific, weighted phylogenetic profiles based on an algorithm called PSIC in connection with their structure-based predictions (69). Although they assign a discrete threshold for judging whether an nsSNP has functional consequences, their parameter might be interpreted as a continuously valued measure of the degree of functional perturbation caused by amino acid substitution.

5   CHOICE OF A STRUCTURAL MODEL

To be sure, having a crystallographic model for every polymorphic protein would optimize structure-based analysis, and the current structural genomics initiatives have this goal as a long-term objective (see in this volume the Introduction and Chapters 4, 5, and 7). Until these ambitious undertakings come to fruition, crystallographic models will exist for only a modest proportion of protein sequences. However, for about 30–35% of known protein sequences, the structure of a protein sharing at least 30% amino acid identity in sequence will likely be available from the PDB (Refs. 25 and 28 and this volume). These structures almost surely represent the correct fold, and in many cases the relative positions of backbone atoms and β-carbon atoms will deviate only slightly from their true positions. Models based on the structures of homologous proteins need only map the sequence of the polymorphic protein onto the homologous structure through the residue correspondence established by a sequence alignment, e.g. BLAST (70). For features that do not require precise models, the structures of these homologous proteins are likely to be sufficient, e.g., as has been found for lac repressor mutations modeled using the structure of the homologous purine repressor (56). Experimental models derived from NMR (see Chapter 5) either of target proteins or of their homologs will also be sufficient for features requiring only moderate structural precision. For features that require a precise structural model, computational models based on the structures of the homologous proteins can provide reliable information about the conformation and disposition of polymorphic residues. Software for constructing these models is widely available (e.g., SwissModel, Modeler,

WhatIf, and ICM methods; see Refs. 25, 26, 29, and 71 and this volume). Once the structural model has been identified from the PDB or constructed, a phylogenetic description of each residue from a multiple sequence alignment can be mapped onto the structure for evaluation of sequence conservation in the structural neighborhood of the polymorphic residue, for example, through the HSSP database (33,72).

No matter how the model is obtained, it is also important to record a parameter that estimates the model's accuracy (73). This value can be as simple as the proportion of amino acids shared either by the sequence of the entire polymorphic protein and the protein that provides the structural information or more accurately by the residues in the structural neighborhood around the polymorphic residue (see Chapter 10 and Ref. 33).

6 A PROFILE OF FEATURES FOR EACH POLYMORPHISM

Once the structural model has been constructed, the structural, phylogenetic, and crystallographic features can be evaluated and used to annotate each polymorphism rapidly by standard computational methods. These annotations—especially when combined with a graphical representation of the structural model—can provide the expert structural biologist with a "sense" for judging the potential functional consequences of the amino acid substitution caused by an nsSNP. For application to the vast numbers of nsSNPs from the genome sequencing projects, the entire process can be automated. And the annotations can be integrated into algorithms for predicting an effect on function. This step requires evaluating the features for their predictive strength on large data sets of suitable mutations.

7 DATA SETS FOR VALIDATION OF STRUCTURE-BASED ANALYSIS

In principle, any collection of amino acid substitutions in proteins that have known functional effects and adequate structural representations can serve as a validation data set for structure-based predictions. Through completely automated methods, a model can be made for each polymorphic residue and the values of its structure- and sequence-based features collected. Then the feature values can be compared with the known effects on function—either discrete or continuous—for analysis by standard statistical methods to judge their signficance as predictors of effects on function (74). For example, in the study of human nsSNPs, Wang and Moult derived a validation data set from nsSNPs in the Human Genome Mutation Database (see Table 5) known to be associated with disease (75). Of 557 candidate proteins, 157 were found to have the requisite structural information (35). Similarly,

Table 5 Databases of Genetic Variation and Mutation

Database name	Database description	Web access
Genome-wide human genetic variation		
ALFRED	Allele frequencies and DNA polymorphisms	http://alfred.med.yale.edu/alfred/index.asp
HGBASE	Intragenic sequence polymorphisms	http://hgbase.cgr.ki.se
Human Gene Mutation Database (HGMD)	Known (published) gene lesions underlying human inherited disease	http://www.uwcm.ac.uk/uwcm/mg/hgmd0.html
Online Mendelian Inheritance in Man	Catalog of human genetic and genomic disorders	http://www.ncbi.nlm.nih.gov/Omim/
dbSNP	Single-nucleotide polymorphisms	http://www.ncbi.nlm.nih.gov/SNP/
Human locus specific		
Androgen Receptor Gene Mutations Database	Mutations in the androgen receptor gene	http://www.mcgill.ca/androgendb/
Cytokine Gene Polymorphism Database	Cytokine gene polymorphisms, in vitro expression and disease-association studies	http://www.pam.bris.ac.uk/services/GAI/cytokine4.htm
Database of Germline p53 Mutations	Mutations in human tumor and cell line p53 gene	http://www.lf2.cuni.cz/win/projects/germline_mut_p53.htm
GRAP Mutant Databases	Mutants of family A G-Protein-Coupled Receptors (GRAP)	http://tinyGRAP.uit.no/GRAP/
HIV-RT	HIV reverse transcriptase and protease sequence variation	http://hivdb.stanford.edu/hiv/
Haemophilia B Mutation Database	Point mutations, short additions, and deletions in the Factor IX gene	http://www.umds.ac.uk/molgen/haemBdatabase.htm
Human PAX2 Allelic Variant Database	Mutations in human PAX2 gene	http://www.hgu.mrc.ac.uk/Softdata/PAX2/
Human PAX6 Allelic Variant Database	Mutations in human PAX6 gene	http://www.hgu.mrc.ac.uk/Softdata/PAX6/
Human Type I and Type III Collagen Mutation Database	Human type I and type III collagen gene mutations	http://www.le.ac.uk/genetics/collagen/
KinMutBase	Disease-causing protein kinase mutations	http://www.uta.fi/imt/bioinfo/KinMutBase/
NCL Mutations	Mutations and polymorphisms in neuronal ceroid lipofuscinoses (NCL) genes	http://www.ucl.ac.uk/ncl/
PAHdb	Mutations at the phenylalanine hydroxylase locus	http://www.mcgill.ca/pahdb/
PHEXdb	Mutations in PHEX gene causing X-linked hypophosphatemia	http://data.mch.mcgill.ca/phexdb
PTCH1 Mutation Database	Mutations and SNPs found in PTCH1	http://www.cybergene.se/PTCH/ptchbase.html
RB1 Gene Mutation Database	Mutations in the human retinoblastoma (RB1) gene	http://www.d-lohmann.de/Rb/

SV40 Large T-Antigen Mutant Database	Mutations in SV40 large tumor antigen gene	http://bigdaddy.bio.pitt.edu/SV40/
iARC p53 Database	Missense mutations and small deletions in human p53 reported in peer-reviewed literature	http://www.iarc.fr/p53/
p53 Databases	Mutations at the human p53 and hprt genes; rodent transgenic lacI and lacZ mutations	http://metalab.unc.edu/dnam/mainpage.html
Variation associated with specific human disease		
Asthma Gene Database	Linkage and mutation studies on the genetics of asthma and allergy	http://cooke.gsf.de/asthmagen/main.cfm
Atlas of Genetics and Cytogenetics in Oncology and Haematology	Chromosomal abnormalities in cancer	http://www.infobiogen.fr/services/chromcancer/
BTKbase	Mutation registry for X-linked agammaglobulinemia	http://www.uta.fi/laitokset/imt/bioinfo/BTKbase/
CASRDB	CASR mutations causing FHH, NSHPT and ADH	http://data.mch.mcgill.ca/casrdb/
KMDB	Mutations in human eye disease genes	http://mutview.dmb.med.keio.ac.jp/mutview3/kmeyedb/index.html
Natural and synthetic amino acid changing		
PMD (Protein Mutation Database)	Compilation of protein mutant data	http://pmd.ddbj.nig.ac.jp/

Source: The database issue of Nucleic Acids Research (2001) NAR (2001) 29(1) (http://www3.oup.co.uk/nar/database/cat/9).

Sunyaev et al. extracted about 500 amino acid substitutions from SwissProt (76) annotations indicating an effect on function (34). They also compiled a data set of functionally inert mutations (their "divergence set") with structural models from sequence differences between human proteins and their close mammalian orthologues found in the HSSP database (72). Almost all of the deleterious mutations in both studies are likely to be severe, and no attempt was made to estimate the magnitude of the effects on function. In our study, we exploited the saturation mutagenesis of the lac repressor (~4000 mutations) and lysozyme (~2000 mutations), in which the effect of each mutation was measured in a standardized assay (33,62). These data sets provide mutations both with and without effects on function. Remarkably, the function of each protein would tolerate the same proportion of mutations, about 60%, in spite of their radically distinct biophysical properties. Alternative data sets could be derived from other databases of mutations (Table 5). Some may be particularly useful for assessing mutations in specific protein classes (e.g., G-protein-coupled receptors) or for analyzing specific kinds of functional effects (e.g., effects on stability, interactions with other proteins).

8   SOME STATISTICAL PROPERTIES OF THE FEATURES

The association of a collection of structure- and sequence-based features with each polymorphism and its known effect on function in a reference data set allows statistical analysis of some intrinsic properties of the features and their utility as predictors of effects on function (33). It is well known that the environment features (solvent accessibility, crystallographic B-factor, and phylogenetic entropy; see earlier) are correlated. For the case of the lac repressor and lysozyme, we determined the correlation values explicitly. They ranged from a high of 0.96 for the comparison of the relative solvent accessibility feature and the solvent accessibility feature in the lac repressor model, to a low of 0.09 for the comparison of the neighborhood relative B-factor feature and the neighborhood relative entropy feature in the lysozyme model. Principal component analysis of the correlation between all pairs of features implied that, data permitting, the most complete parameterization of the environment of a polymorphic residue would include three features: one of the two accessibility features, one of the two crystallographic B-factor features, and one of the two phylogenetic entropy features. Similar results were found in a large database of residues and their structural neighborhoods from the PDB (33).

In our work, the continuously valued environment features were verified to discriminate strongly between polymorphisms with or without effects on function by standard analysis of variance (ANOVA) (Table 6) (33). For

Table 6 Discrimination of Effects on Function by Structure-Based Features

Feature name	Lac repressor mutations		Lysozyme mutations
	LacI model	PurR model	Lysozyme model
ANOVA F-test for continuously valued environment features[a]			
Accessibility	9.12E-117	1.43E-45	1.39E-28
Relative Accessibility	**1.14E-147**	8.22E-44	**2.15E-29**
Relative Entropy	4.32E-73	**1.00E-112**	2.45E-17
Nbhd. Relative Entropy	7.07E-68	4.85E-94	2.80E-09
Relative B-Factor	3.03E-95	1.04E-75	1.72E-24
Nbhd. Relative B-Factor	2.86E-106	1.53E-58	2.77E-24
Chi-squared test for categorical features[b,c]			
Unusual amino acid	1.49E-16 +	1.29E-29 +	1.32E-05 +
Unusual amino acid by class	9.13E-69 +	1.46E-50 +	3.30E-09 +
Rare amino acid	ND	2.53E-25 −	ND
Buried charge	1.48E-83 +	6.31E-50 +	4.40E-18 +
Turn breaking	3.63E-08 −	1.02E-06 −	5.52E-01 +
Helix breaking	2.14E-10 +	4.70E-11 +	5.01E-01 −
Conserved position	4.00E-24 +	1.37E-10 +	3.90E-14 +
Near conserved position	2.82E-11 +	2.65E-32 +	7.00E-10 +
Near het atom	1.19E-50 +	1.94E-11 +	ND
Interface	1.19E-12 +	2.80E-21 +	ND

[a]ANOVA (analysis of variance) test compares the feature variance for mutations with or without effects on function to the feature variance for all mutations. Values indicate probability that the computed F statistic will occur by chance, given the null hypothesis. Features with highest level of discrimination are indicated with boldface type.
[b]Test compares the number of mutations with or without the feature to the number of mutations with or without effects on function.
[c]"+" indicates that the feature is predictive of an effect on function; "−" indicates that the feature is predictive of no effect on function.
Source: Ref. 33.

the case of the lac repressor mutations, the ability of the features to discriminate was preserved when the model for the lac repressor was taken to be the X-ray structure of the purine repressor structure, sharing only 34% amino acid identity in sequence (Table 6). Similarly, χ^2 tests demonstrated that the discrimination of functional effects by most of the categorical features for the lac repressor and lysozyme mutations was also quite strong, although some of the structural features for polymorphisms that were tested, e.g., "turn breaking," were not particularly good predictors of effects on function (Table 6). Again, the categorical features discriminated between polymorphisms with and without effects on function when the structural model for the lac repressor mutations was derived from the purine repressor.

9   APPROACHES TO PREDICTING EFFECTS ON FUNCTION FOR POLYMORPHISMS

As mentioned earlier, the features can be more than annotations, and the published reports have proposed two distinct approaches for relating feature values to predictions about effects on function. In the first approach, only categorically valued features are used, each of which alone signifies an effect on function. The prediction rules specify that the structural model for a polymorphism meeting at least any one of categorical criteria is predicted as having an effect on function (34,35). More elaborate versions of this approach might involve classification with respect to function based on a hierarchy of features. This variation might be useful for predicting the magnitude of an effect, especially if the selected features involve inspecting different classes of intra- or intermolecular interactions caused by the polymorphism, e.g., hydrogen bonding, van der Waals interactions, or solubility.

Our alternative is to describe each polymorphism in terms of a probability of an effect on function where the estimate of the probability is determined empirically from the observed effects on function caused by modeled polymorphisms (mutations) in a reference data set that have feature values similar to those of the test polymorphism (33). This approach can integrate the categorically valued features with continuously valued features, and the probabilistic aspect can reflect all of the sources of the indeterminacy of a prediction. For example, polymorphisms that are characterized as "unusual amino acids" or those that are modeled with residues that have a low crystallographic B-factor will be viewed as more likely to affect function than polymorphisms that are not "unusual amino acids" or are modeled with residues that have high B-factors (Fig. 1). The approach is amenable to the application of statistical methods for identifying reduced subsets of predictive features that are optimal for making predictions about functional effects in a reference data set of polymorphisms, e.g., by maximum-likelihood and other parameter-reduction methods (11,33,74). Although our study assumed a linear relationship between the proportion of suitable mutations in the reference data set with effects on function and the predicted probability of an effect on function, other, nonlinear relationships are possible.

The accuracy of predictions using either approach validates structure-based methods for anticipating functional effects of polymorphisms. In their data set of modeled disease mutations, Wang and Moult's rule-based predictions yielded a false-positive rate of about 10% (35). Using a rule-based procedure with a different set of features, Sunyaev et al. (34) found a 10–30% misclassification rate for mutations with known functional disorders or

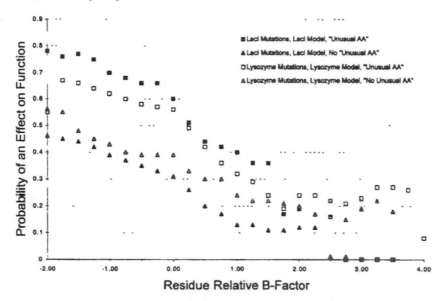

Figure 1 Example of the probabilistic approach to predicting effects on function for nsSNPs using two features, "residue relative B-factor" and "unusual amino acid" (see also Table 3), in the lac repressor (Refs. 56 and 57) and lysozyme (Ref. 62) mutation data sets. For each value of the continuously varying relative B-factor, a probability was computed as the fraction of mutations with an effect on function from among those having a relative B-factor within 1σ of the specified value and the appropriate value of the "unusual amino acid" feature. For mutations in both proteins, the dependence of the probability on the two features is very similar. The greater discrimination provided by the "unusual amino acid" feature for the lac repressor is likely due to the larger number of sequences from the public databases closely homologous to lac repressor (Ref. 20) than to lysozyme (Ref. 5). (From Ref. 33.)

a contributing role in disease. In their "divergence" data set of presumed inert amino acid differences in closely related sequences, they recorded an 8–9% false-positive misclassification rate. Using the probabilistic approach, we found predictions with 3–28% overall misclassification rates when the reference mutations for computing probability values, and the validation mutations were derived from the same protein, either lac repressor or lysozyme (33). When the reference data and the validation mutations were from different proteins, the misclassification rate increased to 10–30% (Table 7). For all of these studies, comparable accuracy in prediction was found with

Table 7 Cross-Validation Test in a Probabilistic Model for Predicting Effects on Function

Training data:		Lysozyme mutations, lysozyme model (PDB: 7lzm)[a]					lac Repressor mutations, lac repressor model (PDB: 1lbh)[b]					Lysozyme mutations, lysozyme Model (PDB: 7lzm)[c]				
Test data:		Lac Repressor mutations, lac repressor model (PDB: 1lbh, Minimum prediction probability					Lysozyme mutations, lysozyme model (PDB: 7lzm) Minimum prediction probability					lac Repressor mutations, pur repressor model (PDB: 2pua) Minimum prediction probability				
Prediction	Experiment	.9	.8	.7	.6	.5	.9	.8	.7	.6	.5	.9	.8	.7	.6	.5
Effect	Effect	68	227	358	483	551	30	70	156	271	341	5	9	20	45	69
	No effect	10	33	101	233	345	8	13	49	108	166	0	1	1	76	79
No effect	No effect	101	259	515	666	786	232	368	436	534	644	201	328	631	654	667
	Effect	9	27	109	132	182	90	135	183	233	328	68	107	262	283	299
Overall misclassified fraction:		0.10	0.11	0.19	0.24	0.28	0.27	0.25	0.28	0.30	0.33	0.25	0.2	0.29	0.34	0.34
False-positive fraction:		0.13	0.13	0.22	0.33	0.39	0.21	0.16	0.24	0.28	0.33	0.00	0.10	0.05	0.63	0.53
False-negative fraction:		0.08	0.09	0.17	0.17	0.19	0.28	0.27	0.30	0.30	0.34	0.25	0.25	0.29	0.30	0.31

The environment features for all tests were "relative accessibility," "residue relative phylogenetic entropy," and "neighborhood relative B-factor."

[a]The categorical features selected by a maximum-likelihood procedure were "buried charge," "unusual amino acid by class", "helix breaking," and "near conserved position."

[b]The categorical features selected by a maximum-likelihood procedure were "buried charge," "unusual amino acid by class", and "turn breaking".

[c]The categorical features selected by a maximum-likelihood procedure were "buried charge", "unusual amino acid by class", "helix breaking", and "near conserved position."

See Ref. 33 for details.

feature values determined from an experimental model of the polymorphic protein and from a structural model derived from a protein homologous to the polymorphic protein.

Often the misclassified mutations in these studies can be understood in retrospect. In some cases, sufficient structural information exists in the PDB for making an accurate prediction, but the automated modeling procedures neglect to use all of it. For example, polymorphism in a residue that is solvent exposed in one PDB entry might be at the interface with another subunit in a complex from a second PDB entry. The first model might not suggest an effect on function, while the second almost certainly would (34). Similarly, polymorphisms that occur near binding pockets for ligands may not be recognized unless the structural model explicitly includes a bound ligand. Wang and Moult (35) also draw attention to a potential discrepancy between effects of polymorphisms on protein stability and their effects on phenotype, i.e., their effects on biology. Some of their rule-based features signify loss of an estimated 1–3 kcal/mole of stability, which may not be sufficient to alter biological function. Similarly, none of the methods to date attempt to predict a magnitude of an effect, but, as mentioned earlier, either of the predictive approaches could be adapted for this challenge. Then some of the misclassifications might be resolved further. Finally, some predictions will fail because either the predictive rules or the reference training data are simply not appropriate for particular classes of proteins. For example, many of the prediction rules for effects on function of polymorphisms in soluble, globular proteins are doubtless inappropriate for membrane proteins. Nevertheless, it should be possible to define and validate features on structures and mutation data sets for individual classes of proteins that would yield accurate predictions for the effects of nsSNPs on function through the structure-based formalism that has been developed.

10 APPLICATION OF PREDICTION METHODS TO SURVEYS OF nsSNPs

The motivation of automated structure-based predictions was to begin to understand the functional nature of large numbers of nsSNPs, and all three groups developing structure-based methods applied their predictions to nsSNPs in the public databases. Sunyaev et al. (34) examined nsSNPs from HGBase, SwissProt, and dbSNP, while the other two groups (33,35) focused on nsSNPs in recently published surveys of genetic variation in clinically relevant genes. Our study (33) found sufficient structural information for predictions with 23% (46/200) and 39% (58/148) of the nsSNPs in two different data sets, respectively (6,7), while the study from Wang and Moult (35) found sufficient structural information for about 28% (157/557) of the nsSNPs they examined. All three groups are in agreement about the proportion of human nsSNPs with effects on function. Wang and Moult estimate this value at 30%, Sunyaev et al. estimate it at about 20%, and our studies estimate an average probability of an effect on function of 26–32%. A second estimate of the proportion of nsSNPs with an effect on function of about 18–25% can be derived from our data by making predictions based on whether the predicted probability of an effect on function is greater or less than .5. Our approach also allowed comparison of the prevalence of nsSNPs with their predicted probability of an effect on function as a histogram to reveal, as expected, that most but not all nsSNPs are unlikely to affect function (Fig. 2). With the caveat that the accuracy of structure-based

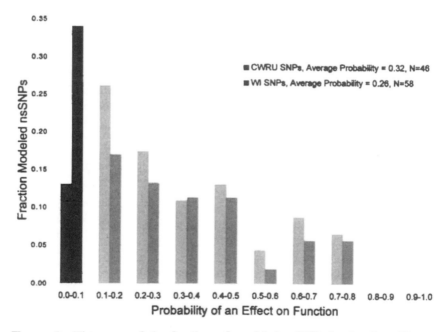

Figure 2 Histogram of the fraction of modeled nsSNPs in the Case Western (CWRU) (Ref. 7) and Whitehead Institute (WI) (Ref. 6) data sets versus the predicted probability of an effect on function. The probability values were estimated using the continuously valued features "relative accessibility," "residue relative phylogenetic entropy," and "neighborhood relative B-factor" and the categorical features "buried charge," "unusual amino acid," "unusual amino acid by class," and "turn breaking." (From Ref. 33.)

predictions may require additional validation, these preliminary studies indicate that an appreciable fraction of nsSNPs appear to be functionally nonneutral. A recent statistical analysis comparing the frequency spectrum of synonymous and nsSNP alleles in the same data sets we studied concluded that an even higher proportion of nsSNPs is likely to affect function (36), as had other, earlier and also purely genetic studies (37).

There was further agreement on predictions of functional effects for individual nsSNPs that were examined in all three studies. These nsSNPs encode a proline-to-leucine change in annexin III, a glutamatic acid–to-glycine change in prostoglandin synthase 2 (the COX-2 enzyme), and a histidine-to-leucine change in aldose reductase (Fig. 3). Only the first of these SNPs has not been confirmed by sequencing, and none of them has been examined by experiment. Others among the predictions by Sunyaev et al. have a confirmed association with disease, including nsSNPs in the haemochromatosis gene product, the β-1 adrenergic receptor, apolipoprotein E, insulin receptor subunit-I, cholinesterase, and alcohol dehydrogenase. An alanine-to-serine change at residue 304 of dopamine β-hydroxylase caused by an nsSNP was identified in our study as having an effect on function, and reports indicate that there may be a functional change associated with this variation (77–79). In spite of the many years spent by the medical genetics community on the identification of mutations associated with disease, the functional consequences of most common nsSNPs remain unknown, and the rest of the predictions in the three studies will have to await experimental confirmation.

11 IMPLICATIONS FOR HUMAN POPULATION GENETICS

The prediction of nsSNP effects on function allows revisiting the link between allele frequency and allele function from a new perspective. Purely genetic analysis of nsSNPs inferred their effects on function through their lower allele frequency and lower heterozygosity compared with synonymous SNPs and SNPs in noncoding sequences (Table 1). By comparing allele frequencies for structurally modeled nsSNPs, Sunyaev et al. found that, on average, polymorphisms predicted to affect function also had lower allele frequency (p-value $= .0004$). Similarly, our analysis found a higher probability of an effect on function among lower-frequency alleles but only with marginal statistical significance. The statistics in both cases were limited by the quantity of nsSNPs analyzed and the accuracy of the allele frequency data. Notwithstanding the evidence that some nsSNPs affecting function are maintained at moderate to high frequency (33,36), the trend of lower allele frequencies for alleles predicted to affect function

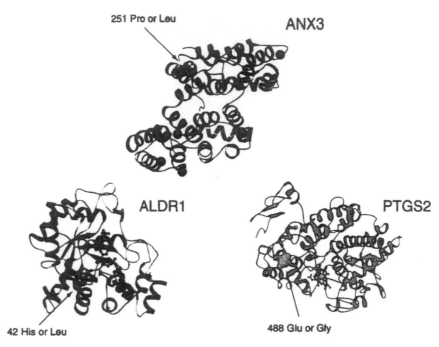

Figure 3 Three amino acid polymorpisms encoded by nsSNPs that are predicted to affect function by all three groups (Refs. 33–35; see text). ANX3: a model for annexin III based on PDB entry 1axn. The proline/leucine polymorphism is buried in the protein (relative accessibility 0.13) and in a structural neighborhood that has a relatively low B-factor (-3.5σ). But the polymorphic residue is not strongly conserved among 51 proteins homologous to Annexin III. However, the leucine represents an "unusual amino acid" and it is near the conserved residue aspartate 287. Calcium atoms (dark spheres) in the crystal structure are also shown. ALDR1: a model for aldose reductase based on PDB entry 2acs. The histidine/leucine polymorphism is inaccessible to solvent and has low relative phylogenetic entropy and B-factors for both the polymorphic residue and its structural neighborhood. The histidine represents a "buried charge," while the leucine does not, and neither represents an "unusual amino acid." The polymorphic residue is, however, part of the aldose reductase active site determined by a match to a PROSITE pattern (67). The ligand molecule (ball-and-stick representation) in the structure is NADP. PTGS2 (or COX2): a model for prostoglandin synthase 2 based on PDB entry 1cx2. The glutamate/glycine polymorphism occurs in a solvent-inaccessible residue that is also a "conserved position" in a structural neighborhood with a low relative B-factor (-1.5σ). The ligand molecule (ball-and-stick representation) in the structure is the heme cofactor.

is likely to be verified as the ongoing resequencing efforts elucidate the scope of human genetic variation.

Even if the more strongly deleterious nsSNPs are preferentially associated with lower allele frequency, measures of the heterzygosity still imply that a typical person will have a substantial number of polymorphic proteins encoded by his or her diploid genome. Cargill et al. estimate this value at 25,000–40,000 (6). Their numbers are derived from an estimated 100,000 protein sequences in the genome, but the revised estimates of about 30,000 proteins (or protein encoding loci) suggest 7,500–12,000 heterozygous sites. Of these, the structure-based predictions estimate 20–30% will have functional consequences. Therefore, the *functional* heterozygosity of a typical person due to nsSNPs is likely 1,500–3,600 loci (or possibly a fewfold less, since alleles with functional consequences are more rare than alleles that are functionally inert). Using slightly different arguments, Sunyaev et al. found about 1,000–2,000 functionally heterozygous loci per individual due to nsSNPs. Purely statistical arguments, again from genetics alone, lead to slightly lower estimates of the numbers of nsSNPs having substantial effects on function, about 500–1,200 (36). Based on an estimate of the number of essential proteins in the genome and fecundity in first cousin marriages, Sunyaev et al. argue that only a small proportion of functionally significant polymorpisms will lead to a total loss of function. Wang and Moult would concur, since their modeling indicates relatively small differences in the free energy of protein stability caused by most of the nsSNPs they examined.

12 CONCLUDING REMARKS

It has long been recognized that protein structure can provide insights into effects on function caused by amino acid substitutions. The validation of the structure-based computational methods reviewed here extends the analysis of natural amino acid polymorphisms into a genomic scale. Application of these methods to initial data sets of nsSNPs suggests that a remarkably large proportion of nsSNPs will affect biological function. Reflecting the comprehensiveness of the structure-based approaches, natural polymorphisms are predicted to alter function for a multitude of reasons, with bases in structure, chemistry, and phylogenic relationships. Today, the methods are limited only by the number of experimentally determined structures. But as new structures are determined through structural genomics initiatives and as modeling techniques improve, the structure-based analysis of nsSNPs will be increasingly applicable and powerful. Perhaps the methodology in structure-based analysis of nsSNPs should become part of the Critical Assessment of Structure Prediction contests (CASP) (see Ref. 80). In the postgenomics era, the methods will have widespread application in association studies linking nsSNPs to disease and drug response. And they will be invaluable for helping to understand both the extent and the nature of molecular functional diversity in human populations.

ACKNOWLEDGEMENTS

I thank Ann Ferentz, Jim Freeman, S. Roy Kimura, and Al Lau for critical readings of the manuscript.

REFERENCES

1. ES Lander. The new genomics: global views of biology. Science 274:536–539, 1996.
2. ES Lander, LM Linton, B Birren, C Nusbaum, MC Zody, et al. Initial sequencing and analysis of the human genome. Nature 409:860–921, 2001.
3. JC Venter, MD Adams, EW Myers, PW Li, RJ Mural, et al. The sequence of the human genome. Science 291:1304–1351, 2001.
4. JG Hacia, JB Fan, O Ryder, L Jin, K Edgeman, et al. Determination of ancestral alleles for human single-nucleotide polymorphisms using high-density oligonucleotide arrays. Nat Genet 22:164–167, 1999.
5. R Sachidanandam, D Weissman, SC Schmidt, JM Kakol, LD Stein, et al. A map of human genome sequence variation containing 1.42 million single nucleotide polymorphisms. Nature 409:928–933, 2001.
6. M Cargill, D Altshuler, J Ireland, P Sklar, K Ardlie, et al. Characterization of single-nucleotide polymorphisms in coding regions of human genes. Nat Genet 22:231–238, 1999.
7. MK Halushka, JB Fan, K Bentley, L Hsie, N Shen, A Weder, R Cooper, R Lipshutz, A Chakravarti. Patterns of single-nucleotide polymorphisms in candidate genes for blood-pressure homeostasis. Nat Genet 22:239–247, 1999.
8. SR Sunyaev, WC Lathe 3rd, VE Ramensky, P Bork. SNP frequencies in human genes: an excess of rare alleles and differing modes of selection. Trends Genet 16:335–337, 2000.
9. D Housman, FD Ledley. Why pharmacogenomics? Why now? Nat Biotechnol 16:492–493, 1998.
10. GJ Chin, T Appenzelter. Computers in biology. Science 273:585, 1996.
11. R Durbin, S Eddy, A Krogh, G Mitchison. Biological Sequence Analysis. Cambridge, UK: Cambridge University Press, 1998, p 356.
12. C Gibas, P Jambeck. Developing Bioinformatics and Computer Skills. Cambridge, MA: O'Reilly, 2001, p 427.
13. SJ Spengler. Techview: computers and biology. Bioinformatics in the information age. Science 287:1221, 1223, 2000.
14. L Holm, C Sander. Dali/FSSP classification of three-dimensional protein folds. Nucleic Acids Res 25:231–234, 1997.

15. L Lo Conte, B Ailey, TJ Hubbard, SE Brenner, AG Murzin, C Chothia. SCOP: a structural classification of proteins database. Nucleic Acids Res 28:257–259, 2000.
16. CA Orengo, AD Michie, S Jones, DT Jones, MB Swindells, JM Thornton. CATH—a hierarchic classification of protein domain structures. Structure 5:1093–1108, 1997.
17. A Bateman, E Birney, R Durbin, SR Eddy, KL Howe, EL Sonnhammer. The Pfam protein families database. Nucleic Acids Res 28:263–266, 2000.
18. JY Huang, DL Brutlag. The EMOTIF database. Nucleic Acids Res 29:202–204, 2001.
19. JG Henikoff, S Henikoff. Blocks database and its applications. Methods Enzymol 266:88–105, 1996.
20. S Henikoff, JG Henikoff, S Pietrokovski. Blocks+: a nonredundant database of protein alignment blocks derived from multiple compilations. Bioinformatics 15:471–479, 1999.
21. JS Fetrow, J Skolnick. Method for prediction of protein function from sequence using the sequence-to-structure-to-function paradigm with application to glutaredoxins/thioredoxins and T1 ribonucleases. J Mol Biol 281:949–968, 1998.
22. MA Andrade et al. Automated genome sequence analysis and annotation. Bioinformatics 15:391–412, 1999.
23. L Holm, C Sander. Mapping the protein universe. Science 273:595–603, 1996.
24. D Vitkup, E Melamud, J Moult, C Sander. Completeness in structural genomics. Nat Struct Biol 8:559–566, 2001.
25. N Guex, A Diemand, MC Peitsch. Protein modeling for all. Trends Biochem Sci 24:364–367, 1999.
26. G Vriend. WHAT IF: a molecular modeling and drug design program. J Mol Graph 8:29, 52–26, 1990.
27. MA Marti-Renom, AC Stuart, A Fiser, R Sanchez, F Melo, A Sali. Comparative protein structure modeling of genes and genomes. Annu Rev Biophys Biomol Struct 29:291–325, 2000.
28. R Sanchez, U Pieper, F Melo, N Eswar, MA Marti-Renom, MS Madhusudhan, N Mirkovic, A Sali. Protein structure modeling for structural genomics. Nat Struct Biol 7 Suppl:986–990, 2000.
29. T Cardozo, M Totrov, R Abagyan. Homology modeling by the ICM method. Proteins 23:403–414, 1995.
30. MF Perutz. Structure and function of haemoglobin. I. A tentative atomic model of horse oxyhaemoglobin. J Mol Biol 13:646–668, 1965.
31. JU Bowie, JF Reidhaar-Olson, WA Lim, RT Sauer. Deciphering the message in protein sequences: tolerance to amino acid substitutions. Science 247:1306–1310, 1990.
32. S Sunyaev, W Lathe 3rd, P Bork. Integration of genome data and protein structures: prediction of protein folds, protein interactions and "molecular phenotypes" of single-nucleotide polymorphisms. Curr Opin Struct Biol 11:125–130, 2001.

33. D Chasman, RM Adams. Predicting the functional consequences of nonsynonymous single-nucleotide polymorphisms: structure-based assessment of amino acid variation. J Mol Biol 307:683–706, 2001.

34. S Sunyaev, V Ramensky, I Koch, W Lathe 3rd, AS Kondrashov, P Bork. Prediction of deleterious human alleles. Hum Mol Genet 10:591–597, 2001.

35. Z Wang, J Moult. SNPs, protein structure, and disease. Hum Mutat 17:263–270, 2001.

36. JC Fay, GJ Wyckoff, CI Wu. Positive and negative selection on the human genome. Genetics 158:1227–1234, 2001.

37. M Kimura. The Neutral Theory of Molecular Evolution. Cambridge, UK: Cambridge University Press, 1983, p 353.

38. N Takahata. Neutral theory of molecular evolution. Curr Opin Genet Dev 6:767–772, 1996.

39. A Eyre-Walker, PD Keightley. High genomic deleterious mutation rates in hominids. Nature 397:344–347, 1999.

40. GJ Wyckoff, W Wang, CI Wu. Rapid evolution of male reproductive genes in the descent of man. Nature 403:304–309, 2000.

41. SA Sawyer, DL Hartl. Population genetics of polymorphism and divergence. Genetics 132:1161–1176, 1992.

42. AR Templeton. Contingency tests of neutrality using intra/interspecific gene trees: the rejection of neutrality for the evolution of the mitochondrial cytochrome oxidase II gene in the hominoid primates. Genetics 144:1263–1270, 1996.

43. E Zuckerkland, L Pauling. Molecular disease, evolution, and genic heterogeneity. In: M Kasha, B Pullman, eds. Horizons in Biochemistry. New York: Academic Press, 1962, pp 189–225.

44. S Kawashima, H Ogata, M Kanehisa. AAindex: Amino Acid Index Database. Nucleic Acids Res 27:368–369, 1999.

45. K Nakai, A Kidera, M Kanehisa. Cluster analysis of amino acid indices for prediction of protein structure and function. Protein Eng 2:93–100, 1988.

46. K Tomii, M Kanehisa. Analysis of amino acid indices and mutation matrices for sequence comparison and structure prediction of proteins. Protein Eng 9:27–36, 1996.

47. PC Ng, S Henikoff. Predicting deleterious amino acid substitutions. Genome Res 11:863–874, 2001.

48. R Grantham. Amino acid difference formula to help explain protein evolution. Science 185:862–864, 1974.

49. G Wyckoff. PhD dissertation, University of Chicago, Chicago, 2001.

50. N Goldman, Z Yang. A codon-based model of nucleotide substitution for protein-coding DNA sequences. Mol Biol Evol 11:725–736, 1994.

51. SV Muse, BS Gaut. A likelihood approach for comparing synonymous and nonsynonymous nucleotide substitution rates, with application to the chloroplast genome. Mol Biol Evol 11:715–724, 1994.

52. AK Pedersen, C Wiuf, FB Christiansen. A codon-based model designed to describe lentiviral evolution. Mol Biol Evol 15:1069–1081, 1998.

53. RM Adams, S Das, TF Smith. Multiple-domain protein diagnostic patterns. Protein Sci 5:1240–1249, 1996.

54. JG Henikoff, S Henikoff. Using substitution probabilities to improve position-specific scoring matrices. Comput Appl Biosci 12:135–143, 1996.

55. K Sjolander, K Karplus, M Brown, R Hughey, A Krogh, IS Mian, D Haussler. Dirichlet mixtures: a method for improved detection of weak but significant protein sequence homology. Comput Appl Biosci 12:327–345, 1996.

56. J Suckow, P Markiewicz, LG Kleina, J Miller, B Kisters-Woike, B Muller-Hill. Genetic studies of the Lac repressor. XV: 4000 single amino acid substitutions and analysis of the resulting phenotypes on the basis of the protein structure. J Mol Biol 261:509–523, 1996.

57. P Markiewicz, LG Kleina, C Cruz, S Ehret, JH Miller. Genetic studies of the lac repressor. XIV. Analysis of 4000 altered *Escherichia coli* lac repressors reveals essential and nonessential residues, as well as "spacers," which do not require a specific sequence. J Mol Biol 240:421–433, 1994.

58. WA Lim, RT Sauer. Alternative packing arrangements in the hydrophobic core of lambda repressor. Nature 339:31–36, 1989.

59. T Alber, DP Sun, JA Nye, DC Muchmore, BW Matthews. Temperature-sensitive mutations of bacteriophage T4 lysozyme occur at sites with low mobility and low solvent accessibility in the folded protein. Biochemistry 26:3754–3758, 1987.

60. S Dao-pin, DE Anderson, WA Baase, FW Dahlquist, BW Matthews. Structural and thermodynamic consequences of burying a charged residue within the hydrophobic core of T4 lysozyme. Biochemistry 30:11521–11529, 1991.

61. BW Matthews. Studies on protein stability with T4 lysozyme. Adv Protein Chem 46:249–278, 1995.

62. D Rennell, SE Bouvier, LW Hardy, AR Poteete. Systematic mutation of bacteriophage T4 lysozyme. J Mol Biol 222:67–88, 1991.

63. C Lee, M Levitt. Accurate prediction of the stability and activity effects of site-directed mutagenesis on a protein core. Nature 352:448–451, 1991.

64. CM Topham, N Srinivasan, TL Blundell. Prediction of the stability of protein mutants based on structural environment-dependent amino acid substitution and propensity tables. Protein Eng 10:7–21, 1997.

65. B Rost, C Sander. Conservation and prediction of solvent accessibility in protein families. Proteins 20:216–226, 1994.

66. TD Schneider, GD Stormo, L Gold, A Ehrenfeucht. Information content of binding sites on nucleotide sequences. J Mol Biol 188:415–431, 1986.

67. K Hofmann, P Bucher, L Falquet, A Bairoch. The PROSITE database, its status in 1999. Nucleic Acids Res 27:215–219, 1999.

68. SR Sunyaev, F Eisenhaber, P Argos, EN Kuznetsov, VG Tumanyan. Are knowledge-based potentials derived from protein structure sets discriminative with respect to amino acid types? Proteins 31:225–246, 1998.

69. SR Sunyaev, F Eisenhaber, IV Rodchenkov, B Eisenhaber, VG Tumanyan, EN Kuznetsov. PSIC: profile extraction from sequence alignments with position-specific counts of independent observations. Protein Eng 12:387–394, 1999.

70. SF Altschul, TL Madden, AA Schaffer, J Zhang, Z Zhang, W Miller, DJ Lipman. Gapped BLAST and PSI-BLAST: a new generation of protein database search programs. Nucleic Acids Res 25:3389–3402, 1997.

71. A Fiser, RK Do, A Sali. Modeling of loops in protein structures. Protein Sci 9:1753–1773, 2000.

72. C Sander, R Schneider. Database of homology-derived protein structures and the structural meaning of sequence alignment. Proteins 9:56–68, 1991.

73. T Cardozo, S Batalov, R Abagyan. Estimating local backbone structural deviation in homology models. Comput Chem 24:13–31, 2000.

74. DC Montgomery, EA Peck. Introduction to Linear Regression Analysis. 2nd ed. New York: John Wiley, 1992, p 525.

75. M Krawczak, DN Cooper. The human gene mutation database. Trends Genet. 13:121–122, 1997.

76. A Bairoch, R Apweiler. The SWISS-PROT protein sequence database and its supplement TrEMBL in 2000. Nucleic Acids Res 28:45–48, 2000.

77. B Li, S Tsing, AH Kosaka, B Nguyen, EG Osen, C Bach, H Chan, J Barnett. Expression of human dopamine beta-hydroxylase in *Drosophila* Schneider 2 cells. Biochem J 313:57–64, 1996.

78. A Ishii, K Kobayashi, K Kiuchi, T Nagatsu. Expression of two forms of human dopamine-beta-hydroxylase in COS cells. Neurosci Lett 125:25–28, 1991.

79. JF Cubells, K Kobayashi, T Nagatsu, KK Kidd, JR Kidd, F Calafell, HR Kranzler, H Ichinose, J Gelernter. Population genetics of a functional variant of the dopamine beta-hydroxylase gene (DBH). Am J Med Genet 74:374–379, 1997.

80. J Moult. Predicting protein three-dimensional structure. Curr Opin Biotechnol 10:583–588, 1999.

Index